Organic & Wholefoods

Naturally delicious cuisine

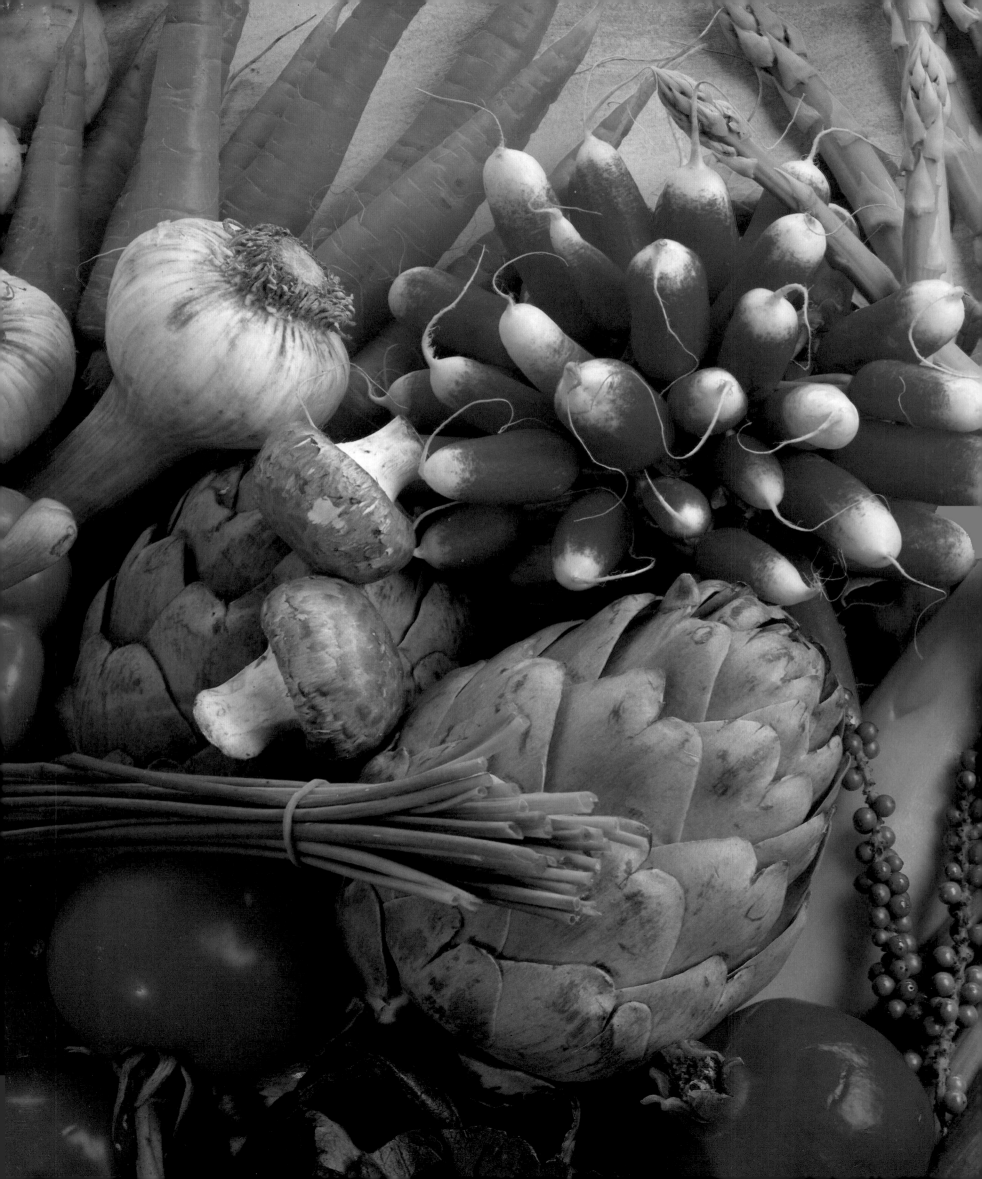

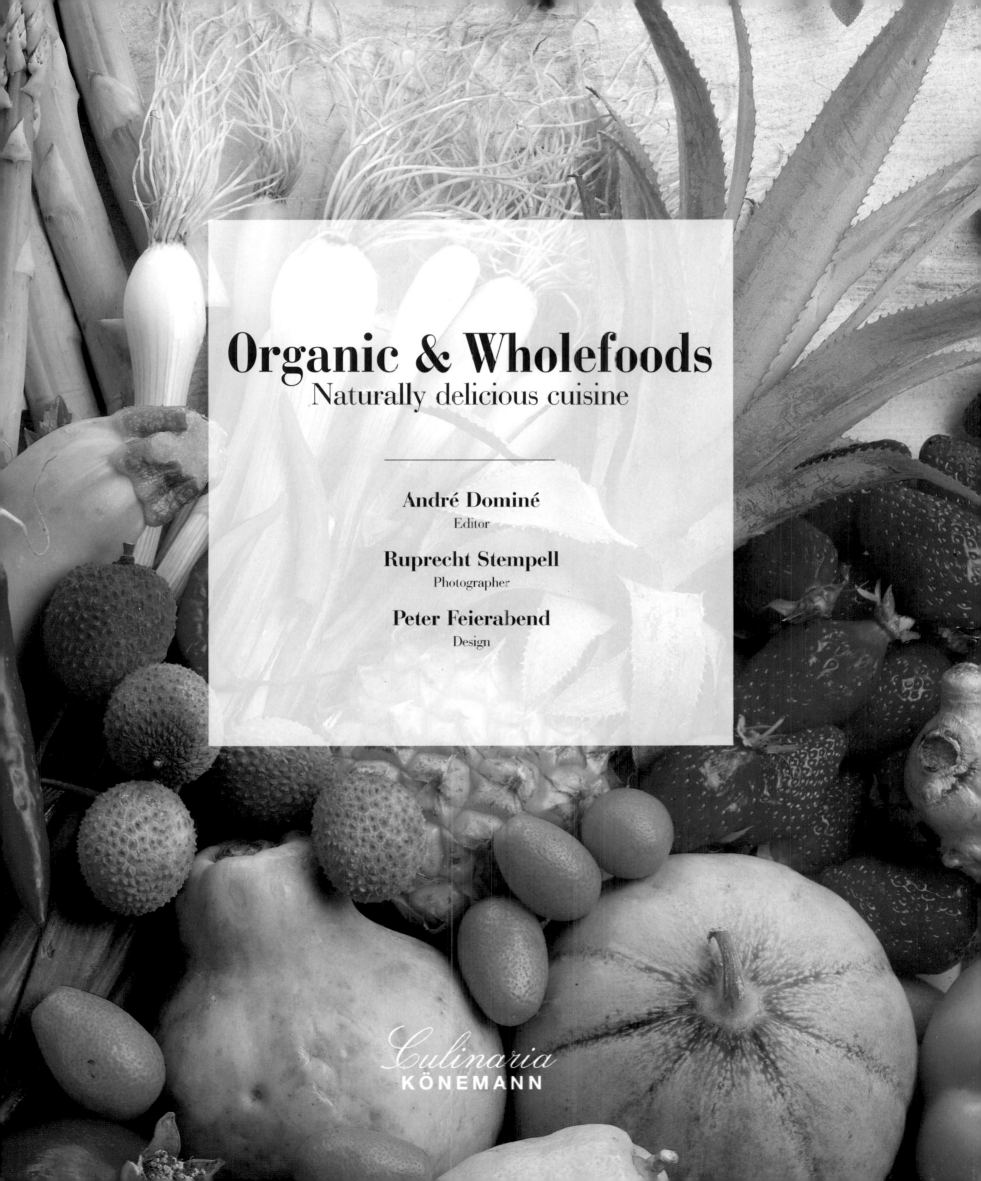

Organic & Wholefoods
Naturally delicious cuisine

André Dominé

Editor

Ruprecht Stempell

Photographer

Peter Feierabend

Design

Culinaria
KÖNEMANN

Abbreviations and Quantities

1 oz	1 ounce	$1/16$ pound
1 lb	1 pound	16 ounces
1 cup		8 ounces with solids* (see below); 8 fluid ounces with liquids
1 cup		4 ounces with flour and powdered sugar
1 cup		6 ounces with uncooked rice
1 cup		7 ounces with dried fruit
1 fl oz	1 fluid ounce	$1/16$ pint
1 pt	1 pint	16 fluid ounces
1 qt	1 quart	32 fluid ounces
1 gall	1 gallon	3.9 quarts
1 Tbs	1 level tablespoon	$1/12$ ounce with solids; 15–20 grams with solids; $1/2$ fluid ounce with liquids; 15 ml with liquids
1 tsp	1 level teaspoon	$1/6$ ounce with solids; 3–5 grams with solids; $1/6$ fluid ounce with liquids; 5 ml with liquids

Spoon measurements always apply to prepared ingredients
e.g. 1 Tbs chopped onion but 1 onion, peeled and chopped

Recipe portions
If not otherwise stated, the recipes serve four. To avoid any
misunderstanding, when a double page spread of recipes serves
different numbers of people, the number of portions that each recipe
makes is stated on each recipe, even when the recipe serves four.

Ingredients
These recipes use the highest quality ingredients, which are the richest
in nutrients, such as freshly milled flour, whole wheat flour, baking
powder, cold pressed, extra virgin olive oil, the zest of unwaxed citrus
fruits, honey, coarse salt, etc.

Nutritional information
All nutritional information is based on $3^1/2$ ounce (100 gram)
quantities of ingredients.

*Where feasible, quantities in recipes have been rounded up or down
for convenience. Metric conversions may therefore not correspond
exactly. It is important to use either American or metric
measurements within a recipe.

© 1997 Könemann Verlagsgesellschaft mbH
  Bonner Straße 126, D-50968 Cologne

Coordination:	Michael Ditter
Editing:	Christine Westphal (pp. 10–251); Ralph Fischer (pp. 252–293, 348–383, 396–443); Daniela Kumor (pp. 294–347, 384–395)
Home economists:	Astrid Öwermann, Uschi Stender-Barbieri
Help with recipes:	Yvonne Bauer, Andreas Köthe, Andreas Willius
Appendix:	Sabine Bleßmann
Photographic assistant:	Martin Kurtenbach, Yonca Norgaz
Studio:	Food Foto Köln – Brigitte Krauth and Jürgen Holz
Food styling:	Stephan Krauth
Translation from German:	Philip Jenkins; Lucy Morgan, Janet Richmond, and Jackie Smith for Hart McLeod, Cambridge
Copy-editing of the English edition:	Rosalind Horton for Hart McLeod, Cambridge
Typesetting:	Goodfellow & Egan, Cambridge
Production manager:	Detlev Schaper
Production:	Michael Ditter, Birgit Beyer
Reproductions:	Günnewig Produktions GmbH
Printed and bound by:	Neue Stalling, Oldenburg

Printed in Germany
ISBN 3-89508-472-7

Contents

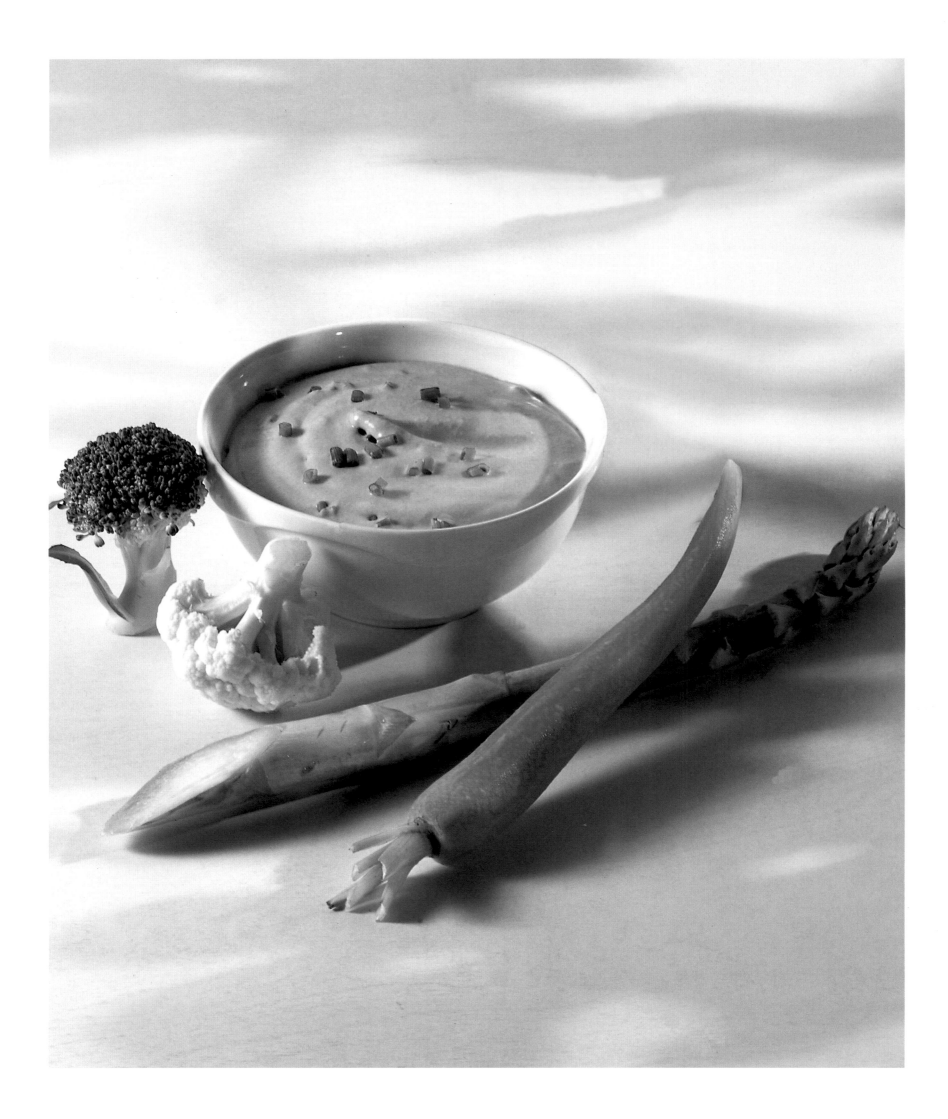

Not least because of numerous food scandals, consumers' awareness of the importance of a healthy diet has increased, and the eating habits of many people have changed for good. It has increasingly been recognized that fresh fruit and vegetables – if they are grown on living soil, fertilized with compost, protected from pests by natural means, and harvested when fully ripe – contain a wealth of vital substances which are of central importance for our well-being. Ecological farming and the wholefood trade have profited from this trend towards naturally grown, quality products. These products are now available everywhere – just around the corner or a few miles away out in the country where organic gardeners and farmers offer their products for sale: at markets, in stores, on the farm or through Box Schemes where goods are delivered to the door at no extra charge. The range of organic foods is now exceptionally large, not only with regard to fruit and vegetables. It also includes "wonder grains" such as spelt and amaranth, untreated rice from the Camargue, and hand-made pasta as well as virgin olive oil, exquisite vinegars, and organic bread, cakes, and pastries. All the products and ingredients presented and used here were produced in harmony with nature and provide food of the highest quality. Their health benefits, harvesting and production methods are highlighted as central themes. How the farm and orchard are run, on what soil something thrives, how to create the necessary conditions, which principles are taken into account so that plants and animals can develop in the best possible way – these are of great interest to all those who are concerned with the subject of wholefood. The organic pioneer Hans-Peter Rusch once pointed out: "Our own constitution will never be better than the constitution of our biological predecessors that provide us with food." If you eat organic food you are not only promoting your own health but also that of plants and animals, and the environment generally. The fact that a whole world of flavors and pleasures can be (re)discovered at the same time will also totally satisfy the gourmet.

**Preface by
André Dominé**

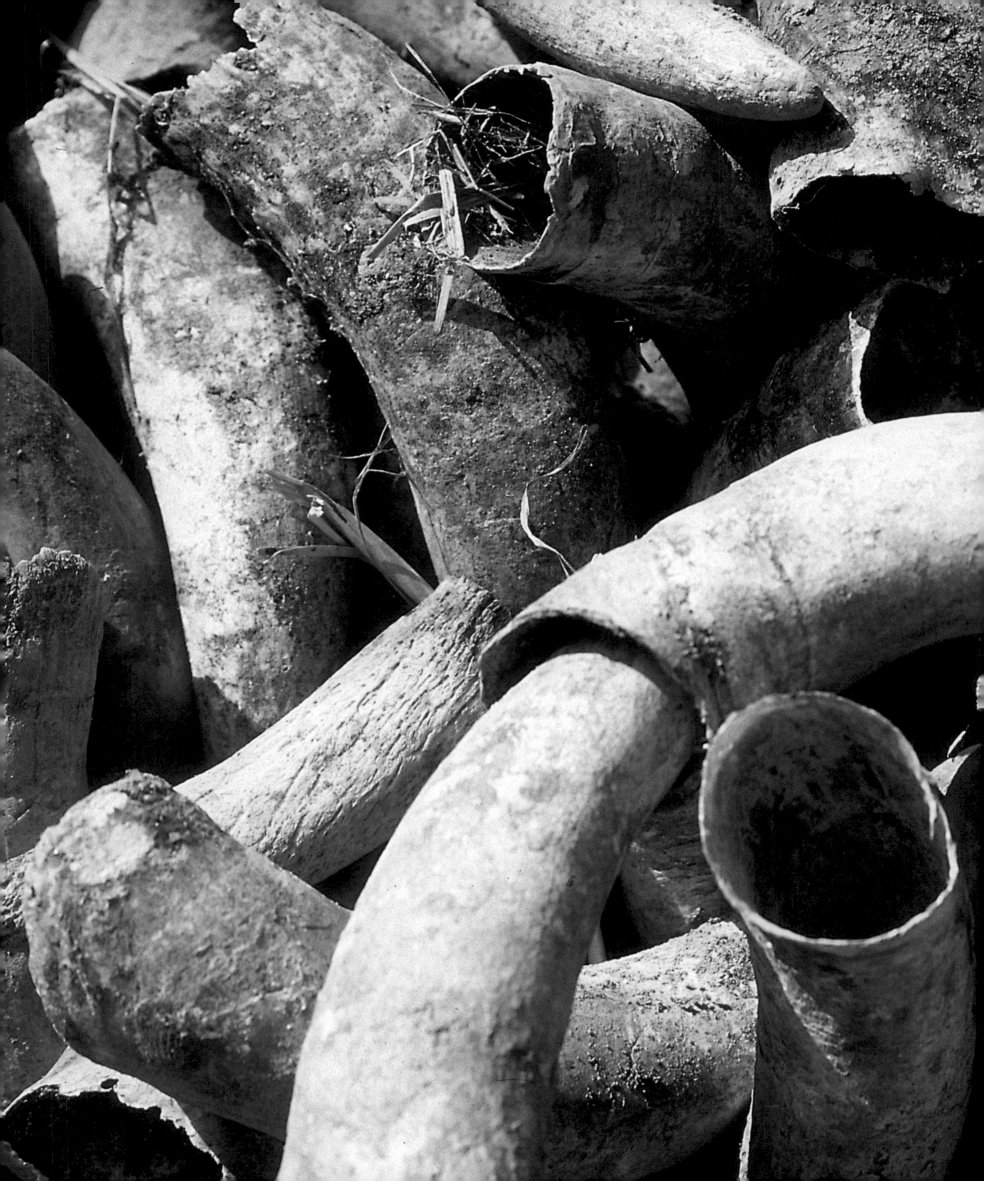

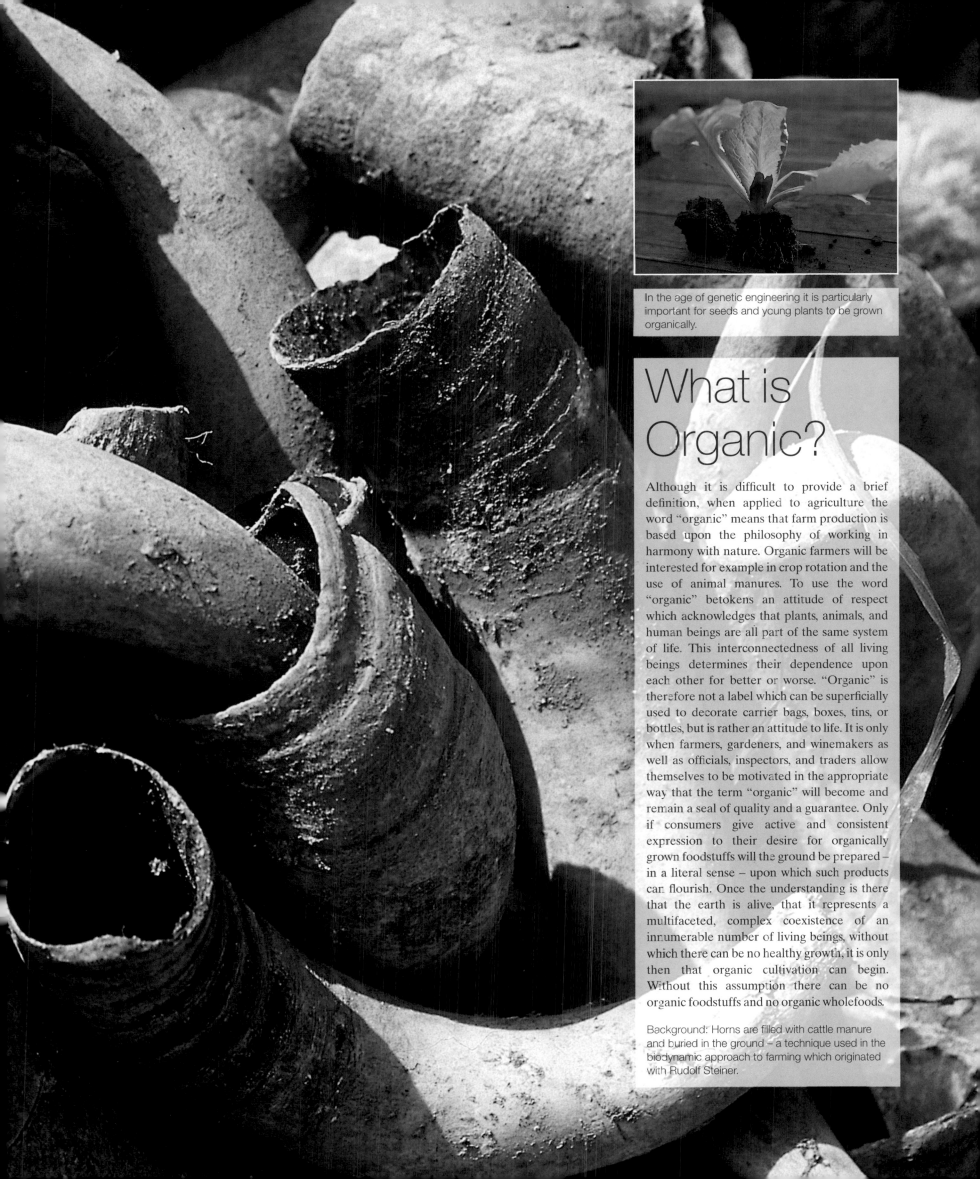

In the age of genetic engineering it is particularly important for seeds and young plants to be grown organically.

What is Organic?

Although it is difficult to provide a brief definition, when applied to agriculture the word "organic" means that farm production is based upon the philosophy of working in harmony with nature. Organic farmers will be interested for example in crop rotation and the use of animal manures. To use the word "organic" betokens an attitude of respect which acknowledges that plants, animals, and human beings are all part of the same system of life. This interconnectedness of all living beings determines their dependence upon each other for better or worse. "Organic" is therefore not a label which can be superficially used to decorate carrier bags, boxes, tins, or bottles, but is rather an attitude to life. It is only when farmers, gardeners, and winemakers as well as officials, inspectors, and traders allow themselves to be motivated in the appropriate way that the term "organic" will become and remain a seal of quality and a guarantee. Only if consumers give active and consistent expression to their desire for organically grown foodstuffs will the ground be prepared – in a literal sense – upon which such products can flourish. Once the understanding is there that the earth is alive, that it represents a multifaceted, complex coexistence of an innumerable number of living beings, without which there can be no healthy growth, it is only then that organic cultivation can begin. Without this assumption there can be no organic foodstuffs and no organic wholefoods.

Background: Horns are filled with cattle manure and buried in the ground – a technique used in the biodynamic approach to farming which originated with Rudolf Steiner.

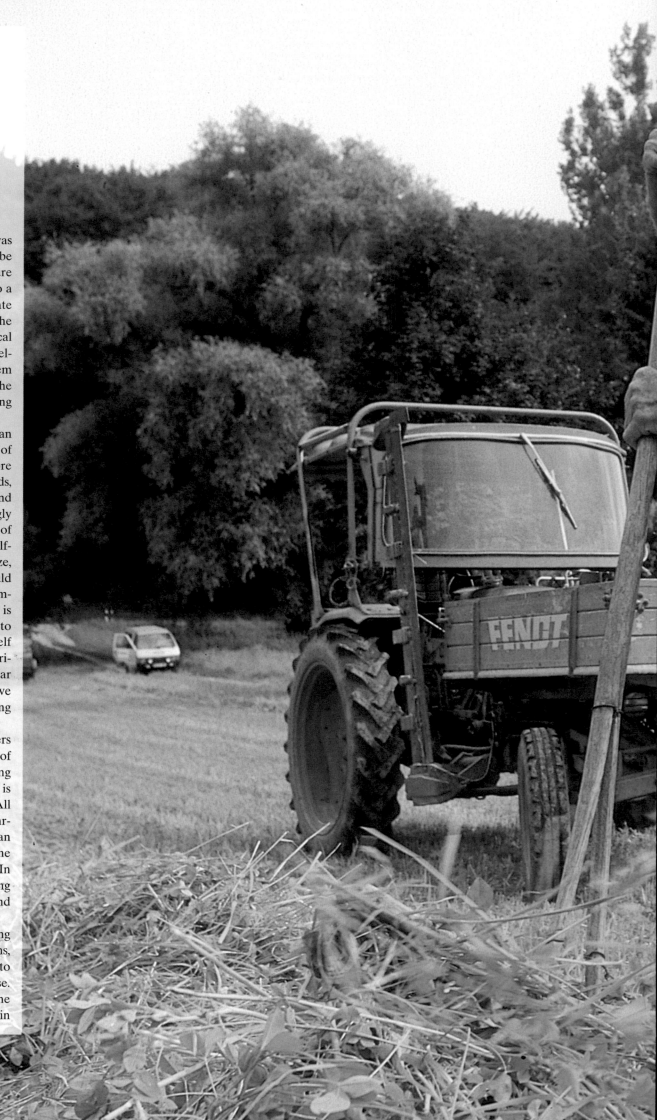

Organic Farming

The Biodynamic Approach to Farming

The oldest school of organic farming was founded in 1924 by Rudolf Steiner. It can be traced back to the lectures on agriculture which Steiner gave during the same year to a group of farmers on the Koberwitz estate near Wrocław in what is now Poland. The basis of this approach is the philosophical system of anthroposophy which was developed by Steiner. According to this system cosmic forces exercise an influence upon the earth which is itself understood as a living organism.

According to this view a farm is also an organism which reflects the diversity of nature. A biodynamic farm will therefore ideally consist of meadows and pasture, fields, vegetable plots and orchards, hedges and forest. The farming itself is correspondingly diverse. The aim is that the natural cycle of soil, plants, and animals should remain as self-enclosed as possible. According to the size, climate, and location of the farm there should be enough animals present so that the compost which is created from their manure is sufficient for fertilizing and contributing to the humus from which their feed is itself produced. Great importance is thereby attributed to animal husbandry, and in particular the raising of cattle, meaning that exclusive specialization in horticulture or the growing of fruit is not what is intended.

Synthetic means such as chemical fertilizers or poisons have no place in such a system of natural harmony, in which both human being and cosmos are included. In their place use is made of the influence of cosmic rhythms. All activities such as sowing, planting, or harvesting take place in accordance with an annual lunar calendar which indicates the most fruitful days and times for them. In contrast to the precepts of organic farming the earth is plowed in order to "open" it and make it receptive to cosmic powers.

Great significance is attributed to "imbuing the earth with life." Special preparations, which are made on every farm according to precise guidelines, are used for this purpose. They have a stimulating effect in the same way that homeopathic medicines have in

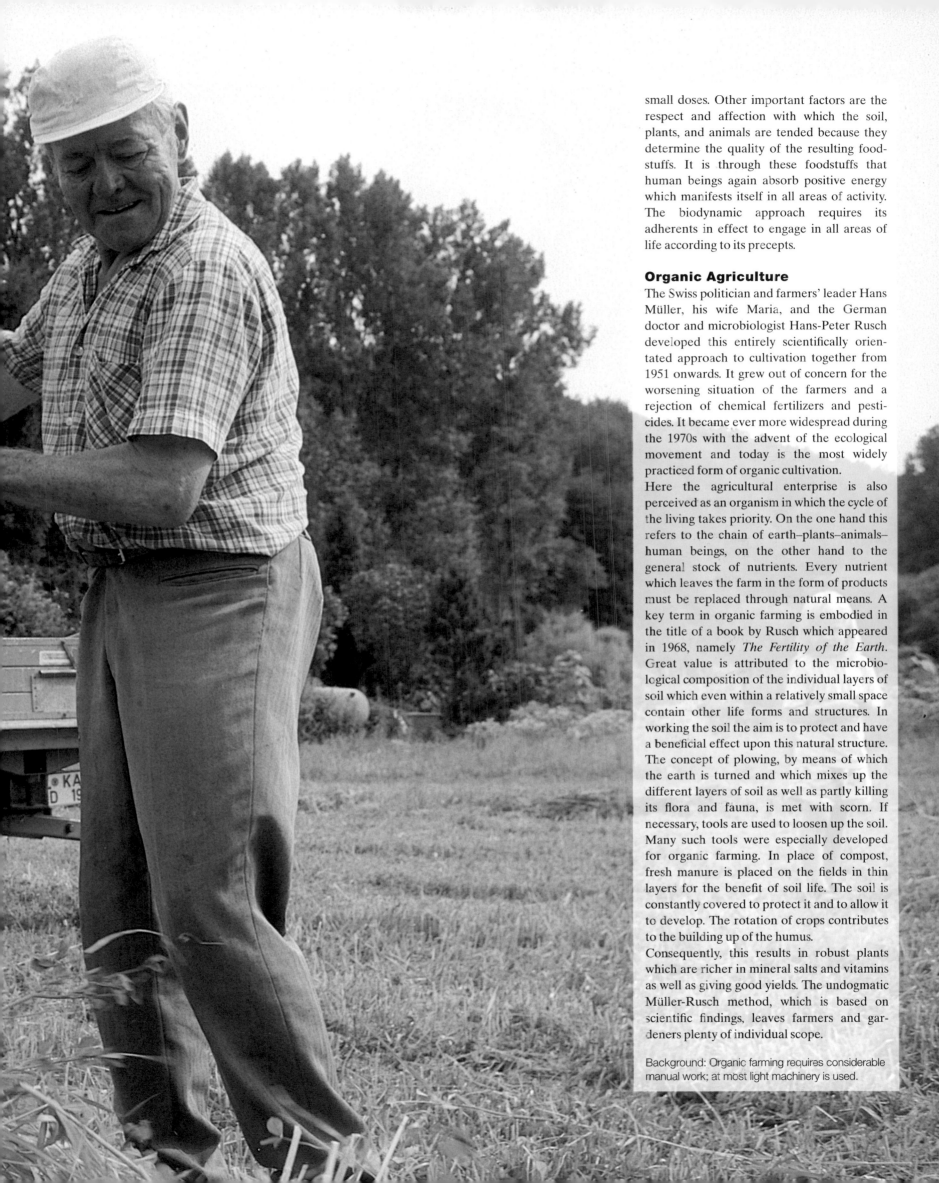

small doses. Other important factors are the respect and affection with which the soil, plants, and animals are tended because they determine the quality of the resulting foodstuffs. It is through these foodstuffs that human beings again absorb positive energy which manifests itself in all areas of activity. The biodynamic approach requires its adherents in effect to engage in all areas of life according to its precepts.

Organic Agriculture

The Swiss politician and farmers' leader Hans Müller, his wife Maria, and the German doctor and microbiologist Hans-Peter Rusch developed this entirely scientifically orientated approach to cultivation together from 1951 onwards. It grew out of concern for the worsening situation of the farmers and a rejection of chemical fertilizers and pesticides. It became ever more widespread during the 1970s with the advent of the ecological movement and today is the most widely practiced form of organic cultivation.

Here the agricultural enterprise is also perceived as an organism in which the cycle of the living takes priority. On the one hand this refers to the chain of earth–plants–animals–human beings, on the other hand to the general stock of nutrients. Every nutrient which leaves the farm in the form of products must be replaced through natural means. A key term in organic farming is embodied in the title of a book by Rusch which appeared in 1968, namely *The Fertility of the Earth*. Great value is attributed to the microbiological composition of the individual layers of soil which even within a relatively small space contain other life forms and structures. In working the soil the aim is to protect and have a beneficial effect upon this natural structure. The concept of plowing, by means of which the earth is turned and which mixes up the different layers of soil as well as partly killing its flora and fauna, is met with scorn. If necessary, tools are used to loosen up the soil. Many such tools were especially developed for organic farming. In place of compost, fresh manure is placed on the fields in thin layers for the benefit of soil life. The soil is constantly covered to protect it and to allow it to develop. The rotation of crops contributes to the building up of the humus.

Consequently, this results in robust plants which are richer in mineral salts and vitamins as well as giving good yields. The undogmatic Müller-Rusch method, which is based on scientific findings, leaves farmers and gardeners plenty of individual scope.

Background: Organic farming requires considerable manual work; at most light machinery is used.

The Pioneers

Forerunners of Organic Farming in England, France, Switzerland, and Germany

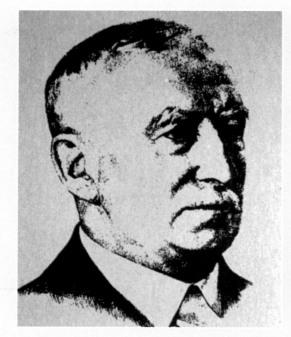

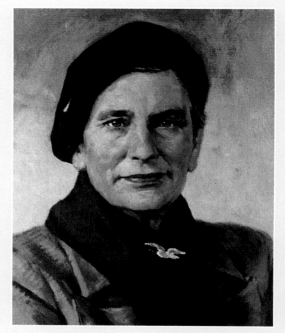

Albert Howard

Sir Albert Howard (1873–1947) was one of the first agricultural biologists who spoke out expressly against the use of chemical fertilizers and recognized their negative effects. Howard spent his childhood on a farm in Wales and after studying he worked in the British colonies. From 1905 he worked in India at the Agricultural Research Institute in Pusa. With his first wife Gabrielle, who was an outstanding botanist, he developed a series of wheat and hemp varieties for which he won international recognition.

He founded the Institute for Plant Cultivation in the Indian city of Indore and researched the traditional Indian methods of cultivation which had kept the soil there fertile for generations. In close collaboration with Indian farmers he developed the "Indore Method" of composting, as it is known, which was introduced in the 1930s on many plantations in Asia, Africa, and South America. His book *An Agricultural Testament*, published in 1940, shows the relationship between the health of the soil and that of plants and animals and explains the law of the return of nutrients. It not only had a great influence upon Lady Eve Balfour but also inspired Hans Müller and Hans-Peter Rusch. In the years before he died this highly respected scientist, who nonetheless had often been treated with hostility, became a wholehearted supporter of organic farming.

Eve Balfour

Even at the age of twelve Lady Eve Balfour (1899–1990) wanted to become a farmer. When she was 17 she enrolled at the University of Reading which she left with a degree in agriculture. She founded a jazz band in which she played the saxophone, wrote three detective novels, and gained a pilot's license. Such details are already a testimony to her independence, strength of will, and energy. She was 20 years old when she bought New Bells Farm near Haughley in Suffolk. Together with the neighboring farm which belonged to her friend Alice Debenham she had over 150 acres (60 hectares) of land at her disposal upon which she later began to experiment with organic cultivation. Inspired by the work of Albert Howard and an investigation into the connection between health and diet in rats, as well as on the basis of her own studies, she published her book *The Living Soil* in 1943. Its publication brought together farmers and interested academics and led to the founding of the Soil Association in 1952 with Balfour as its first president.

Diet and health in relation to the soil and the working of the soil were her lifelong concerns. She was convinced of the need for scientific research and on her own farmland initiated the "Haughley Experiment," in which various methods of cultivation were explored. To finance this project she founded the magazine *Mother Earth*, the predecessor of today's *Living Earth*. In 1970 this courageous project came to an end for financial reasons and the farm had to be sold in order to repay the debts.

Her lecture tours of the USA and Australia were received with great interest. As a founding member of the Soil Association, an organization of which she was general secretary for many years, as manager of the research farm, and as an author, Lady Eve Balfour stood at the beginning of the organic movement in England.

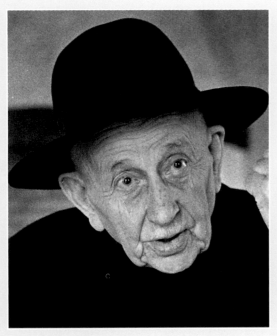

Raoul Lemaire

Raoul Lemaire (1884–1972) was already working in the wine and grain trade at the age of 14. In a few years he had become the largest wine and grain trader in the Somme, his native region of France. Since France was only producing mediocre wheat at that time and had to import wheat which was rich in gluten from the USA and Canada, Lemaire decided to devote himself to genetic research and cultivation of wheat. His investigations, for which he received a prize in Paris in 1928, lead to the development of imports of superior varieties of wheat. The nutritional scientist Paul Carton suggested that he create bread from natural ingredients. In 1931 Lemaire founded the first business selling natural products in Paris. Bakers could obtain stoneground flour from Société Lemaire and bake Pain Lemaire according to the company recipe. Today it is available in nearly 2,000 bakeries and foodstores.

Lemaire had already been studying the problem of using fertilizers since 1924. He approved of natural fertilizers and later experimented with magnesium fertilizers. In 1959 he discovered the advantages of calcified seaweed which contains calcium carbonate and magnesium, and propagated its use in organic farming. His acquaintance with Jean Boucher, a specialist on the subject of humus, led to the Lemaire-Boucher Method, which many French farmers began to use. The process is primarily based on five principles, which are as follows. 1. Natural balance of the soil thanks to the cultivation of cereals; 2. A deep loosening of the soil without breaking up soil stratification; 3. The creation of compost using organic fertilizers; 4. Mixed cultivation; 5. The use of the "calmagol alga as an organic catalyst. The method developed by Lemaire and Boucher and their definitions of farming laid the foundation stone for organic agriculture in France.

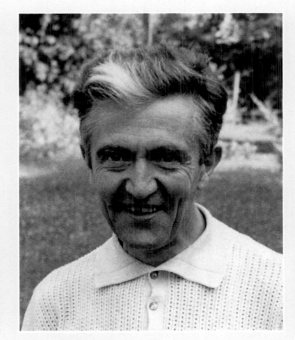

Jean Boucher

Jean Boucher was already specializing in soil life in 1936 during his studies in Versailles. When he was later working as the chief of the Department for Plant Protection in Loire-Atlantique and Vendée he objected to the officially recognized methods of pest control and despite their use increasingly attacked them. For this reason he made humus the focus of his scientific investigations at the beginning of the 1950s. Once he determined that the humus which was created on farms and in nurseries was often of poor quality, Boucher studied ways of improving it. He took as his starting points the work of Albert Howard as well as biodynamic viewpoints. By making skillful use of farm machinery he developed a technology for making compost which could also be practiced on larger farms. He personally stood up for an agriculture which made no use of toxins or artificial fertilizers. Together with Raoul Lemaire he worked on the Lemaire-Boucher method of organic farming and took over the technical management of Société Lemaire in 1963. He was a tireless campaigner for organic principles in agriculture.

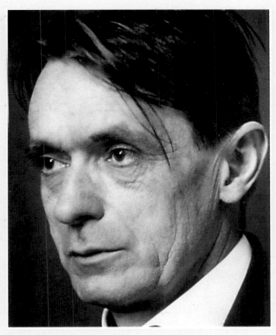

Rudolf Steiner

Rudolf Steiner (1861–1925) began studying at the Technical University in Vienna in 1879. He also studied literature and in 1882 edited Goethe's scientific writings. In 1890 Steiner moved to Weimar, where he wrote *The Philosophy Of Freedom* in 1894, one of his most important works. He was concerned with various aspects of philosophy although a tendency towards a reckoning with spiritual themes increasingly began to emerge.

In 1897 Steiner went to Berlin where amongst other things he gave courses in history which were well attended—proof of his great gift as a teacher. In Berlin he also came into contact with the theosophists, to whom he gave esoteric lectures. In 1902 he visited Annie Besant, the head of the Theosophical Society in London, who appointed him as their leader in Germany. Intensive work for the Theosophical Society became the preliminary step in the development of his own spiritual teaching, anthroposophy. In 1913 he founded the Anthroposophical Society and laid the foundation stone in the same year for its center, the Goetheanum, in Dornach in Switzerland.

From 1905 onwards Steiner's lecturing activities had increased enormously but were interrupted by war. He resumed them in 1921, following the foundation of the Waldorf School in 1919 and the opening of the Goetheanum in 1920. In the first nine months of 1924 Steiner increased the number of courses he was giving and devoted himself particularly to specialized areas such as special education, medicine and the formation of language. At the invitation of Carl Graf Keyserling who was aware of the fact that he was concerned with relevant questions, Steiner gave the lectures on agriculture on Keyserling's estate near Wrocław before over 100 farmers. The course became the founding moment of the biodynamic approach to farming (see p. 12).

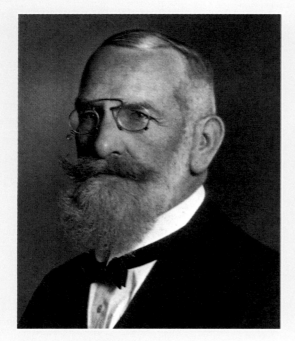

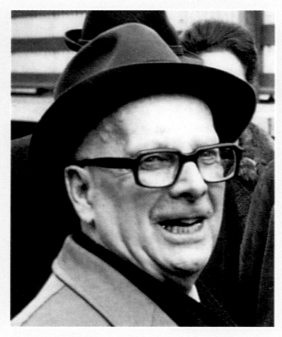

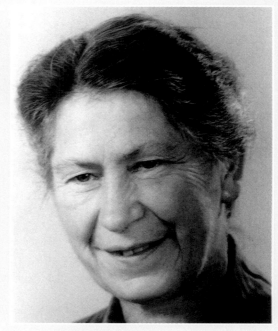

Maximilian Oskar Bircher-Benner

The Swiss doctor Maximilian Oskar Bircher-Benner (1867–1939) made an early study of the healing power of fresh plants which were able to absorb the energy of the sun and transform it. He was inspired in this respect due to his own frail health which was attributable to a congenital heart defect. At a time when the entire world believed that the best diet consisted of white bread and plenty of meat, he researched the healing properties of raw fruit and vegetables. In 1891 he opened a medical practice in Zurich and founded his own clinic there in 1895 in order to put his discoveries into practice.

Around 1900 he began to recommend to his patients that they ate a dietary meal made with apple for dinner. This became famous under the name "Bircher Muesli." To make this 3 tablespoons per person of oat flakes with cereal germ were soaked for twelve hours in three times their volume of water, then mixed with a little lemon juice, 2 tablespoons of honey and 3 tablespoons of light cream or milk and an unpeeled apple grated over the top. Finally freshly ground nuts are sprinkled over the granola. It quickly became popular everywhere. Soon companies began to manufacture and market it in a dried version. However a freshly prepared "Bircher Muesli" has little in common with the commercially packaged granola mixtures.

Bircher-Benner's successful cures attracted people from all over the world – Rainer Maria Rilke, Hermann Hesse, and Thomas Mann as well as Mahatma Gandhi with whom he corresponded. After the First World War the doctor made an intensive study of psychoanalysis and Eastern Asian teachings and attempted to discover the psychological causes of physical illnesses. He collected together a resumé of his work amongst other things in his book *A New Dietary Doctrine*, which was already in its sixth edition by 1937.

Hans Müller

Hans Müller (1891–1988) grew up in Switzerland on a large farm in the Emmental and from 1908 studied to be a teacher in Hofwil near Berne. After working as a teacher for three years he began studying biology, gaining his doctorate in 1921. He married Maria Bigler in 1914.

He was acquainted with the difficulties of the farmers at first hand. Industrial society, which was expanding, was threatening many farms and many farmers were seeking consolation in homemade schnapps. Influenced by the charitable example of his mother, who not only brought up seven of her own children but also 14 orphans, Müller founded the Swiss Association for Abstinent Farmers. He recognized that it was only through receiving a better education that the farmers would have greater opportunities and in 1926 he initiated week-long courses in cultural education. Whilst his wife ran a school for housekeeping on the Möschberg, Müller founded an educational center there modeled on the Danish system of adult education.

In 1946 Müller, together with like-minded people, founded the Co-operative for Cultivation and Utilization which still exists today, as well as the journal *Culture and Politics*. These initiatives were intended to propagate and further the cause of quality in foodstuffs. For he and his wife had since become preoccupied with a quite different set of problems. Migration from the countryside to the towns was consistently on the increase and the use of chemical fertilizers and pesticides in agriculture had, in the meanwhile, become alarming. Through a study of the relevant literature, contact with the advocates of the biodynamic approach to agriculture and their own studies, they were seeking a path which was in harmony with nature. With Hans-Peter Rusch, the German microbiologist, Müller and his wife developed the organic approach to agriculture. Möschberg became a training center and Hans Müller gave courses there for farmers until he died.

Maria Müller-Bigler

Hans Müller's work would be inconceivable without his wife Maria Bigler (1894–1969). Like him she also came from a farm in the Emmental. She received her education at the School of Horticulture and Home Management. After marrying in 1914 and giving birth to a son she made an intensive study of literature concerning diet, health, and agriculture. Through doing this she gained a specialized knowledge which she passed on to hundreds of young women farmers, most of whom came from modest backgrounds, in the small home management school on the Möschberg from 1933 onwards. As well as giving them a general education, which was unusual elsewhere, and teaching infant care, household, and garden management, Maria Müller laid stress on the teaching of dietary principles, drawing here on the work of pioneers such as Bircher-Benner. In 1959 she gathered together her experiences and insights in a publication called *What the Farmer's Family Needs to Know About Modern Diets*.

Maria Müller made her own important contribution to the principles of organic cultivation from the 1940s onwards. Reading through the night she researched all the available literature and discussed its contents with her husband. She tried out the knowledge that she had acquired in her own garden and on the Möschberg. The result of these practically-oriented investigations was a series of sound discoveries concerning organic farming and methods for maintaining the fertility of the soil, which formed the basis of Müller's approach, when the couple joined forces with Hans-Peter Rusch. Maria Müller's legacy is the *Practical Instructions for Organic Horticulture*. Shortly after it appeared she died at the age of 75.

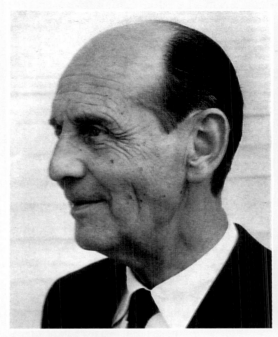

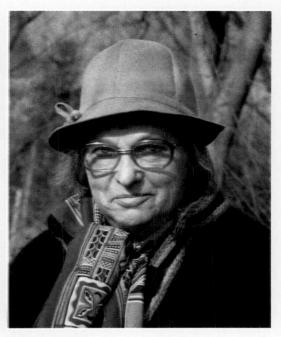

Hans-Peter Rusch

Hans-Peter Rusch (1906–1977) was born in East
Prussia and spent his childhood there. He studied
medicine in Giessen and from 1932 until the
Second World War he worked there in gynecology
in the University Clinic. Once he had qualified as
a university lecturer he was appointed as lecturer
in gynecology and obstetrics. However, before he
could take up his teaching appointment he was
ordered to Sicily to serve as a military medical
officer.

After the war Rusch found a position as a doctor
at the cancer clinic in Lehrbach and with the
bacteriologist A. Becker he researched the function of bacteria with the aim of developing new
medicaments. In the process, Rusch made discoveries which he published in an article in a
medical journal in 1950 entitled *The Cycle of
Bacteria as Life Principle*. In this article Hans
Müller found the scientific approach which was
lacking in organic farming. Müller sought out
Rusch, and when Rusch was given notice by the
clinic, Hans Müller urged him to found a
laboratory for which a friendly drugstore owner in
Herborn placed a garage at his disposal. Over the
years a significant medical institute evolved from it.
In this laboratory Rusch investigated the microbiological condition of the soil and developed a
test which was named after him and which gave
farmers and gardeners who were working
organically precise information about the fertility
of the soil. At the same time Rusch acted as
scientific adviser to the Swiss Co-operative for
Cultivation, gave courses on the Möschberg and
explained the scientific principles of organic
agriculture in lectures and in regular contri-
butions to *Culture and Politics*. The publications
Science of Tomorrow (1955) and *Fertility of the
Soil – A Study of Organic Thinking* (1968) are
textbooks for the Müller–Rusch approach to
cultivation.

Maria Thun

Maria Thun, née Jung, was born in Marburg an
der Lahn, Germany in 1922. She grew up in
nearby Grossfelden on a farm and as a child had
to keep watch over geese and cows. It was through
this that she learnt which plants animals preferred
and which they disliked. During the Second
World War she worked in nursing and it was here
that she became acquainted with her future
husband Walter Thun, who was a painter and
pupil of Rudolf Steiner. Through Walter Thun she
came into contact with anthroposophy and the
principles of the bio-dynamic approach to
farming. Through shared observations their attention was drawn to the striking differences in the
development of plants which occurred despite
apparently similar growing conditions. In 1952 she
first began to think that the cosmos around us,
represented by the sun, the moon, and the planets
could have an influence on the growth of plants,
and she began a series of experiments aimed at
exploring this idea.

She published her findings in 1963 in the article *A
Nine Year Investigation into Cosmic Influences
upon Annual Plants*. It met with lively interest
amongst both gardeners and farmers, offering
them concrete recommendations concerning seeds,
husbandry, and harvesting. The same year saw the
publication of the first sowing calendar which has
since appeared in more than 20 languages and
entered its 34th edition in 1996.

In 1964 Maria Thun also began to research the
way in which biodynamic preparations work. At
her research institute for the influence of the
constellations on the cultivation of plants, which is
located in Biedenkopf in Germany, she carried
out experiments with all European cultivated
plants. She has at her disposal twelve acres (five
hectares) of gardening land, her own laboratory
for soil and plant analysis, and baking facilities for
the investigation of bread quality. Her son and
grandson now provide her with support in her
work.

The Basis of a Healthy Diet

Nutrients and Vitamins

There is no life without food. Malnutrition is seriously damaging to one's health whilst over-eating also leads to grave health problems. This suggests that a correct diet is not only a matter of eating the correct amount of food. It seems reasonable to assume that for many patients, incorrect eating and drinking habits and/or poor quality foodstuffs are responsible for their suffering. For this reason it is important to understand the ways in which the most fundamental elements of our diet work.

Nutrients

Carbohydrates

Photosynthesis is one of the most miraculous things which happen on our earth. Plants absorb carbon dioxide and water and under the influence of sunlight and with the help of chlorophyll, the green pigment in plant leaves, they produce glucose, a carbohydrate. From material that is inorganic and low in energy they produce a substance which is organic and rich in energy. Put another way, thanks to plants sunlight is transformed into energy which living beings can absorb. And in the process another element is released, without which life could not exist, namely oxygen.

Carbohydrates, by which we mean sugars or saccharides, constitute the mainstay of any diet in volume terms. A distinction is made between the following:
• Monosaccharides or simple sugars such as glucose and fructose,
• Disaccharides, which are compounds of two monosaccharides such as maltose and lactose or cane sugar and beet sugar, the latter also being made into household sugar,
• Polysaccharides such as starch, cellulose, or pectin.

The body can use only glucose and fructose directly. All other carbohydrates must be broken down by the metabolism and turned into glucose. Glucose is broken down into carbon dioxide and water in the body thus releasing the energy which is created during photosynthesis. Generally this energy is required for all bodily activities and body temperature. Furthermore, it is essential for the functioning of the brain, red corpuscles, and the nervous system. However this process of transformation can only take place through the influence of vitamin B1, thiamin.

As a rule, nature itself will provide any necessary supplements. However, when for example in the manufacture of household sugar B vitamins are

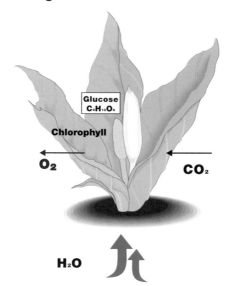

Sunlight

Glucose C₆H₁₂O₆

Chlorophyll

O₂ ← → CO₂

H₂O

The process of photosynthesis: with the help of light and chlorophyll, green plants make glucose, which is organic and rich in energy, from inorganic carbon dioxide (CO_2) and water (H_2O) and release oxygen (O_2).

removed, this can cause severe problems, particularly in the nervous system. The same is true of white flour because the removal of minerals from it has a negative effect on teeth and bones. Disaccharides such as maltose by contrast, which is widespread in cereal germ and lactose, which is used in infant and dietary food, have positive characteristics.

When two monosaccharide molecules combine, the product is a disaccharide. If the reaction involves numerous molecules the resulting sugar complexes can consist of hundreds or even thousands of molecules. One of these polysaccharides, which are not sweet in taste, is starch. It is stored in plants and is particularly concentrated in seeds and tubers. So that organisms can make use of starch, enzyme molecules must be split up. Since these processes require time, glucose is only released gradually and the body is continuously supplied with energy. Fiber (see p. 31) is also one of the polysaccharides, but is generally not broken down and therefore not absorbed.

If more carbohydrates are consumed than are needed to fulfil the body's energy requirements there are two possibilities. Either the energy is transformed into glycogen, which is stored in the liver and muscles as reserves which can be easily drawn upon. Their capacity for absorption is limited to approximately 12 ounces (350 grams). Anything in excess of this turns into fat. This is also stored and can be drawn upon, assuming that no glucose, which is easier to metabolize, is absorbed first.

Fat

Carbohydrates, protein, and fat constitute together the so-called three primary nutrients,

since they supply the organism with energy. Once plants have created carbohydrates, the same basic elements – carbon, water, and oxygen under the further influence of the energy of the sun – combine to produce fat, which has the important function of transporting vitamins which are fat-soluble. Fat consists mainly of three different fatty acids and glycerine. A distinction is made between saturated, monounsaturated, and polyunsaturated fatty acids. Saturated fatty acids such as butyric acid, occur predominantly in animal foodstuffs but can also be produced by the body itself. They are water-soluble, are directly absorbed into the bloodstream during digestion, and are of use only as a source of energy.

The situation is otherwise with unsaturated fatty acids which are able to combine with other substances such as vitamins. Olive oil consists predominantly of monounsaturated fatty acids which prevent the occurrence of arteriosclerosis. Polyunsaturated fatty acids are essential, that is to say that the body needs them in order to function properly but is unable to produce them itself. The most important are linoleic and linolenic acid, from which further essential fatty acids can be formed. These have a variety of effects, are a constituent part of cell structure and of nervous tissue as well as being the starting point for indispensable tissue hormones and also influencing metabolism. Furthermore they also reduce any excess cholesterol. Essential fatty acids are produced by plants; they can also be absorbed from fish or meat. At their best however they produce edible oils, the quality of which depends upon the content of essential fatty acids.

Protein

The third principal nutrient is protein which at the same time is part of the fabric of the body. Whether it is hair or skin, muscles or bone, organs or blood, they all primarily consist of protein. Once again it is plants which produce protein in a spectacularly simple way by absorbing another element, namely nitrogen. From nitrogen, carbon, hydrogen, and oxygen they form proteins, which are macromolecules. Proteins behave in the most differing ways and their spheres of influence are correspondingly differentiated. So, for example, enzymes, hormones, hemoglobin, or antibodies are all proteins. Proteins fulfil functions such as stimulation, transformation, transportation, resistance, but also the transmission of nerve impulses, the storage of trace elements and tissue support.

Although the different number of proteins in existence is quite enormous and many of them remain unresearched, they are made up of only 20 amino acids which can be characterized as the "alphabet of life." Eight amino acids are essential, whilst the body can synthesize the remaining twelve itself. The fact that all eight essential amino acids are contained in meat has led to a disproportionate emphasis being placed on the eating of meat and as a consequence the intake of protein is too high and is damaging to health. Animal protein moreover has to be converted in the human body, whilst vegetable protein can be utilized more directly. It is certainly true that plants rarely contain all essential amino acids and those that they do contain are present in differing degrees of concentration, but by combining them with various ingredients – and this is most patently the case with cereals and legumes – the biological valence of vegetable protein is increased. This is even more the case when plant and milk protein are combined. As the nutritional scientist and founder of the wholefood approach to eating, Werner Kollath, demonstrated, there is a substantial difference between raw, living protein and protein which has been heated to a temperature in excess of 110 °F (43 °C), which loses important living factors such as enzymes. For this reason vegetables when eaten raw, despite the proportionately low protein content are particularly valuable sources of protein.

Vitamins and Other Vital Substances

Vitamins are organic substances which are essential to life and which, with the exception of vitamin C, occur and function in tiny amounts. Their sphere of influence lies particularly in the metabolism which converts carbohydrates, fats, and protein. Without vitamins, which are often constituent parts of enzymes and which act as catalysts, this conversion process cannot take place, or only takes place in a disturbed fashion. Since vitamins cannot be formed sufficiently by the body itself, we have to absorb them from food. They are therefore essential. Vitamins, which represent sensitive and extremely complicated structures, show a poor level of tolerance where oxygen, light, and heat are concerned. It therefore follows that foodstuffs which are rich in vitamins

Essential Amino Acids

All protein in our bodies consists of 20 building blocks, the amino acids. We have to absorb eight of them from food, so that the body can produce the remaining twelve itself. These eight amino acids are described as "essential." What is important is that the essential amino acids are all absorbed at the same time, because it is only then that they can be transformed into proteins according to current need. Since there is a high protein requirement during growth in particular, a deficiency can lead to considerable health problems and deformities. Two amino acids, arginine and histidine, are described as "semiessential" because they are only necessary as part of an infant diet; they are to be found in breast milk.
Aside from meat and fish, countless other foodstuffs also contain all eight essential amino acids, for example eggs, milk, cheese, quark and other milk products, as well as several varieties of grain and various vegetables and fruits.
Several varieties of vegetables and fruit do not contain all of the amino acids, but contain some of them in noteworthy amounts.

must be handled with the greatest of care when it comes to storage and preparation. Meals which are prepared raw from fresh ingredients guarantee the highest intake of vitamins. Foodstuffs show a marked reduction in vitamin content when they are processed and stored for longer periods of time or are preserved by the use of heat. The most recent research has determined that there is a high degree of differentiation amongst vitamins. However it is still customary to follow the preexisting system of classification according to which vitamins are divided into two large groups, namely the fat-soluble and the water-soluble.

Fat-soluble Vitamins

• Vitamin A (retinol) – In foods from an animal source as retinol in liver and protein; in vegetables and fruit, as its active precursor betacarotene in carrots, pumpkins, apricots etc; component of the pupil of the eye, indispensable for vision; protective function for cells, their membranes, for skin and mucous membrane.

• Vitamin D (calciferol) – In food from an animal source in liver, fish, milk products; in those from a vegetable source as its active precursor in mushrooms, wheat germ oil, spinach, yeast etc; necessary for the regulation of calcium in bones, teeth, skin; deficiency leads to rickets.

• Vitamin E (tocopherol) – Present in small amounts in foods from an animal source, high incidence in soybean, sprouts, germ oils, nuts, and plants that produce oils; protects vitamins A, D, and C as well as fatty acids from oxidation, thus protecting cell membranes and the nervous system, thereby maintaining healthy blood vessels and countering blood clotting.

• Vitamin K (phyloquinone) – In milk products, liver, and fish, in cress, leafy vegetables, and salads, cabbage, sauerkraut; indispensable for clotting of the blood, protection against strokes.

Water-soluble Vitamins

• Vitamin B1 (thiamin) – In pork, poultry, and milk; above all in whole wheat, untreated rice, yeast, wheat germ, kernels; important role as an enzyme in metabolism, having an effect on the brain, nerves, mental state; severe problems where deficient (beri beri).

• Vitamin B2 (riboflavin) – In milk, milk products, egg yolk, meat; brewer's yeast, legumes, nuts, whole wheat; indispensable to metabolism as a constituent of various enzymes, important for the blood, eyes, skin, hair, and aids sleep.

• Vitamin B3 (niacin) – In lean meat, poultry, game, fish, eggs; in vegetables and whole wheat; indispensable to the metabolism and as a constituent part of cells and enzymes; ensures psychological balance, works against heart attacks; a deficiency causes severe weakness.

• Vitamin B5 (pantothenic acid) – In offal, blue-veined cheese; in legumes, various vegetables, and whole wheat; activates fatty acids; important constituent part of the energy giving coenzyme A

and other coenzymes, limits inflammation, reduces stress, counteracts rheumatism.

• Vitamin B6 (pyridoxine) – In fish and meat; above all in whole wheat, legumes, leafy vegetables, potatoes, also in honey and various fruits; necessary in metabolism for conversion of essential fatty acids and amino acids, blood formation, and for various hormones; works against psychological irritability, arteriosclerosis, and asthma; deficiency causes far-reaching problems.

• Vitamin B12 (cyanocobalamin) – In foods derived from animals; otherwise in soy sauces, sauerkraut, brewer's yeast, rare in plants; with enzymes builds up amino acids and nucleic acids and breaks down fatty acids; counters illnesses of the stomach and intestines; deficiency leads to anemia and nervous disorders.

• Folic Acid – In meat; above all however in vegetables, salads, sprouts, whole wheat, and brewer's yeast; indispensable for cell formation, transmission of the genetic code, red corpuscles, metabolizing of protein; counters anemia and is regenerative; deficiency manifests itself in anemia, illnesses of the stomach and intestine, tissue damage; most widespread vitamin deficiency in Europe.

• Biotin (Vitamin H) – In egg yolk, offal, cheese; in soybean, whole wheat, nuts, spinach, and green herbs; stimulates metabolic processes, particularly in the breaking down and conversion of saccharides; good for the skin and hair; deficiency manifests itself in dry, inflamed skin and nervousness.

• Vitamin C (ascorbic acid) – In liver and kidneys; above all in fruit and vegetables; extraordinarily diverse roles in metabolism, formation of connective tissue and stroma, hormones and antibodies; promotes iron absorption; highly diversified role as protection against pathogens and toxins, regenerative, strengthens the immune system.

Free Radicals

Chemical reactions are constantly taking place in the human body. The metabolism consists of processes which are to a great extent highly complicated and which furthermore happen extraordinarily quickly. These do not always proceed as is to be hoped. This is particularly the case if the negative consequences of nicotine or alcohol, radiation or environmental toxins, smog or ozone, infections or wrongly prescribed medicines are experienced, since these are all factors which enhance oxidation. The result is the separation of atoms or molecules which remain chemically unattached – the result being the creation of so-called free radicals. They react in an extremely aggressive fashion. As they combine forcibly with atoms or molecules, they attack other molecules as well as cells and cell nuclei, thus damaging and altering them. Free radicals are thought to be carcinogenic. However, they also have a preference for combining with fatty acids, and when modified these can lead to arteriosclerosis, heart attacks, and strokes. Vitamins are antagonistic towards free radicals, protecting against oxidation.

Living Topsoil

The Soil

The soil is the wafer thin weathered skin of the earth, consisting of stones which have been ground into dust and humus. It grows naturally at a rate of only one tenth of a millimeter per year and is constantly formed, transformed, and enriched by billions of microorganisms from minerals and plant remains, the air, and water. The living topsoil is the most valuable possession in the field and in the organic garden. The chemical and physical characteristics of soil – whether it is acidic or alkaline, sticks heavily to the spade or crumbles easily from the hoe – depend upon the varieties of rock from which it is derived. The composition of soil is always different, broadly consisting of the following:

- Primary or igneous rocks such as granite, basalt, greenstone, or porphyry – the result of volcanic eruptions which took place billions of years ago;
- Sedimentary rocks such as sandstone and clay, gravel and morainal rock;
- Metamorphic rocks such as slate, gneiss, phyllite, and argillite – the result of major events such as the formation of mountains at high temperature and great pressure;
- Limestones such as Jura, chalk, marble, or dolomite – formed by lime in water or from the skeletons and shells of mussels, corals, and snails.

All four types of rock help to make up the subsoil. They are important as a means of storing water, as drainage, and as a sieve and a filter.

Soil Types

Sandy Soil

Sandy soil grows warm quickly and cools down equally quickly. It can be worked without effort. Its level of water retention is low, which makes watering more often necessary. Organic fertilizers rot quickly, it is a poor retainer of nutrients which are quickly washed into the subsoil. The humus content is low. Sandy soil of a fine consistency is easily carried away by the wind.
Soil care: With sandy soil it is above all the humus component which must be increased by adding compost. In order to improve water retention and to keep nutrients for longer in the topsoil, a filler such as bentonite with a high content of clay minerals is suitable. Covering the soil with a layer of mulch will prevent it from drying out quickly.

Loamy Soil

Loamy soil is ideal for the garden. It retains water and nutrients very well and aeration is good.
Soil care: Loamy soil is rich, regularly requiring the addition of organic matter via compost, so that the humus content remains intact. If it is given the proper organic treatment, this soil will present few problems.

Clay Soil

Clay soil is heavy, wet, and sticky. It warms up only slowly in the spring and must be dug over often with a hoe, so that it does not become rock hard and tear when dry. Clay soil retains nutrients well, but aeration is poor.
Soil care: Clay soil must be broken up, and for this it is best to use sand. So that the sand does not form dry pockets in the clay, compost is added with the sand. Deep-rooting plants loosen clay soil. A covering of mulch prevents it from drying and cracking.

Humus – Retainer of Water and Source of Nutrients

It is humus which makes fertile topsoil out of soil which contains minerals. Humus is the organic substance, the connecting link between living things and minerals, storing water and providing nutrients. Billions of things which live in the soil nourish themselves on organic substances, are converted into something else, die, and themselves become a source of organic nutrition. For this they need air, water, and heat. If the soil has hardened, has been spoilt by mismanagement, or if the layer of decomposing organic matter and accompanying microorganisms are buried below the reach of spade or plough then organic material will go rotten rather than decompose. The activity of the soil is responsible for its humus content, its suitability for cultivation and the degree to which it crumbles. In the uppermost 6 inches (15 centimeters) of soil which is used for growing plants there live in one hectare (2.5 acres) approximately 22,000 pounds (10,000 kilograms) of bacteria, 22,000 pounds (10,000 kilograms) of fungi, 815 pounds (370 kilograms) of protozoa, 306 pounds (140 kilograms) of algae, 37 pounds (17 kilograms) of insects and 13 pounds $3^1/_2$ ounces (6 kilograms) of springtails.

The Life of the Soil

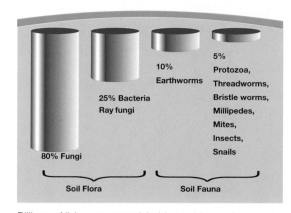

80% Fungi

25% Bacteria
Ray fungi

10%
Earthworms

5%
Protozoa,
Threadworms,
Bristle worms,
Millipedes,
Mites,
Insects,
Snails

Soil Flora   Soil Fauna

Billions of living creatures inhabit a cubic centimeter of healthy soil, renewing it by means of their complex interaction with it.

Soil Life

In the natural cycle of matter it is soil life which transforms all organic material into nutrients for the next generation of plants. In the garden and the field, compost, solid manure, and plants which fertilize organically provide additional nutrition for the living things in the soil. According to the fundamental principle of fertilizing in organic farming and horticulture it is not the plants which are fed, but rather the soil. Plants obtain their nutrients from soil life, therefore receiving them in a natural, harmonious form.

The Earthworm as Organic Indicator

Particularly important in nature's recycling system – the layer of decomposing organic matter – is the earthworm. Up to 8,800 pounds (4,000 kilograms) of earthworms live in one hectare (2.5 acres) of farmland. Earthworms dig deep into the soil down to the layer of minerals and from there they fetch weathered rock up – 13 tons per acre (30 tonnes per hectare) of grazing land per year. Earthworms are geophages, earth eaters. They swallow the earth through which they tunnel and eat the dead parts of plants. In their digestive tracts organic and mineral substances are digested and knitted together. The resulting tiny piles of excrement are mixtures of clay and humus with a high concentration of nutrients, they contain seven times as much nitrogen, six times as much magnesium, three times as much potash, and twice as much phosphorus and lime as firm garden earth. Earthworms are infallible organic indicators. The more the soil is inhabited by them, the healthier it is.

Optimal Suitability of the Soil for Cultivation

Fertile soil has as many cavities as a sponge and even when subjected to quite heavy demand will remain crumbly and loose. Soil which is tended organically can store twice its own weight in water: just under four pints (two liters) of water to two pounds (one kilogram) of earth. It is extremely well suited to cultivation – the ideal conditions for growing.

Ecological Working of the Soil Through the Seasons

Living things in the soil have quite different requirements for light, air, and heat. Each will live in the layer of soil which provides it with optimal conditions. If a spade or plow breaks into this ordered world, digs out clods of earth, and stands them on their heads, this will be a fatal shock for billions of living things. The rest is taken care of by frost. Gardeners and farmers who work organically do not turn the soil but loosen it at a deeper level. For this the farmer uses a grubber, whilst the gardener uses a digging fork. The digging fork is inserted into the soil every 4 inches (10 centimeters) and moved backwards and forwards energetically. The soil is loosened immediately after the harvest or after the first frost. An exception is made for extremely hard soils or newly cultivated surfaces. Here spades and plows are used until the soil is alive and suitable for planting.

If the soil is to be worked, it is covered with a layer of rough compost, rotted straw, or fruit tree leaves approximately 2 inches (5 centimeters) thick. Beneath this warm cover the living creatures of the soil continue to work long after beast and man no longer can. In the spring the covering of mulch is removed. Then all that is required to make the soil ready for sowing and planting is the crumbling of the surface. As an alternative, plots and fields are sown in the late summer with plants which fertilize organically. These expanses are then broken up in the spring. Over the winter the organic fertilizer forms a vital protective layer.

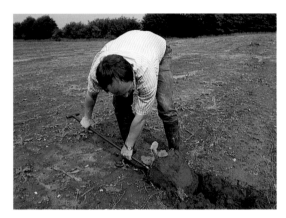

To carry out the spade test a flat spade is inserted vertically into the soil. A portion of soil is lifted clear in order to take the sample.

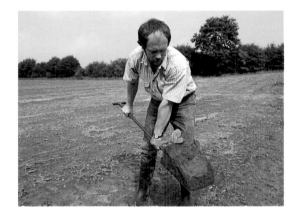

The sample – as a rule it is fixed initially with a board – shows a clean cut profile of the soil approximately 12 inches (30 centimeters) deep.

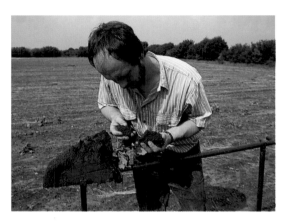

Two wooden supports, upon which the spade and the soil sample can be placed, allow the test to be carried out comfortably whilst standing.

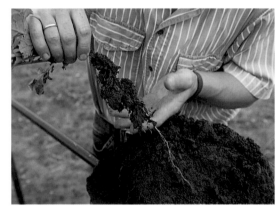

Close scrutiny of the sample provides information about the condition of the soil. Long roots which reach deep are a good sign.

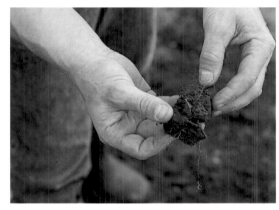

Finally the sample is thrown to the ground and falls apart. The size of the lumps of soil as well as the existence of living creatures both provide further information.

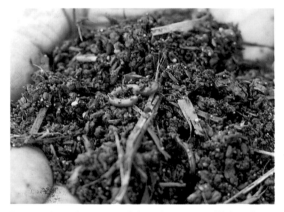

The gardener has every right to be content if his soil displays such a teeming mass of different living things and such a loose structure.

The Spade Test

(Illustrations above)

The spade test was developed after the First World War by Johannes Görbing. It was Gerhardt Preuschen who restored its respectability above all for organic farming and brought it to the attention of many young farmers, gardeners, and advisers.

- 1. To carry out the test you will need a flat spade, one which has either been molded flat or made from flat steel, with a blade 4 inches (10 centimeters) wide and 12 inches (30 centimeters) long; you will also require a garden spade, a simple nail, and a small board the size of the blade of the spade. It is also useful to have two wooden supports at hand, on which to place the spade and earth so that the sample can be inspected whilst standing.
- 2. The flat spade is inserted vertically into the soil at an angle of 90°. If it can be inserted easily then the soil is rich in humus and loose. If it is difficult to penetrate the soil the spade is driven into the earth with a hammer.
- 3. A portion of soil approximately 20 inches (50 centimeters) long, the width of the spade but slightly deeper is then lifted clear with the garden spade holding it in place. The flat spade is now free, is carefully removed and the soil sample is fixed with a small board. A cube of earth about 4 to 8 inches (10 to 20 centimeters) large should then be cut out, lifted clear – as quickly as possible and ideally with help from somebody so that it does not crumble – and should be placed on the floor or the wooden supports.
- 4. The soil sample should now be scrutinized quite closely:
– How deep are the roots? Are the roots narrow ones which reach up to a depth of 12 inches (30 centimeters) or is it only the main roots which have managed to force their way through soil which has become compressed?
– Is there any evidence of earthworms in the soil sample or was the hard subsoil too difficult for earthworms to penetrate?
– Do the roots break off horizontally because they have reached a layer of soil that they could not penetrate?
– Does the soil break up into proper rounded clumps rather than losing its form?
– Is there only a thin surface layer of soil suitable for cultivation whilst the remainder is rock hard?
– Do any parts of the soil give off a foul smell and are there any areas lacking in oxygen where sludge gases have formed?
- 5. Finally, the lump of earth is inspected as a whole. It is broken open with the nail, thrown into the air and when it has landed it is inspected once again.

The spade test provides many valuable pointers and information but ideally also proof of the value of tending the soil according to organic principles.

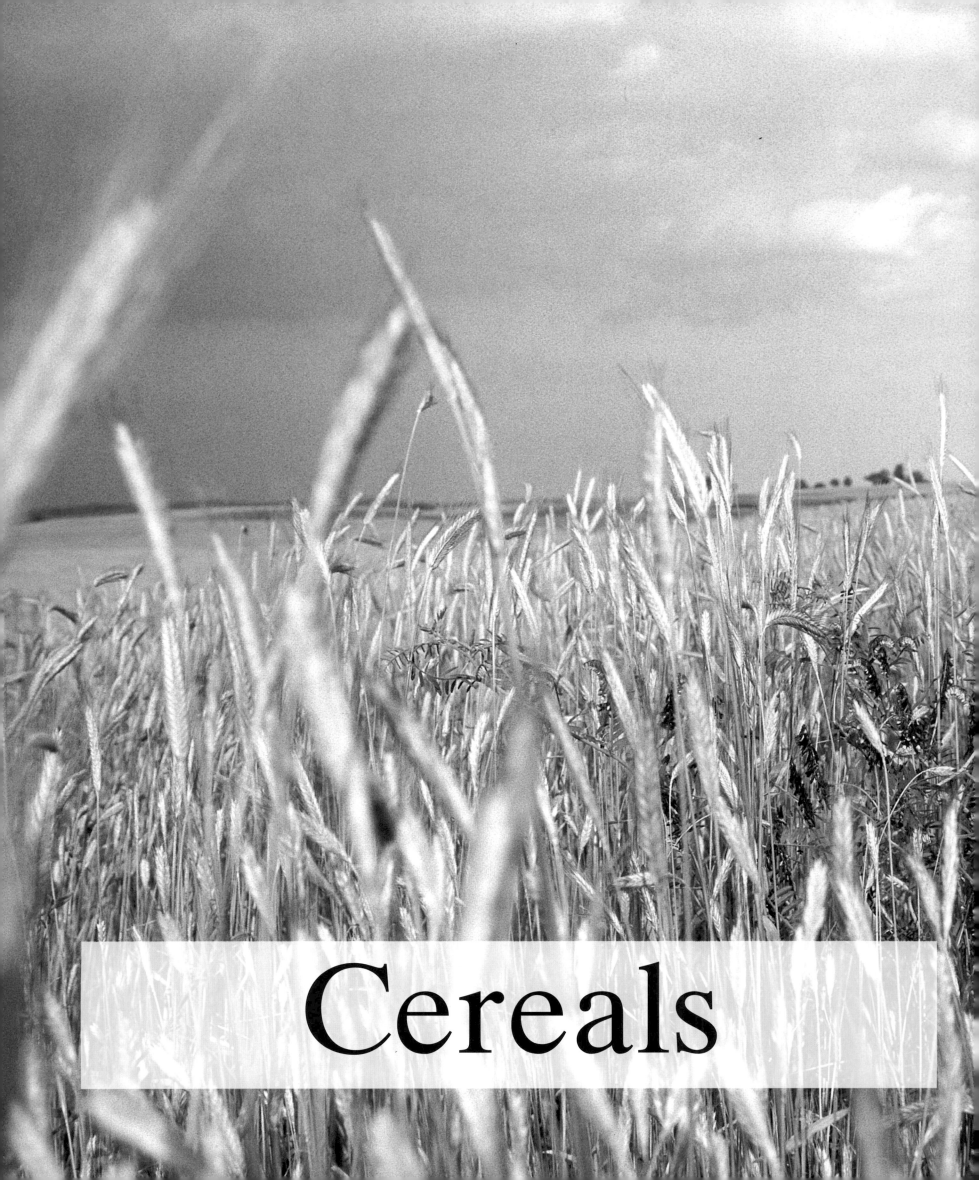

Cereals

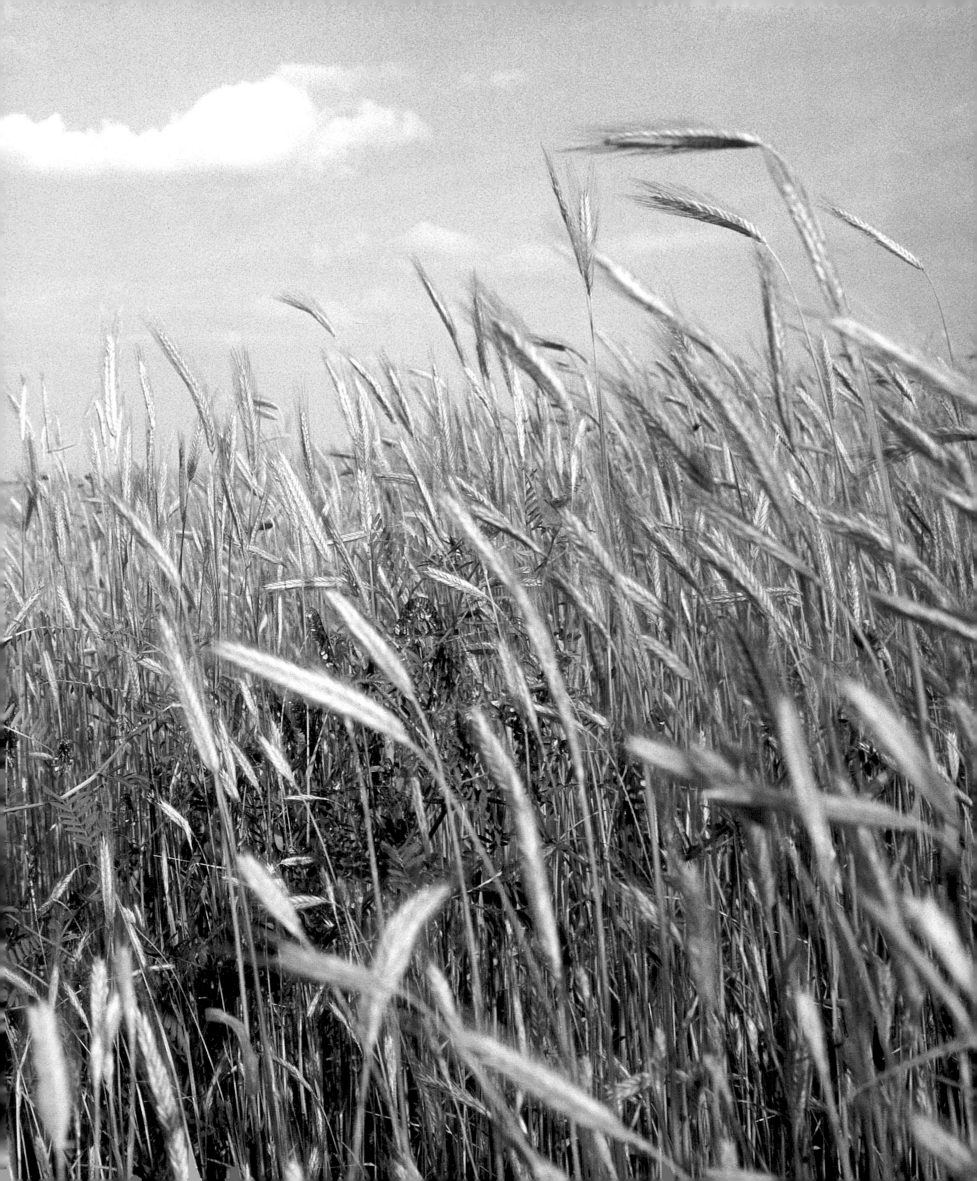

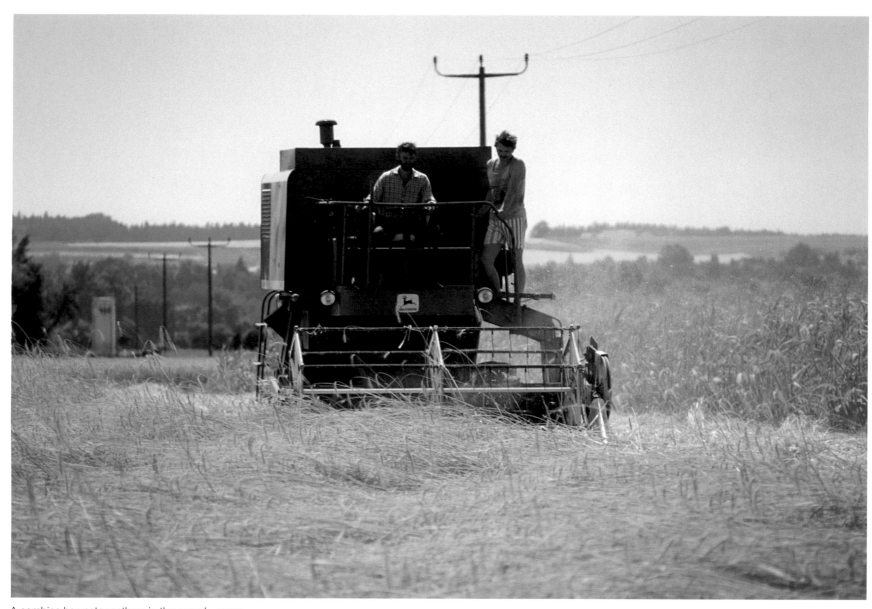

A combine harvester gathers in the cereal – even organic farming cannot do without technical equipment entirely.

Previous double page: Grain waving beneath the broad skies of northern Europe.

Cereals have been the basis of the human diet since our forebears succeeded thousands of years ago both in growing wild grasses and in improving them by cultivation. In Europe the prevailing varieties are wheat, rye, barley, and oats. In Asia rice dominates, whilst in Africa it is millet and in Central and South America it is corn. Groats, soup, and oatmeal represent the oldest forms of preparation. It was not long before cereals were being mixed with other ingredients giving rise to highly nutritious meals, particularly when combined with legumes or nuts. Where the prevailing varieties of cereal play a marginal role or no role at all in the manufacture of bakery products they are, to this day, the principal factor in shaping the diet. This is particularly the case for rice, millet, and corn. An inevitable by-product of kneading ground cereals and water into dough and baking it was the discovery of the positive effect of leavening. It was this that allowed the art of baking bread to develop. However it was only in more temperate climates that bread became a basic item of food. Primarily the whole grain was used. However, from about 1850 onwards white bread made from finely ground and more heavily filtered flour became a kind of status symbol in Europe, with those parts of the grain which contained the most minerals and vitamins serving as animal feed. Patent flour, which is lacking in bran and deficient in flavor, vitamins, and nutrients began its triumphal progress, and so that it satisfies the requirements of industrial processing, bakers today have more than 150 additives at their disposal. These are to a certain extent damaging to health but their use is nonetheless permitted by law. It is one of the absurdities of the modern diet that it sets such little store by whole grain products. In view of the fact that unhulled cereals contain such an abundance of nutrients it is absurd that such energy is extended in removing precisely the most nutritious part. It is not only from the standpoint of a healthy diet however that the whole grain has so much to offer, but also with regard to flavor. Excellent breads and cakes which will last for some time can be made from it, as well as delicious spreads and dumplings, excellent crêpes and waffles, as well as couscous, rice, and pasta dishes.

The Wide Variety of Cereals

Amaranth

One of the oldest cereal varieties cultivated by man and the principal foodstuff of the Aztecs and Incas. It is extraordinarily healthy as a cereal or foliage plant because of the high protein content of 16 percent – its leaves are popular either as a vegetable or as seasoning; as flour it is used to make bread, cookies, and pastries, whilst its seeds are used to make a variety of dishes (popcorn).

Barley

A hardy cereal which is quick to ripen. Husked barley loses virtually all its germ during threshing unlike naked barley, which contains many B vitamins and silicic acid. Even polished grains of pearl barley still contain a significant proportion of nutrients. Used in the manufacture of beer and liquor; major ingredient in wholefood cooking.

Buckwheat

This is not a cereal but a simple variety of bistort with triangular grains whose contents are nonetheless like those of a cereal; contains highly nutritious protein and many minerals as well as lysine, an essential amino acid which rarely occurs in cereals. Easily digestible and a versatile ingredient in the kitchen (blinis, pancakes, dumplings). Wash before use and do not cook for too long.

Corn

Sacred plant of the Aztecs, Mayas, and Incas, used in Europe as cattle feed as well as in the industrial production of starch, semolina, molasses, and oil. Cleanses the kidneys and contains a good deal of fiber. As polenta, a primary foodstuff in Italy. Rarely grown organically.

Durum Wheat

Derives from the emmer and einkorn wheat varieties, the latter being rarely cultivated today. The latter has the same positive features as spelt. Cultivated above all in Italy and France to make pasta and semolina for couscous and bulghur wheat. Only whole grain products are high in nutritional value.

Kamut

An unadulterated older cereal variety from Ancient Egypt with grains often three times the size of wheat. High protein content as well as being rich in amino acids and vitamins. Particularly suitable for baking providing a robust, nutty semolina.

Millet

The oldest cultivated variety of cereal in the world, an important basic foodstuff above all in Africa and Central Asia; millet with panicles was previously also widespread in Europe. Very rich in unsaturated fatty acids and vitamins. Tasty as couscous, as a rice substitute in risotto dishes and in puddings.

Oats

Previously a basic foodstuff in northern Europe. Because of its high protein content it is regarded as the greatest source of energy amongst cereals, contains easily digested carbohydrates, many unsaturated fatty acids, and vitamin B1. Not very suitable for baking, used primarily in flake form. Naked oats are a strain without husks and a recent phenomenon.

Quinoa

A plant which grows in the Andes at altitudes in excess of 13,000 feet (4,000 meters). Nutritious as a leaf vegetable and having small seeds rich in vitamins and nutrients which were much prized by the Incas. Prepared either sweet or savory, only to be used as a flour in small amounts because of the bitter substance saporin. Mostly available in health food shops.

Rice

Asia's main foodstuff loses the mainstay of its vitamins and nutrients when milled and polished to produce white rice. Only hulled natural, brown, or whole grain rice contain all eight essential amino acids, vitamins, and minerals. Because of the extensive use of pesticides it is advisable only to use organic whole grain rice.

Rye

Straightforward grain which is particularly popular in northern Europe. It is lacking in gluten and is primarily used for whole grain flour. Doughs which have been leavened produce grainy, tasty, long-lasting breads.

Spelt

Sometimes known as large spelt, this form of wheat is low-yielding, robust and has grains which grow together with the husks. Thanks to its highly nutritious gluten content it is very well suited to use in baking and has an excellent flavor (bread, cakes and pastries, pasta and dumplings.) Practically speaking virtually all spelt is grown organically.

Unripe Spelt

Unripe spelt is still green and has a high water content. Once dried it has a subtle but nonetheless distinctive aroma. Not suitable for baking, but excellent in soups and piquant dishes.

Wheat

Worldwide the most important cereal variety because of its balanced content of vitamins and nutrients. Because of its high gluten content, soft wheat is very well suited to baking. Minerals and vitamins are, for the most part, concentrated in the outer layers, for which reason only whole wheat is to be recommended.

Wild Rice

Not a cereal but rather a variety of grass whose seeds were the principal foodstuff of the North American Indian; growing wild in lake and river marshes wild rice was harvested from the canoe; today it is cultivated. The long black grains which are regarded as a delicacy have a high vitamin and nutrient content.

Storing Cereals and Cereal Products

- Homemade flour or whole meal: 3 weeks in a sealed container; should however always be ground freshly
- Home crushed flakes: 4 weeks in a sealed container; oats are the exception as they should only be used fresh
- Home cooked cereals: approximately 5 days in the refrigerator
- Roasted cereals: approximately 3 months*
- Cereals stored at home: approximately 6 months*
- Whole grain flour (commercially produced): approximately 12 months*
- Flakes (commercially produced): approximately 18 months*
- Couscous (commercially produced): approximately 18 months*
- Pasta (commercially produced): approximately 24 months*

*depending upon various factors which affect storage including moisture, heat and the container; with commercially produced products consumers should be guided by the "use by" dates given on the packaging

Cross Section of a Cereal Grain

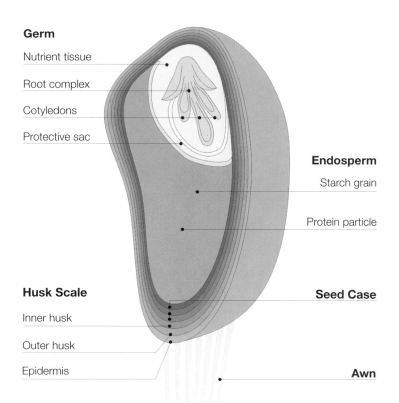

Germ
Nutrient tissue
Root complex
Cotyledons
Protective sac

Endosperm
Starch grain
Protein particle

Husk Scale
Inner husk
Outer husk
Epidermis

Seed Case

Awn

Why Cereals are Good for Your Health

Cereal grains contain virtually all essential nutrients.

• Starch represents the largest part of the grain, accounting for between 60 and 75 percent.

• Highly nutritious protein makes up between 7 and 15 percent of the grain and is therefore the second largest component. The cereal germ also contains a lot of protein (oats contain six essential amino acids, rice all eight).

• Unsaturated fatty acids are to be found particularly in the nutrient tissue. Germ oil can account for up to 7 percent of the grain.

• Minerals are primarily contained in the outer layers. Amongst them are salts of potassium which strengthen the nerves and tissue, and of calcium which are indispensable for bones and teeth as well as those of magnesium, a necessary component of blood and tissue, which are thought to act as a protection against cancer.

• There is a high incidence of trace elements, including iron for the absorption of oxygen and the formation of blood, zinc for conferring powers of resistance and the healing of wounds, fluorine to harden enamel and to counter caries. Also of some importance is the silicic acid content which is often high. This has a positive effect upon bones, teeth, hair, and skin, and on the elasticity of tissue as well as upon powers of concentration and vision.

• Vitamins are similarly found mainly in the outer layers. The most important are the following: vitamin B1 fortifies the nerves and tissues and stimulates metabolism whilst vitamin B2 promotes cell renewal. Vitamin E functions as an antioxidant in cell tissue and has a rejuvenating function. Folic acid (vitamin M) activates blood and cell renewal. Pantothenic acid (vitamin B5) prevents stress symptoms. Niacin (vitamin B3) is beneficial to the metabolism.

In addition the outer layers provide over 12 percent of fiber (see p. 31).

Most of the contents of cereals which are beneficial to health are sacrificed during the modern milling process. For patent flour and hulled cereals in particular the outer layers and cereal germ are removed and it is precisely these parts of grain that contain the most vitamins and minerals. It is only in the whole grain that their undiminished presence is guaranteed. Since pesticides penetrate the outer layers of the grain and chemical fertilizers adulterate their contents, only organically cultivated whole cereals can be fully satisfactory.

1 Corn	6 Unripe spelt	12 Rye
2 Wheat	7 Durum wheat	13 Naked oats
3 Wild rice	8 Millet	14 Amaranth
4 Untreated rice, medium grain	9 Naked barley	15 Spelt
5 Quinoa	10 Buckwheat	16 Kamut
	11 Untreated rice, round	

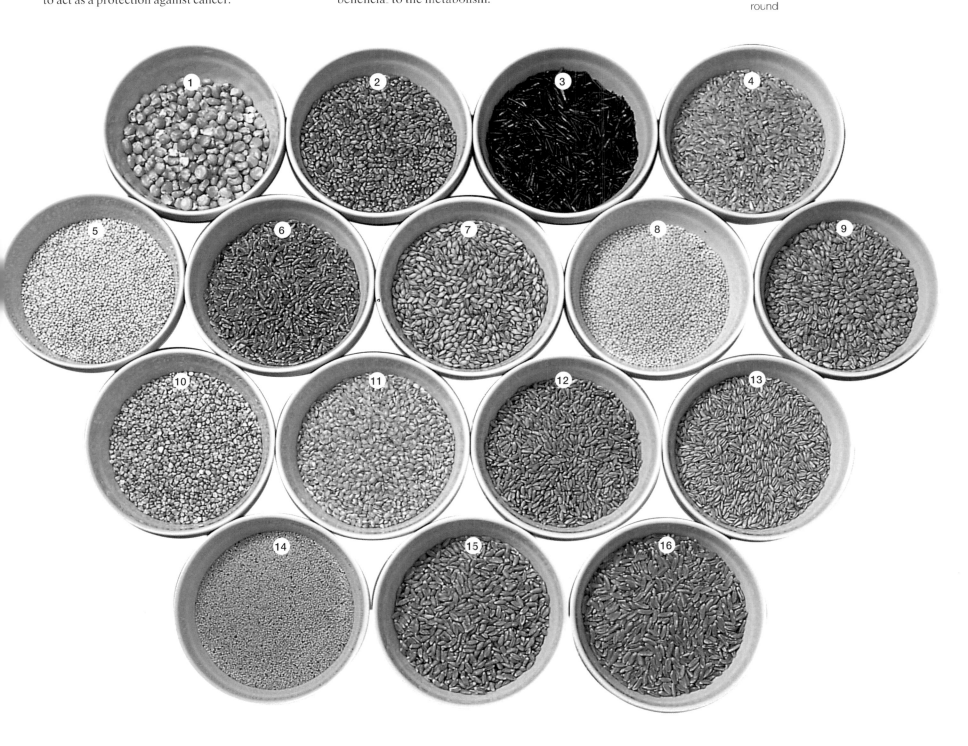

29

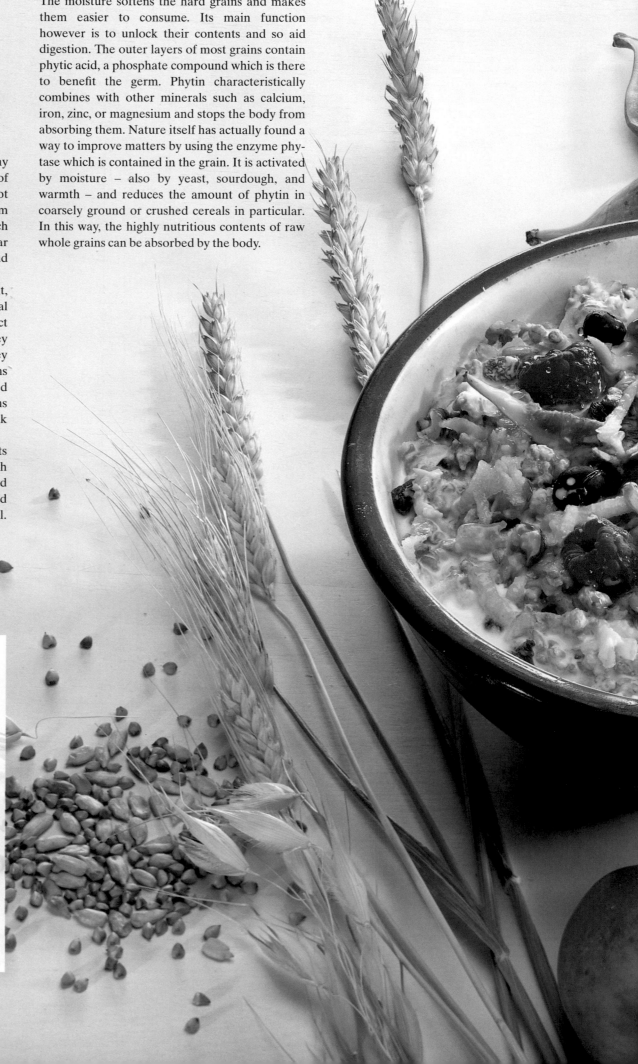

A Healthy Breakfast

Freshly Ground Granola

The word "granola" has come to apply to any mixture containing cereals – mostly in the form of flakes – dried fruit, seeds, or nuts. In order not simply to enjoy granola but also to benefit from the wealth of vitamins and trace elements which organically grown cereals have to offer, it is far better to make granola at home from freshly and coarsely milled grain.

The most suitable grains are oats, wheat, spelt, barley, rye, kamut, and rice. Oats occupy a special position. If coarsely ground oats remain in contact with liquid for longer than 30 minutes they become bitter. Since oats are relatively soft they can be soaked without grinding. Other grains must be ground coarsely, immediately covered with water in order to protect essential vitamins and nutrients from oxidation and left to soak overnight.

Whilst yogurt or other fermented milk products are also suitable for use in soaking grains, fresh milk or juices should not be used. Adding dried fruit to cereal which has been soaked, ground coarsely, or crushed is problematic as well.

Lactose and fructose can cause fermentation to take place.

The moisture softens the hard grains and makes them easier to consume. Its main function however is to unlock their contents and so aid digestion. The outer layers of most grains contain phytic acid, a phosphate compound which is there to benefit the germ. Phytin characteristically combines with other minerals such as calcium, iron, zinc, or magnesium and stops the body from absorbing them. Nature itself has actually found a way to improve matters by using the enzyme phytase which is contained in the grain. It is activated by moisture – also by yeast, sourdough, and warmth – and reduces the amount of phytin in coarsely ground or crushed cereals in particular. In this way, the highly nutritious contents of raw whole grains can be absorbed by the body.

Fiber

The fibers and fibrous structures which are particularly found in whole grain, vegetables, fruit, and nuts are not just useless baggage. Fiber is formed by a group of carbohydrates of which cellulose and pectin are the most widely known. These substances are not broken down in the human digestive system. For this reason they create an enhanced feeling of fullness (which stands those conscious of their figure in good stead) and furthermore they are absorbent, combining with water and the harmful substances which are found in the intestine, cholesterol being an example. Their primary function is to regulate the absorption of digestible carbohydrates and intestinal activity in general.

Because of these characteristics, fiber is effective in preventing diabetes, intestinal difficulties, cancer of the large intestine, heart conditions, and high blood pressure. Since these fibers which are beneficial to health are primarily to be found in the shells and outer layers, it is obvious that untreated foodstuffs are to be preferred.

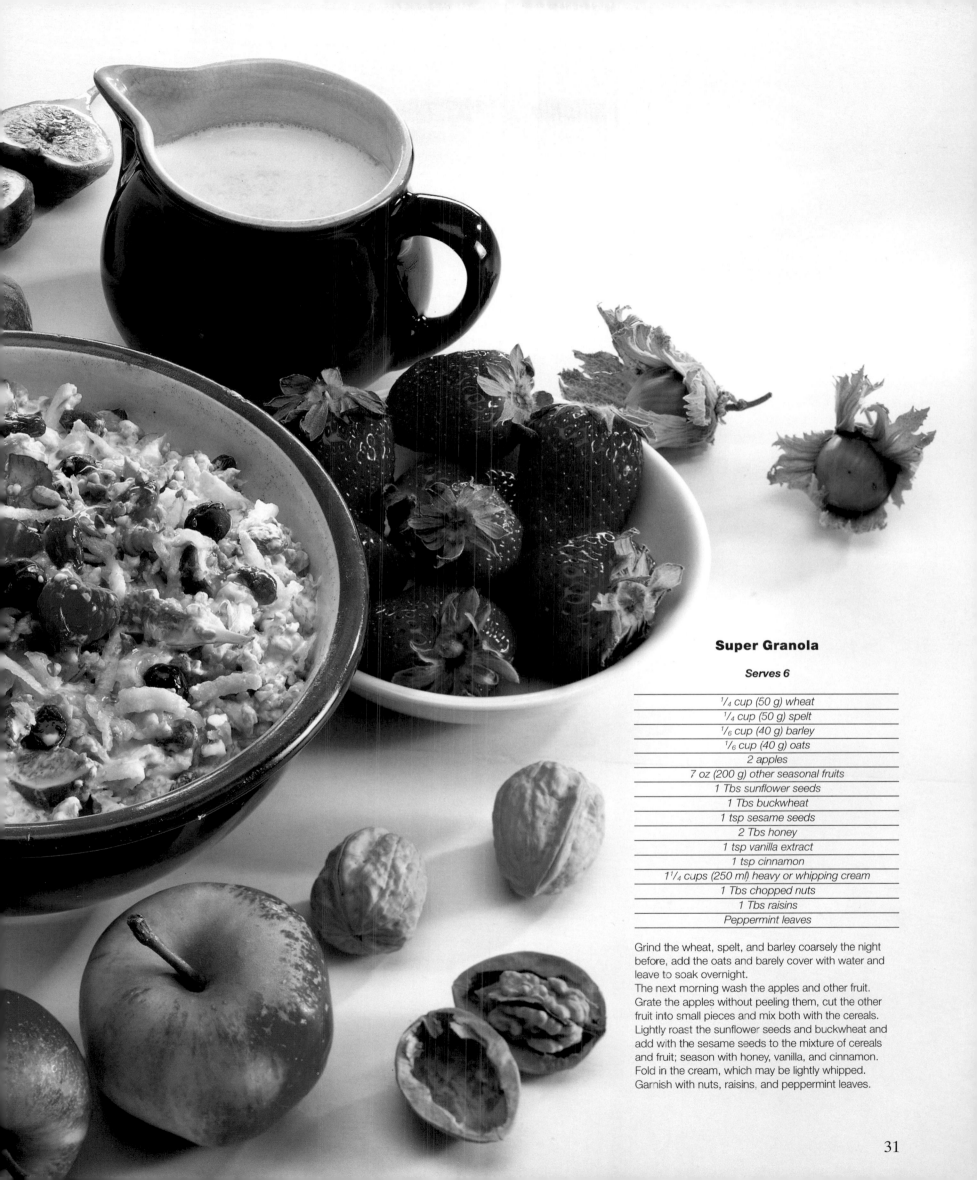

Super Granola

Serves 6

$1/4$ cup (50 g) wheat	
$1/4$ cup (50 g) spelt	
$1/6$ cup (40 g) barley	
$1/6$ cup (40 g) oats	
2 apples	
7 oz (200 g) other seasonal fruits	
1 Tbs sunflower seeds	
1 Tbs buckwheat	
1 tsp sesame seeds	
2 Tbs honey	
1 tsp vanilla extract	
1 tsp cinnamon	
$1^{1}/4$ cups (250 ml) heavy or whipping cream	
1 Tbs chopped nuts	
1 Tbs raisins	
Peppermint leaves	

Grind the wheat, spelt, and barley coarsely the night
before, add the oats and barely cover with water and
leave to soak overnight.
The next morning wash the apples and other fruit.
Grate the apples without peeling them, cut the other
fruit into small pieces and mix both with the cereals.
Lightly roast the sunflower seeds and buckwheat and
add with the sesame seeds to the mixture of cereals
and fruit; season with honey, vanilla, and cinnamon.
Fold in the cream, which may be lightly whipped.
Garnish with nuts, raisins, and peppermint leaves.

1 Wheat
2 Wheat flakes
3 Millet
4 Millet flakes
5 Barley
6 Barley flakes
7 Spelt
8 Spelt flakes
9 Durum wheat
10 Durum wheat
   flakes

11 Oats
12 Rolled oats
13 Rye
14 Rye flakes

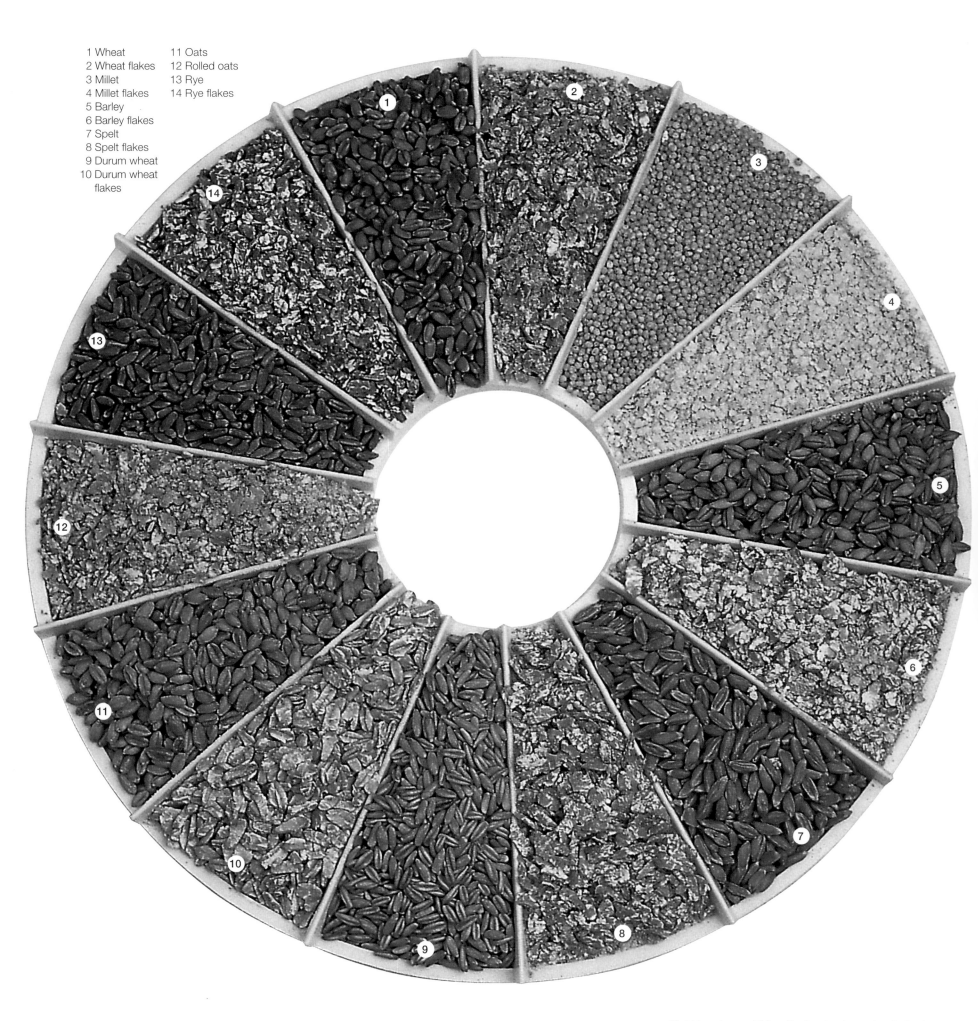

Right hand page: This mill will not only crush rolled oats, wheat flakes, and other flakes, but can also be used to produce smaller amounts of whole meal and flour.

Flakes and
Mills

The same is true of cereal flakes as is the case with the complete grain. Only when they are fresh or to be precise when they have been freshly milled do flakes offer the full richness in vitamins and nutrients which cereals offer. Commercially produced flakes from the packet have already lost an important part of their highly nutritious contents, since the flakes are heated with steam and are therefore more or less cooked. There is even less of the original vitamins and nutrients in cornflakes and in sugar-coated breakfast flakes. They are made from mashes with a high sugar content (up to 28 percent) which have been subjected to pressure and heat to produce the flakes. Flavorings and vitamins are then added.

Anyone who likes to eat granola regularly should obtain a grain mill. As with the machines discussed later in this chapter (see p. 34) the various available models differ primarily with regard to the material from which the grinders are made, be it stainless steel, ceramic, or even stone. A mill which has a gentle stone grinding mechanism to crush the grain will have rollers made from Naxos basalt by using magnesite cement. It is suitable for all dry varieties of cereal whose grains are approximately the size of wheat. Modern grinders can even be used for high-fat oats. Stainless steel or ceramic grinders can also be used to process seeds such as sesame, poppy, and linseeds, which would gum up a stone grinding mechanism. Similarly spices such as fennel, aniseed, coriander, or caraway seeds can be fed through a mill to release properly the full force of their flavor. A mill can also be used to make small amounts of whole meal or flour. The grains are crushed several times until the required degree of fineness is reached. An important criterion for selecting a mill which will as a rule be fixed firmly to the table is its maneuverability, something which is best ascertained by prospective purchasers trying them out for themselves.

Oats can be ground without prior soaking, but all other varieties of corn should be soaked briefly beforehand for at least an hour so that their skins become soft and should then be left to dry. As with whole meal, freshly milled cereal flakes should – with the exception of oatflakes – then be soaked in water or yogurt to make them more digestible and to make their minerals easier to absorb. If the flakes are to be used at breakfast, the grains should be milled the night before and soaked for at least three hours before being eaten. Flakes are also suitable for making bread, cakes, and pastries, giving both texture and flavor.

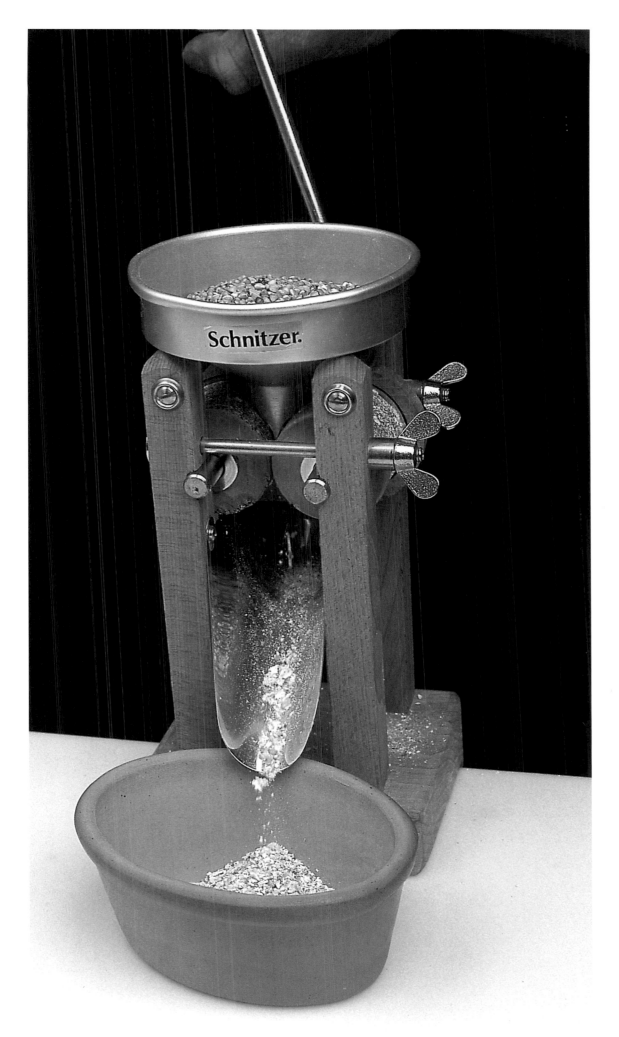

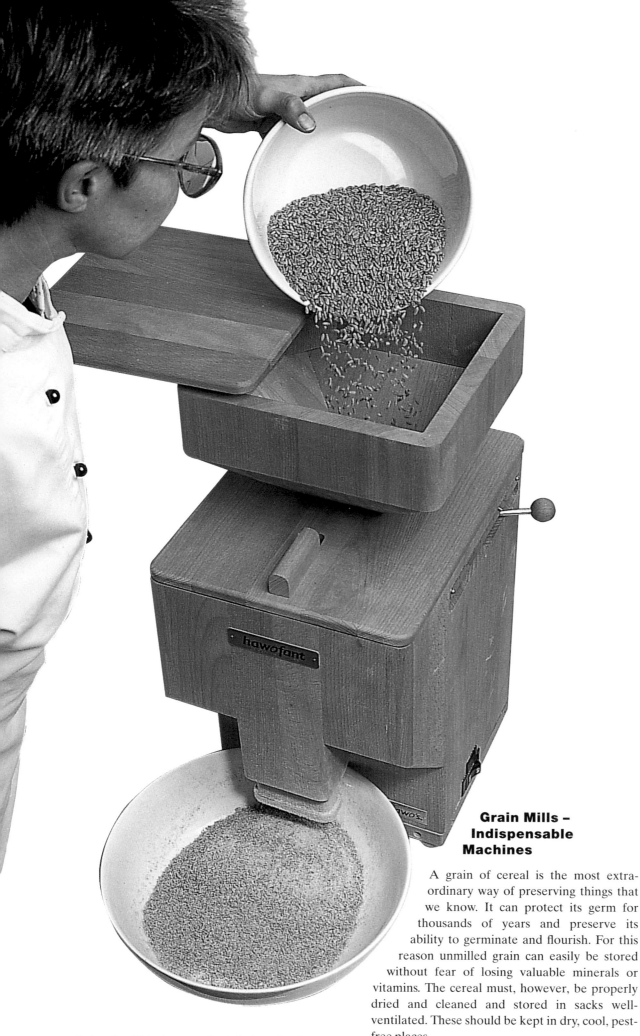

are exposed to the air. Such contact with oxygen is particularly bad for vitamins and flavors. They oxidize quickly and thereby deteriorate in quality. Their natural fats begin to turn rancid after a few weeks' storage. Because of the methods used to produce flour, most conventional flours moreover contain only a fraction of their original vitamins and nutrients.

Anyone who values the undiminished natural richness of cereals has only one option, namely that of milling the cereal themselves immediately before use.

There is by now a wide range of mills for domestic use on the market. They differ principally in being either hand operated or mains powered as well as in the different grinding mechanisms available. Mills operated by hand are to be recommended if only small amounts are to be milled or ground coarsely, for instance for granolas.

With mains powered mills the differences are to be found in the motor and in the grinding mechanism. Smaller mills and food processors which can be fitted with extensions for the purpose of milling have universal motors. They are very loud and unsuitable for constant use since they wear out relatively quickly. Permanent magnet motors by contrast last somewhat longer. All larger mills which are intended to be used often have an industrial motor – also known as a condenser motor – which is quiet, long-lasting, and maintenance-free.

As far as grinding mechanisms are concerned, the main difference is between two different types, namely cone and disc mills. Cone grinders, whether they are steel, ceramic, or stone, mill cereal into flour of different consistencies ranging from the granular to the extremely fine-grained. Steel and ceramic grinders are appropriate if a lot of seeds are going to be milled.

Cast stone has become the norm for disc mills. Such discs are based on magnesite, which consists of the natural mineral salts magnesium carbonate and magnesium chloride. When water is added to it, it behaves like cement. Magnesite is mixed with sharp-edged granules of the hard mineral corundum or of Naxos basalt, moulded into the desired shape and then fired. This process results in extremely hard grinding stones which are self-sharpening. When such grinding stones are used, the minimal loss of mass consists of trace elements. Mills which are equipped with these stones can grind corn into very finely flaked flour.

The fineness of flour is calculated by means of special sieves. The smallest of these has a mesh which is 0.3 of a millimeter across. More than 80 percent of flour passes through these sieves with fine adjustment. In this way such grain mills provide not only whole meal but also flour which is suitable for high-quality pasta, bread, cakes, and pastries.

Grain Mills – Indispensable Machines

A grain of cereal is the most extraordinary way of preserving things that we know. It can protect its germ for thousands of years and preserve its ability to germinate and flourish. For this reason unmilled grain can easily be stored without fear of losing valuable minerals or vitamins. The cereal must, however, be properly dried and cleaned and stored in sacks well-ventilated. These should be kept in dry, cool, pest-free places.

Unlike cereal, flour is more sensitive. As soon as the grains of corn have been milled, their contents

Grain mills of this size are suitable for large families or restaurants. Their stone grinding mechanisms can be adjusted for any grain, including the smallest.

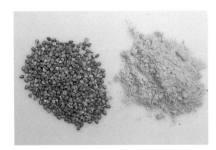

Buckwheat – Buckwheat Flour
Suitable for baking bread only when mixed with flours rich in gluten; attractive flavor in fancy cakes and pastries

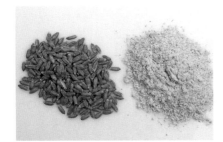

Spelt – Spelt Flour
Excellently suited for bread, cakes, crêpes and home-made pasta; delicious and easily digested

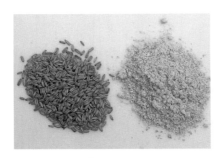

Oats – Rolled Oats
Unsuitable for baking since it lacks gluten; is used as an additional ingredient (c. 10%) in bread and cake doughs

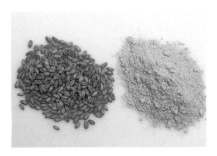

Durum Wheat – Durum Wheat Flour
Ideal for home-made pasta; is used above all to make semolina

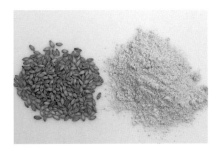

Barley – Barley Flour
Fortunately for the allergic contains little gluten; traditionally used to bake unleavened bread or with natural yeast to make bread

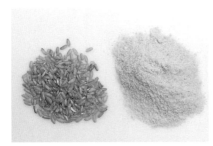

Whole Grain Rice – Rice Flour
Flour made from the slightly sweet whole grain rice is particularly suitable for desserts and creams or as a thickener for sauces. Milling rice cleans the grinding stones

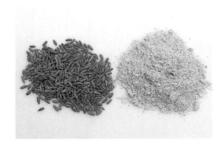

Rye – Rye Flour
Basis for sourdough bread rich in mineral salts; has a pronounced taste and fine-grained texture

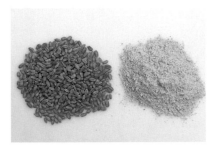

Wheat – Wheat Flour
As whole grain flour this has an excellent flavor. The high proportion of gluten creates a light dough; highly versatile when used with other flours

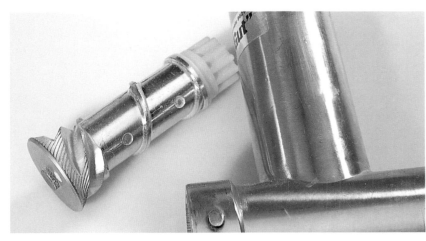

Steel grinding mechanisms, with which many food processors are also equipped, have the advantage of being able to mill seeds, although not the finest flour.

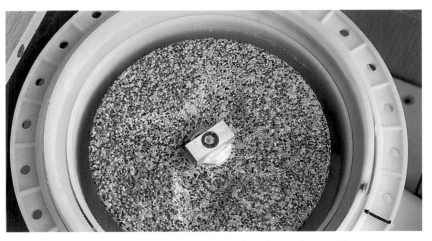

Disc grinders are cast using magnesite and granules of natural stone. They are very hard and self-sharpening. Any loss of mass during grinding is not detrimental to health.

Flour

In seeking to provide an overview of flour one thing is certain. There is a lack of absolute global conformity in the way in which flour is graded and classified. This is also true of countries within the European Union despite the trend to harmonization there. There is of course good reason for this lack of uniformity. Consumers in each country have different expectations of bread and other bakery products and the varieties of flour used will naturally vary to a lesser or greater extent in the light of those expectations. This in turn may lead to different systems of classification. As far as some European countries are concerned, bakers in Italy for example tend to use wheat flours with a lower protein and gluten content than is normal elsewhere in Europe. French wheat flour usually contains less protein than flours common in Germany. Flour production in the United Kingdom is geared to the expectations of the larger producers who dominate the bread manufacturing sector.

Speaking in very broad terms, there are three factors which differentiate flour. These are the protein, ash, and moisture content. In terms of end use, flour is also considered from the point of view of how much of the original wheat grain remains in it. The fineness of the grind is an indication of what percentage of the original grain weight is contained in the finished product. Therefore if whole grain meal or flour has a value of 100 percent, with wheat flour which is used to make patisserie, the fineness of the grind would range between a very small proportion of the original weight and about half. A greater proportion of the original grain would be required for making bread. It should be noted however that the more the cereal is milled, the more the outer layers of the grain are removed and it is here that the greatest share of vitamins and nutrients are found. German flour grades indicate how many milligrams of mineral salts remain if 100 grams of flour were to be burnt to ashes. In the case of the German wheat flour grade 405 an average of only 405 milligrams would remain, namely only 0.4 percent of the original content. The finest rye flour contains on average 610 milligrams of mineral salts, the frequently used rye flour grade 1740 between 1.64 and 1.84 percent. In other countries the details of the calculation where it is made will not be identical but the principle will be the same. No distinction according to mineral salt content is made in the United Kingdom.

Anyone who mills their own flour should only use organically grown cereals, since in conventional agriculture a wide range of chemical substances are used, which all leave a residue on and in the outer layers of the corn.

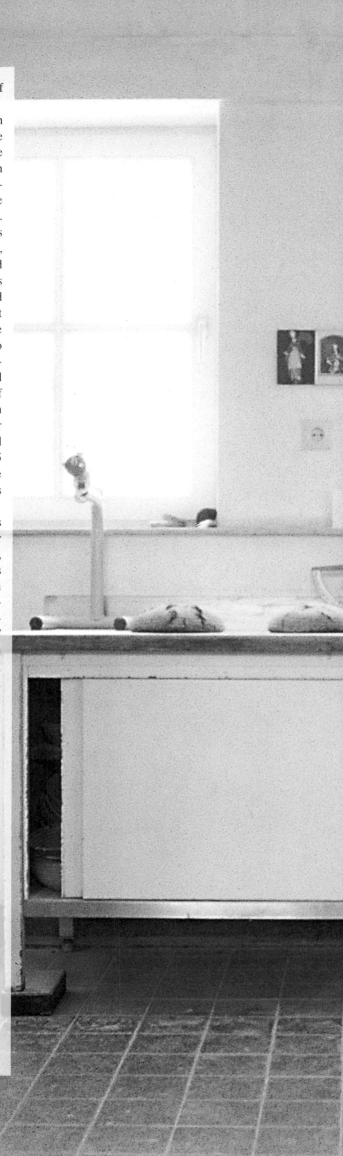

The Organic Farm Bakery

It used to go without saying that, on a working farm, bread would be baked from the cereal grown in the fields, even if it was only for home use. In organic agriculture baking has taken on a new significance. If the fields are managed organically and a conscious decision is thereby made to forego the use of artificial fertilizers, pesticides, and preparations used to shorten the height at which grain stands, the latter being particularly harmful, the yields will inevitably remain below the highest which are made possible by using chemicals. Organic farmers should therefore receive proportionately higher prices for their grain. However, even if such compensation were guaranteed – which it is certainly not – it would often be insufficient to pay for the increase in labor.

Many farms which find themselves in this situation have dared to make the leap forward and have begun to refine their grain. A useful first step in this respect can be the purchase of a grain cleaner which removes the soil, stones, or other pollutants from the grain which has been brought in by the combine harvester. Once it has been sieved and cleaned it is ready for milling. The farm can then sell the grain itself or process it further. A grain cleaner, however, is an expensive piece of equipment and for this reason the majority of farm bakeries have their grain cleaned at the mill. It is rather a matter of honor on an organic farm to mill the grain on the premises. Baking bread and selling it from the farm has proved itself to be an attractive form of refinement and has led to the creation of a loyal clientele.

The oven naturally becomes the centerpiece of the farm bakery. Organic farmers who bake prefer to use wood-fired brick ovens. The amount of wood required depends upon the size of the oven and the temperature at which baking takes place. For a medium-sized oven approximately 110 pounds (50 kilograms) of wood is required to reach a temperature of 480 °F (250 °C) in two hours. Larger ovens, which can hold about 70 loaves weighing just over two pounds (one kilogram) each are quite often heated to temperatures above 575 °F (300 °C), which takes about three hours. If the fire burns down, the ashes and embers have to be swept out. The heat will immediately begin to fall away slowly and steadily. The loaves of bread are placed in the oven at a temperature of around 480 °F (250 °C).

By far the most widely used form of leaven in organic farm baking is sourdough. The sourdough starter will often date from the early days of the bakery and will have been treated with a great deal of care and attention. It is used each time baking takes place and time and again a portion is taken from it. It goes without saying that every baker has developed their own recipe for baking bread, but in principle the following method should be followed. First of all, a good 24 hours before baking, the sourdough starter is mixed with rye flour and lukewarm water and left for twelve hours. Then flour and water are both added twice and the dough is left to develop for five to six hours on both occasions. This allows the leavening of the bread to take place more gently than it would if everything was added at once. Aside from sourdough, water, and coarse salt, a popular loaf made from rye and wheat flour will consist of 65 to 70 percent rye and 30 to 35 percent wheat, milled into flour with the farm's own stone grain mill. The dough is usually mixed mechanically at a slow speed.

Whilst the fire is burning and the oven is slowly warming up, the bread is prepared for baking. The baker weighs off the dough, works each lump individually by hand, places them in small round baskets made from willow rods and places these in the fermentation cupboard for 40 minutes. The temperature there is always between 79 and 82 °F (26–28 °C) – the ideal temperature for the entire process of making sourdough. When the temperatures of the bread and the oven are correct the loaves are placed in the oven on the hot bricks and, as the temperature falls, they will be baked in 60 to 80 minutes. Sourdough bread which is baked in a wood-fired oven has an incomparable flavor and keeps extremely well.

Farm bakeries largely confine themselves to a small range of bread, cakes, and pastries, which are essentially made using a sourdough base, but which also make use of other flours and seeds such as linseeds or sesame and sunflower seeds as well as herbs and spices. When making wheat or spelt yeast bread it is popular by contrast to use a preparatory dough which is mixed the night before using a third flour and a third yeast. Yeast not only makes bread lighter, it also intensifies its flavor.

Background: If bread becomes important economically, shrewd farmers will equip their farm with model bakehouses.

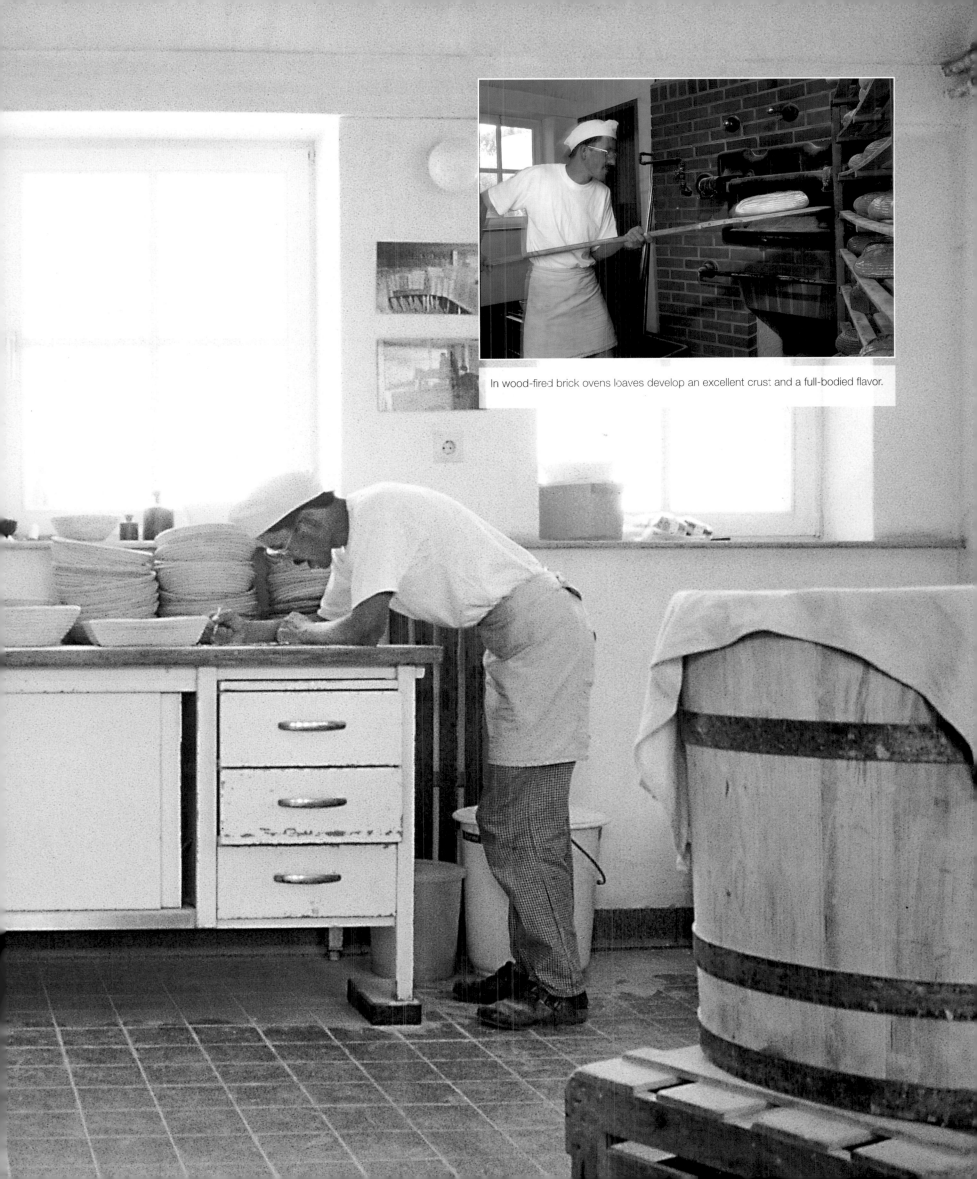

In wood-fired brick ovens loaves develop an excellent crust and a full-bodied flavor.

How Animal Husbandry and the Farm Bakery Promote Each Other

After years in Tuscany, Klaus and Christel Dörr took over a farm in 1984 in the Taunus region of Germany. Since the farm mainly consisted of pasture land as well as fields for cultivation, albeit of poor quality, and steep hillsides which could be leased as pasture above the village, the idea of raising cattle suggested itself – and so the Dörrs decided to do exactly that. The result was a splendid herd of between 80 and 100 animals. The problem arose as to where the animals were to spend the winter without small plots of pasture becoming completely overmanured. A cowshed and straw were therefore necessary. According to modern farming practice farmers expect to use 27 pounds (12 kilograms) of straw as bedding for every 1,100 pounds (500 kilograms) of animal per day. But the farm was unable to produce this because of its poor soil. The Dörrs did not want to buy the straw in, because straw produced on conventional farms is of questionable value from an ecological point of view as it has been sprayed with chemical substances to reduce the height at which the grain stands.

Hence the two farmers constructed a special cowshed which only requires nine pounds (4 kilograms) of straw per day which they were able to produce themselves since the fields which possessed comparatively good soil and which were located relatively close to the farmhouse were being cultivated on the basis of crop rotation. Since the soil is acidic and poor, the principal crop to flourish is rye. Although rye produces a lot of straw it is very expensive to cultivate with low yields. Since selling the grain would not cover the costs, the Dörrs stumbled upon the idea of refining it. The Dörrs explain the resulting necessity of the principle "From Manure to Bread" as follows: "We need the straw for the manure, and so we bake. That is the philosophy." The Dörrs built a bakehouse which buys the grain from the farm "at prices which are so low they are crazy" – so that the bakehouse subsidizes the farm. And because the excellent organic bread is in great demand the cattle in the cowshed are comfortable.

Different Types of Bread

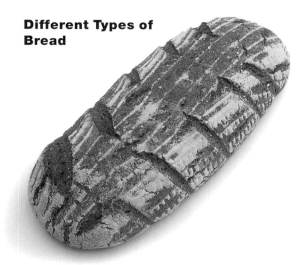

Spelt Bread
Finely ground rye flour and a little sourdough provide additional flavor

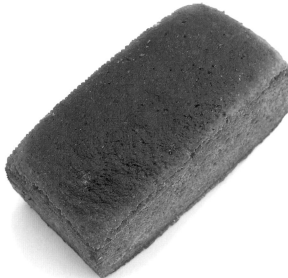

Sourdough Bread
The classic loaf – a pure sourdough bread made from finely and coarsely ground rye flour

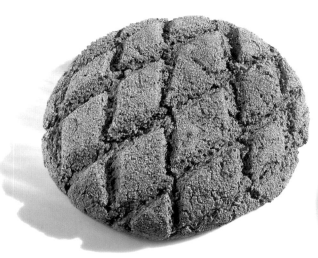

Natural Yeast Bread
Made from both barley and spelt this type of bread is both light and aromatic and also very easy to digest

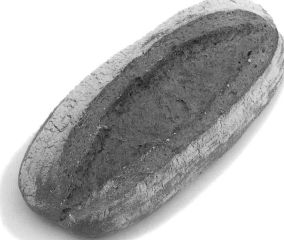

Black Forest Bread
A robust bread made from a mixture of wheat and rye flour with an attractive crust

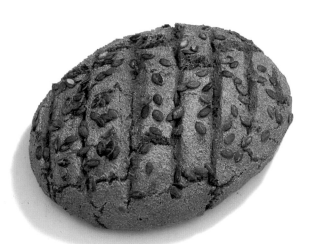

Rye Meal Bread with Pumpkin Seeds
Bread seasoned with coriander and cumin

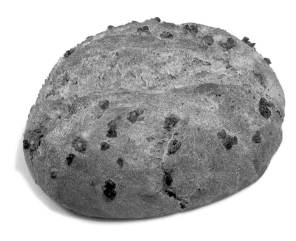

Walnut Bread
Bread made with a large amount of spelt flour, yeast, and chopped walnuts

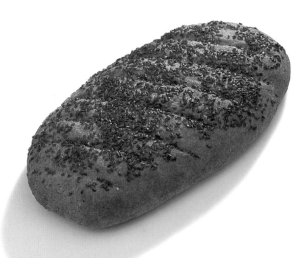

Linseed Bread
Another loaf made with yeast; linseeds contain unsaturated fatty acids and highly nutritious protein

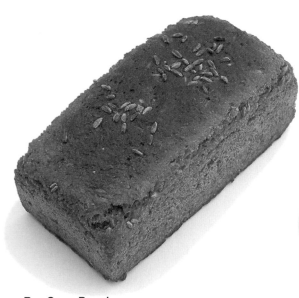

Rye Germ Bread
Fresh rye germ and wheatgerm enrich this sourdough bread with vitamins and nutrients and give it bite

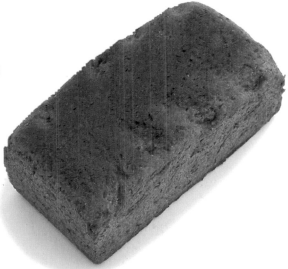

Rye and Linseed Bread
Linseeds and pear syrup give this bread, which also contains a little wheat flour, a mild spicy flavor

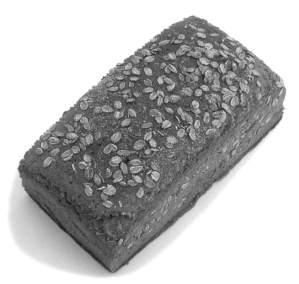

Mixed Grain Bread
Bread made from a mixture of rye and wheat flour with corn, barley, oats, and millet

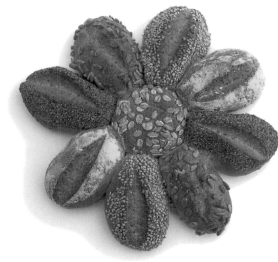

Whole Grain Wheat Sunburst
Rolls seasoned with various kernels and seeds, made from a light yeast and butter dough

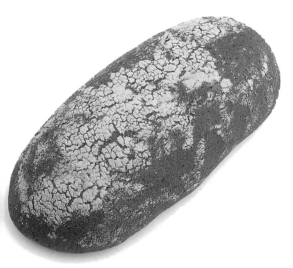

Rye Bread
A very light sourdough bread made with wheat flour and additional yeast

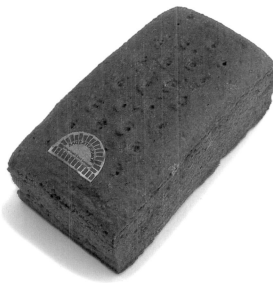

Sunflower Seed Bread
Sourdough and yeast, spelt and rye as well as sunflower seeds give this bread a robust yet refined flavor

Problems in Switching to Whole Grain Products

Whole grain bread is a difficult proposition for inexperienced stomachs. That it should cause some upset in the intestine – above all when it contains whole grains – is quite natural because the gastrointestinal tract needs a certain amount of training in order to be able to digest whole grains or fresh grain without difficulties. Therefore people who are switching to food which contains more fiber would be wise to follow certain guidelines.
• Bread made from cereals such as wheat or spelt which are easier to digest should be eaten for preference;
• Choose bread which is made from more finely ground flour;
• Eat bread which is made with natural yeast;
• Avoid eating oven fresh whole grain bread, cakes, and pastries and allow wheat bread one day to mature, sourdough bread at least three days;
• Avoid spreads and drinks which contain sugar as sugar can trigger fermentation in the intestine;
• Allow time to eat and to chew thoroughly.
In this way it is possible to adapt one's body carefully to the changes in diet. For older people who have not eaten any grainy foodstuffs the transition can last for months. It is well worth the effort however, since it is the outer layers of the intact grain which contain the most minerals and flavor as well as vitamins. The body's requirement for essential vitamins and nutrients can largely be met by consuming whole grain products.

Spicy Bread

Sourdough
Rye flour and water in a ratio of 1:1
1 cup (200 ml) buttermilk
10 cups (1.2 kg) freshly ground rye
3¹/₂ oz (100 g) sourdough
1³/₄ oz (50 g) yeast
1 tsp honey
5 tsp (25 g) coarse salt
1 oz (30 g) spices (caraway, coriander, fennel)

Mix the ingredients for the sourdough in a deep clay bowl. Cover the bowl and put in a warm place. Stir the mixture both morning and evening; on the third day small bubbles should be in evidence. On the evening of the third day add rye flour and water in a ratio of 2:1; put in a warm place until the following day.
To make the spicy bread mix 7¹/₂ cups (900 g) rye flour with the sourdough and 2¹/₂ cups (500 ml) lukewarm water; leave to rise for 4 hours.
Mix the yeast with 1 cup (200 ml) lukewarm water and the honey, add the salt and spices and knead everything together.
Make loaves from the dough and leave these to rise once again for about 60 minutes.
Preheat the brick oven to 575 °F (300 °C). Brush the loaves with water and bake them for 15 minutes, then reduce the temperature to 425 °F (220 °C) and bake for a further 90 minutes.

Sourdough

Sourdough is probably the oldest leaven used for making bread dough. It comes into being quite naturally from milled rye and water. A small miracle takes place in the process, since rye flour, which is lacking in the gluten necessary to produce good doughs, is held together by the resulting lactic acid bacteria and forms a light texture. At the same time the bacteria protect the bread once it has been baked from being attacked by mold and make it keep well without the need for any further additives. Most importantly, after several days of maturing they give rye bread its powerful flavor and its easy digestibility.

The classic development of natural sourdough takes place in three stages. Caraway not only provides an extra flavoring but also has a positive effect on the development of the leavening process.

Basic Starter

| 3¹/₂ cups (400 g) medium to fine rye meal |
| 1 tsp ground caraway seeds |

Mix 3¹/₂ oz (100 g) rye meal with the caraway seeds and ³/₄ cup (150 ml) lukewarm water and stir until you achieve the consistency of oatmeal, cover and leave to rise in a warm place for 1–2 days. As soon as the mixture begins to smell slightly sour, is light in consistency, and small bubbles have begun to appear, work in a further 3¹/₂ oz (100 g) meal with ¹/₂ cup (100 ml) lukewarm water. Cover and leave to rise in a warm place for a further day.
On the third day stir in the remaining meal with 1 cup (200 ml) lukewarm water, cover and leave overnight.

Starter For 2 Loaves

| 11 cups (1.3 kg) rye, ground moderately coarsely |
| 1¹/₃ cups (300 g) basic starter |

Mix the rye meal and basic starter thoroughly with 3³/₄ cups (750 ml) lukewarm water, which should give a relatively moist dough. Cover and leave to rise for 12 hours.
Remove 1¹/₃ cups (300 g) sourdough, place in a preserving jar or a jar with a screw top and keep in the refrigerator as a starter for the next 2 loaves.

Whole Rye Bread with Pumpkin Seeds
(Illustration below)

| 9 cups (1 kg) coarsely ground or finely milled rye |
| 1 Tbs honey |
| 2 Tbs pumpkin seeds |
| 1 Tbs coriander |
| 1 Tbs cumin |
| 1 Tbs ground caraway seeds |
| 3 Tbs coarse salt |
| 1 Tbs herb salt |

Mix all the ingredients with the sourdough starter from the previous day as well as 3³/₄ cups (750 ml) water. If the dough is too dry add a little more water.
Divide the dough into two halves and place in two large baking pans which have been greased and sprinkled with flour. Smooth the surface of each loaf with wet hands, sprinkle with pumpkin seeds, cover, and leave the dough to rise in a warm place for 30 minutes.
Place a small bowl of water in the preheated oven and bake the bread for about 50 minutes at 375 °F (190 °C), spraying occasionally with water. Then remove the loaves from the baking pans and bake for a further 15 minutes. The way to tell if the loaves are done is to tap them. If this produces a hollow sound, they are done.
Tip: Pure sourdough bread lasts for a long time and has a lasting freshness and a firm crust which is smooth and firm on top. When stored in a dry place it will keep just as well in wood, earthenware, or metal containers.

Multigrain Bread with Sourdough

Follow the recipe for *Whole Rye Bread with Pumpkin Seeds*, but in place of pure rye meal use a mixture of rye, unripe spelt, wheat, and barley meal. Suitable seasonings are paprika, cardamom, caraway seeds, cumin, pimiento, fennel seeds, nutmeg, coarse or herb salt. In addition the dough can be enriched with coriander or sesame seeds, linseeds, kernels, and nuts to taste.

Bread Seasoning
1 Pimiento
2 Herb salt
3 Cardamom
4 Cumin
5 Nutmeg
6 Coriander seeds
7 Pumpkin seeds

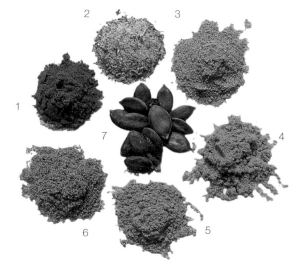

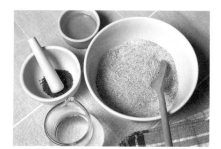

Ingredients for the basic starter: rye meal and water, caraway seeds and a little honey to taste.

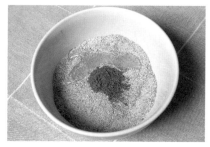

Caraway seeds, which react more quickly with honey, serve as a leaven to raise the meal.

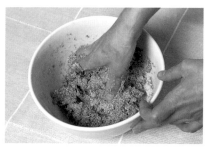

The ingredients are thoroughly kneaded together, covered, and put in a warm place for 1–2 days.

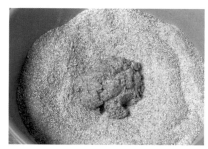

Meal and water are added on two further occasions, until bubbles appear. The basic starter can then be worked on further.

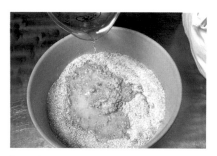

To make sourdough bread, finely or more coarsely ground rye, basic starter, and water are used.

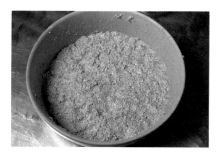

The starter dough which must be left alone for 12 hours should be really moist. It forms the basis for the next loaf.

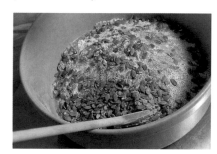

Pumpkin seeds give rye meal bread a nutty and refined flavor; they are mixed into the bread dough.

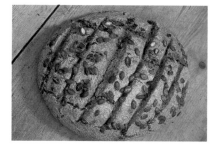

Before baking, the bread is sprinkled with more pumpkin seeds. They make for an attractive crust.

Yeast Dough

Yeast – originally a by-product in beer brewing – is regarded today as a valuable form of food because of the nutritious vitamins and essential amino acids that it contains. Amongst natural leavens it is to a certain extent regarded as a "speedy worker" and merely requires a little patience. Its influence is best shown at a temperature of about 77 °F (25 °C), and it is for this reason that any water that it is mixed with really should be only lukewarm. It is better to use cold water than water which is too warm and which will kill the yeast bacteria.

Yeast will have no difficulties in making whole grain flour rise. Sugar is not needed and it is also possible to make do without honey, although it does encourage the activity of the yeast. Although yeast makes all flour rise – with the exception of rye flour – it is recommended that wheat flour or spelt flour are always added when making mixed grain breads. It is usual to make a preparatory yeast dough. To do this the yeast is mixed with a third of the liquid and a third of the flour. The preparatory yeast dough is best left overnight in a warm place. However even if only 30 minutes are allowed for the dough to rise this will increase the effect of the yeast. Furthermore a preparatory yeast dough has a beneficial effect on the flavor.

Tasty rolls can be baked from yeast dough. The dough should be prepared the night before and even made into roll shapes which are then placed overnight in the refrigerator. When refrigerated they rise slowly so that the dough becomes particularly light. It is then merely necessary to brush them with a little water or milk the next morning and to bake them in a preheated oven.

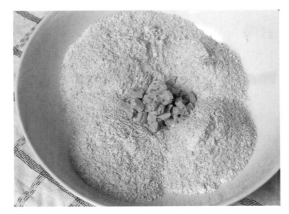

To make a yeast dough the flour is passed through a sieve into a bowl and a hollow is made in the center into which the yeast is crumbled.

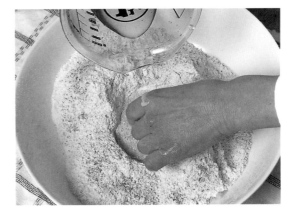

A little cold or lukewarm water is added and the yeast is mixed with a little flour, starting at the outside and working inwards.

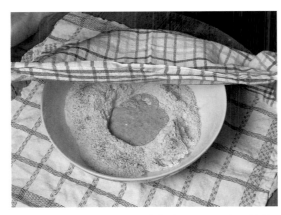

This simple preparatory dough is then covered and left to rise in a warm place for 30 minutes.

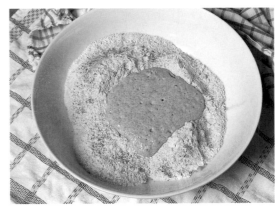

The preparatory dough has risen well, having more than doubled in size. Salt is then added.

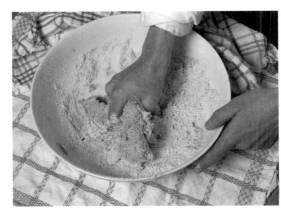

Flour, preparatory dough, other ingredients, and butter are now kneaded together until the dough comes away from the bottom of the bowl.

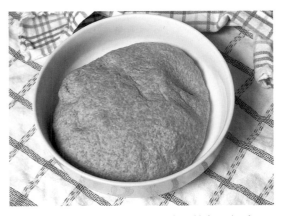

Once the dough has been covered and left to rise for 30 minutes it can be shaped and baked.

Toasting Bread

For 2 loaves

1¹⁄₂ oz (42 g) yeast
2 tsp each coarse salt and herb salt
1 Tbs honey
3¹⁄₂ cups (400 g) freshly milled wheat
3¹⁄₂ cups (400 g) finely ground spelt
¹⁄₃ cup (80 g) butter

Stir the yeast, salt, and honey together with a little lukewarm water and mix with both portions of flour, adding 2¹⁄₂ cups (500 ml) water. Add the butter and work it into the dough. Thoroughly knead the dough for 10 minutes, cover and leave to rise in a warm place for 30 minutes.

Grease two rectangular loaf pans and sprinkle with flour. Thoroughly knead the dough again, divide into two and place in the pans. With wet hands smooth the top of each loaf, cover and leave to rise for a further 20 minutes. Preheat the oven to 425 °F (220 °C). Spray the loaves lightly with water and bake for about 10 minutes. If baking at 350 °F (180 °C) bake for about 30 minutes.

Walnut Bread

2 Tbs yeast
2 tsp coarse salt
4 tsp herb salt
1 Tbs acacia honey
2¹⁄₂ cups (300 g) finely ground spelt
1³⁄₄ cups (200 g) freshly ground wheat
¹⁄₂ cup (120 g) walnuts
¹⁄₄ cup (50 g) butter

Stir the yeast, salt, and honey together with a little lukewarm water and mix with both portions of flour adding 1¹⁄₄ cups (250 ml) water. Knead the dough

thoroughly for 10 minutes, cover and leave to rise for 20 minutes in a warm place.

Chop the walnuts, melt the butter and knead both ingredients into the risen dough for 10 minutes. Shape the dough into a loaf and place on a greased baking tray. Leave to rise for a further 15 minutes. Preheat the oven to 425° F (220 °C) and place a bowl of water in the oven. Make parallel incisions on the surface of the loaf and spray lightly with water. Bake for 25 minutes.

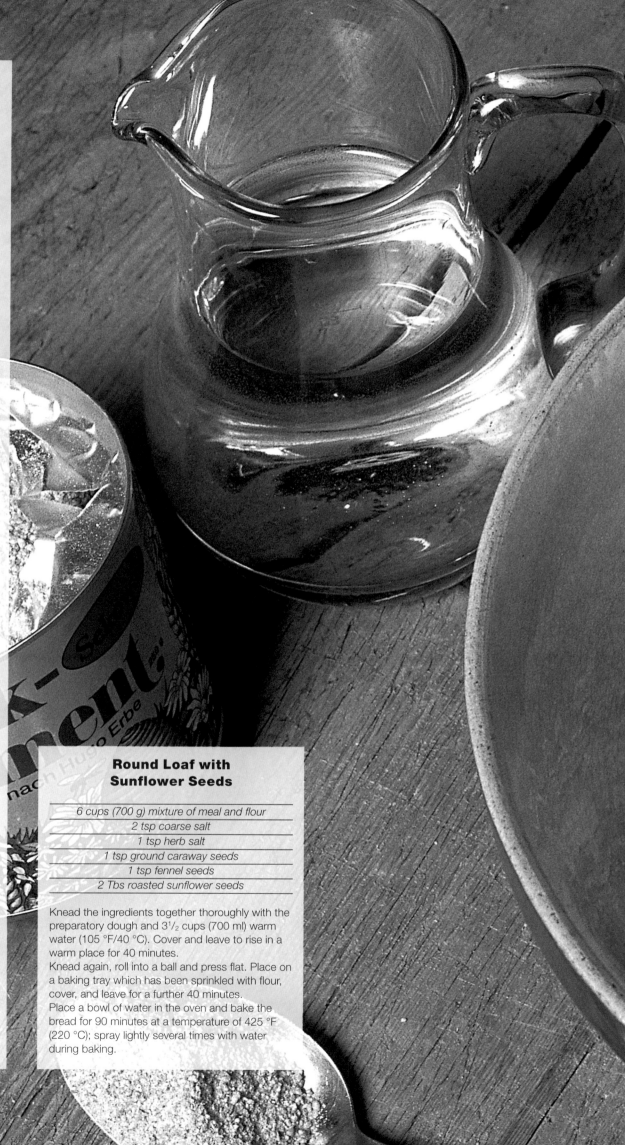

Honey Leaven Dough

Honey leaven is based on honey and wheat. Its power as a raising agent is a result of the spontaneous fermentation which turns honey and water into mead. Whilst making a basic starter is certainly a lengthy undertaking it is only necessary to take the trouble to make it occasionally because it will last for months in the refrigerator.

The advantage of honey leaven is that it can be used with any flour and any mixture of flour and that it produces bread which is light, full-flavored, and easily digestible. If the basic starter is available – it is also possible to buy it prepackaged in granules – the rest of the baking process will pose no difficulties. The one thing to observe is that the minimum times for dough to rise should be observed; the dough will not be harmed at all by allowing longer.

Basic Starter

Stage 1

4 tsp honey leaven
A mixture of ³/₄ cup (100 g) wheat meal and the same of wheat flour

Stir the ingredients together adding 1 cup (200 ml) of warm water (105 °F/40 °C), cover and leave the dough to stand for 12–18 hours at a temperature of 82–86 °F (28–30 °C). After this time has elapsed, small bubbles should be appearing on the surface.

Stage 2

A mixture of 1¹/₄ cups (150 g) wheat meal and 1¹/₄ cups (150 g) wheat flour

Stir the mixture together with ¹/₂ cup (100 ml) warm water (105 °F/40 °C) and the basic starter from the first stage. Cover and leave the dough to stand for a further 5–10 hours at a temperature of 82–86 °F (28–30 °C). After this time has elapsed the dough should have roughly doubled in size.

This basic starter can be kept in a jar with a screw top in the refrigerator for approximately 6 months.

Preparatory Dough

2 tsp basic starter
A scant tsp (3 g) honey leaven
3 cups (350 g) meal

Stir the basic starter and honey leaven together with a little water. Then add the meal and about 1³/₄ cups (350 ml) warm water (105 °F/40 °C); mix everything together thoroughly.

Cover and leave the dough to stand for at least 12 hours at a temperature of 82–86 °F (28–30 °C).

Round Loaf with Sunflower Seeds

6 cups (700 g) mixture of meal and flour
2 tsp coarse salt
1 tsp herb salt
1 tsp ground caraway seeds
1 tsp fennel seeds
2 Tbs roasted sunflower seeds

Knead the ingredients together thoroughly with the preparatory dough and 3¹/₂ cups (700 ml) warm water (105 °F/40 °C). Cover and leave to rise in a warm place for 40 minutes.

Knead again, roll into a ball and press flat. Place on a baking tray which has been sprinkled with flour, cover, and leave for a further 40 minutes.

Place a bowl of water in the oven and bake the bread for 90 minutes at a temperature of 425 °F (220 °C); spray lightly several times with water during baking.

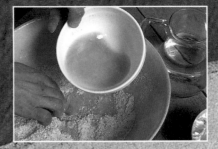

A basic starter is made in two stages. In the first stage honey leaven is dissolved in water and mixed with the cereal. The dough is then left to rise for 12–18 hours.

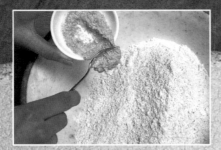

Once the dough has risen, the meal, flour, and water are added in the second stage.

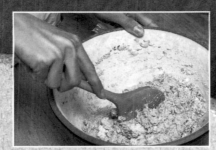

These ingredients must be mixed well. The dough needs up to a further 10 hours in order to rise.

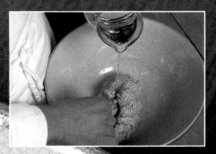

To make a preparatory dough, a small amount of basic starter is mixed with honey leaven and water.

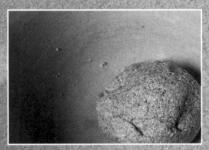

After 12 or more hours the preparatory dough will have risen well and breadmaking can continue.

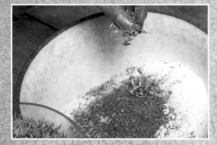

To make a loaf, 1 lb 9 oz (700 g) mixed meal, 3 tsp salt, and various spices are added to the preparatory dough.

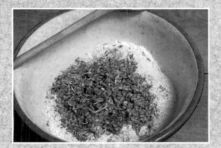

2 tablespoons of sunflower seeds (to taste) are then added to the mixture, into which 3½ cups (700 ml) of warm water are stirred.

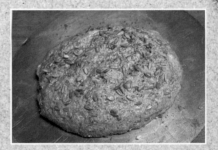

After the dough has risen for 40 minutes it is shaped into a loaf which is left for a further 40 minutes before being baked at 425 °F (220 °C).

The Village Bakery

In no other European country has the vegetarian movement reached the size it has in England. There is scarcely a pub, café, or restaurant which does not offer at least one vegetarian meal. Organic farming however is (still) rarely found, since English agriculture adheres too inflexibly to forms of production which have been handed down and is now, as before, programmed to produce the highest possible yields. By contrast there are an increasing number of small holdings which are cultivated according to organic principles and an ever increasing number of gardens run along similar lines.

One of the most striking examples of the British organic movement is the result of the initiative of Andrew Whitley who previously produced Russian language broadcasts for the BBC. He owes his love of Russia and of Russian rye bread to this time in his life. In Melmersby, a quiet village built out of red sandstone which nestles at the foot of the Pennines in the North of England, Whitley founded a bakery which used organically cultivated grain in 1976. To do this he converted a 200 year-old barn and opened a restaurant attached to the bakery. The "soul" of the business was the brick oven which was constructed according to an old Scottish model. It was wood-fired since there was no high-voltage current or gas at all and oil was too expensive. Whitley discovered the advantages of the brick oven which collects heat which it then radiates gently, giving the bread a special flavor and delicious crusts. Soon his passion for baking took him beyond his excellent Russian sourdough bread. Other varieties were added, including Greek olive bread, Italian tomato bread, and bread in the French country style, as well as a dozen other variations. They also produce gingerbread, oatcakes, and Dundee Cake; organic plum and Christmas pudding are very popular specialties.

When some old stables burnt down in 1986 the chance arose to build a new bakehouse with a gigantic French brick oven as its focus. A greenhouse was added to make good use of surplus heat. The oven which is 13 feet (4 meters) high offers an optimal use of heat. This giant can simultaneously hold 500 pan loaves each weighing 14 ounces (400 grams) and is to a certain extent heated along environmentally friendly lines being fired with wood and briquettes made from sawdust.

The enterprise currently employs 45 men and women – and this in an isolated village in an economically disadvantaged region. Whilst the Village Bakery flourishes, is famous throughout the whole country, and dispatches its products, which number about 60, by post, Andrew Whitley is giving something back to Russian culture in recognition of what he has borrowed. He is supporting the building of a village bakery in a small town near Moscow. It is not only creating jobs which are much sought after but is also returning to the Russians their nutritious rye bread, which had gone out of fashion under the Soviet system because of egalitarian state-run enterprises.

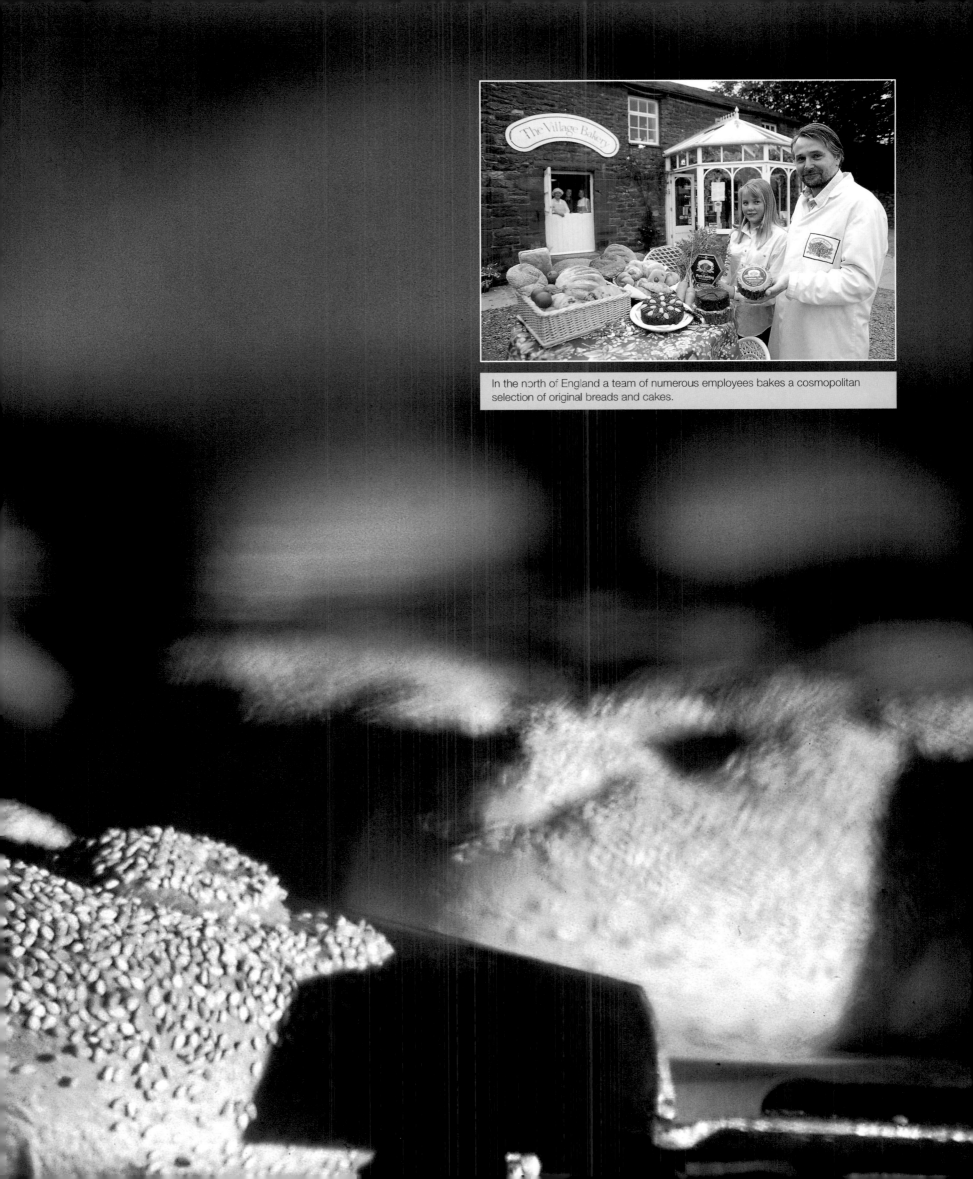

In the north of England a team of numerous employees bakes a cosmopolitan selection of original breads and cakes.

Dundee Cake
(Illustration below)

For a cake 9 inches (24 cm) in diameter

1 cup (250 g) butter
1/2 cup (125 g) cane sugar
6 Tbs orange juice
4 Tbs lemon juice
Grated peel of 1 orange and 1 lemon
Just over 4 cups (500 g) sifted whole wheat flour
2 tsp baking powder
5 eggs
1 cup each (175 g) of currants and light raisins
1/2 cup (100 g) raisins
1/2 cup (100 g) candied pineapple
1/3 cup (75 g) candied lemon and orange peel
1/2 cup (100 g) ground almonds
1/3 cup (75 g) candied cherry halves
Halved blanched almonds
Milk

Grease a spring form 9 inches (24 cm) in diameter. Preheat the oven to 350 °F (180 °C).
In a large bowl cream the butter and sugar until it is pale, then add the citrus juice and rind.
Mix the flour and baking powder together. Stir into the butter and sugar mix alternating with the eggs. Stir in the remaining ingredients with the exception of the blanched almonds and the milk. Put the mixture into the form. Dip the blanched almonds in milk and cover the surface of the cake with them.
Bake the cake for 60 minutes, then reduce the oven temperature to 300 °F (150 °C) and bake for a further 60 minutes. If the cake becomes too brown, cover it with aluminum foil.
Remove the cake from the oven and leave it to cool in the form, then place on a wire rack.
Dundee Cake is very substantial and will last for several weeks in an airtight container.

White Bread Dough

4 cups (500 g) sieved whole wheat flour
4 tsp yeast
4 tsp coarse salt

Mix the ingredients with just under 1 1/2 cups (275 ml) water and knead into a smooth dough. If possible finish kneading with the dough at a temperature of approximately 81 °F (27 °C).
Cover the dough and leave to rise until it has doubled in volume.

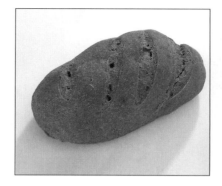

Caraway Rye Bread

For 4 loaves each weighing 14 ounces (400 g)

3 cups (650 g) sourdough (see p. 42)
2 1/2 cups (300 g) sieved rye flour
4 1/8 cups (500 g) sieved wheat flour
1 1/4 cups (150 g) whole wheat flour
2 tsp caraway seeds
1 Tbs coarse salt
2 tsp yeast

Prepare the sourdough according to the recipe.
Add the remaining ingredients as well as about 1 1/4 cups (250 ml) of water and work everything into a relatively firm dough.
Divide the dough into 4 equal portions and shape these into round loaves or sticks. Place them on a greased baking tray, cover and leave to rise for 60 minutes. Then score the tops of the loaves diagonally with a sharp knife several times.
Preheat the oven to 435 °F (225 °C) and put the loaves into the oven. After 10 minutes reduce the temperature to 400 °F (200 °C) and bake the loaves for a further 20 minutes.

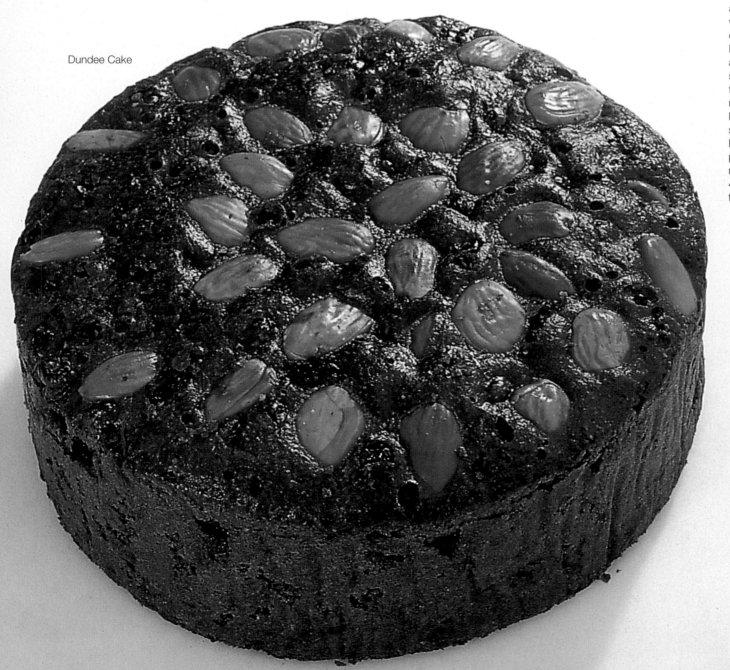

Dundee Cake

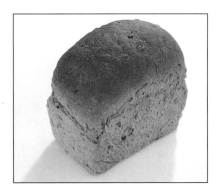

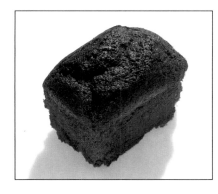

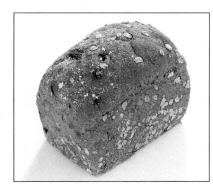

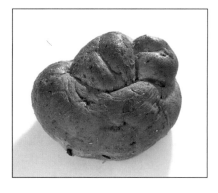

| **Maltgrain Bread** | **Gingerbread** | **Oat and Olive Bread** | **Wild Mushroom and Garlic Bread** |

Maltgrain Bread

*For 4 loaves each weighing
14 ounces (400 g)*

2 Tbs malted barley syrup
1/2 cup (125 g) malted wheat flakes
4 cups (500 grams) sieved whole wheat flour
4 cups (500 g) whole wheat flour
1 Tbs palm oil
5 tsp coarse salt
5 tsp yeast

Dissolve the barley syrup in just over 3 cups (approximately 650 ml) water. Add the remaining ingredients and work everything into a soft, smooth dough. Cover and leave to rise for 60 minutes until it has doubled in volume.
Divide the dough into 4 equal portions, knead each one of them thoroughly and shape into loaves. Place these into greased rectangular baking pans and leave to rise once again until they have doubled in size.
Preheat the oven to 425 °F (220 °C) and put the loaves into the oven. After 10 minutes reduce the temperature to 400 °F (200 °C) and bake the loaves for a further 20 minutes.

Gingerbread

*For 2 loaves each weighing
18 ounces (500 g)*

1/4 cup (50 g) cane sugar
3/4 cup (150 ml) molasses
A large pinch of cinnamon
1 Tbs ground ginger
Nutmeg
3 eggs
3/4 cup (150 ml) sunflower oil
4 tsp powdered milk
2 tsp baking powder
3 cups (350 g) whole wheat flour

Mix the sugar, molasses, and spices and heat in a saucepan, then add about a cup (200 ml) cold water and stir. Mix in the eggs and the oil. Sieve the powdered milk and the baking powder into the flour and sprinkle into the molasses mixture whilst stirring.
Line two cake forms with parchment paper, divide the dough into two portions and put into the forms. Each portion should only fill the form up halfway.
Bake for approximately 40 minutes at 325 °F (170 °C).

Oat and Olive Bread

*For 4 loaves each weighing
14 ounces (400 g)*

2 cups (500 g) white bread dough (see left hand page)
1 cup (200 g) coarse rolled oats
5 cups (600 g) whole wheat flour
Pinch coarse salt
1 Tbs olive oil
4 tsp yeast
1/2 cup (100 g) chopped onions
1 1/4 cups (150 g) pitted olives

Prepare the white bread dough according to the recipe.
Put just under 1/2 cup (50 g) of rolled oats aside.
Mix the remaining ingredients together and knead them into the white bread dough adding 1 3/4 cups (350 ml) water to achieve a smooth consistency.
Without allowing it to rise again divide the dough into 4 equal portions. Shape the portions of dough into loaves and roll the top of each loaf in the coarse rolled oats which were put to one side.
Place the loaves in greased baking pans and leave them to rise well.
Preheat the oven to 425 °F (220 °C) and put the loaves into the oven. After 10 minutes reduce the temperature to 400 °F (200 °C) and bake the loaves for a further 20 minutes.

Wild Mushroom and Garlic Bread

*For 4 loaves each weighing
9 ounces (250 g)*

1 1/4 cups (300 g) white bread dough (see left hand page)
1/4 cup (50 g) dried mushrooms
3 tsp dried wild mushrooms
2 tsp garlic purée (made from crushed garlic cloves and sunflower oil mixed together)
2 1/2 cups (300 g) sieved whole wheat flour
1 cup (100 g) whole wheat flour
2 Tbs olive oil
Large pinch of coarse salt
Just over 2 tsp (12 g) yeast
1/4 cup (50 g) pumpkin seeds

Prepare the white bread dough according to the recipe. Pour about 3/4 cup (150 ml) boiling water over the dried mushrooms and leave them to soak for 30 minutes. Then place them in a sieve and press out any excess moisture, making sure to collect it.
Put half the garlic purée to one side. Keeping aside the white bread dough, mushrooms, and pumpkin seeds, mix all the other ingredients together in a large bowl with the liquid from the mushrooms and about 1/2 cup (100 ml) water. Knead everything into a soft dough.
Then add the white bread dough. Knead both doughs together thoroughly until they have become one. Finally work the pumpkin seeds and mushrooms in carefully. Leave the dough to rise for 60 minutes.
Divide the dough into 4 equal portions, shape these into round loaves, place on a greased baking tray and leave to rise to twice their former size.
Preheat the oven to 425 °F (220 °C) and put the loaves in the oven. After 10 minutes reduce the temperature to 400 °F (200 °C) and bake the loaves for a further 10 minutes. Remove them from the oven and brush them with the garlic purée which has been put to one side.

Barley

Barley was probably the first grass to be cultivated intentionally by mankind and thus to become a cereal. Two characteristics of barley support this assumption in particular. In comparison with all other cereal varieties it requires the least time to grow and is a very undemanding crop. The Himalayas are regarded as its home. Tsampa, the traditional basic foodstuff of the Tibetans, is roasted barley. It was equally highly regarded in China and Egypt and Homer praised it in his *Odyssey* as "the marrow of men."

Regardless of the state of the soil and the climatic conditions, barley grows everywhere. It is still the fourth most important cereal variety in the world today after wheat, rice, and corn. In Europe, however, it has virtually lost its earlier importance as part of the diet and is primarily used as fattening feed, particularly in raising pigs, and in brewing beer.

A distinction is made between winter and summer barley. Varieties of modern winter barley produce high yields, are short-stalked, and delicate. They are not well suited to organic cultivation. Summer barley by contrast has retained the cereal's original positive characteristics and adapts very well to crop rotation. Husked barley is the main crop. In order to prevent the germ from being lost during threshing and the grain being damaged great care is necessary. This problem is not encountered with naked barley. By its very nature it has no husk and therefore provides intact grain which is capable of germinating. Since yields of naked barley are considerably lower than those of the husked varieties it is today a specialty of organic agriculture.

Barley contains little gluten and is only suitable for the baking of unleavened bread, unless flour milled from barley is mixed with other varieties of flour. It was and is eaten in many countries as oatmeal. It is mostly used in flake or coarsely ground form. Pearl barley is also popular, being polished grains of barley which have lost some of their vitamins and nutrients and therefore can no longer be regarded as whole grain.

Greater interest is certainly being taken in barley. It contains several B vitamins and vitamin E as well as many minerals. In folk medicine it is highly regarded for the gruel which is formed when it is boiled. It is used as a stomach remedy and also as an infusion for treating fever, as in the case of barley water, for which the English are famous.

Oats

In contrast to barley, which became widespread in the most diverse parts of the world, oats were predominantly regarded as a weed. It is thought that oats made their way to Europe hidden in barley and the original strains of wheat. Ignored in all warmer climates it found fame in northern Europe where there is little sun and heat. In Scandinavia and Russia, northern Germany and the Alps, as well as in the British Isles, husked oats brought food, strength, and health. Oatmeal or groats, porridge or *rømme-grøt* nourished the ancient Germanic peoples and the Vikings, the Scots, and the Irish. It was only after the arrival of the potato that oats became less important, often being used merely as animal feed. In the wholefood kitchen it is most widely used in flake form and also as flour mixed with other flours.

Oats became best acclimatized in a damp and cold climate. They make few demands on the soil, putting down a thick network of roots, but they do require a good and regular supply of water as they have a poor tolerance of drought. Oats have panicles with many branches and on each small branch there are usually two grains protected by husks, of which the outer one is always clearly the larger. In the case of husked oats the grains are completely enclosed. As with barley the danger arises that grain and germ are damaged as the cereal is hulled. There is also a naked variety of oats. The husk protects the grain in naked oats just as much but is not firmly attached and so can be removed without any difficulty. Its disadvantage lies in producing a yield one third lower, its advantage being its germ, if undamaged, and also enjoying better suitability for storage.

Oats are considered to be an energy-giving food. In the harsh regions in which they were most widespread people needed physical strength. And in many ways oats are indeed truly outstanding amongst cereals. They contain by far the most fat at 7 percent, of which 80 percent is accounted for by poly-unsaturated fatty acids, above all linoleic acid (see pp. 20–21). It has the highest protein content of all European cereals and contains six essential amino acids. Oats also contain a lot of vitamin B1 and the starch it contains is particularly easily digested thanks to the effect of an enzyme. However it is the roughage contained in oats which is very absorbent and which works miracles, removing unwanted bacteria, toxins, and acids from the intestinal tract.

Gluten

The suitability of a cereal for use in baking is dependent upon the quality and amount of the gluten that it contains. Gluten occurs in spelt, barley, oats, rye, and wheat but not in millet, corn, or rice. It is also absent from buckwheat, amaranth, and quinoa. Only spelt and wheat contain a sufficiently high amount of gluten to be able to produce light bread when combined with yeast. Gluten is found in the endosperm of a grain of cereal, actually between the grains of starch which form the bulk of that part of the grain. It consists of glutelin and gliadin, two proteins of which the body can make only restricted use but which are highly absorbent in contrast to starch. For this reason they absorb water – like the fiber contained in the outer layers of the grain – and give the dough volume. If the grain has not been milled at all or if it has, only coarsely, then this process will need time. If the flour is of a fine consistency and if the gluten has been ground into the smallest particles and reacts immediately, then the flour will swell up quickly. Whilst the dough is being kneaded the proteins glutelin and gliadin have the opportunity of attaching themselves to complex molecules and of enclosing grains of starch. The action of the yeast bacteria ensures furthermore that any bubbles which form during fermentation are integrated. In this way the dough initially becomes loose and elastic as does the bread during the process of baking.

Silicic Acid

Silicic acid is present in the earth's crust as an anhydride or more precisely as silicum dioxide in crystalline form, as quartz or pebbles and in the form of silicates. It also plays an important role in the human body as part of connective tissue – as does the chemical element silicon. As far as diet is concerned, cereals in particular contain the trace element silicon in the form of silicic acid, spelt and millet being first and foremost in this respect. It not only nourishes and strengthens connective tissue but also has the same effect upon skin, hair, and nails. In the first years of life a sufficient supply of silicic acid is of central importance. This can easily be guaranteed by eating cereal products.

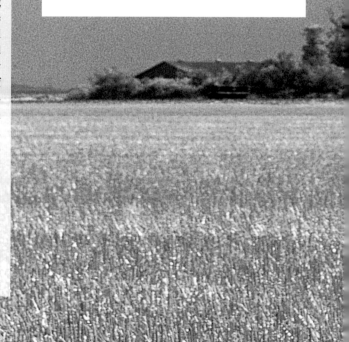

Rye

Rye originates from the Middle East. There are often droughts there, the soil is poor and stony and cereals are also cultivated at high altitude. Rye can cope well with such difficult conditions. It spreads its roots out widely and drives them deep into the soil to find the nutrients it needs. It therefore flourishes in places where a more delicate crop such as wheat would fail. This is why farmers in the Middle East remained loyal to it.

Winter rye should be sown at the end of September or the beginning of October. Frost has no effect upon it. Whenever the temperature rises just above freezing point, rye will resume growth. This gives it a sufficient advantage over weeds in the early spring, and as it is a long-stalked crop it can also survive well later on. Summer rye is planted in March and ripens a mere two weeks later.

Rye remained the predominant cereal for baking bread into the present century. Whilst it is certainly heavier to handle than wheat as a dough, it nonetheless forms lactic acid bacteria of its own accord three days after simply being mixed with water, making it light, digestible, and long-lasting. It was however the dark color of rye flour and its strong, robust character which concealed great advantages for health, that brought about its decline in social status. The upper classes were already firmly in favor of the lighter wheat. When modern milling techniques brought about the phenomenon of white bread, which is low in vitamins and nutrients, this became a status symbol and even the poorest members of society no longer wanted to eat dark bread. This can be seen as the beginning of grave diseases of modern civilization in the more northerly countries. For rye – which was practically always used as a whole grain as indeed it still is today – supplies the body with vitamins B1, B2, E, and niacin, important minerals and trace elements. Furthermore it provides a relatively large amount of lysine, the amino acid which is vital to the metabolism and essential for growth, something which gives rye a greater biological valence than wheat. It is for this reason that sourdough bread assumes such importance in wholefood cuisine, although other flours are often added to rye flour since it contains no gluten. Whilst rye certainly finds its principal use in bread, it is also an excellent ingredient for granola and makes a delicious addition to salads or vegetable dishes such as sprouts.

Wheat

Central Asia is regarded as the cradle of wild wheat. Since wheat exists with two, three, and six chromosome arrangements, it began its career as the most widely cultivated cereal in the world with an extraordinary variety of possibilities for variation. Wheat varieties are counted in their thousands and classified in three main groups: einkorn, emmer, and spelt. The low-yielding einkorn is of little importance today, being cultivated organically only very rarely. It could assume new importance, however, as an unadulterated strain of cereal in the future. The most widely known example of an emmer wheat is durum wheat, which has become widespread because of its suitability for making pasta and semolina. Aside from spelt, the dominant bread wheat also belongs to the third group.

Wherever wheat is cultivated there are varieties which suit the specific characteristics of the region. It is however for this very reason that wheat remains the most demanding cereal. It has a preference for warmth and needs a good supply of water, particularly in late spring. The soil it grows upon must be deep and rich in nutrients if good yields are required. Since it is precisely this that has become overly important in conventional agriculture, strains have been bred which produce a high yield but which are very susceptible to diseases and correspondingly dependent upon chemical fertilizers and treatment. A distinction is made generally between winter and summer wheat. The former can be sown from the middle of October whilst the latter can be sown in January. If winter wheat has the advantage of producing slightly higher yields than summer wheat it is surpassed by the latter in gluten content. Summer wheat therefore is more suitable for baking. For a long time central European wheat contained so little gluten that it had to be combined with wheat from the USA to make it viable for baking purposes. In the meantime suitable strains have also appeared in Europe. Aside from spelt, its close relative, wheat is the most easily handled cereal from the point of view of baking, being also the most flavorful. It produces fine bread, cakes, and pastries on its own but can also be mixed with many other cereals, its gluten giving them the structure that they lack. Furthermore it is used in granola as coarse meal or flakes. Wheat germ acts as a supplement which is rich in vitamins and minerals for sweet or hearty meals, and oil which is derived from wheat has therapeutic properties.

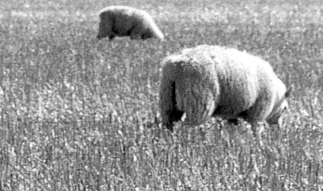

The Miraculous Seed of the Aztecs

Amaranth

This miraculous seed once fortified the peoples of the advanced Indian civilizations of Central and South America, giving them powers of resistance and extraordinary health. Amaranth was sacred at least to the Aztecs. They made sacrificial offerings which were consumed at religious ceremonies by mixing its flour with honey and blood. Not only did the conquistadores and missionaries regard these rites with suspicion, they were also suspicious of the effect that these tiny seeds had on the constitution of the Indians, something which was clearly almost magical. As a result the cultivation and consumption of amaranth were forbidden with infringements of the law punishable by death. It was only in isolated villages that farmers dared continue to cultivate it. Amaranth did, however, cease to have any significance whatsoever in its country of origin for centuries.

Amaranth was brought to Europe as an ornamental plant because of its decorative red inflorescence. It also became widespread as a foodstuff in the mountainous regions of Asia. It is popular in many tropical and subtropical countries because of its bright red color and as a tasty foliage plant which is prepared like spinach. Its particular strength lies however in its tiny seeds. One single inflorescence can easily conceal 30,000 seeds which will still only have a total weight of just under 1 ounce (25 grams).

The revival in the fortunes of amaranth is due in large part to North American research in the 1980s which demonstrated scientifically its outstanding characteristics as a foodstuff and led to the development of strains which were suitable

for cultivation. By now there are a large number of wild or cultivated varieties. Amaranth plants which are cultivated for their seeds are annuals which can grow to a height of between eighteen inches and ten feet (a half and three meters) and develop broad leaves. As a rule amaranth only blossoms in climates where the days are short in summer. The seeds vary strongly in color and their shape resembles that of lentils, although they are only about half as large.

Despite a preference for warm temperatures, short days, and a great sensitivity to frost, varieties of *Amaranthus cruentus* tolerate the central European climate well. It is possible to plant at least in May at the earliest. If the seeds have germinated then it will be approximately four months before harvesting is possible. In contrast to cereals the plants will not have died off and dried out but will still be a deep shade of green. It is to this that their name refers, meaning "not wilting" or "immortal" in Greek. If the plant is harvested at this stage it must be dried immediately. A more economical alternative is to wait for the first frost, assuming that it is accompanied by dry weather.

Although amaranth, like buckwheat and quinoa, is not a cereal, it contains many of the things that cereals contain. It has an extraordinarily high protein content at 75 percent which exceeds that of all other cereals both in terms of quantity and quality and is even higher than that of milk (see table). The essential amino acid lysine which otherwise occurs very rarely in plants is the reason for the abundance of protein in amaranth. It also has a clear advantage over other types of cereal in its calcium, magnesium, and iron content (see table). The ways in which the miraculous seeds are beneficial to health are manifold but it fortifies the nervous system, the brain, and the metabolism above all.

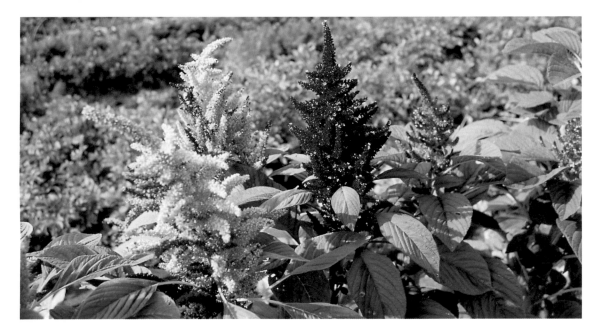

Amaranth was brought to Europe by the victorious Spanish from South America because of its attractive flowers. Today its nutritional value has been rediscovered.

Amaranth Mash for Babies

For 1 small child

2 Tbs amaranth
1/4 cup (50 ml) light cream
1/2 tsp honey
1 apple

Mill the cereal finely and mix with 3/4 cup (150 ml) water. Bring to the boil in a small saucepan whilst stirring continuously and allow it to boil briefly. Remove from the stove and allow to cool slightly. Stir the cream and honey into the mixture. Grate the apple and mix in as well.

Note: Other fruit can be used according to the season.

Frothy Amaranth and Vegetable Soup

7 oz (200 g) carrots
1 onion
1 Tbs butter
1/4 cup (50 g) amaranth
3 cups (600 ml) vegetable stock
1/2 cup (100 ml) whipping cream
Coarse salt, pepper
2 Tbs finely chopped seasonal herbs

Grate the carrots coarsely, chop the onions into small pieces and braise both ingredients lightly in the butter. Roast the amaranth seeds lightly, grind as finely as possible and sprinkle into the skillet through a sieve. Add the vegetable stock.
Bring the soup to the boil, leave to simmer for 10 minutes and then purée. Whip the cream and stir most of it into the hot soup. Season to taste with salt and freshly ground pepper. Garnish with the herbs and the remaining cream.

Red Berry Pudding with Amaranth

1/2 cup (100 g) amaranth
2 1/4 cups (450 ml) apple juice
Grated peel of 1 lemon
1 cinnamon stick
2 1/4 cups (500 g) fresh berries
2 Tbs acacia honey
1/2 cup (100 ml) whipping cream
2 oz (50 g) sliced almonds

Grind the amaranth coarsely and bring it briefly to the boil in the apple juice with the lemon peel and cinnamon stick. Leave to soak over a low heat for 10 minutes. Remove the cinnamon stick and stir in the berries and honey.
Pour the pudding into small bowls and put in a cool place. Whip the cream, top each pudding with some of the cream and garnish with the sliced almonds.

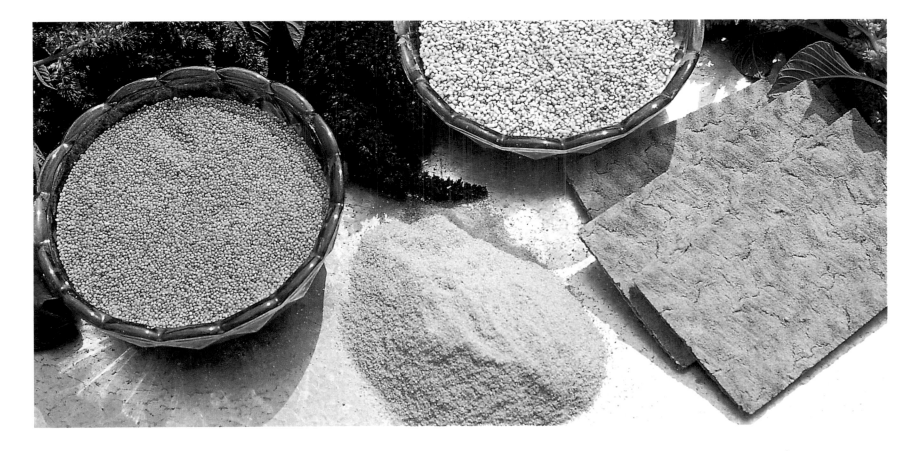

Inca Cake

¹/₄ cup (50 g) soft butter
3 Tbs honey
2 eggs
Grated peel of 1 lemon
4¹/₂ oz (125 g) amaranth popcorn (see right)
1 cup (120 g) wheat flour
Pinch of coarse salt
1¹/₂ tsp baking powder
1 tsp vanilla extract
³/₄ cup (150 ml) milk
¹/₄ cup (50 g) chopped hazelnuts

Beat the butter in a bowl with the honey until it is fluffy. Mix in the eggs and lemon peel. Mix the amaranth popcorn with the wheat flour, coarse salt, baking powder, and vanilla and slowly stir into the butter mixture alternating with the milk. Finally mix in the hazelnuts. Place the dough in a rectangular baking pan which has been greased and sprinkled with flour. Bake for about 45 minutes in a preheated oven at 350 °F (180 °C). Then turn the cake out of the form and leave to cool.

Amaranth Products and Recipes

• Flakes: Soak the seeds, allow them to dry, then grind them and use like rolled oats.
• Germinated seeds: Wash the seeds well and leave them to germinate at a temperature of at least 77 °F (25 °C); rinse daily with fresh water. Use in granolas, salads, vegetable dishes, or bread. Germination releases vitamins and nutrients in the optimal fashion.
• Popping: Heat a pan with a lid without adding any fat. Briefly lift the lid, throw in 1 tablespoon of amaranth seeds and replace the lid very quickly; remove from the heat. Wait for a moment and then move the pan backwards and forwards. When the popping has ceased, place the popcorn in a sieve in order to separate it from the seeds which have not popped. These can be ground coarsely or milled.
• Cooking: Bring the grains to the boil in water three times their volume. Add salt and seasoning

Above: Amaranth products – whole grain flour (center front), meal (left), popcorn (top), crispbread (right).

to taste. Cover and simmer for 30 minutes, then leave them to soak for 10 minutes. Alternatively, boil coarse meal for 5 minutes and then leave to soak for a short while. Can be used as a side dish, in soups and oven baked dishes and in desserts.
• Sauces and soups: Particularly when roasted and freshly milled, amaranth is an aromatic thickener for sauces or creamy soups.
• Desserts: Coarsely milled amaranth can be used to produce delicious puddings with fruit, nuts, and honey.
• Baking: Grind the seeds coarsely or mill them into fine flour in a household grain mill either untreated, roasted, or popped, then process immediately. For pancakes or flat cakes; for bread or cakes mix amaranth flour with flours rich in gluten in a ratio of 1:2.

Biological Valence of Protein

Amaranth	75%
Milk	72.2%
Soybeans	68%
Barley	62%
Wheat	56.9%
Peanuts	52%
Corn	44%

Nutritional Values (Amount per 100 g)

	Amaranth	Wheat	Corn	Rice	Oats
Protein	16.0 g	13.3 g	7.8 g	7.6 g	14.2 g
(of which) **Lysine**	0.89 g	0.32 g	0.27 g	0.31 g	0.43 g
Fat	7.5 g	2.0 g	2.6 g	0.3 g	7.4 g
Carbohydrates	62.0 g	71.0 g	76.0 g	79.4 g	68.2 g
Fiber	4.2 g	2.3 g	0.7 g	0.2 g	1.2 g
Iron	15.0 mg	3.4 mg	1.8 mg	0.8 mg	4.5 mg
Calcium	250.0 mg	47.4 mg	6.0 mg	24.0 mg	53.0 mg
Magnesium	310.0 mg	110.0 mg	90.0 mg	120.0 mg	120.0 mg
Energy	370 kcal/ 1,554 kJ	333 kcal/ 1,399 kJ	368 kcal/ 1,546 kJ	362 kcal/ 1,520 kJ	390 kcal/ 1,638 kJ

Note: 1 g = 0.0353 oz; 1 mg = 0.001 g

The Original Cereal

Spelt

Spelt is an old cereal which developed from the original wheat varieties of einkorn and emmer. Since it makes few demands of the soil, is not susceptible to diseases, and also flourishes under the most difficult climatic conditions, it was widespread in mountainous regions. It was particularly popular in certain areas of Germany, also being cultivated in Switzerland, Austria, France, and Spain, mostly at high altitudes. Since crop yields are significantly lower than those of wheat, and the hulling of spelt is a costly exercise, it has fallen out of favor in the present century. Spelt also responds poorly to synthetic fertilizers, showing no increase in yield. It was this that finally rendered it unsuitable for modern agriculture so that it had to give way to "progress."

Hildegard of Bingen, mystic and abbess who was skilled in the art of healing in the 12th century, regarded spelt as the best cereal. She not only treasured its positive effects on the body, blood, and digestion, but also recognized that it imparted "a relaxed disposition and the gift of cheerfulness." Spelt exceeds most varieties of wheat in its content of essential amino acids. It contains seven of the eight essential building blocks of protein, more than the normal soft wheat. It also contains a higher than average amount of vitamins and minerals. What is unusual is a considerable presence of silicic acid. It is to this that spelt's positive effect upon the intellectual faculties is attributed as is its effect upon skin and hair. As far as using spelt is concerned, it stands out for its protein content, containing as it does much excellent gluten. As a result it is very well suited to baking, producing light doughs and excellent, easily digestible pasta. It is slightly nutty in flavor.

The revival in the fortunes of spelt may rest upon the fact that the cereal generally has a reputation for being healthy – spelt diets are especially regarded in the medicine of Hildegard as a kind of universal remedy – whilst its culinary attractions have won it a steadily growing band of admirers. The demand for bread and pasta made with spelt is increasing constantly. In this respect spelt is also excellently suited to being mixed with other cereals which lack gluten.

The expense of spelt has not hindered this phenomenon. There are indeed good reasons for the cost. Firstly it produces rather modest yields. What makes it particularly costly however is its husk. Its grains, which are almost twice the size of wheat grains, are firmly attached to the husk. Threshing alone is not enough, a special shelling procedure being necessary to remove them. This is something that can only be accomplished by special mills or organic farmers who have a shelling machine at their disposal.

The husk makes up one third of the weight of spelt, but it can be put to medicinal uses, something which Hildegard of Bingen already indicated. Sleeping on a mattress, or at least a pillow full of spelt husks will result in the alleviation of pain, relaxation, and in various instances a therapeutic effect thanks to spelt's high silicic acid content.

Green spelt, as its name suggests, is spelt which has been harvested early and which whilst already being fully developed is still green. The exact moment of harvesting must be timed very carefully. Green spelt is then dried at 230 °F (110 °C) or more which destroys its ability to germinate but it is then ready for milling. The role of green spelt in the revival of interest in the grain is not inconsiderable.

Whole Wheat Spaghetti with Green Spelt "Bolognese"

$^1/_2$ cup (100 g) green spelt
1 onion
1 garlic clove
2 tomatoes
3 Tbs olive oil
Pinch of cayenne pepper
$^1/_2$ tsp coarse salt
$^1/_2$ tsp sweet paprika
1 Tbs oregano
1 Tbs marjoram
1 Tbs basil
1 Tbs vegetable stock granules
5 oz (150 g) whole wheat spaghetti
Parmesan cheese

Grind the green spelt moderately coarsely. Chop the onion and garlic into small pieces. Prepare the tomatoes in the same way, purée them and then pass through a sieve. Heat the oil, braise the onion and garlic in it lightly. Add the unripe spelt meal and fry it whilst stirring. Add 2$^1/_2$ cups (500 ml) water and cook the cereal, stirring often. Add the tomatoes and season the mixture to taste with salt, seasoning, herbs, and vegetable stock.
Cook the spaghetti in salted water until it is "al dente", serve with the green spelt "Bolognese" and sprinkle with freshly grated Parmesan.

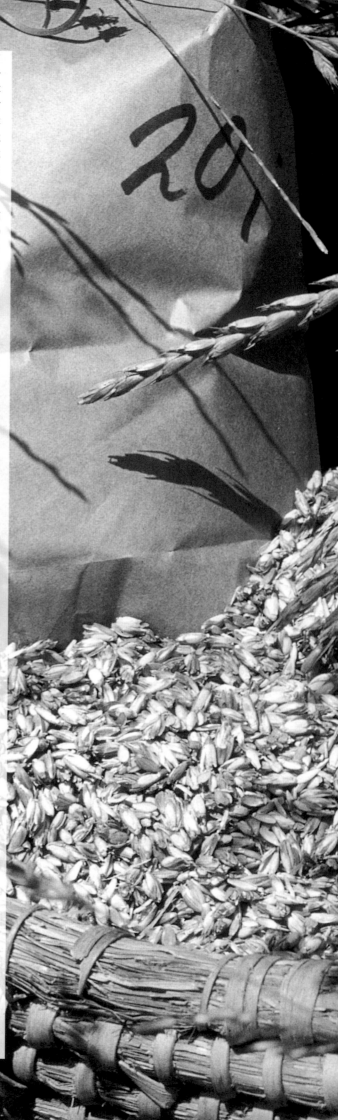

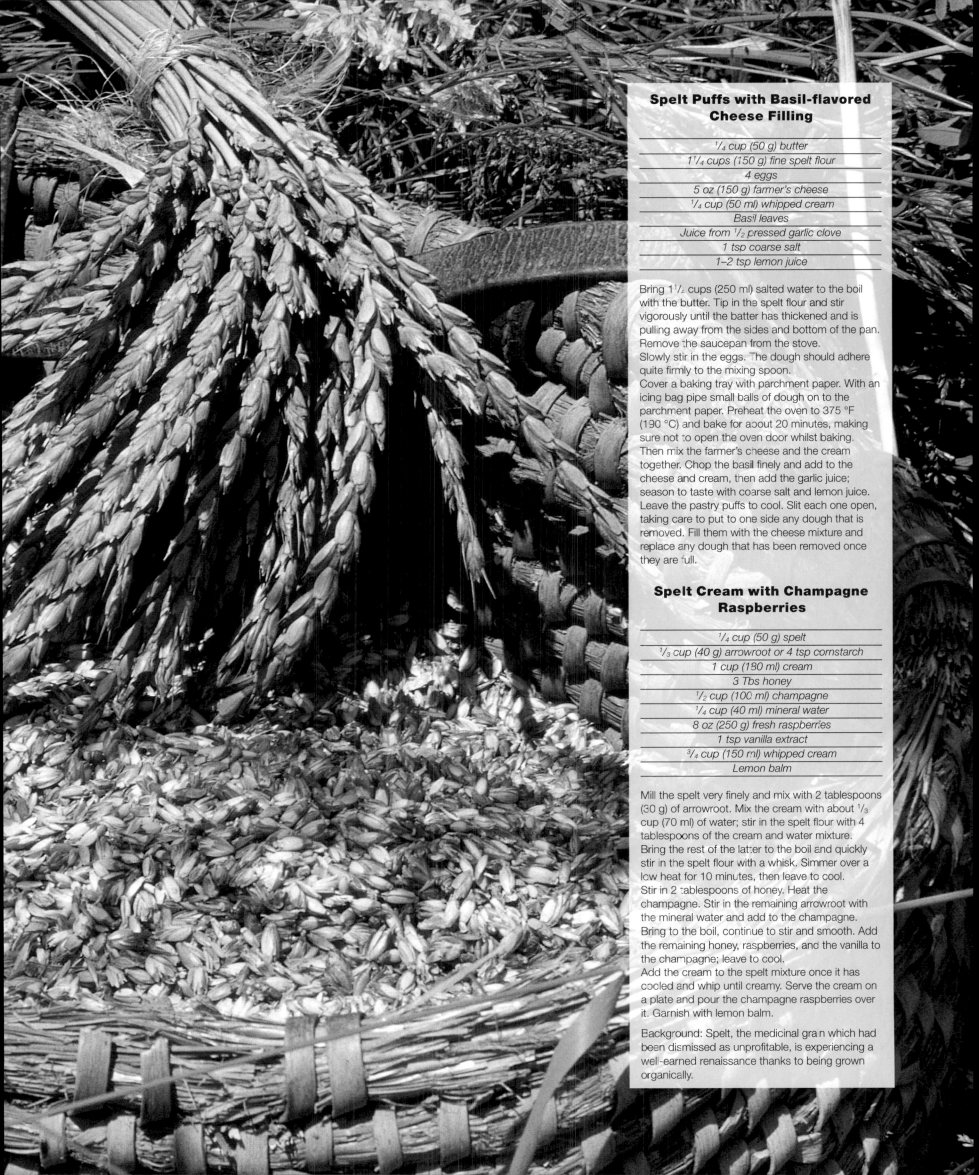

Spelt Puffs with Basil-flavored Cheese Filling

¹/₄ cup (50 g) butter
1¹/₄ cups (150 g) fine spelt flour
4 eggs
5 oz (150 g) farmer's cheese
¹/₄ cup (50 ml) whipped cream
Basil leaves
Juice from ¹/₂ pressed garlic clove
1 tsp coarse salt
1–2 tsp lemon juice

Bring 1¹/₂ cups (250 ml) salted water to the boil with the butter. Tip in the spelt flour and stir vigorously until the batter has thickened and is pulling away from the sides and bottom of the pan. Remove the saucepan from the stove.
Slowly stir in the eggs. The dough should adhere quite firmly to the mixing spoon.
Cover a baking tray with parchment paper. With an icing bag pipe small balls of dough on to the parchment paper. Preheat the oven to 375 °F (190 °C) and bake for about 20 minutes, making sure not to open the oven door whilst baking. Then mix the farmer's cheese and the cream together. Chop the basil finely and add to the cheese and cream, then add the garlic juice; season to taste with coarse salt and lemon juice. Leave the pastry puffs to cool. Slit each one open, taking care to put to one side any dough that is removed. Fill them with the cheese mixture and replace any dough that has been removed once they are full.

Spelt Cream with Champagne Raspberries

¹/₄ cup (50 g) spelt
¹/₃ cup (40 g) arrowroot or 4 tsp cornstarch
1 cup (180 ml) cream
3 Tbs honey
¹/₂ cup (100 ml) champagne
¹/₄ cup (40 ml) mineral water
8 oz (250 g) fresh raspberries
1 tsp vanilla extract
³/₄ cup (150 ml) whipped cream
Lemon balm

Mill the spelt very finely and mix with 2 tablespoons (30 g) of arrowroot. Mix the cream with about ¹/₃ cup (70 ml) of water; stir in the spelt flour with 4 tablespoons of the cream and water mixture. Bring the rest of the latter to the boil and quickly stir in the spelt flour with a whisk. Simmer over a low heat for 10 minutes, then leave to cool.
Stir in 2 tablespoons of honey. Heat the champagne. Stir in the remaining arrowroot with the mineral water and add to the champagne. Bring to the boil, continue to stir and smooth. Add the remaining honey, raspberries, and the vanilla to the champagne; leave to cool.
Add the cream to the spelt mixture once it has cooled and whip until creamy. Serve the cream on a plate and pour the champagne raspberries over it. Garnish with lemon balm.

Background: Spelt, the medicinal grain which had been dismissed as unprofitable, is experiencing a well-earned renaissance thanks to being grown organically.

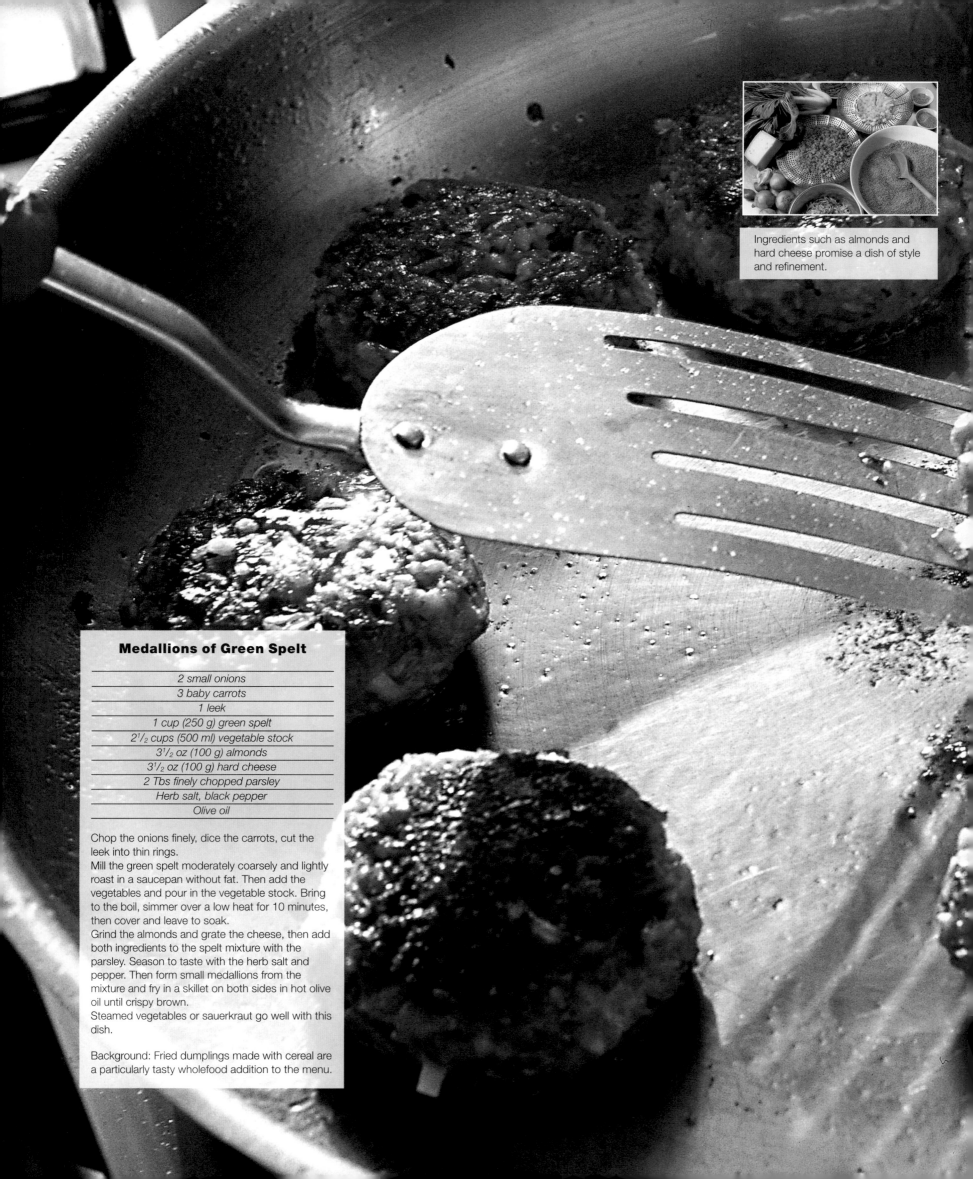

Ingredients such as almonds and hard cheese promise a dish of style and refinement.

Medallions of Green Spelt

2 small onions
3 baby carrots
1 leek
1 cup (250 g) green spelt
2$\frac{1}{2}$ cups (500 ml) vegetable stock
3$\frac{1}{2}$ oz (100 g) almonds
3$\frac{1}{2}$ oz (100 g) hard cheese
2 Tbs finely chopped parsley
Herb salt, black pepper
Olive oil

Chop the onions finely, dice the carrots, cut the leek into thin rings.

Mill the green spelt moderately coarsely and lightly roast in a saucepan without fat. Then add the vegetables and pour in the vegetable stock. Bring to the boil, simmer over a low heat for 10 minutes, then cover and leave to soak.

Grind the almonds and grate the cheese, then add both ingredients to the spelt mixture with the parsley. Season to taste with the herb salt and pepper. Then form small medallions from the mixture and fry in a skillet on both sides in hot olive oil until crispy brown.

Steamed vegetables or sauerkraut go well with this dish.

Background: Fried dumplings made with cereal are a particularly tasty wholefood addition to the menu.

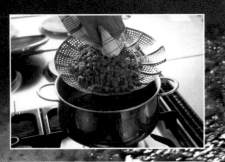

After the green spelt has been lightly roasted without using fat, the raw vegetables are added.

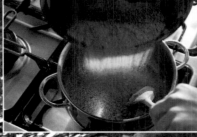

Having added the vegetable stock, the green spelt simmers and soaks until it is cooked.

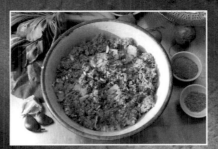

By using ground almonds and freshly grated hard cheese a juicy, firm, spicy dough is produced.

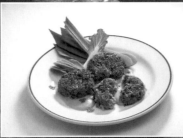

Fried crispy brown on both sides in hot olive oil, medallions of green spelt are a delight.

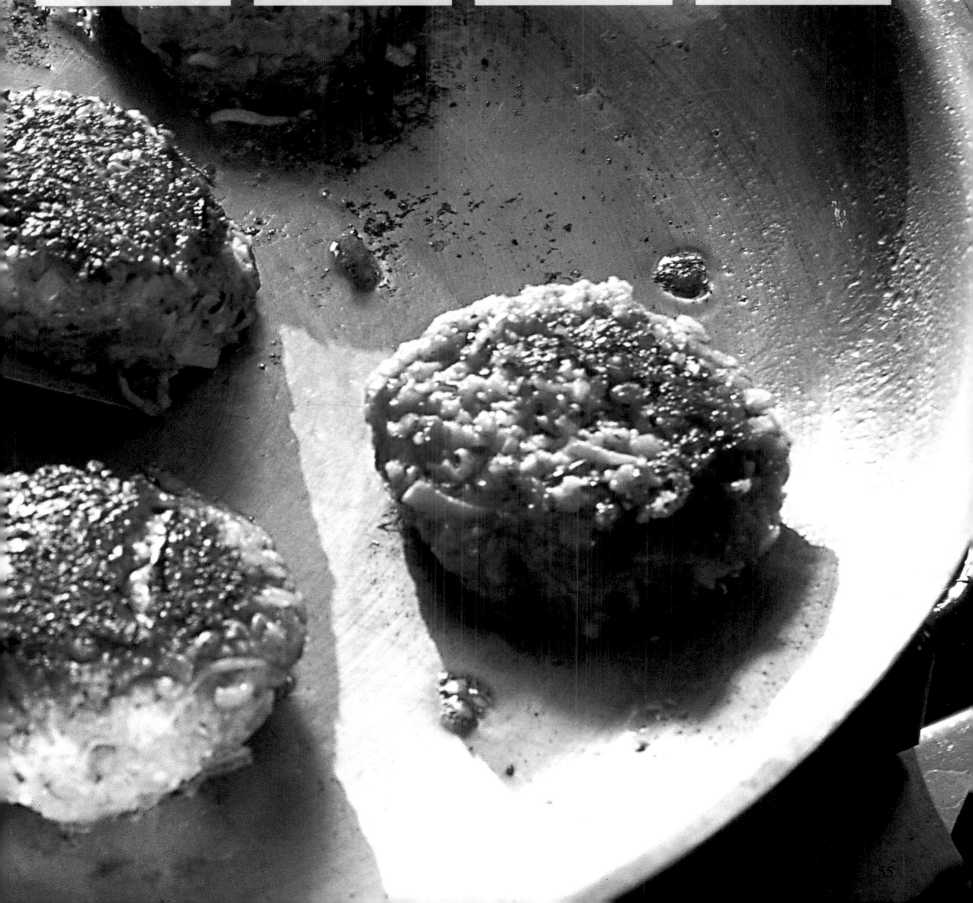

Buckwheat

Rather than being a grain as such, buckwheat is actually the fruit of any cereal plant of the genus *Fagopyrum*. Buckwheat has been rediscovered for wholefood cooking and can be used in the same way as a cereal despite not being one. Since it contains no gluten, buckwheat flour must always be mixed with other flours which are rich in gluten such as that of spelt to produce bread, cakes, and pastries. Buckwheat has a mild, nutty flavor and contains the essential amino acid lysine which rarely occurs in most grains.

How to Handle Buckwheat

Buckwheat is sold in various ways:
• Untreated seeds: as sprouts after 15 hours soaking in about 4 days or after 10 or more days if they have seed leaves; also cooked – pour away the red precipitate which forms during cooking – served with vegetables, as a rice substitute in risottos, used for dumplings;
• Flakes: for granolas and desserts;
• Roasted coarse groats, Russian kasha, or as semolina. Heat with twice its own volume of water, stock, or milk and leave to soak for 15 minutes; served with vegetables, as a rice substitute in risottos, for oven baked dishes, soups, fried dumplings, or desserts;
• Flour: used to make pancakes, crêpes, or blinis.

Hearty Buckwheat Dishes

Buckwheat Soup with Winter Vegetables
(Illustration below right)

³/₄ cup (150 g) buckwheat
1 large onion
³/₄ oz (20 g) butter
5 cups (1 l) vegetable stock
1 small carrot
1 small parsnip
1 small celery stalk
Coarse salt, black pepper
1 small leek
1 Tbs finely chopped parsley
1 Tbs finely chopped lovage
Tamari

Cover the buckwheat in hot water, leave to drain well then roast lightly in a saucepan without adding fat. Chop the onion finely, add to the buckwheat with the butter and fry lightly. Add the vegetable stock. Dice the carrot and parsnip. Cut the celery into small pieces, putting the leaves to one side.
Add the vegetables to the stock, leave to simmer gently, and season with salt and pepper to taste. Cut the leek into thin rings and chop the celery leaves finely. Shortly before serving add the herbs to the soup and season with the tamari.

Below: Buckwheat Bake with Hazelnuts and Sauerkraut

Buckwheat Bake with Hazelnuts and Sauerkraut
(Illustration below)

1 cup (200 g) buckwheat
3¹/₂ oz (100 g) hazelnuts
1¹/₂ cups (300 ml) vegetable stock
2 onions
2 Tbs olive oil
1 bayleaf
2 apples
14 oz (400 g) sauerkraut
¹/₄ cup (50 g) raisins
²/₃ cup (125 ml) white wine or apple juice
Coarse salt, white pepper
1 tsp ground caraway seeds
Pinch of cinnamon
Pinch of ground cloves
1¹/₄ cups (250 ml) heavy cream

Rinse the buckwheat, leave to dry, and roast lightly. Chop the nuts finely, add to the buckwheat and roast them together briefly. Add the stock and cook everything over a low heat for about 15 minutes.
In the meantime, cut the onions into thin slices and braise lightly in the olive oil. Crumble the bayleaf into the pan, cut the apples into small pieces and add to the onions with the sauerkraut and raisins; braise briefly. Add the white wine and leave to simmer gently for 10 minutes. Mix the buckwheat and sauerkraut together. Season with salt, pepper, caraway, cinnamon, and cloves. Grease a baking pan with olive oil, place the buckwheat and sauerkraut mixture in it, pour the cream over the top, and cook in a preheated oven at 350 °F (180 °C) for about 30 minutes.

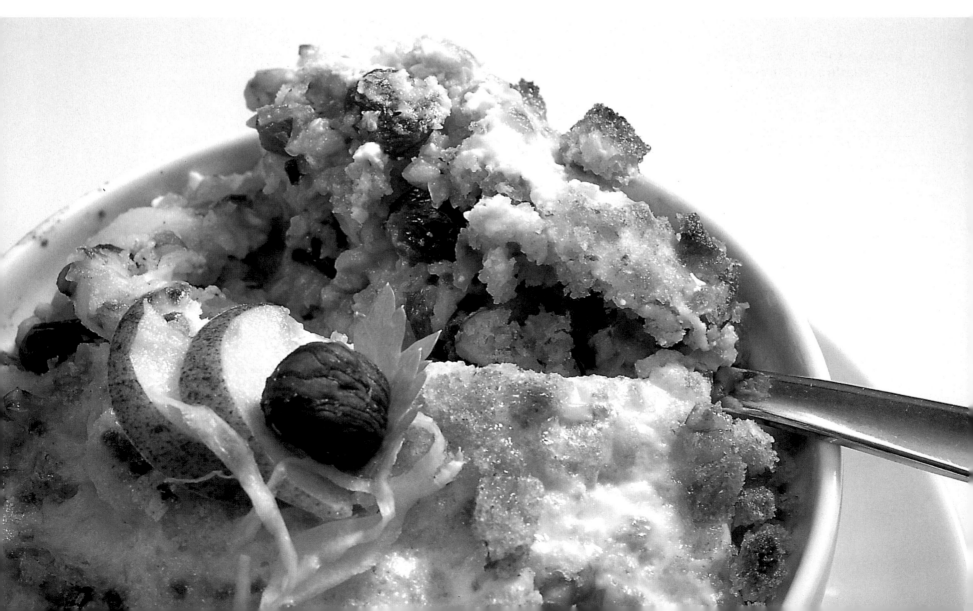

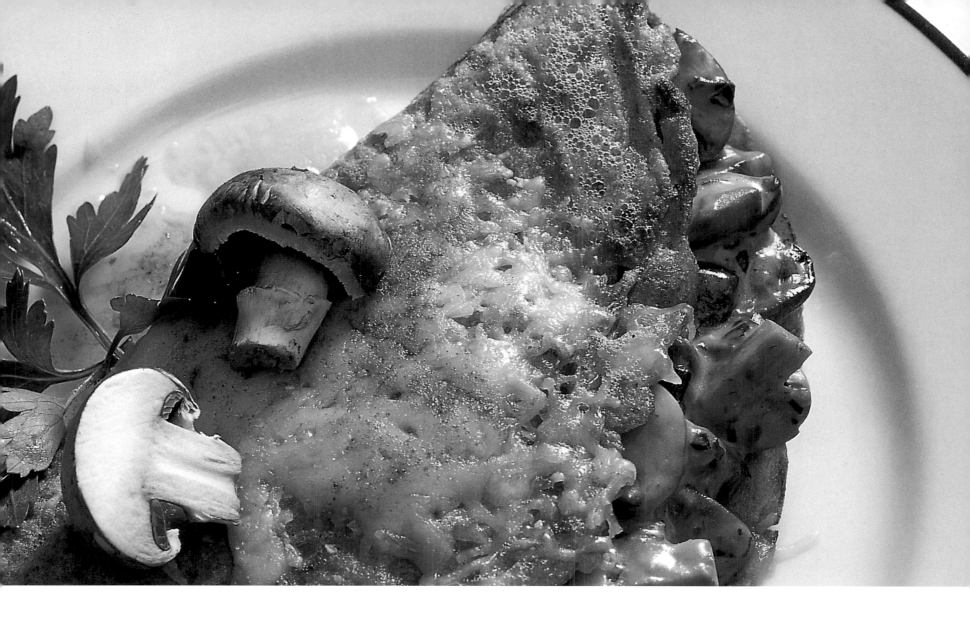

Buckwheat Pancakes with Mushroom Filling

(Illustration above)

Dough
³/₄ cup (100 g) fine buckwheat flour
¹/₂ cup (50 g) fine spelt flour
1 tsp coarse salt
1 tsp herb salt
1¹/₄ cups (250 ml) mineral water
2 eggs

Filling
11 oz (300 g) fresh mushrooms
1 small onion
1 Tbs butter
1 garlic clove
Just over ¹/₂ cup (120 ml) sour cream
1 tsp vegetable stock granules
2 Tbs finely chopped parsley
Herb salt, black pepper
¹/₄ cup (50 g) each of grated Parmesan and Swiss cheese

To make the dough mix the buckwheat flour and the spelt flour with the salt and mineral water, achieving a smooth consistency and leave to rise for 30 minutes. Beat in the eggs and cook the pancakes in batches.
To make the filling cut the mushrooms into quarters and dice the onion. Melt the butter, add the mushrooms and onion, and press the garlic into the pan. Braise everything lightly and add the sour cream. Stir in the stock and parsley; season to taste with salt and pepper.

Fill the pancakes with the mushroom mixture and roll them up. Mix the Parmesan and Swiss cheese together. Top the pancakes with the cheese and brown lightly under the broiler.

Buckwheat Groats

1 cup (250 g) buckwheat

Cover the buckwheat in hot water, drain and dry it again then mill it very coarsely. Cook with about 1³/₄ cups (350 ml) water over a low heat for about 15 minutes.
The groats can be served either spicy or sweet. To make spicy groats add some vegetable stock granules and season to taste with fresh herbs and a little garlic. 2–3 tablespoons of grated cheese can also be mixed in.
To make sweet groats add a little honey and vanilla extract. Fold in ordinary cream or whipped cream to taste.
Variation: 1–2 grated apples make the groats light and airy. It is also possible to add a number of different berries.

Whether in pancakes with mushrooms (above), soup with winter vegetables (below) or baked with hazelnuts and sauerkraut (left hand page) – buckwheat can be prepared in quite a number of different ways.

Above: Buckwheat Pancakes with Mushroom Filling
Right: Buckwheat Soup with Winter Vegetables

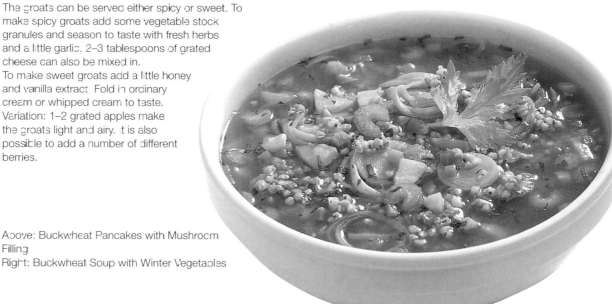

A Gift from the Middle East

Bulgur Wheat and Couscous

Everywhere in the Middle East dishes based on semolina are numbered amongst traditional specialties. To make bulgur wheat, wheat is steamed in order to precook it sufficiently, and is then shelled, dried, and finally milled finely or coarsely. Bulgur wheat is primarily used in pilaf dishes and fillings or for the popular kibbehs. To make the latter it is mixed with ground meat, onions, and seasoning. It also tastes good in salads. Burghul, to give it its Armenian name, lost its central position in the Middle East as by far the most important foodstuff when rice was introduced from India and Persia.

Wheat based semolina maintained its position as a national dish by contrast in the countries of the Maghreb, which includes Tunisia, Algeria, and Morocco. It is known as couscous there, a refined version of bulgur wheat which probably even dates back to the Ancient Egyptians. Couscous was traditionally made in the home by every family, the women of the neighborhood helping each other. Coarsely ground and milled wheat was mixed in large flat dishes with high sides, sprinkled with water and then rubbed with the flat of the hand in a circular movement to make tiny little pellets. These were then poured into sieves to obtain small grains of equal size. The couscous was then steamed over boiling water, spread out on cloths, and dried in the sun. This provided the basic ingredient for many dishes, which when stored in a dry place would keep without any difficulty until the next harvest.

Regardless of which of the many different ragouts were prepared as an accompaniment, cooks always used the traditional utensil which is known by its French name of *couscousière*. It was originally made of clay but is now also made from aluminum and stainless steel. The kitchenware consists of a deep braising pan, in which meat and vegetables are cooked, whilst the couscous itself is cooked over the pan in a type of sieve in the rising steam. A tight fitting lid preserves the flavors.

This relatively time consuming process has been sacrificed to the pace of modern life. Couscous and bulgur wheat are sold today commercially in precooked form, as well as being cultivated organically. France, with its particular historical links to north Africa, is one of the main producers. Bulgur wheat is the somewhat coarser version as well as being the more substantial wholefood. Couscous is manufactured by passing grains of durum wheat through a grinding mechanism. After each grind the grains are sorted into large groat particles and then passed once again through the grinding mechanism which is set to produce a finer grind; particles which are too fine are excluded. The semolina which is eventually produced by this procedure has granules of equal size which contain 70 percent of the vital substances of whole wheat. The precooking which follows will also make subsequent use easier in the case of organic durum wheat semolina. In contrast to conventional products which, mixed with and left to soak in water or stock, are ready for consumption, it is recommended that organic bulgur wheat or couscous is placed in boiling salted water and cooked for about 10 minutes. The semolina can be used in a number of different ways, whether it be in hearty or sweet dishes, in salads, traditionally steamed over ragouts, or as excellent dumplings.

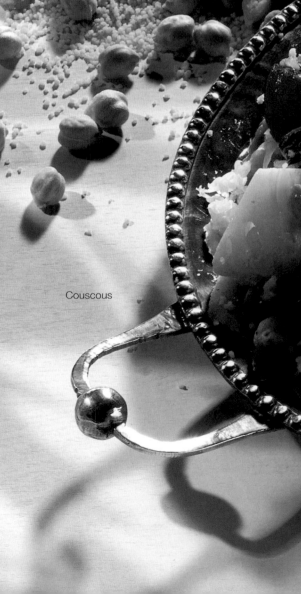

Couscous

Couscous
(Illustration)

1²/₃ cups (300 g) couscous
1 tsp herb salt
1 lb 10 oz (750 g) vegetables (such as white cabbage, carrots, zucchini, leek, tomatoes, cauliflower, broccoli)
2 shallots
2 garlic cloves
6 Tbs garbanzo beans, germinated
4 Tbs olive oil
1¹/₂ cups (300 ml) yogurt
¹/₂ cup (100 ml) sour cream
1 tsp cumin
1 tsp harissa (strong spicy paste)
¹/₂ tsp coarse salt
Peppermint leaves
Chives, Parsley, Chervil

Soak the couscous in 2¹/₂ cups (500 ml) water for 30 minutes, adding the herb salt. Then place in a sieve, cover, and cook over the steam from the water.
Chop the vegetables into small pieces in the meantime; slice the shallots and garlic finely.
Cook the vegetables, shallots, garlic, and garbanzo beans in 3 tablespoons of olive oil until they are firm, then add some water. Stir the yogurt, sour cream, the remaining olive oil as well as the seasoning, and finely chopped herbs together to make a sauce. Serve the couscous with the vegetables on a large plate, adding the yogurt sauce.

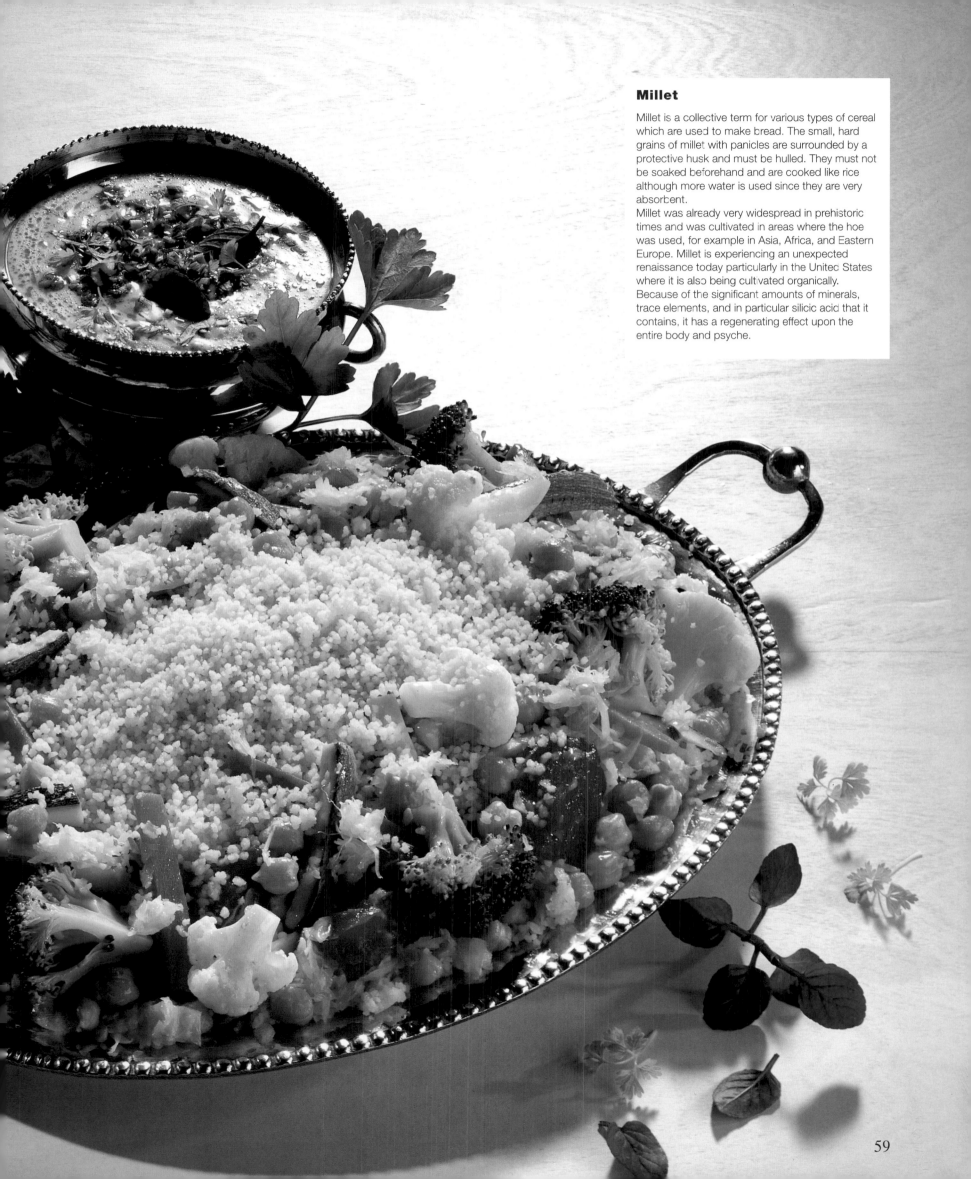

Millet

Millet is a collective term for various types of cereal which are used to make bread. The small, hard grains of millet with panicles are surrounded by a protective husk and must be hulled. They must not be soaked beforehand and are cooked like rice although more water is used since they are very absorbent.

Millet was already very widespread in prehistoric times and was cultivated in areas where the hoe was used, for example in Asia, Africa, and Eastern Europe. Millet is experiencing an unexpected renaissance today particularly in the United States where it is also being cultivated organically. Because of the significant amounts of minerals, trace elements, and in particular silicic acid that it contains, it has a regenerating effect upon the entire body and psyche.

59

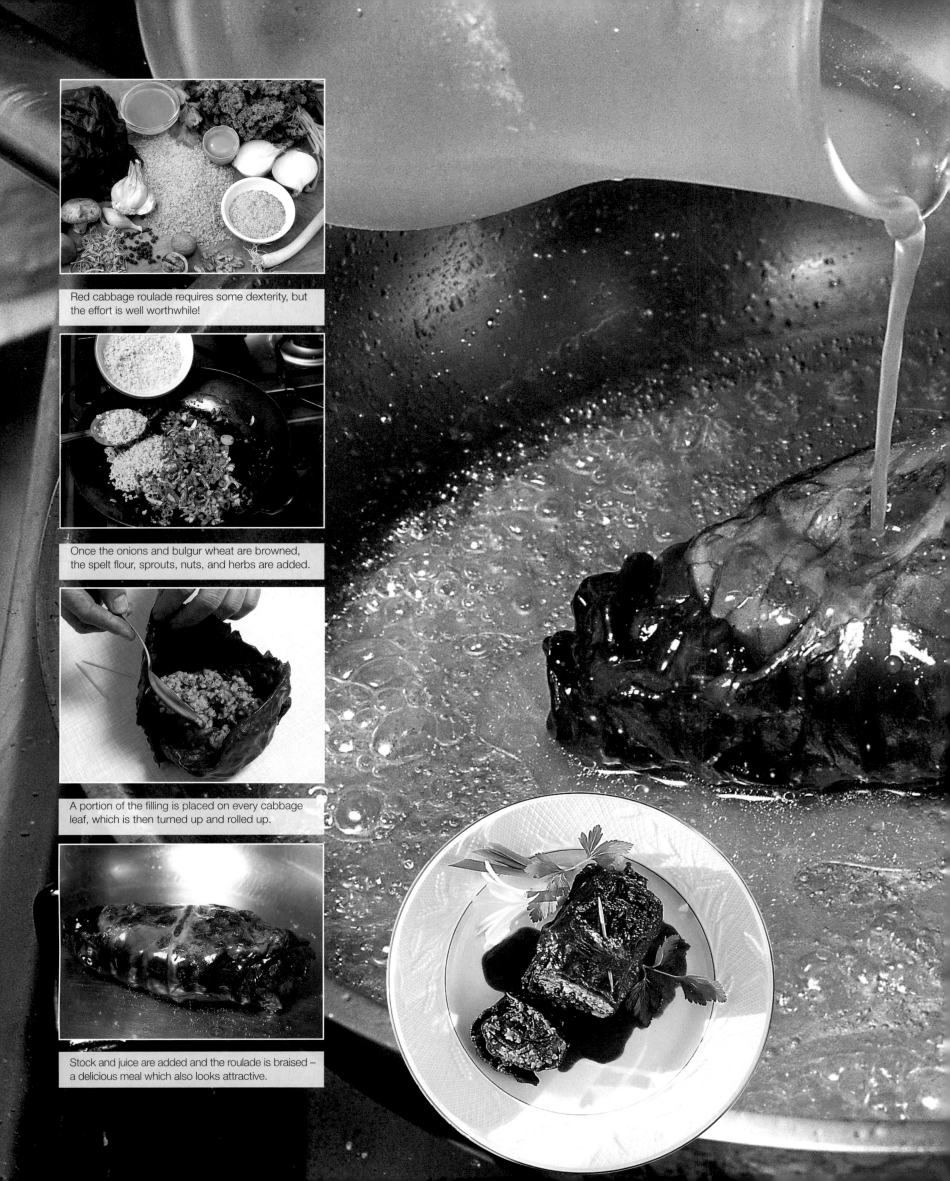

Red cabbage roulade requires some dexterity, but the effort is well worthwhile!

Once the onions and bulgur wheat are browned, the spelt flour, sprouts, nuts, and herbs are added.

A portion of the filling is placed on every cabbage leaf, which is then turned up and rolled up.

Stock and juice are added and the roulade is braised – a delicious meal which also looks attractive.

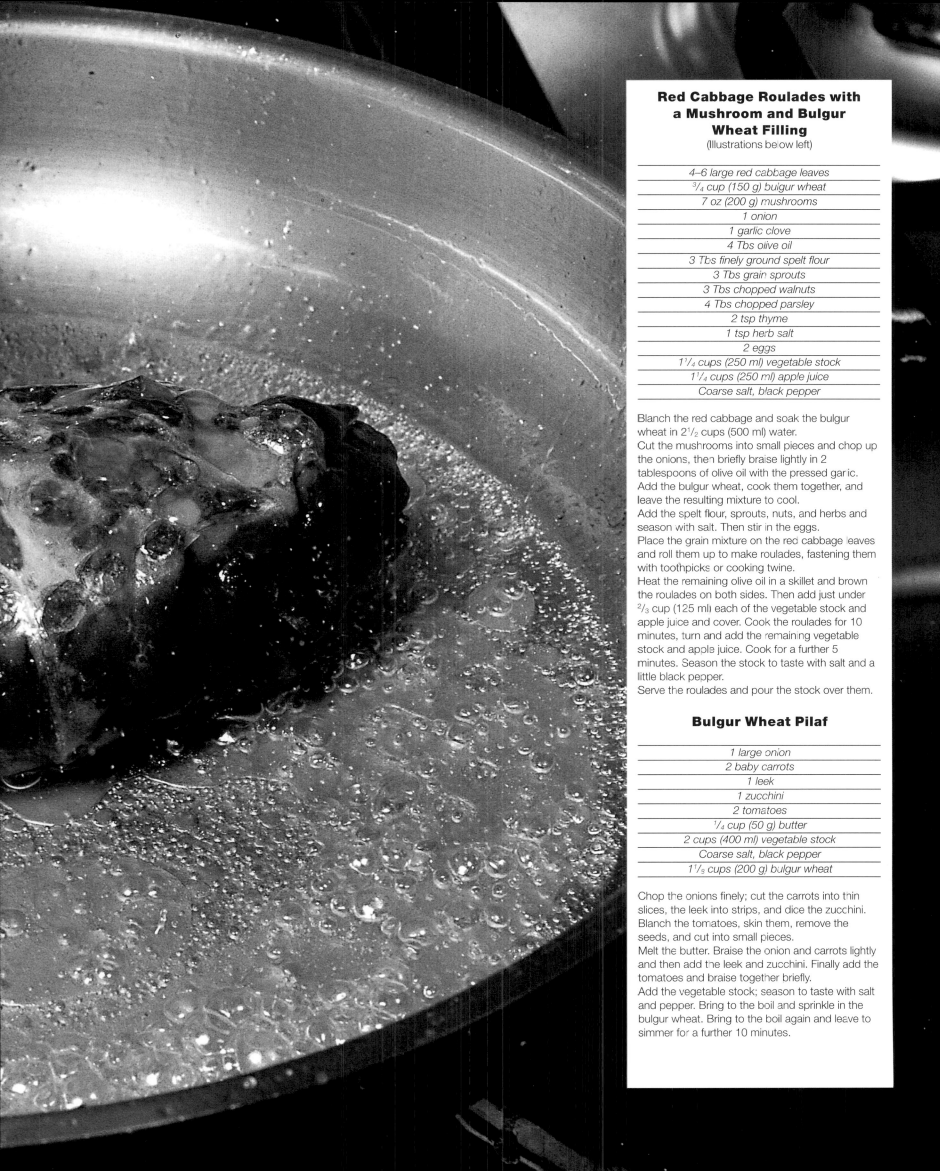

Red Cabbage Roulades with a Mushroom and Bulgur Wheat Filling

(Illustrations below left)

4–6 large red cabbage leaves
³/₄ cup (150 g) bulgur wheat
7 oz (200 g) mushrooms
1 onion
1 garlic clove
4 Tbs olive oil
3 Tbs finely ground spelt flour
3 Tbs grain sprouts
3 Tbs chopped walnuts
4 Tbs chopped parsley
2 tsp thyme
1 tsp herb salt
2 eggs
1¹/₄ cups (250 ml) vegetable stock
1¹/₄ cups (250 ml) apple juice
Coarse salt, black pepper

Blanch the red cabbage and soak the bulgur wheat in 2¹/₂ cups (500 ml) water.

Cut the mushrooms into small pieces and chop up the onions, then briefly braise lightly in 2 tablespoons of olive oil with the pressed garlic. Add the bulgur wheat, cook them together, and leave the resulting mixture to cool.

Add the spelt flour, sprouts, nuts, and herbs and season with salt. Then stir in the eggs.

Place the grain mixture on the red cabbage leaves and roll them up to make roulades, fastening them with toothpicks or cooking twine.

Heat the remaining olive oil in a skillet and brown the roulades on both sides. Then add just under ²/₃ cup (125 ml) each of the vegetable stock and apple juice and cover. Cook the roulades for 10 minutes, turn and add the remaining vegetable stock and apple juice. Cook for a further 5 minutes. Season the stock to taste with salt and a little black pepper.

Serve the roulades and pour the stock over them.

Bulgur Wheat Pilaf

1 large onion
2 baby carrots
1 leek
1 zucchini
2 tomatoes
¹/₄ cup (50 g) butter
2 cups (400 ml) vegetable stock
Coarse salt, black pepper
1¹/₃ cups (200 g) bulgur wheat

Chop the onions finely; cut the carrots into thin slices, the leek into strips, and dice the zucchini. Blanch the tomatoes, skin them, remove the seeds, and cut into small pieces.

Melt the butter. Braise the onion and carrots lightly and then add the leek and zucchini. Finally add the tomatoes and braise together briefly.

Add the vegetable stock; season to taste with salt and pepper. Bring to the boil and sprinkle in the bulgur wheat. Bring to the boil again and leave to simmer for a further 10 minutes.

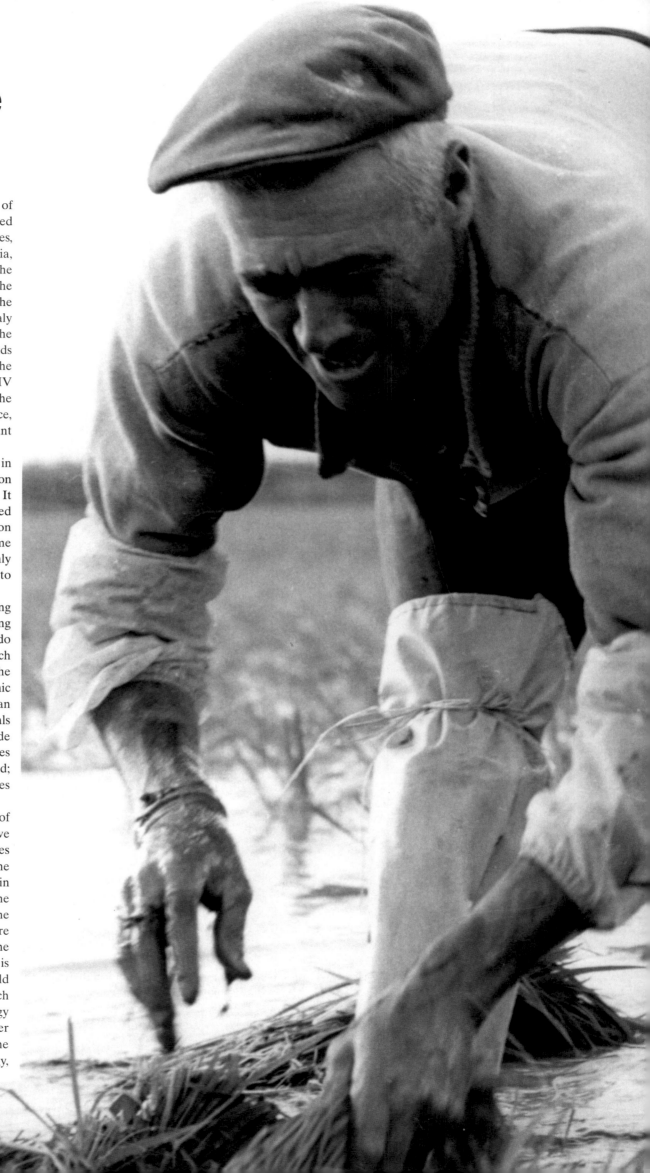

Rice from the Camargue

Rice is the basic foodstuff today for half of the world's population. It has been cultivated for thousands of years in Asian countries, where it spread from Thailand, Cambodia, and southern China. At the time of the Persian Empire around 2,500 years ago the plant made its way to the Middle East. The Moors introduced it to Spain. It came to Italy from there before it reached France at the end of the 13th century. Many paddy fields were created in Provence in the course of the next 200 years. A decree made by Henry IV has survived in which it is laid down that the farmers of the Camargue are to cultivate rice, sugar cane, and a type of madder, the plant which produces a red dye.

As became apparent from various attempts in other regions, the Camargue is the only region in France where rice can be cultivated at all. It was only after the Camargue was equipped with dikes around 1870 that cultivation spread, the dikes causing the fields to become salty. It was the intention of the farmers only to use rice as a temporary crop in order to prepare the soil for vines in particular.

The suspension of deliveries of rice during the Second World War and the increasing independence of the colony of French Indo China led after 1945 to a new initiative which received material assistance through the Marshall Plan, a program for economic reconstruction proposed by the American General George Marshall. Irrigation canals and pumping stations were built. Wine made way for rice, and up until 1960 74,000 acres (30,000 hectares) of rice fields were planted; today there are still around 62,000 acres (25,000 hectares).

Rice cultivation begins with the leveling of the field. This used to be a very expensive procedure involving the insertion of stakes every thirty feet (ten meters) or so. The height of the soil would then be measured in order finally to even out the undulations. The use of laser equipment was introduced in the middle of the 1980s. The measurements are transmitted electronically to bulldozers, the movement of whose digging equipment is regulated by a computer. In this way a field can be leveled exactly to within $3/4$ inch (2 centimeters). This ultramodern technology brings considerable advantages. The water level can remain lower than before on the precisely leveled soil, which saves energy, time, and costs. The water stands a mere two to four inches (five to ten centimeters) deep nowadays. The height of the water has a direct influence on crop yields which are dependent upon the temperature. The lower the water level the sooner the water will become warm. This factor plays a considerable role in the Camargue which is the northernmost area for rice cultivation in Europe – rice is also still grown in the Mediterranean countries of Spain, Portugal, Italy, and Greece.

Time is therefore at a premium. Sowing begins on April 15. Rice is the only cereal which instead of being planted beneath the surface of the soil is sown on top. The fields are flooded four to five days before sowing so that the water can heat up. The Rhône which supplies water to the Camargue takes in the melting snow from the Alps and for this reason its water is cold. Rice requires a temperature of between 59 and 63 °F (15 to 17 °C) to germinate. If this has not taken place within 20 days the seeds will rot and the crop will have to be sown again.

Farmers who grow rice organically use a simple, natural method. They submerge their fields in water before it is time to sow. As soon as the weeds have germinated they drain the fields. Once the weeds have withered and died they are plowed in at a depth of three-quarters of an inch (two centimeters). Then the field is watered again and sown according to the normal practice but with a slightly higher amount of seeds, about 1,200 pounds per acre (225 kilograms per hectare). About a month after sowing the water is gradually drained away so that the small, young rice plants which are still swimming can sink on to the soil and strike root there. They are then submerged in water again.

Rice blossoms in the second half of August. The blossom only lasts for one and a half hours and takes place between noon and two o'clock in the afternoon. If the flowering is a bad one the seed will remain empty. If this is the case the plant will stand upright whilst if the opposite occurs it will bend over. Rice needs a total of between 130 and 150 days to develop from the germinated seed to the harvest and cannot tolerate temperatures below 54 °F (12 °C), which can often cause problems in the fall.

The rice farmers are prevented by law from processing and selling what they harvest themselves. There are three small enterprises in the Camargue that process and market crops from 2,500 acres (1,000 hectares) of paddy fields which are farmed organically. Rice which is ready for harvesting has a moisture level of between 25 and 27 percent, but in order for it to be hulled and shelled this must be reduced to 14 percent. The conventional method consists in drying the rice immediately with the help of special ovens, something which causes a lot of grains to crack. Joseph Bon was the first French rice farmer to switch to organic techniques in 1963. When he built the warehouse of his rice mill the following year he devised a method of drying which was as original as it was efficient. It relies upon the wind known as the Mistral which often blows strongly in the Rhone delta. The rice which is still damp from being harvested is stored in leveled heaps about twenty feet (six meters) high in ten compartments made of wood, each of which is capable of holding 275 to 330 tons (250 to 300 tonnes) of rice. Four powerful ventilators suck in the dry air of the Mistral and blow about three cubic feet (one cubic meter) per second into each compartment.

Untreated rice, so called "paddy," is enclosed in a hard husk. When this coarse, inedible outer shell is removed brown whole grain rice is obtained with the germ and a protective skin. This contains the majority of rice's extremely nutritious contents. These are the B vitamins 1, 2, and 3, as well as other vitamins and all eight of the essential amino acids (see p. 21). Whole grain rice is broadly comparable to vegetables. Its optimal storage temperature is 41 °F (5 °C). The cold protects natural rice – and cereals in general – from mites and other undesirable fellow diners, which is why it is best kept in the refrigerator. In the course of processing, the rice is passed through a shelling machine which removes the thin protective skin and germ. The result is white rice which retains very few vitamins and nutrients. Whilst it certainly contains a lot of starch it no longer has enough vitamin B1 to help our bodies digest it. It is for this reason that it became the cause of beri beri, a serious nervous disease in Asia.

The paddy fields of the Camargue are laid out in a way that allows them only to be flooded from one side. The remaining sides are surrounded by ditches which are just over three feet (one meter) deep. All water from the fields in the Camargue flows into the large Etang de Vaccarès. Unfortunately conventional agriculture which uses pesticides, insecticides, and weedkillers and which is predominant has led to an increase in the pollution of its waters. This has resulted in the disappearance of various species of fish there such as the zander which was once much in evidence. In order to preserve the Camargue nature reserve it would be desirable if France's entire rice production were put on an organic footing.

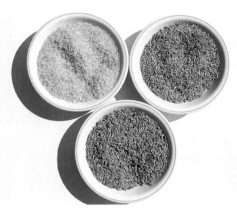

Paddy with husks (below), highly nutritious natural rice (above right), and white rice which contains few vitamins.

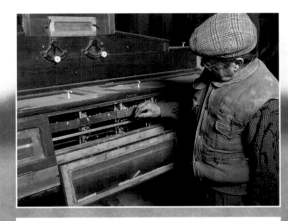

Thanks to the vibration of the separating machine the rough paddy climbs to the top whilst the smooth whole grain slides downwards.

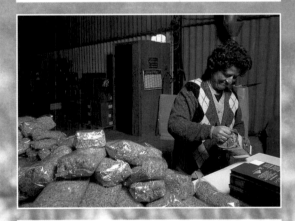

The original rice of the Camargue has round grains. This has however been supplanted to a considerable extent by the rather "fashionable" long grained rice.

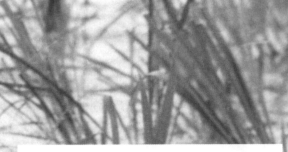

Background: The more popular rice was only planted in the two decades between 1950 and 1970 in the Camargue in nurseries by hand.

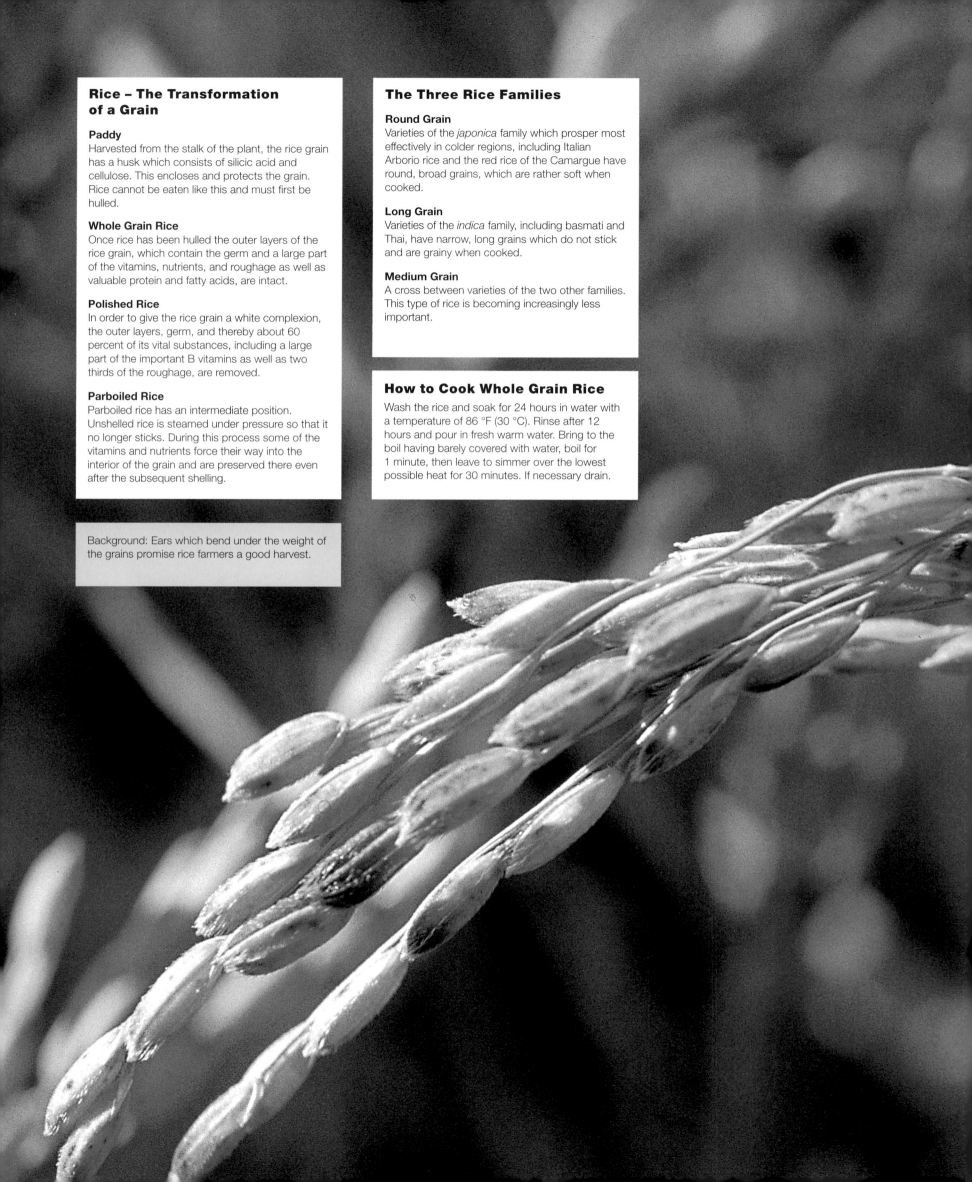

Rice – The Transformation of a Grain

Paddy
Harvested from the stalk of the plant, the rice grain has a husk which consists of silicic acid and cellulose. This encloses and protects the grain. Rice cannot be eaten like this and must first be hulled.

Whole Grain Rice
Once rice has been hulled the outer layers of the rice grain, which contain the germ and a large part of the vitamins, nutrients, and roughage as well as valuable protein and fatty acids, are intact.

Polished Rice
In order to give the rice grain a white complexion, the outer layers, germ, and thereby about 60 percent of its vital substances, including a large part of the important B vitamins as well as two thirds of the roughage, are removed.

Parboiled Rice
Parboiled rice has an intermediate position. Unshelled rice is steamed under pressure so that it no longer sticks. During this process some of the vitamins and nutrients force their way into the interior of the grain and are preserved there even after the subsequent shelling.

Background: Ears which bend under the weight of the grains promise rice farmers a good harvest.

The Three Rice Families

Round Grain
Varieties of the *japonica* family which prosper most effectively in colder regions, including Italian Arborio rice and the red rice of the Camargue have round, broad grains, which are rather soft when cooked.

Long Grain
Varieties of the *indica* family, including basmati and Thai, have narrow, long grains which do not stick and are grainy when cooked.

Medium Grain
A cross between varieties of the two other families. This type of rice is becoming increasingly less important.

How to Cook Whole Grain Rice

Wash the rice and soak for 24 hours in water with a temperature of 86 °F (30 °C). Rinse after 12 hours and pour in fresh warm water. Bring to the boil having barely covered with water, boil for 1 minute, then leave to simmer over the lowest possible heat for 30 minutes. If necessary drain.

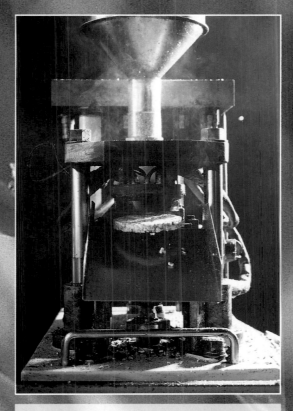

Heated for seconds at 520 °F (270 °C), rice grains puff up and are shaped into rounds in a press.

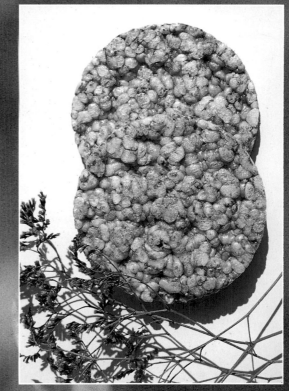

Rice cakes, mixed with other grains and spices, are a featherlight specialty.

Turkish Lamb and Rice Casserole

11 oz (300 g) lamb
4 red onions
3 Tbs olive oil
4 large slicing tomatoes
1¹/₂ cups (250 g) untreated rice
¹/₂ tsp Turkish paprika
¹/₂ tsp ground cumin
6 cups (1.2 l) vegetable stock
12 dried apricots
Coarse salt, white pepper
1 small bunch dill
1 Tbs lemon juice
7 oz (200 g) strained yogurt

Remove any fat and tendons from the lamb and cut into small cubes. Cut the onions into small pieces and brown with the meat in the olive oil. Blanch the tomatoes, skin and also cut into cubes; add to the meat with the rice. Season with paprika and cumin. Heat the vegetable stock and pour in. Add the apricots and cook the mixture for 45 minutes.

At the end of the cooking time the rice should be dry. Season with salt and pepper. Chop the dill finely, putting some tips aside for decoration purposes. Stir into the yogurt with the lemon juice and season to taste with salt and pepper.

Serve the Lamb and Rice Casserole on preheated plates, decorate with dill tips, and serve the yogurt sauce separately.

Saffron Rice with Oyster Mushrooms

6 cups (1.2 l) vegetable stock
¹/₄ cup (50 g) butter
1 Tbs finely chopped shallots
1¹/₂ cups (250 g) untreated round grain rice
1 small packet of saffron
1 Tbs olive oil
1 crushed garlic clove
1 lb 2 oz (500 g) oyster mushrooms
2 Tbs parsley
White pepper
2¹/₂ oz (60 g) freshly grated hard cheese

Bring the vegetable stock to the boil. Melt half the butter and cook half the shallots in it until they are a golden-yellow color. Add the unwashed natural rice and cook until transparent. Pour in the boiling stock and add the saffron. Leave to soak for 30 minutes over a very low heat.

Put the rest of the butter and the olive oil in a skillet and braise the remaining shallots and the garlic lightly. Wash the mushrooms, cut them into strips, and place in the skillet. Braise whilst stirring constantly for 15 minutes. Add the parsley, season the mushrooms with pepper and cook for a further 30 minutes. Add to the saffron rice, cover, and cook for a further 15 minutes.

Remove from the stove and mix in 1¹/₂ oz (40 g) cheese. Place on preheated plates, sprinkle with the remaining cheese, and serve.

Organic Pasta

There are as many different types of pasta made with flour from organically grown cereals today as there are traditional ones. When the first pioneers began to manufacture organic pasta in the early 1980s, spelt was not available and durum wheat was the main ingredient used by pasta makers. From 1985 onwards spelt was discovered anew and was quickly on the way to becoming extremely popular. It is not unusual for spelt to account for two thirds of the cereals used to make pasta in northern Europe today, and it is rapidly gaining in popularity in Switzerland and France as well. Other cereals such as amaranth, buckwheat, or millet are also added in smaller amounts to make special types of pasta. In order to secure their supplies of highly nutritious spelt varieties, many pasta producers have signed delivery contracts with organic farmers. Great stress is also laid on preserving the nutritious content of the ingredients when it comes to the way in which craftsmen work when making organic pasta.

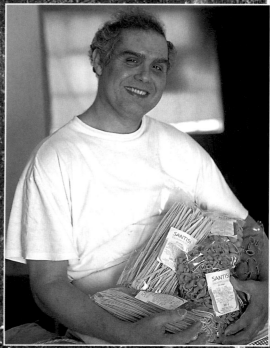

Master pasta maker Giuseppe Santisi swears by the traditions of his craft and by organic cereals.

Background: Pressed through nozzles with fine holes, strips of dough are cut off to make pasta.

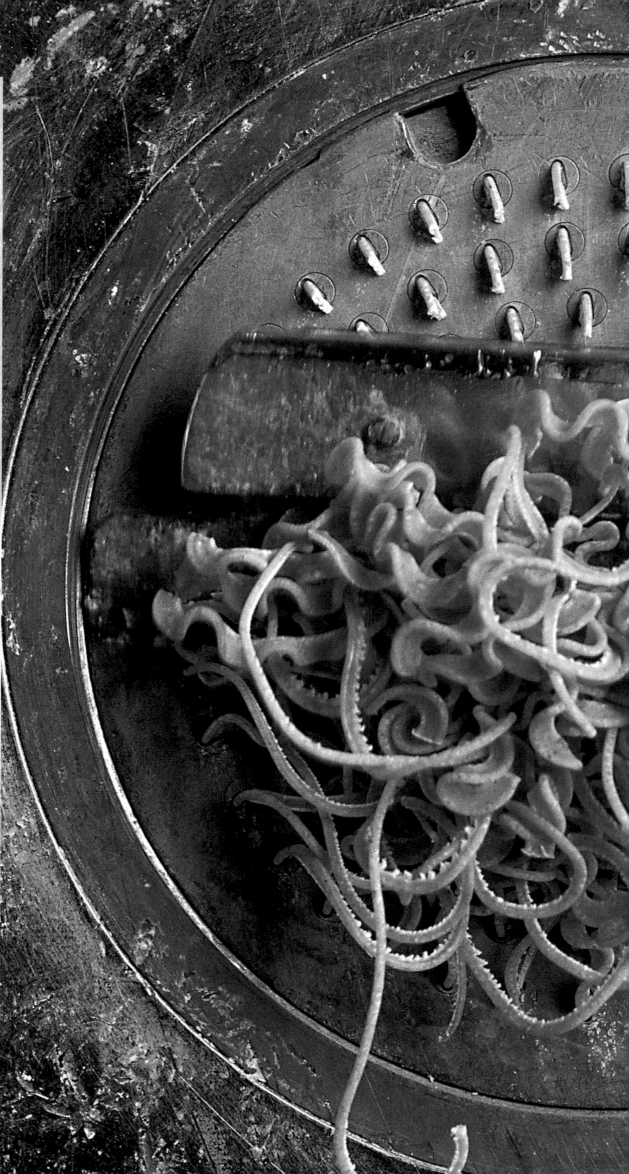

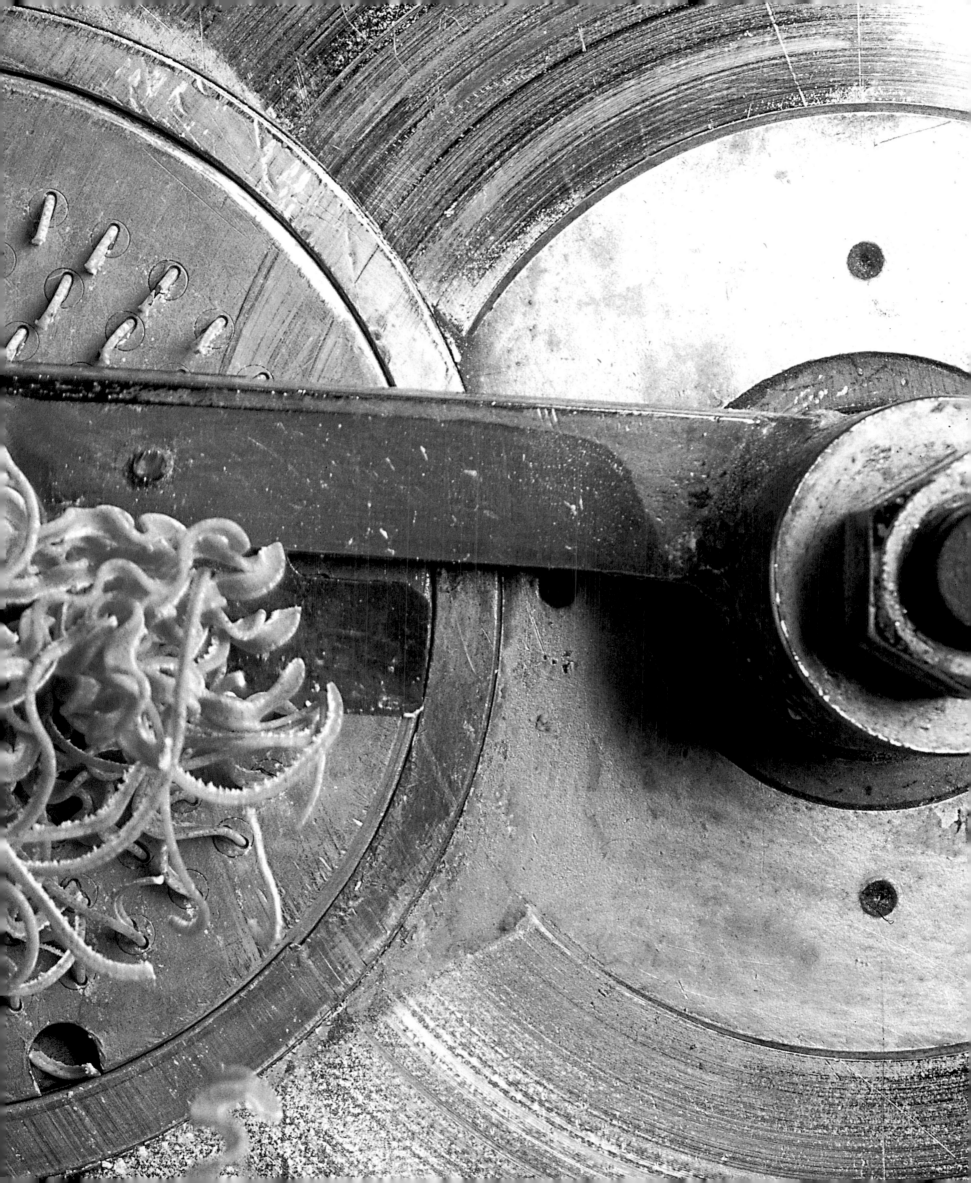

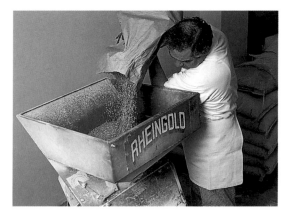

Every morning this hammer mill grinds the cereal for the day's pasta production.

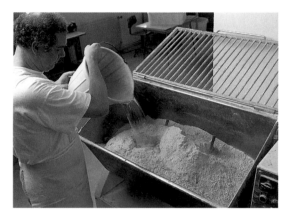

Only flour and water produce the dough, only experience guarantees the correct consistency.

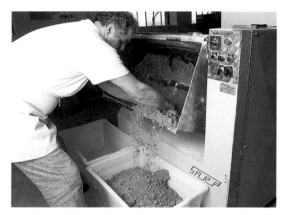

The pasta dough which comes out of the kneading trough is crumbly and elastic. It is then pressed or rolled.

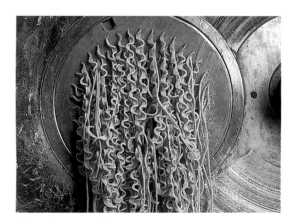

All smaller types of pasta are pressed through nozzles which give them shape and are cut to measure.

When stored in a cool and dry place organic pasta will last for months and can therefore be easily integrated into the everyday diet.

In the small factories where organic pasta is produced the working day begins with the fresh milling of the daily requirement of flour. Opinions differ as to the choice of mill. Hammer mills produce an equally small grind in one go whilst stone mills require an additional grind. This procedure is also recommended for making flour for pasta dough in the home.

The kneading machine resembles a trough in which fixed arms turn. It is made from stainless steel and can hold 200 pounds (90 kilograms) of flour to which 42 pints (20 liters) of water are added. After 10–15 minutes of kneading, the master pasta maker adds water again. The amount depends on the weather and the quality of the grain because whole grain flour will never react in the same way twice. The finished dough feels crumbly and elastic but does not drip between the fingers.

During the next stage the pasta receives its shape. To make smaller types of pasta such as rigatoni, pasta shells, and spirals the dough is placed into the press in which blades are constantly turning and which cut up the dough. The latter must be continually in motion and be at a temperature of 113 °F (45 °C) if possible. It is then passed through filters whose openings shape the dough with an 80 gram force pressure. If for example spirals are being made a knife rotates in front of the press which accurately cuts off strips of pasta in appropriate lengths. The fresh pasta then falls into sieves, beneath which ventilators are located. Shaken and dried at the same time in this way the pasta shapes do not stick to each other.

To produce longer types of pasta another manufacturing procedure is used. The pasta maker places the dough in a rolling mill which works at a temperature of 77 °F (25 °C). It is for this reason that rolled pasta is lighter in color even using the same dough to begin with. A wide, thin, light brown strip of pasta only one fifth of an inch (five millimeters) thick comes out of the machine and is rolled up like a fitted carpet. Placed in a second rolling mill its thickness is reduced and it is cut into the required width by knives. A constant stream of pasta strips pours out of the machine. At exactly the right moment a steel rod is pushed beneath the strips of dough to raise the pasta slightly. After every 16 inches (40 centimeters) or so the ends are then severed. Now fresh spaghetti hangs over the rod which is then dried.

Finished pasta has to dry. It is a legal requirement that it should contain no more moisture than the cereal from which it was made, namely 11 to 13 percent. The water which was added to the flour must therefore be removed again. It is an adage amongst pasta experts that moisture is required to dry it. This is particularly successful if the drying takes place slowly. Damp weather is therefore ideal. Racks upon which longer types of pasta are hung and sieves containing the smaller varieties are placed in a drying room. Warm air is blown in on one side at a temperature of 113 °F (45 °C) and moist air is drawn off on the other side. Within 24 hours the pasta is dry.

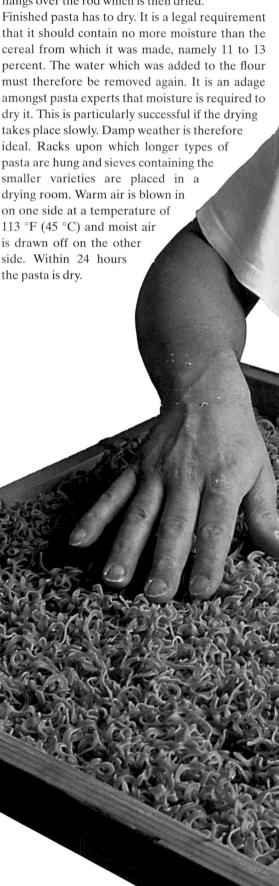

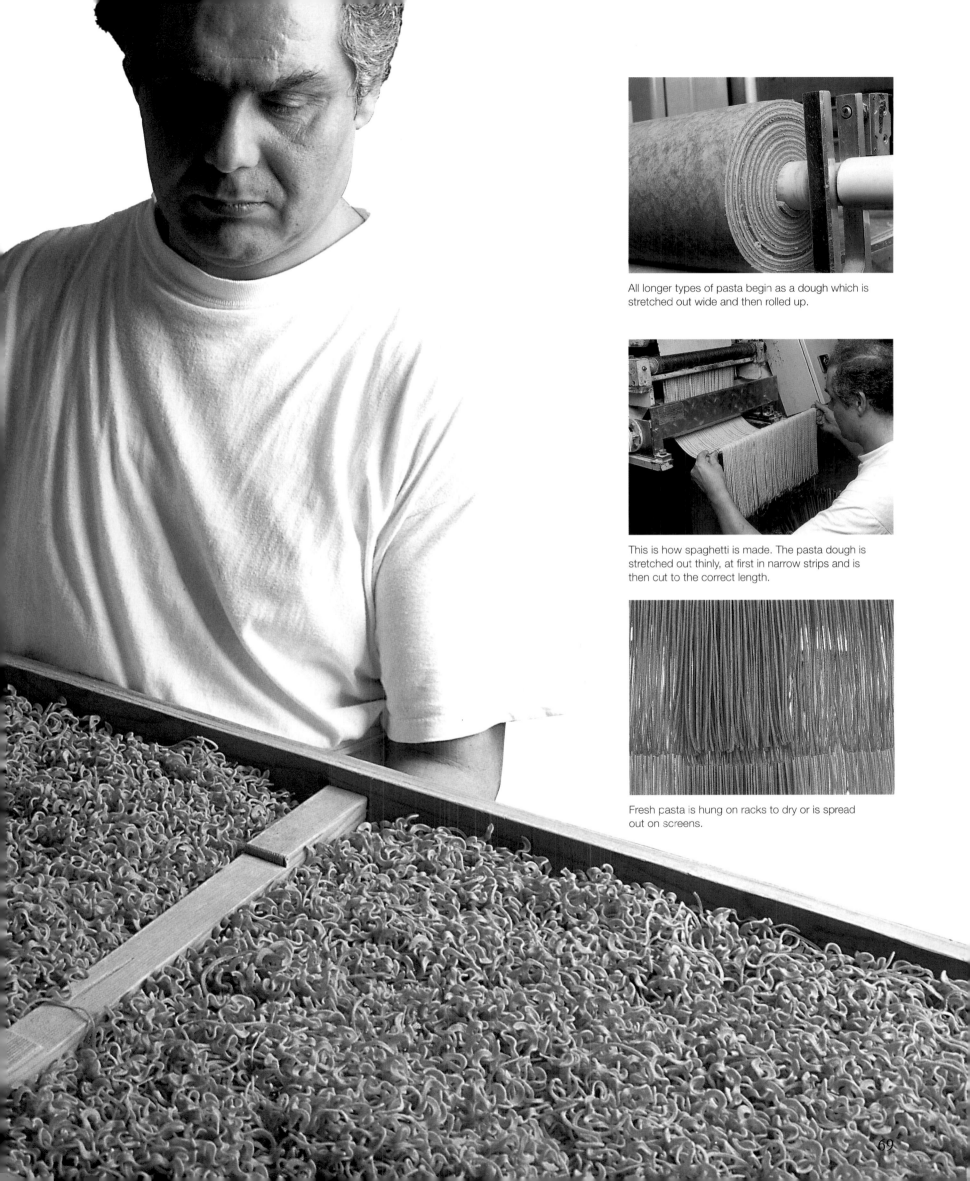

All longer types of pasta begin as a dough which is stretched out wide and then rolled up.

This is how spaghetti is made. The pasta dough is stretched out thinly, at first in narrow strips and is then cut to the correct length.

Fresh pasta is hung on racks to dry or is spread out on screens.

Pasta Made From Organically Grown Cereal

Lasagna
Sheets of lasagna made from whole grain wheat semolina and eggs, for the traditional dish with tomato and béchamel sauce.

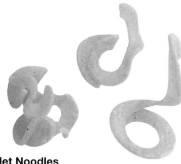

Millet Noodles
These can be served with many dishes and are the easiest way of including this valuable grain in one's diet.

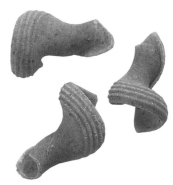

Spelt Santisi
A small, ribbed, almost funnel like pasta shape which turns in on itself, made by Giuseppe Santisi – real designer pasta with medium absorbency.

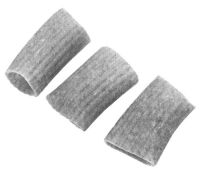

Spelt Rigatoni
Short, thick, ribbed tubes of pasta with a nutty taste; especially good with cream sauces.

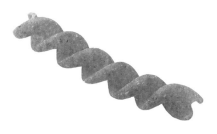

Spelt Whole Grain Spirals
Spirals absorb plenty of sauce and are also very well suited to pasta bakes.

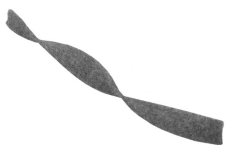

Spelt Whole Grain Tagliatelle
Spelt is excellently suited to make pasta doughs; as a whole grain it gives these tagliatelle their dark color.

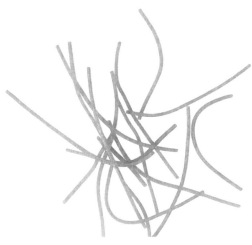

Whole Wheat Soup Noodles

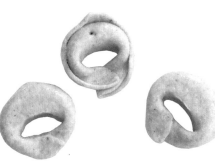

Tortellini with Tofu Filling
Small round parcels of dough, originally a specialty of Bologna, shown here with a spicy tofu filling.

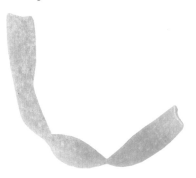

Soybean Noodles
Noodles made from soybean flour which enriches these noodles with protein.

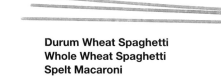

Durum Wheat Spaghetti
Whole Wheat Spaghetti
Spelt Macaroni
Spelt and Buckwheat Spaghetti

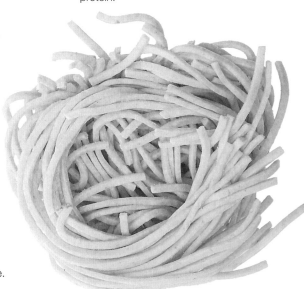

Spaghetti with Turmeric
Turmeric is an Asian ginger plant which contains a yellow dye.

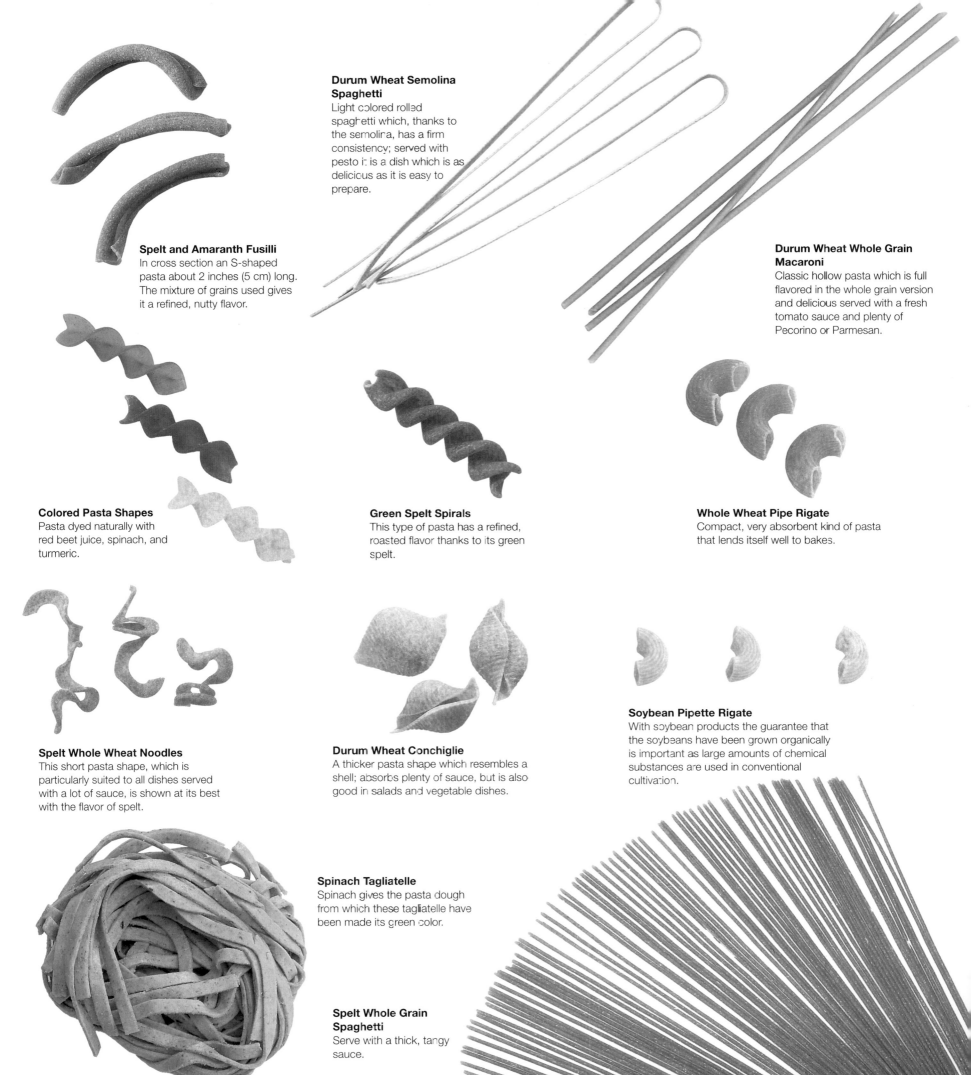

Spelt and Amaranth Fusilli
In cross section an S-shaped pasta about 2 inches (5 cm) long. The mixture of grains used gives it a refined, nutty flavor.

Durum Wheat Semolina Spaghetti
Light colored rolled spaghetti which, thanks to the semolina, has a firm consistency; served with pesto it is a dish which is as delicious as it is easy to prepare.

Durum Wheat Whole Grain Macaroni
Classic hollow pasta which is full flavored in the whole grain version and delicious served with a fresh tomato sauce and plenty of Pecorino or Parmesan.

Colored Pasta Shapes
Pasta dyed naturally with red beet juice, spinach, and turmeric.

Green Spelt Spirals
This type of pasta has a refined, roasted flavor thanks to its green spelt.

Whole Wheat Pipe Rigate
Compact, very absorbent kind of pasta that lends itself well to bakes.

Spelt Whole Wheat Noodles
This short pasta shape, which is particularly suited to all dishes served with a lot of sauce, is shown at its best with the flavor of spelt.

Durum Wheat Conchiglie
A thicker pasta shape which resembles a shell; absorbs plenty of sauce, but is also good in salads and vegetable dishes.

Soybean Pipette Rigate
With soybean products the guarantee that the soybeans have been grown organically is important as large amounts of chemical substances are used in conventional cultivation.

Spinach Tagliatelle
Spinach gives the pasta dough from which these tagliatelle have been made its green color.

Spelt Whole Grain Spaghetti
Serve with a thick, tangy sauce.

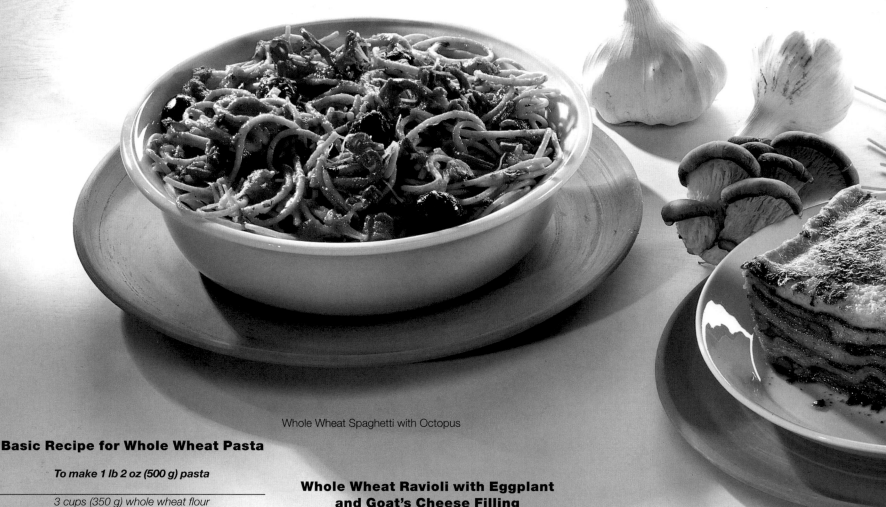

Whole Wheat Spaghetti with Octopus

Basic Recipe for Whole Wheat Pasta

To make 1 lb 2 oz (500 g) pasta

3 cups (350 g) whole wheat flour
3 medium-sized eggs
2 egg yolks
1/4 tsp coarse salt

(If you are going to mill the wheat yourself, grind it quite finely.) Place the flour on a work surface and make a well in the middle. Place the eggs, egg yolks, and the salt in the well and stir with a fork. Then work the flour in starting from the outside. If the dough will not absorb any more flour gradually add 4–6 tablespoons of water. (Only work liquid in spoonful by spoonful. Home milled flour will absorb more liquid than commercially produced varieties.) The dough should be smooth.
Wrap the dough in foil and leave for at least 60 minutes in the refrigerator. According to what sort of pasta is required either roll the dough out thinly in portions on a surface which has been sprinkled with flour or process further with a pasta machine.
The cooking time for pasta is roughly between 6–9 minutes.

Basic Recipe for Buckwheat Pasta

To make about 1 lb 5 oz (600 g) pasta

1 1/4 cups (300 g) buckwheat
1 1/8 cups (200 g) wheat
3 eggs
1/2 tsp coarse salt
1 Tbs olive oil

Mill the buckwheat and wheat finely. Mix the two flour varieties and with the eggs, salt, oil, and 3–5 tablespoons of water knead into a dough. Roll the dough out thinly on a surface which has been sprinkled with flour and cut into short pieces the width of a finger with a sharp knife.
Leave the pasta to stand for 15 minutes and then cook until "al dente" in salted water for about 10 minutes.

Whole Wheat Ravioli with Eggplant and Goat's Cheese Filling

(Illustration right hand page)

8 oz (250 g) eggplant
Coarse salt
1 lb 2 oz (500 g) whole wheat pasta dough as in basic recipe (see left)
4 Tbs olive oil
3 1/2 oz (100 g) coarsely chopped walnuts
3 1/2 oz (100 g) Parmesan
7 oz (200 g) goat's curd cheese
1 Tbs finely chopped basil
2 Tbs finely chopped parsley
3 egg yolks
Tomato sauce (see recipe for Buckwheat Noodles with Beans)
2 Tbs butter
2 1/2 oz (60 g) freshly grated Parmesan

Dice the eggplant, sprinkle with salt, and leave for 60 minutes so that the bitter juices can drain away. Roll the dough out into large rectangular sheets on a surface which has been thoroughly sprinkled with flour. Place between paper towels which have been sprinkled with flour until needed again.
Rinse the eggplant and press thoroughly. Heat the olive oil, fry the eggplant cubes thoroughly in it and leave to drain on paper towels.
Then mix together with the nuts, Parmesan, goat's cheese, herbs, and egg yolks.
Place a sheet of pasta on the flour-sprinkled work surface and with a teaspoon place the eggplant and goat's cheese mixture on it at intervals of about about 1 1/4 inch (3 cm). Brush the dough around the filling with water using a pastry brush. Cover with a second sheet of pasta. Using your fingers press the dough down around the filling. Using a pastry wheel cut out rectangular or square ravioli. Cook the ravioli in boiling salted water for about 15–20 minutes. Heat the tomato sauce and stir in the butter. Cover the ravioli with the tomato sauce and Parmesan and serve.

Whole Wheat Lasagna with Ceps and Pesto

Whole Wheat Spaghetti with Octopus

(Illustration above left)

3 garlic cloves
2 Tbs olive oil
2 anchovy fillets
14 oz (400 g) small ready-prepared octopuses
1/2 cup (100 ml) white wine
14 oz (400 g) tomatoes
1 small red pepperoni
1 Tbs finely chopped parsley
1 Tbs finely chopped basil
Coarse salt
10 black olives
14 oz (400 g) whole wheat spaghetti

Chop the garlic cloves and braise lightly in the olive oil. Chop the anchovy fillets finely and place in the oil with the octopuses, stir and add the white wine. Reduce over a high heat.
Blanch the tomatoes, skin them, and cut them into pieces, also cutting the pepperoni into thin strips. Add to the octopuses and leave to simmer for 30 minutes. Add the parsley, basil, and olives and season to taste with salt. Cook the spaghetti until it is "al dente", drain and mix in the skillet with the sauce. Serve on preheated plates.

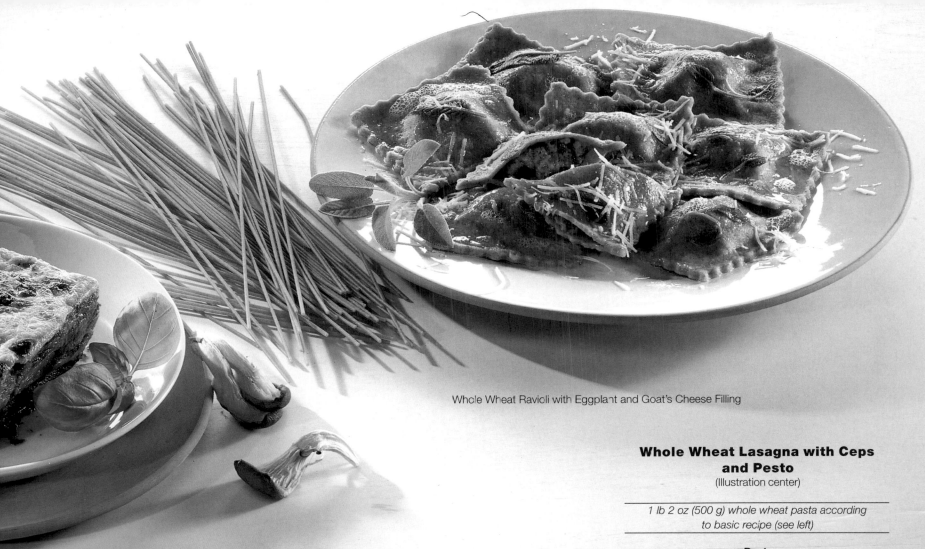

Whole Wheat Ravioli with Eggplant and Goat's Cheese Filling

Whole Wheat Lasagna with Ceps and Pesto

(Illustration center)

1 lb 2 oz (500 g) whole wheat pasta according to basic recipe (see left)

Pesto
1 bunch basil
2 garlic cloves
2 oz(50 g) pine nuts
2 oz (50 g) Parmesan
3 Tbs olive oil
1 lb 2 oz (500 g) mushrooms or oyster mushrooms
1/3 cup (80 g) butter
1 Tbs olive oil
1 garlic clove
1 1/2 oz (40 g) soaked ceps
1 1/4 cups (250 ml) milk
1/2 cup (50 g) whole wheat flour
3 1/2 oz (100 g) Parmesan
Coarse salt, nutmeg
2 Tbs (30 g) butter in flakes

Make sheets of lasagna from the dough and cook these in batches in plenty of salted water for 8 minutes. Remove from the water and set aside until needed. To make the pesto pound all the ingredients into a smooth, homogeneous paste and put to one side. Clean the fresh mushrooms and cut into slices. Heat 2 tablespoons of butter and the olive oil. Press the garlic and place in the fat with the mushrooms. Brown for about 5 minutes over a high heat. Then add the ceps and the strained soaking water. Reduce the liquid by half. Remove from the stove and stir in the pesto. To make a béchamel sauce melt the rest of the butter and stir in the flour. Add the milk gradually and continue to stir until a smooth sauce results. Add half the Parmesan. Season the sauce with salt and nutmeg. Grease an ovenproof dish with butter and in it layer alternately the lasagna, mushroom mixture, and béchamel sauce – finishing with 8 tablespoons of béchamel sauce. Sprinkle with the remaining Parmesan and the flakes of butter. Preheat the oven to 400 °F (200 °C). Cook and brown lightly for about 40 minutes.

Whole Wheat Tagliatelle with Broccoli

2 cups (500 g) whole wheat pasta dough according to basic recipe (see left)
1 lb 2 oz (500 g) broccoli
Coarse salt
3 Tbs olive oil
2 white onions
1 garlic clove
1 small red pepperoni
1 lb 2 oz (500 g) whole wheat tagliatelle
2 oz (50 g) freshly grated Pecorino

Roll the dough out into large sheets 12 inches by 12 inches (30 cm by 30 cm) and cut into wide strips. Place on a cloth which has been sprinkled with flour until needed again and cover. Cut off the broccoli stalks, peel and cut into small pieces; break up the florets and put to one side.
Bring 15 cups (3 l) salted water to the boil in a saucepan. Firstly boil the stalks for 5 minutes, then add the florets for 3 minutes.
In the meantime heat the oil in a skillet. Chop the onions and garlic finely and cook until transparent in the oil. Remove the seeds from the pepperoni and cut into rings. Remove the broccoli from the water and place in the skillet with the pepperoni.
Cook the tagliatelle in the broccoli water until it is "al dente," drain and mix in the skillet with the vegetables. Serve the Pecorino separately.

Buckwheat Noodles with Beans

7 oz (200 g) borlotti beans
1 lb 5 oz (600 g) buckwheat pasta dough according to basic recipe (see left)
4 ripe tomatoes
1 Tbs olive oil
4 tsp butter
1 small white onion
1 garlic clove
1/2 cup (100 ml) white wine
1 Tbs granules vegetable stock
Coarse salt, black pepper
Cayenne pepper
2 1/2 oz (70 g) freshly grated Pecorino

Soak the beans overnight in water, then drain and rinse. Cook in unsalted water for 60–90 minutes and drain. Roll the buckwheat pasta dough out in sheets 8 inches by 3 inches (20 cm by 8 cm) and cutting from the shorter side make noodles which are 3/4 inch (2 cm) across. Place on a cloth which has been sprinkled with flour until needed again and cover.
Blanch the tomatoes, skin, remove the seeds, and dice. Heat the olive oil and butter in a skillet. Chop the onions and garlic up finely and braise lightly. Add the tomato cubes and braise briefly. Add the wine.
Add the vegetable stock and beans and leave everything to simmer for 15 minutes. Season to taste with salt, pepper, and a pinch of cayenne pepper. Cook the noodles until they are "al dente" and mix with the sauce in the skillet. Serve the Pecorino separately.

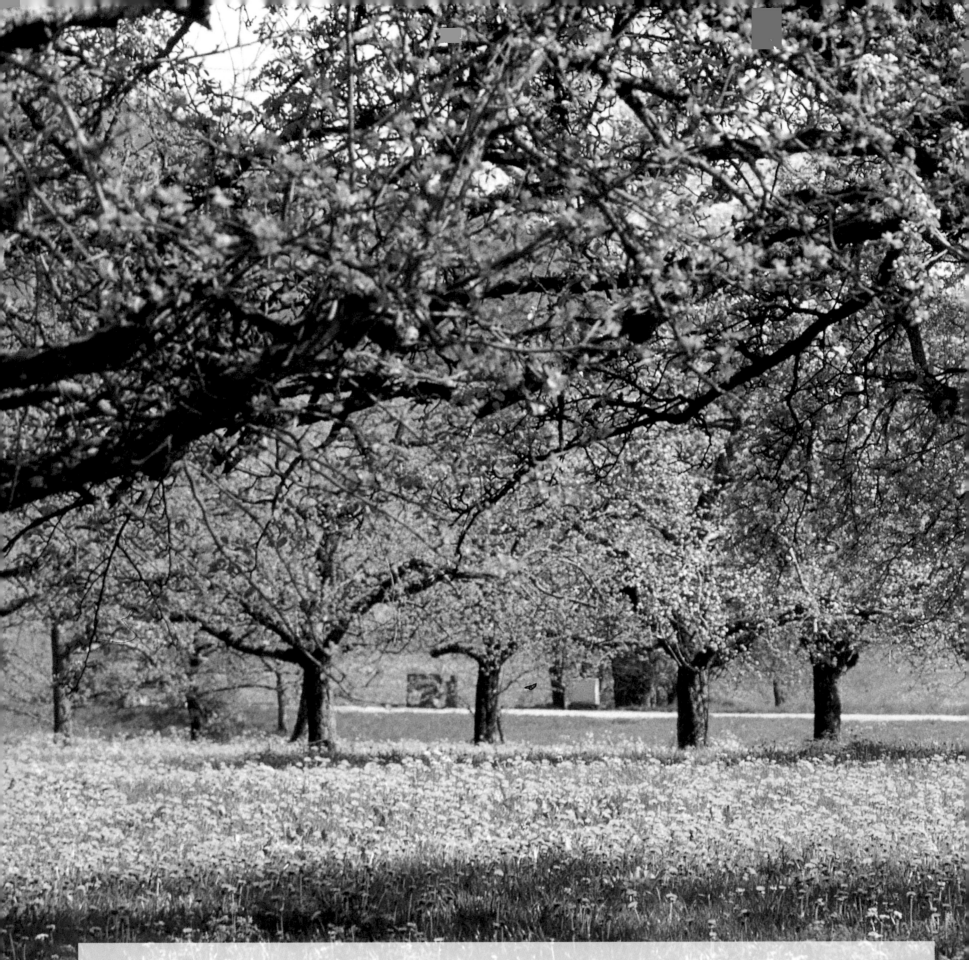

Fruit

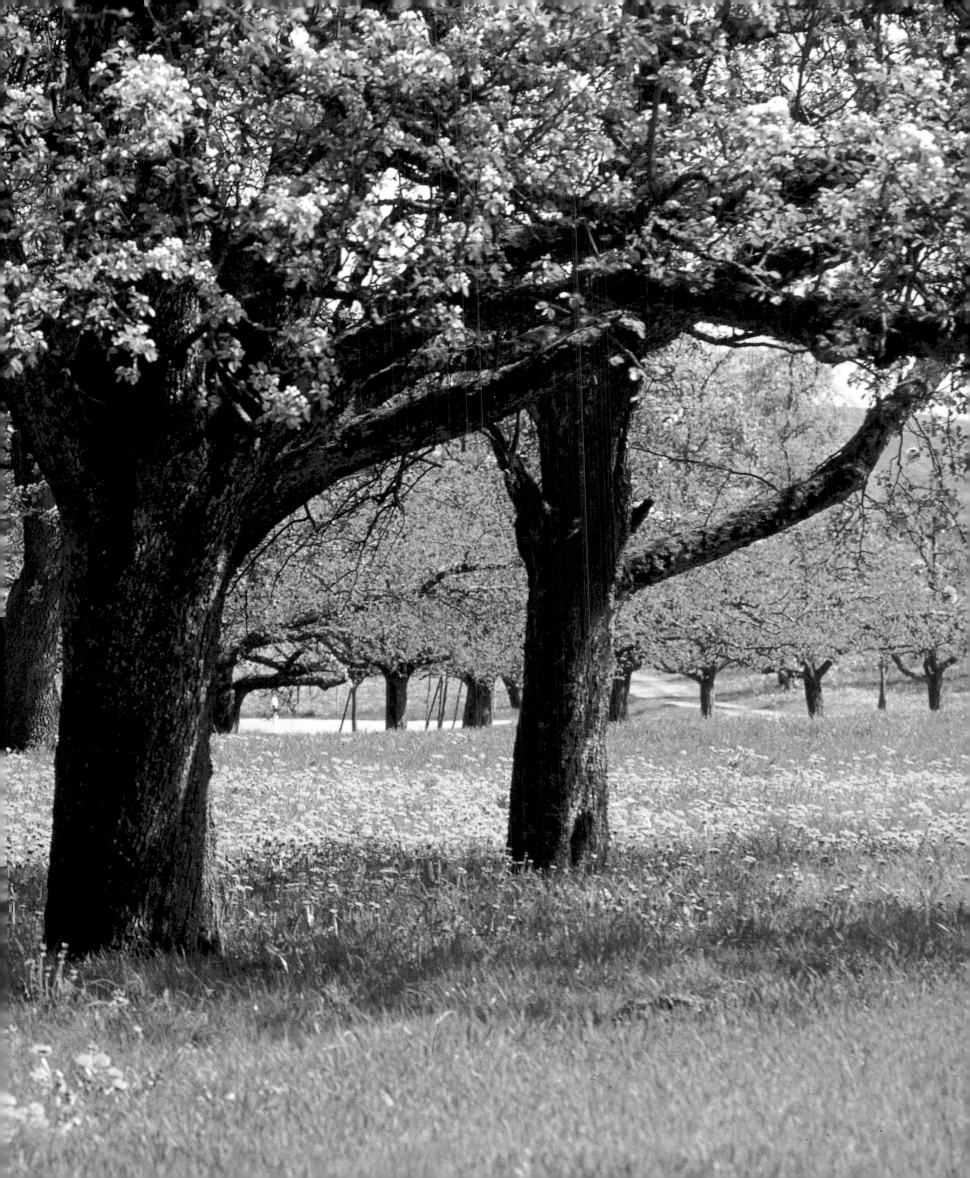

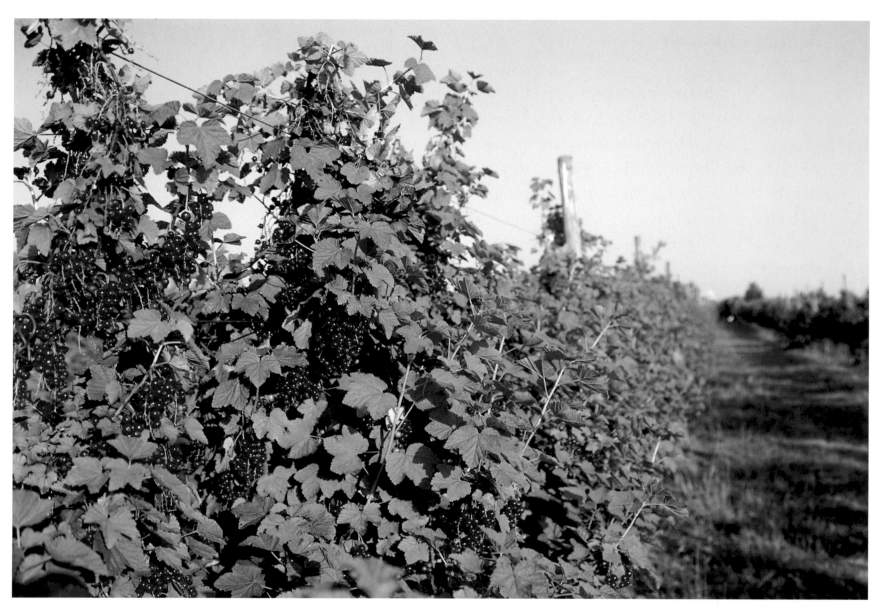

The taste of deliciously bitter-sweet red currants is an
unforgettable experience.

Previous double page: Enchanting apple blossom in an
old, natural orchard on the shores of Lake Constance.

There is something heavenly about fruit. Its appearance, its richness of color and shape alone arouse a feeling of delight and pleasure. It is not by chance that it is considered to be the food of the gods among all cultures. It symbolizes love and seduction, beauty and wisdom.

In the last few decades the range of fruit has increased greatly, and nearly all the popular types of fruit are available all year round. Even many exotic fruits, that we were not familiar with a few years ago, have now become a common sight in stores and on markets. At the same time, consumers have become used to fruit which is externally perfect and uniform in size, something that is guaranteed by laws defining grades of fruit. And to make their choice easier fruit-growing is concentrated on a few varieties. The range of fruit, therefore, gives the impression that a large variety is available, which is no longer the case. Throughout the world fruit is now produced in monocultures which destroy the natural balance – resulting in swarms of insects and tree diseases. So, in order to obtain outwardly perfect fruit geared to market requirements, often up to 20 chemicals are used. You certainly have to be aware of the fact that conventionally-grown fruit contains more chemical residue than vitamins.

Producing organic fruit requires some expense. The fruit farmers firstly have to recreate a natural balance by growing many types and varieties as well as providing space for trees and bushes for beneficial insects. Only a combination of different natural factors guarantees healthy fruit. Harvested when it is ripe, it really does have heavenly qualities and is full of vitamins and minerals, including rare trace elements. Fruit is easy to digest, its carbohydrates are quickly absorbed by the body, and its roughage has a beneficial effect on health. Even citrus and other exotic fruits are now grown organically. In Europe they thrive in temperate and in particular in the more southerly regions.

Pomaceous Fruit
Wild Fruits
Berries
Strawberries
Exotic Fruits
Oranges and Lemons
Melons
Pitted Fruit
Southern Pitted Fruit
Jam
Dried Fruit
Pruneaux d'Agen
Nuts
Avocados

Pomaceous Fruit

Apples, pears, and quinces form the pome family as they have a seed core with small pits. All three belong to the rose family, *Rosaceae*, which was originally indigenous to the Black and Caspian Sea areas. Apples and pears arrived in Europe about 5,000 years ago and since then countless varieties have been developed. Today there is standardization in the market, where high yields, size, and durability are the decisive factors. The Golden Delicious, originally from America, as well as its red variety, the Canadian Summer Red, the internationally-cultivated Granny Smith, and the Starking, grown in many countries, have become dominant together with others. Fortunately, there is a growing interest among producers and consumers in old, almost forgotten varieties. Their advantage is that they are particularly suitable for regional, climatic, and soil conditions and they can develop their own characteristic flavor there. So it is not rare today to find good, organic tree nurseries offering 200 varieties of apple, 80 of pear, and at least half a dozen of quince, a selection of which is given here. Apples and pears are by nature real health foods. This, though, is only the case if they are not sprayed with pesticides and insecticides when they are in blossom, growing, and ripening and if their harvest times are not preprogrammed through the use of hormones. For only then can you eat them unpeeled which is important as most of the vital elements are in and under the skin: provitamin A, B vitamins, vitamin C, many rare trace elements and minerals, tannin, and pectin. Pectin is mainly found in apple skins, as well as in considerable quantities in quinces, and is well-known as a natural gelling agent. It acts against diarrhea, but above all it has a function of cleaning the intestine. It even absorbs carcinogenic substances in the intestine and eliminates cholesterol.

It is of the utmost importance for the development of vital elements that the fruit is picked ripe as the optimum vitamin content is only acquired during the ripening process on the tree. Fruit that is picked unripe for reasons of transportation or so that it will keep longer has a clearly lower vitamin content, as well as much less flavor. Ripe pears, which contain several B vitamins, stimulate growth and improve the nervous system. With their high carbohydrate content, but small amount of fruit acids compared with apples, pears are sweeter in taste and can be used in many recipes without additional sugar. Their thickened juice can even be used as a sweetener.

Quinces spread not only to the Near East, but also to the Mediterranean region. The pleasantly fresh smelling, bright yellow fruit was popular with the ancient Greeks, who called it the "apple of Cydonia" after the town in Crete. The Greeks passed on their liking to the Romans. The undemanding, sun-loving and self-fertile tree even spread to the Iberian Peninsula. In the north, Charlemagne did much to help the spread of the quince but its popularity remained patchy, becoming widely used in England but hardly at all in Germany. In hot countries, soft-skinned fruits are grown which you can simply bite into, but generally quinces have hard skins and can only be eaten cooked. Because of their excellent aroma they were used in all kinds of ways as fragrances and flavorings, for example in liqueurs and wines, or as pomanders in rooms and cupboards. However, the fruits, which have a very high pectin content, are ideal for compote, jam, jelly, and purée.

Background: Only unsprayed apples like these are really rich in vital and protective substances.

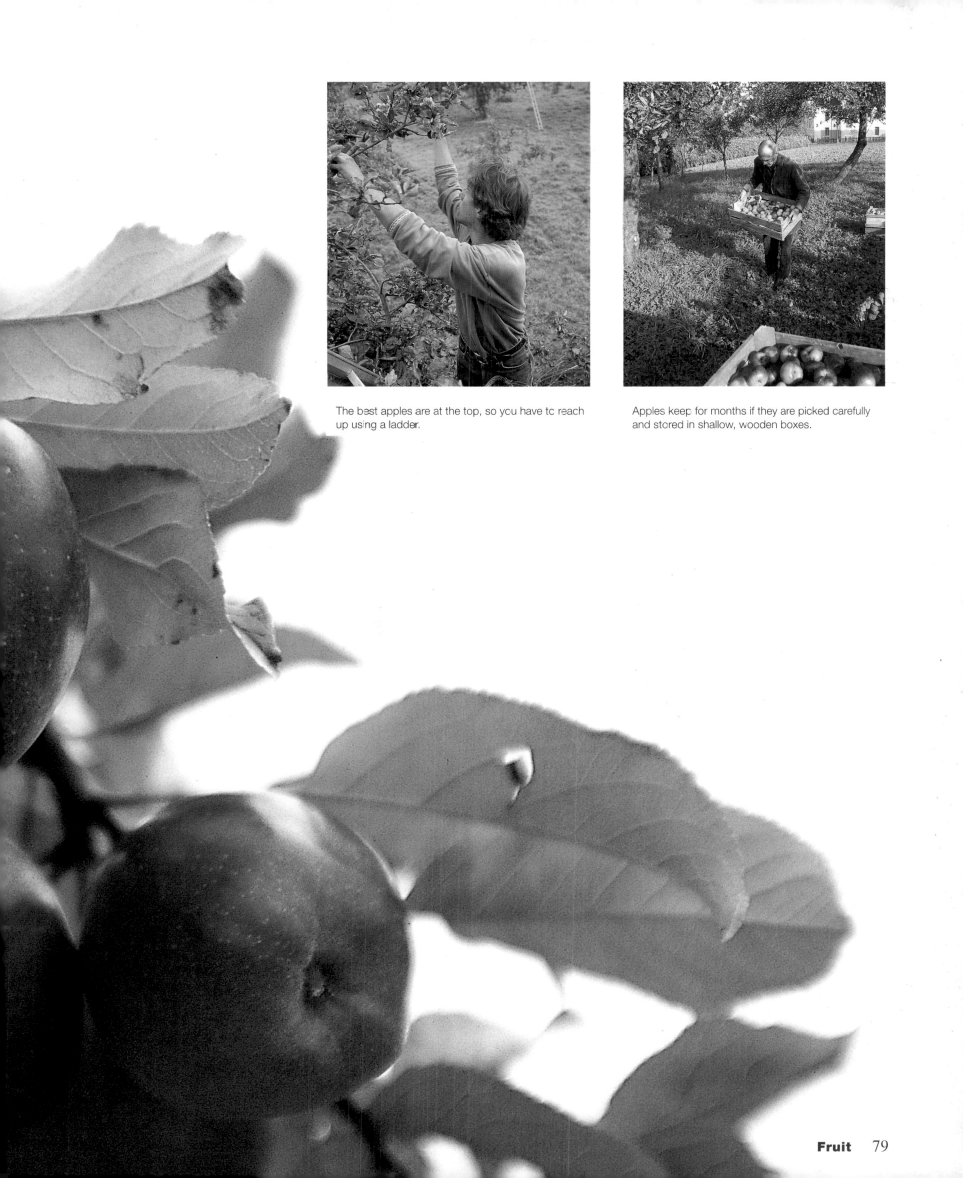

The best apples are at the top, so you have to reach up using a ladder.

Apples keep for months if they are picked carefully and stored in shallow, wooden boxes.

Eating Apples

 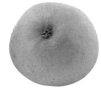

Tumanga
Cultivated from Cox's Orange Pippin crossed with Belle de Nordhausen. A medium-sized, delicate, sweet-and-sour cooking apple with a discreet flavor; keeps until March; soft, with russet speckles, greeny-yellow to slightly reddish skin

 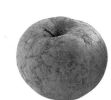

Baumann's Reinette
Also known as Reinette de Bollviller. Pleasantly mild but not very intense flavor, firm, tough skin; varies greatly in size; as it becomes riper it becomes a more intense or dark red

Belle de Boskoop
Produces large, rather irregular fruit with rough, greeny-yellow skin; refreshingly sharp in taste; particularly suitable for cooking and baking

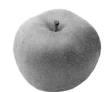

Canada Reinette
Large to very large fruit; at first yellowy-green, later reddish; sometimes a rough skin; aromatic flavor with a discreet sharpness; keeps until April, but does not look so attractive, crunchy when young

Cox's Orange Pippin
Excellent eating apple with outstanding flavor, firm texture, and harmonious sharpness; slightly rough, greeny-yellow skin with reddy-brown marbled cheek; from end of September; keeps well

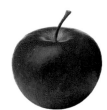

Elstar
Modern cross from Golden Delicious and Ingrid Marie; medium-sized, slightly spotted eating apple with beautiful red cheek; juicy, pleasantly sweet flavor, to be consumed fresh

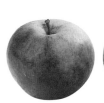

Erwin Baur
Keeps through to January or February, medium to large, yellow apple with red streaks grown high up; firm but not hard skin; fine, acidic flavor; to be consumed and used fresh

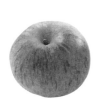

Baron de Berlepsch
Excellent tasting eating apple with golden yellow skin, with orange to reddy-brown cheek, crunchy and juicy; from mid-September, later harvest is recommended if it is to be stored

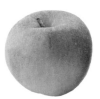

Geheimrat Breuhahn
Late, tapering eating apple grown high up; green to yellow with red watery streaks on cheek; smooth, medium-firm skin; sweet with a delicate sharpness; keeps through February or March

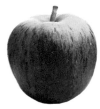

Golden Delicious
Tried and tested variety in warm growing regions; greeny-yellow color, often with dark green or even brownish spots; delicate sweetness when ripe

King of Pippins
Also known as Reine des Reinettes, good eating apple grown widely in France, with beautiful yellow ground and red to dark red streaks; harvested from mid-August in the south

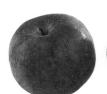

Idared
Delicious eating apple with pleasant sharpness, which often acquires a beautiful dark red color when ripening; does not store well

Jonagold
Beautiful yellow apple, with orange-red ripples on the sunny side. Very good, tangy, aromatic flavor; early-ripening and keeps amazingly well

 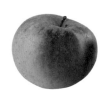

Juno
From an Ontario crossed with London Pepping; harmoniously combines elements of their flavors: aromatic acidity and pleasant sweetness; very late, large, flat apple; keeps well through March or April

Kaiser Wilhelm
Very strong growing tree with at first yellowy-green, then golden yellow fruit with red streaks; often large, firm, very juicy apples with a rather discreet flavor; keeps well

Lessang's Calville
Greeny-yellow, slightly five-ribbed, very late, fine eating apple that grows high up; combines delicate sweetness with elegant sharpness; firm skin; crop may need thinning.

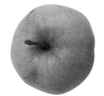

Crispin
Predominantly green skin with some yellow shading and slightly red cheek; fine cell texture and pleasant sweetness

Ontario
Very large, flat, angular apple with smooth yellow skin, rippled on the sunny side; fresh sharpness, very juicy, neutral flavor; keeps very well, versatile

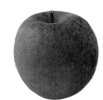

Red Belle de Boskoop
Closely related to the Belle de Boskoop (see left-hand page) and just as strong tasting; orange-red to red fruit, with distinctive sharp flavor; keeps until April if stored in humid conditions

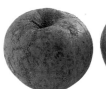

Rubinette (Rafzubin)
Relatively late ripening, very tasty and palatable eating apple; browny-red, slightly rough skin, firm flesh; keeps through early March

Schweizer Orange
Cross between Cox's Orange Pippin and Ontario, which combines a fine, sweet flavor with a delicate acidity and keeps through to April; medium to large fruit with smooth, moderately firm, greeny-yellow to reddy-orange marbled skin

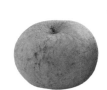

Wober's Rambour
Very old variety with large, wide, robust trees for orchards; wide spherical fruit with distinctive, tasty, moderately sweet-and-sour flavor; from February increasingly floury

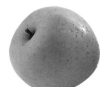

Von Zuccalmaglio's Renette
Late, lemon yellow variety with slightly red cheek, and flavor that is full of character; must be thinned out to produce good fruit; keeps through mid-March

Dessert Pears

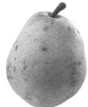 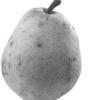

Buerré Alexander Lucas
Large, yellow, often spotted, juicy late pear, which is red on the sunny side and likes warmth; fine, tangy flavor, pleasant sweetness; can be kept through April if harvested late

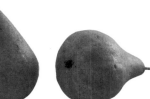 

Calebasse Bosc
Russet, cinnamon-colored, slightly rough skin; good texture with delicate nutmeg flavor; easy to digest, but only keeps for a limited time

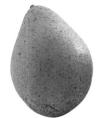

Comte de Paris
Large, greeny-yellow, speckled, juicy winter pear with a pleasant flavor; keeps in the medium-term

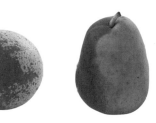

Winter Orange
Firm-skinned, red-cheeked, delicious winter pear with trout-like speckling (known as the Winter Trout in Germany), keeps very well through to March or April; firm, juicy sweet flesh

Quince

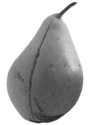 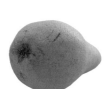

Vicar of Winkfield
Large, bottle-shaped winter pear; greeny-yellow when ripe, tough skin; peel before eating; juicy, slightly sweet flesh; typical flavor with delicate sharpness. Eat from December through March

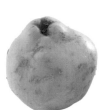

Bereczki
Large, pear-shaped, rich yellow, very sweet fruit; can only be eaten cooked; very good cooking properties and beautiful pink color when a jelly or purée

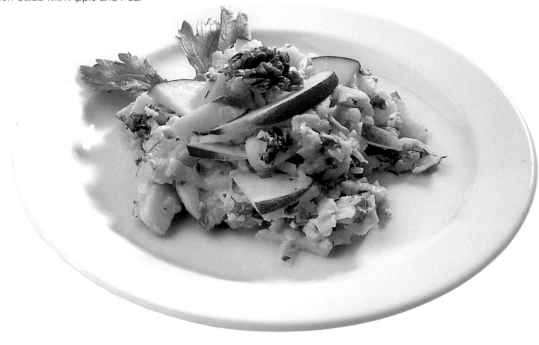

Recipes with Pomaceous Fruit

Waldorf Salad with Apple and Pear
(Illustration right)

1 head celery
Juice of 1 lemon
1 apple
1 pear
2 Tbs walnuts
$^1/_2$ bunch flat leafed parsley
1 Tbs honey
Grated zest of $^1/_2$ a lemon
$^2/_5$ cup (80 ml) heavy cream

Finely chop the celery and immediately squeeze lemon juice over it to stop it discoloring. Chop the apple and pear into slices or small pieces and add to the celery. Roughly chop the walnuts and very finely chop the parsley, add to the fruit and celery mixture along with the honey, lemon zest, and cream. Mix well and serve garnished.

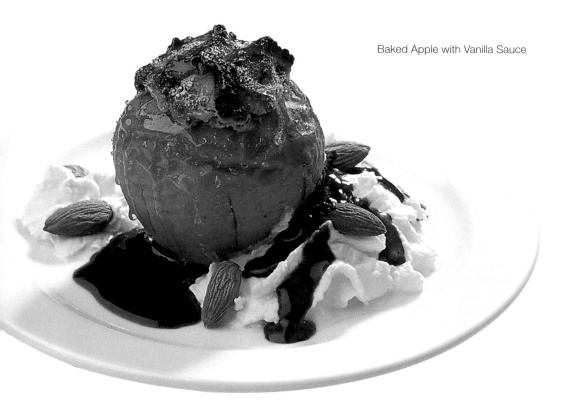

Baked Apple with Vanilla Sauce

Baked Apple with Vanilla Sauce
(Illustration left)

4 medium-sized Boskoops or other tart apples
$3^1/_2$ oz (100 g) farmer's cheese
$^1/_3$ cup (60 ml) cream
1 Tbs cinnamon
1 tsp vanilla extract
2 Tbs raisins or currants
Grated zest of $^1/_2$ a lemon and $^1/_2$ an orange
1 Tbs honey
2 Tbs chopped walnuts
$2^1/_2$ cups (500 ml) white wine or apple juice

Core the apples and run a sharp knife around their middles so they can expand without exploding.
Mix all the ingredients together, except for the wine or juice. Fill the apples with the cheese mixture.
Pour the wine into an ovenproof dish so it comes to almost $^3/_8$ inch (1 cm) high and place the apples in the dish.
Bake in the oven at 400 °F (200 °C) for about 20 minutes.

Vanilla Sauce
$1^3/_4$ cups (350 ml) cream
1 vanilla bean
2 Tbs ground rice
Honey

Mix the cream with $^3/_4$ cup (150 ml) of water and bring to the boil with the vanilla bean. Scrape out the vanilla pulp and discard the bean. Thicken the liquid with the ground rice and add honey to taste.
Tip: The baked apples can also be filled with a mixture of 3 ounces (80 g) marzipan, 1 tablespoon of raisins soaked in rum, and 2 tablespoons of almond pieces.

Cinnamon-flavored Pears with
Chocolate Mousse

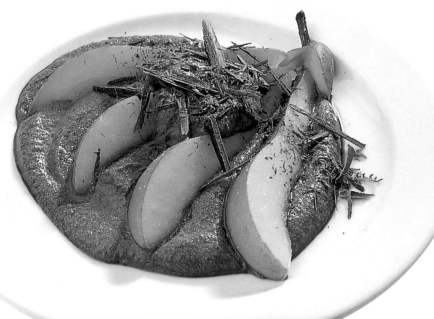

Cinnamon-flavored Pears with Chocolate Mousse

(Illustration below left)

Serves 2
2 pears
Juice of 1 lemon
1 Tbs cinnamon
$^3/_4$ cup (150 ml) heavy cream
3 oz (80 g) Mascarpone
1 Tbs honey
3 tsp cocoa or carob
2 Tbs finely ground roasted almonds

Halve and core the pears, squeeze some lemon juice over them. Mix the rest of the lemon juice with the cinnamon in 2$^1/_2$ cups (500 ml) of water and stew the pears in it until just soft.
Beat the cream with the Mascarpone, honey, and cocoa until stiff, then fold in the almonds.
Drain the pears, cut in a fan-shape and arrange on the chocolate mousse. Decorate with grated chocolate according to taste.

Apple and Orange Chutney

(Illustration right)

2 tart apples
2 oranges
2 medium-sized onions
1 tsp coarse salt
2 tsp finely grated ginger
2 Tbs grated orange zest
1 tsp grated lemon zest
Juice of 1 orange
2 Tbs raisins
1 Tbs honey

Peel the apples and oranges and then core the apples. Chop the apples, oranges, and onions into small pieces. Put all the ingredients in a saucepan, cover and cook on a low heat until a purée.
Serve with salad or poultry.
The purée will keep in the refrigerator for about 1 week in a jar with a screw lid.

Pears with Blue Cheese Cream

(Illustration right)

4 ripe pears
1 tsp lemon juice
5 oz (150 g) not too ripe blue cheese
3$^1/_2$ oz (100 g) cheese made from sour milk
1 Tbs heavy cream
Pinch of cayenne pepper
4 celery leaves

Halve and hollow out the pears, then rub the cut sides with lemon juice so that they do not discolor.
Beat the two cheeses together, then fold the cream into the cheese mixture and season with cayenne pepper.
Arrange the pear halves on the celery leaves and pipe the cheese and cream mixture onto the fruit using a piping bag.

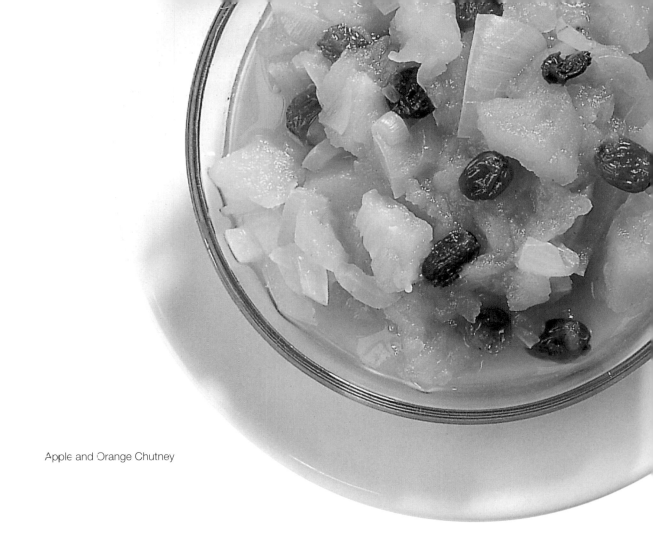

Apple and Orange Chutney

Pears with Blue Cheese Cream

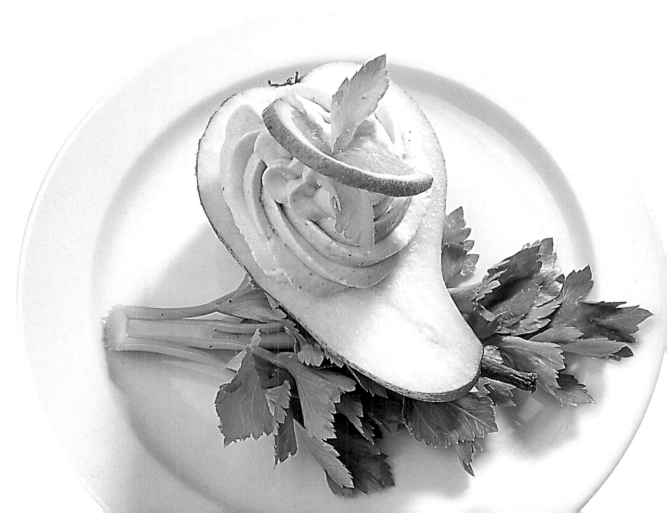

Wild Fruits

Nature always provides a wealth of wild fruits. You should only look for wild fruits in places where meadows and woods are still relatively untouched, in other words not at the side of busy roads, near factories, or conventionally-treated areas of arable land. Radiation exposure following the accident at Chernobyl has now dropped so much that you no longer need to worry about picking fruit.

Every plant prefers a particular location. Many wild plants are found at the edge of woods and in hedgerows, in meadows and in sparse forests. When picking fruit you should take care not to damage the plants or even pull them out. If you come across a solitary bush or tree you should not strip it bare but leave some of the fruit for the birds and other animals. An old rule says that you should not pick up fruit that falls off through clumsiness since it could be damaged and so go bad quicker.

The fruits ripen earlier or later depending on the climatic zone – this also applies to different altitudes. Wild strawberries, which ripen in late spring, are the earliest, while raspberries, wild cherries, and blueberries mark the start of summer. In August nature's supply of fruit increases considerably, as mossberries, rowanberries, elderberries, cranberries, and blackberries arrive. The fall brings ripe sea buckthorn, red and white hawthorn berries, medlars, berberis, and rose hips. Sloes are late arrivals, benefiting from the first frost if they are not in the south, where they are considerably sweeter.

In general, wild fruits should only be picked when they are fully ripe, as only then do they contain the maximum amount of vitamins and minerals. You should only pick what you can eat or use immediately. Wild fruits, especially berries, usually only keep for a short time, and should be put in the refrigerator as soon as you get home. Berries that can be eaten raw freeze very well. Before being used they should be allowed to thaw slowly at room temperature.

Wild fruits keep their intense and often original flavors best when they are made into jam or jelly. The tangy and sharp varieties, which cannot be eaten raw, often improve when they are mixed with apples or pears.

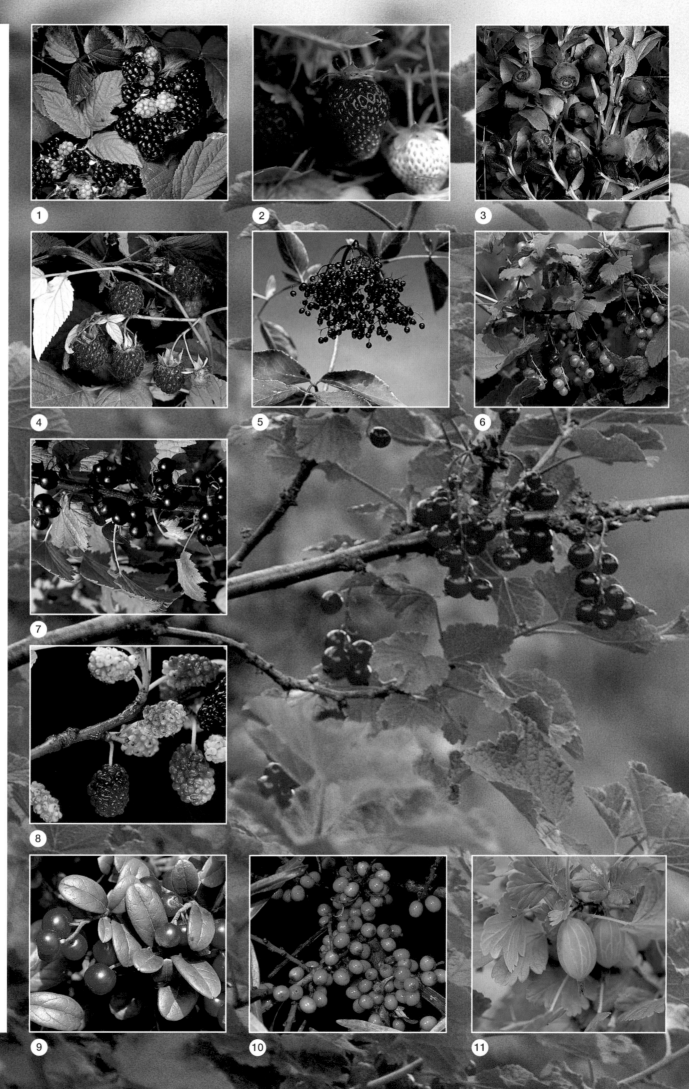

1

2

3

4

5

6

7

8

9

10

11

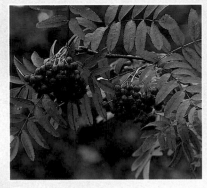

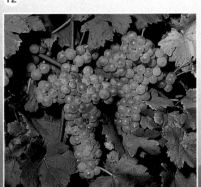

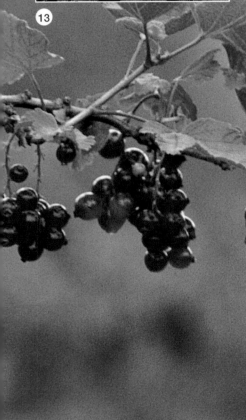

Berries

Blackberries

Common, thorny, wild plants; most cultivated species no longer have thorns, produce more regular crops and larger, juicier fruit which is dark red to ink black in color. Whether fresh or cooked, as jelly or sorbet, blackberries are full of flavor and high in provitamin A and iron. Blackberry and raspberry leaves can be used for herbal teas.

Strawberries

Grown throughout the world in a huge number of varieties. Also wild producing tiny but very aromatic fruit. Exquisite when eaten fresh, but also in numerous recipes (see also pp. 90–91).

Blueberries

As members of the heather family, they love acid soil and grow in spruce and pine woods, often in mountainous regions. The coloring myrtillin, to which a hematinic effect is attributed, is found in their small blue, frosty berries. The fruits, which are laborious to pick, contain a multitude of substances that are beneficial for the intestine and eyes in particular. They are a pleasure eaten fresh with milk. Popular as juice, sorbet, filling for tarts or cakes, as jam and liqueur.

Raspberries

Common throughout the northern hemisphere; wild raspberries also available. Otherwise numerous varieties grown; yellow varieties only in gardens. When ripe they easily come away from their cone-shaped receptacle. Very healthy due to minerals and stimulating acids. Raspberries have an exquisite flavor, and should be consumed or used as quickly as possible as they squash easily; best raw or as a cold sauce; freeze well.

Elderberries

The tall bush, which is often wild and found throughout Europe and Asia, produces umbels with black-purple berries; they are also cultivated now. When unripe the berries are considered to be poisonous, but can certainly be eaten raw if fully ripe, although they are usually cooked and used in iced sweet soup, jelly, juice, wine and liqueur recipes. The flower heads make good sorbet, can be fried or used in herbal tea.

Red and White Currants

Native to more northerly regions where their succinct sharpness is appreciated. High in vitamin C. White varieties are milder and sweeter. The flavorsome berries can be used fresh in fruit salads, otherwise for jams and compotes.

Black Currants

Closely related to the red and white varieties, but also found in more southerly regions. One of their outstanding features is their higher mineral and vitamin C content which makes their juice a real health tonic. Because of the very high vitamin C content the berries oxidize quickly. They should, therefore, be immediately eaten, used, or frozen, for which they are best suited. They have a distinct aromatic flavor; are delicious raw when ripe and make excellent sorbets as well as outstanding jellies, jams, and liqueurs.

Jostaberries

These smooth, black berries are a 20 year old German variety produced from black currants and gooseberries. They grow in pairs on bushes, on thornless shoots, and have a mild gooseberry flavor with a slight hint of cassis. They make excellent jam.

Loganberries

The result of a chance cross between the raspberry and blackberry in the garden of Judge Logan, in California in 1881, then spread quickly and became popular in England too. The fruits are larger and longer than raspberries; wine-red in color when ripe. Striking acidity, slightly sharp, and very intense flavor. Very juicy, keep firm when cooked and therefore excellent for jams. Harvest in August.

Mulberries

If strictly speaking blackberries, raspberries, and strawberries are not berries, but collective fruits, then the very slow-growing mulberry tree belongs to a completely different category. It belongs to the same family, the *Moraceae*, as the fig. However, its fruit is similar in color and appearance to that of the blackberry. It has a delicately fruity, slightly sharp flavor, can be eaten raw, cooked to make juice or jam and can be replaced by blackberries in recipes.

Cranberries

Small berries that ripen to a bright red color; develop a tangy flavor, contain many vital substances and several acids including benzoic acid which relieves rheumatism. They belong to the heather family and thrive on heath and moorland, particularly in the most northerly European countries. They are used to make compote or jelly or with other fruit, such as apples and pears; they traditionally accompany game. Closely related to mossberries.

Sea Buckthorn

This bush or gnarled tree grows wild in many areas of the northern hemisphere, preferring damper regions and coasts. Numerous, sharp thorns protect the small orange or red berries which contain several vitamins, but are exceptionally rich in vitamin C; therefore often sold as a health juice. Their taste is best appreciated in jam or jelly with pomes.

Gooseberries

Many varieties were cultivated by the English and used in different ways, but are originally native to Asia Minor and North Africa. Ripe gooseberries can be extremely sweet. The riper they are, the richer they are in minerals and vitamin C. Red and yellow berries are exquisite raw, white-green varieties taste tangier and tarter and are only suitable for cooking.

Rowanberries

Come from the rowan, a tree or bush often found wild in Europe and the Near East, which is also planted for decoration. Small, often oval, bright orange-red berries grow on their umbels. They are extremely rich in vitamin C; they also have an antiphlogistic effect. Because they are bitter and contain tannin they are unpalatable raw, but make fine compote and jelly to accompany game, as well as cough syrup, and can be used with pomes. The Moravian rowan produces sweet berries.

Grapes

Are one of the most popular fruits and are cultivated throughout the world. A tenth of all grapes harvested are intended as dessert fruit, for which special, particularly flavorsome varieties are grown. Picked ripe, they contain not only glucose which is easy to absorb, but many minerals, vitamins, tannin, and acids which have a stimulating, cleansing, and fortifying effect on the organism. As well as being eaten on their own they are suitable for flan fillings and in salads, for juice and jelly. Grapes, even those grown organically, should always be washed in lukewarm water. Overripe grapes are available dried as raisins, currants, or light raisins; make sure they are unsulfurized, "natural"!

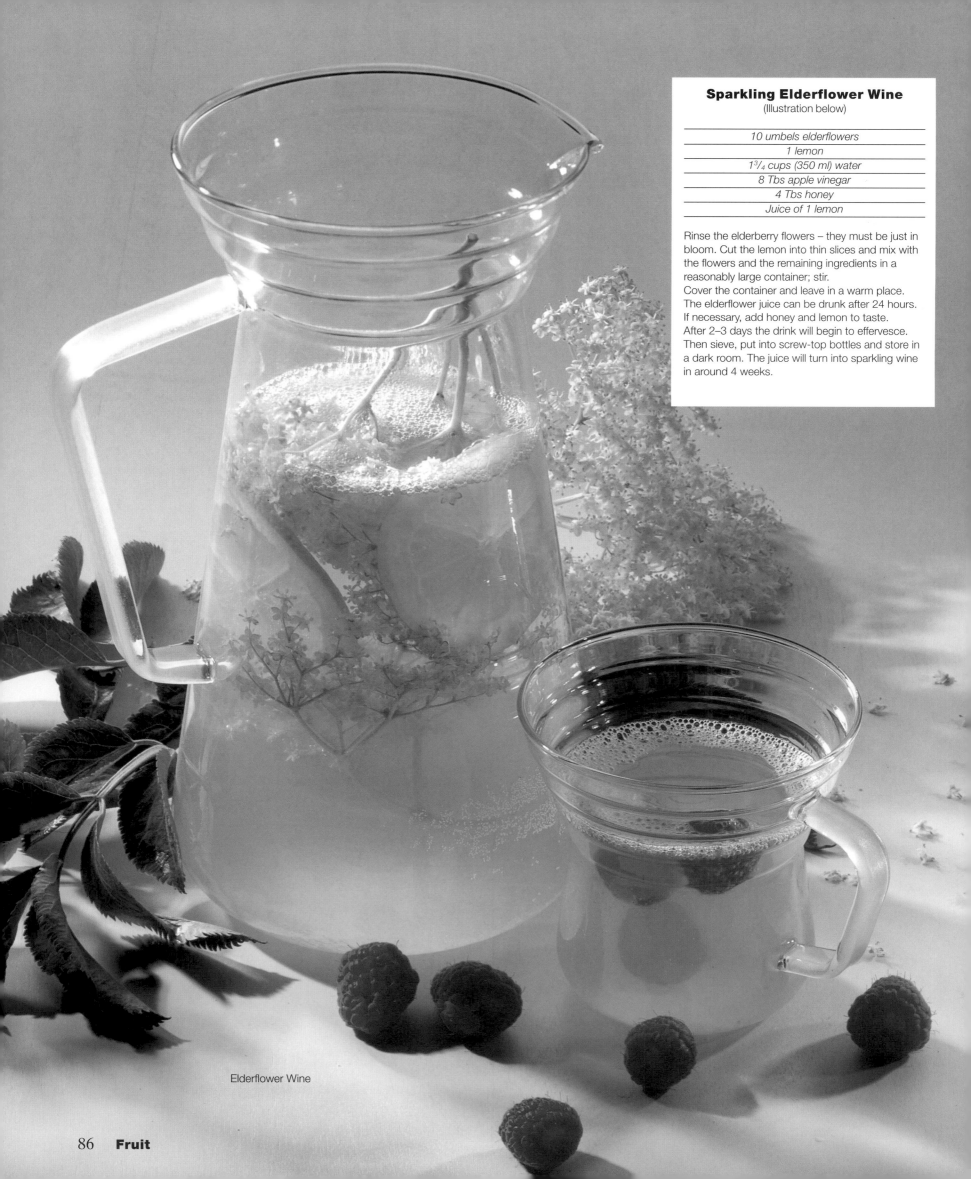

Elderflower Wine

Recipes with Berries

Millet with Raspberries

2/3 cup (125 ml) heavy cream
1 cup (200 g) millet
3 1/2 oz (100 g) raspberries
1 Tbs lemon juice
1 tsp vanilla extract
1 Tbs honey
2 Tbs roughly chopped pistachios
5 Tbs whipped cream

Mix the pouring cream with the same amount of water and cook the millet in this, adding more water if necessary; leave to cool and stir well. Purée the raspberries with the lemon juice, vanilla, and honey and fold into the millet to form a stiff cream. Put into small dishes, decorate with whipped cream and pistachios.

Red Currant Sorbet with Sparkling Wine

1lb 2oz (500 g) red currants
Honey according to taste
1 1/4 cups (250 ml) whipped cream
2 cups (400 ml) sparkling wine

Wash the red currants and remove any stalks, leaving some currants to one side for decoration.
Quickly bring the currants to the boil in a very small amount of water, press through a sieve and collect the juice (about 2 1/2 cups (500 ml)); leave to cool. Mix the honey into the red currant purée and fold in the cream. Put the mixture in a large container in the ice compartment, and every 30 minutes – four times in all – beat to prevent crystals forming. Then leave to freeze for at least 4 hours.
Using a tablespoon put scoops of the sorbet into glass dishes and pour sparkling wine over, decorate with the red currants and serve immediately.
Tip: The sparkling wine can be replaced by a mixture of red currant juice and mineral water.

Gooseberry Tart

Shortcrust pastry
2 cups (250 g) fine spelt flour
2/3 cup (150 g) cold butter in small pieces
2 Tbs honey
Grated zest of 1 lemon
Pinch of coarse salt

Filling
1 lb 12 oz (800 g) gooseberries
2 cups (400 ml) heavy cream
2/3 cup (80 g) potato flour
3 1/2 oz (100 g) honey
5 eggs
2 Tbs pomace
2 Tbs apricot jam

For the pastry, knead the ingredients together well; leave to rest in the refrigerator for 30 minutes.
Grease an 11 inch (28 cm) springform pan with the butter, line with the pastry and make a 1 inch (3 cm) high edge. Prick the base several times with a fork and bake for about 10 minutes at 350 °F (180 °C).
For the filling, wash the gooseberries. Mix the cream, potato flour, honey, eggs, and pomace with a beater. Place the gooseberries in the springform pan and spread over the pastry base.
Put the cream and egg mixture on top and bake at 350°F (180 °C) for 40 minutes, then at 300 °F (160 °C) for a further 30 minutes.
Mix the apricot jam with a little water until it is creamy and spread on the tart.

Crêpes with Blueberries and Vanilla Ice Cream

(Illustration below)

Serves 8–10

Vanilla Ice Cream
1 1/4 cups (250 ml) heavy cream
3 1/2 oz (100 g) honey
2 egg yolks
1/2 tsp vanilla extract

Crêpes
1 lb 2 oz (500 g) blueberries
4 oz (120 g) honey
1 Tbs fruit liquor
1/2 cup (100 ml) milk
1/2 cup (100 ml) light cream
2 eggs
2/3 cup (80 g) fine spelt flour
1/6 cup (40 g) butter
Pinch of coarse salt
Mint to decorate

For the ice cream, whip the cream until stiff, fold in the honey, egg yolks, and vanilla. Put the mixture into a shallow container and freeze. After 60 minutes beat and repeat twice at 30 minute intervals; leave to freeze for 3 hours.
For the crêpes, wash and drain the blueberries. Mix 2 tablespoons (30 g) of honey with the fruit liquor and pour over the berries; leave to stand.
Mix the milk, cream, eggs, flour, salt, and remaining honey into a smooth batter. Melt the butter and mix most of it into the batter. Heat up a pan and add some melted butter.
Cook the pancakes by putting enough batter for one crêpe into the pan, cover and cook on one side, then turn over and cook on the other side without a lid.
Fold each crêpe loosely into a quarter, put ice cream and blueberries around it and decorate with mint.

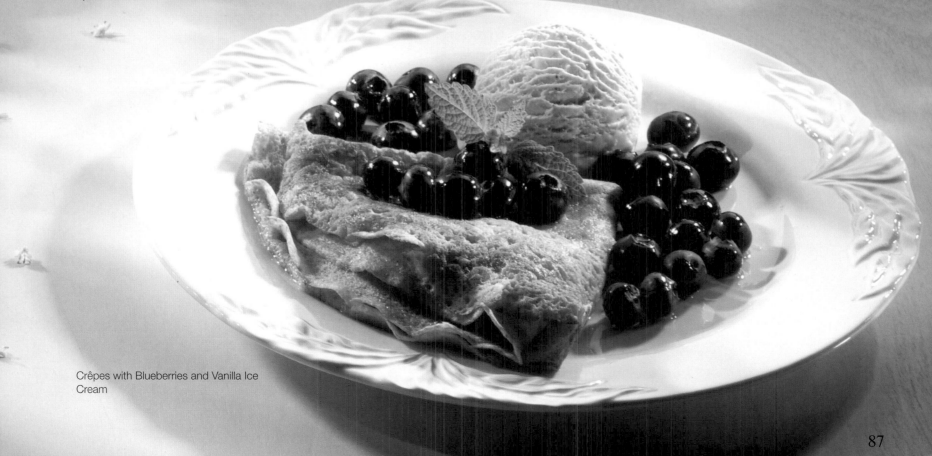

Crêpes with Blueberries and Vanilla Ice Cream

Strawberries

The small herbaceous perennial which lasts for several years and is grown industrially throughout Europe, sometimes in greenhouses, is extremely delicate and accordingly is sprayed often. What is more, in many European Union countries it is quite usual to irradiate strawberries so they will keep longer which, apart from other things, greatly reduces the fruit's vitamin content. Crops that are forced through the use of artificial fertilizers and watering have almost completely lost the real taste of strawberries – reason enough to use strawberries grown organically.

It is important in the organic cultivation of strawberries that the plant can develop in accordance with the natural cycle of the year: in spring it only grows slowly, with few leaves and forms a lot of flowers in relation to its size. In central Europe, strawberries, which are the first fruits of the season, are ready for picking between the first week in June and the first week in July.

At harvest time the small plant is under a lot of stress and is, therefore, very susceptible to disease and parasites. After the fruit has been picked the

Below: When the strawberries are in flower, freshly chopped straw is laid between the rows so that the large fruits will not be touching the ground.

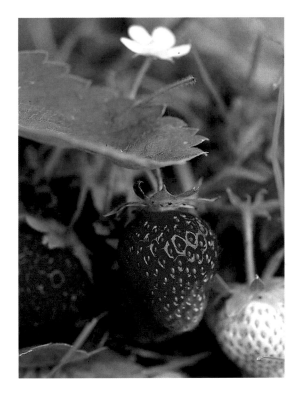

leaves grow so much that it is difficult to see the gaps between the rows. This is also the time when runners form and the plant needs fertilizing with horn meal or well composted cattle manure. Like raspberries, strawberries are grateful for any type of organic fertilizer, having originally developed in forest soil rich in humus.

After the harvest many organic farmers spray the stock with horn manure and ground horn meal three times to help the flowers form. In October

and November an organically-farmed strawberry field is bright red like Virginia creeper, a color which can also be seen in wild strawberries. The color of conventionally-grown strawberry fields is far less intense as frequent spraying of the plants against weeds and fungal diseases prevents the leaves from ripening naturally.

Weeds are, in fact, a major problem. Because they grow low and loosely, strawberry plants cannot suppress weeds. Therefore, four or five times a year hoeing and weeding has to be carried out by hand. Many organic farmers make sure that work on the plants and hoeing only take place on fruit days according to the Thun Sowing Calendar (see p. 19).

When the strawberries are in flower, in mid-May, freshly chopped straw is laid between the rows so that the large fruits will not be touching the ground and rot. The straw also keeps snails and slugs away. An experienced organic farmer always plants four or five varieties to reduce the risk of a poor yield – the yield can vary by up to 200 percent in a year. There is hardly another plant where there is such a fine line between success and failure.

Right-hand page: Organically-grown strawberries have a flavor and taste that has almost disappeared from conventionally-grown ones.

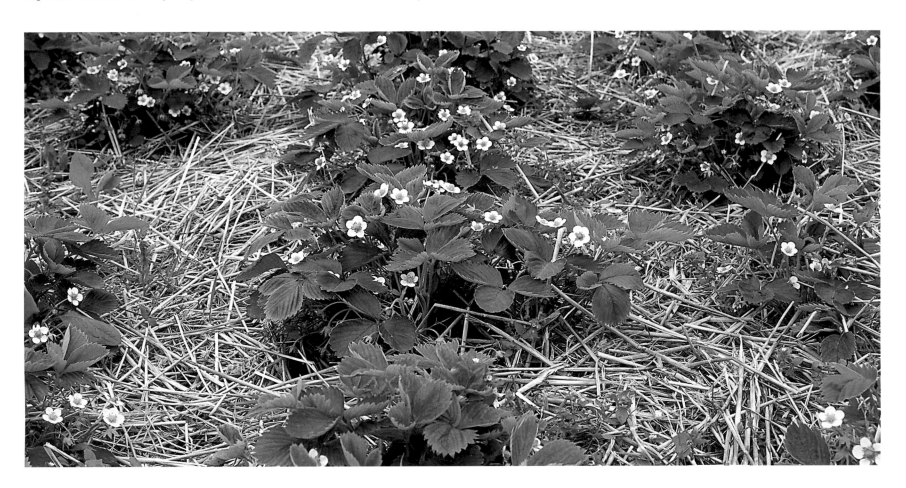

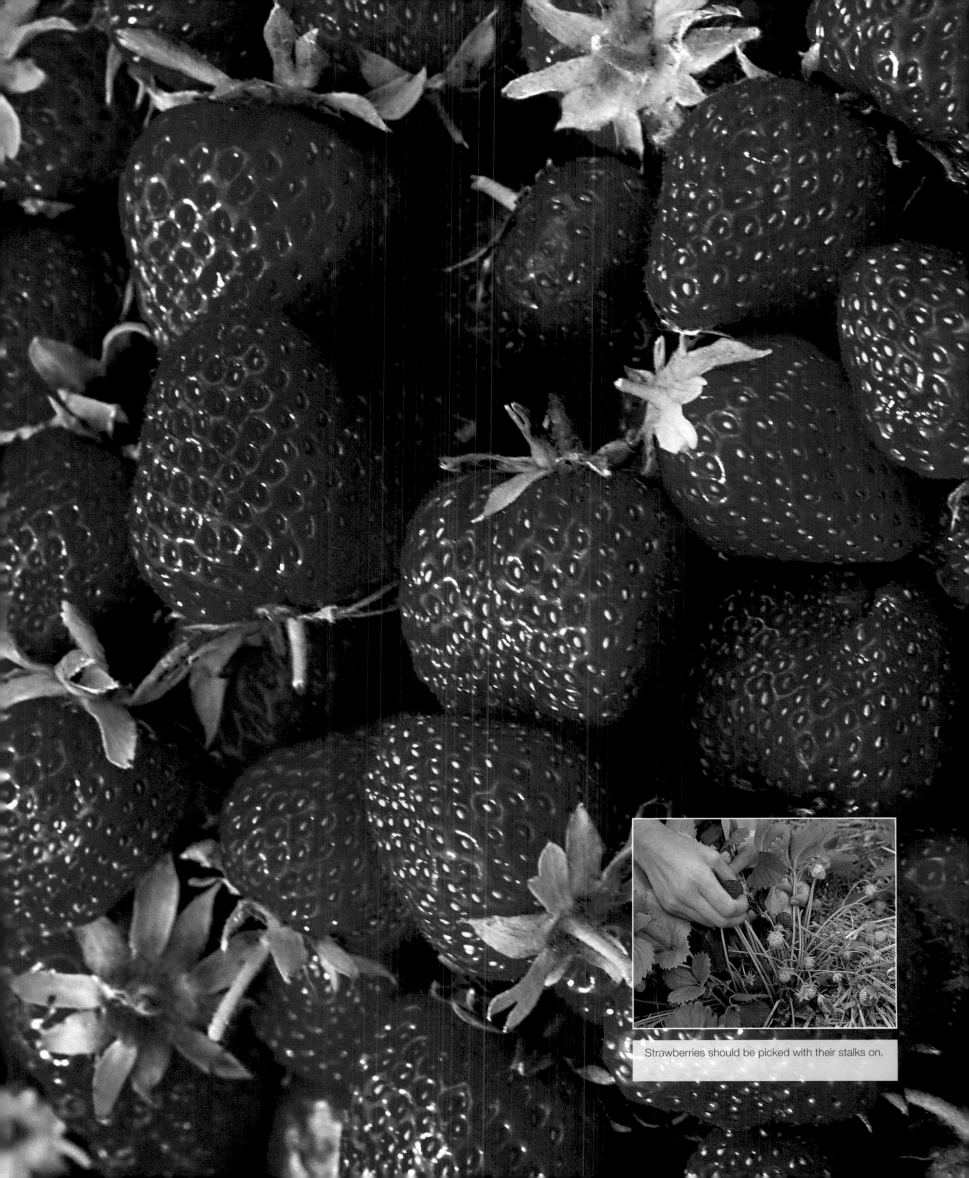

Strawberries should be picked with their stalks on.

Recipes with Strawberries

Marinated Asparagus with Strawberries

11 oz (300 g) green asparagus
9 oz (250 g) strawberries
2 Tbs honey
8 lollo rosso leaves
2 Tbs tarragon vinegar
4 Tbs wheatgerm oil
Coarse salt, white pepper
1 small bunch of tarragon
2 Tbs pistachios

Thinly peel the asparagus and chop into 1 inch (3 cm) pieces; put to one side.
Wash and quarter the strawberries and mix with 1 tablespoon of honey; leave to stand. Wash the lettuce leaves and break into small pieces.
Prepare a vinaigrette from the vinegar, oil, remaining honey, salt, pepper, and 3 tablespoons of water and marinate the asparagus in it for 15 minutes.
Decorate the plates with the lettuce leaves, divide the asparagus and strawberries between them and drizzle over the vinaigrette; decorate with tarragon leaves and pistachios.

Buckwheat Pancakes with Strawberries
Blinis

14 oz (400 g) strawberries
4 Tbs honey
1/2 tsp vanilla extract
2 eggs
5/6 cup (100 g) buckwheat flour
5/6 cup (100 g) fine spelt flour
3/4 cup (150 ml) kefir
Pinch of ground coriander
Pinch of ground cardamom
Wheatgerm oil, clarified butter
Grated zest of 1/2 an orange

Wash and quarter the strawberries and mix with the honey and vanilla; leave to stand.
Separate the eggs, mix egg yolks and flour with 2 1/2 cups (500 ml) water, season the batter with coriander and cardamom.
Beat the egg whites until stiff and fold the beaten whites into the batter. Cook thin pancakes in some oil and butter. Put the strawberries on the pancakes, fold over and serve immediately.

Strawberry Jelly with Mascarpone and Vanilla Sauce

1 lb 2 oz (500 g) strawberries
2 1/2 cups (500 ml) pure fruit juice
1 Tbs lemon juice
Just under 2 tsp agar-agar
3 Tbs honey
5 oz (150 g) Mascarpone
2/5 cup (80 ml) heavy cream
1/2 tsp vanilla extract

Wash and quarter the strawberries and put into small molds which have been rinsed with cold water. Heat up 1 3/4 cups (about 375 ml) fruit juice with the lemon juice. Mix the remaining fruit juice with the agar-agar and add to the hot juice. Continue to heat, stirring constantly, until the liquid has become clear and the agar-agar has dissolved completely. Then stir in 2 tablespoons of honey.
Pour the thickened fruit juice over the strawberries in the molds, cool and leave to set for about 3 hours.
Mix the Mascarpone and cream with the remaining honey and vanilla to form a creamy sauce.
Turn the strawberry jellies out onto plates and pour the sauce over so that it covers half the jelly.

Strawberry Dream
(Illustration right)

1 lb 2 oz (500 g) strawberries
3 Tbs honey
1/2 cup (80 g) brown rice
1 cup (200 ml) heavy cream
Grated zest of 1/2 a lemon
1/2 cup (100 ml) whipped cream

Wash and quarter the strawberries and mix with 2 tablespoons of honey; leave to stand.
Grind the rice into a fine flour. Mix the cream with an equal amount of water and bring to the boil with the lemon zest. Quickly sprinkle in the ground rice, stir until smooth, and continue to cook for about 8 minutes, stirring constantly; leave to cool.
Add the sweetened strawberries and remaining honey to the rice mixture. Carefully fold in the whipped cream, leave to stand for 10 minutes, then serve.

Strawberries with Port Zabaglione

1 lb 12 oz (800 g) strawberries
1 tsp lemon juice
6 Tbs honey
4 egg yolks
8 Tbs red port
Mint to decorate

Wash the strawberries and drain well. Pour the lemon juice and 2 tablespoons of honey over the strawberries and leave to stand for at least 60 minutes.
For the zabaglione, whisk the egg yolks with the remaining honey in a bain-marie until foamy, slowly (as with the oil when making a mayonnaise) add the port and beat into a light zabaglione. Remove from the heat and stir until cold in the bain-marie.
Put the strawberries into individual dishes and cover with the zabaglione. Decorate with the mint and serve.

Strawberry Dream

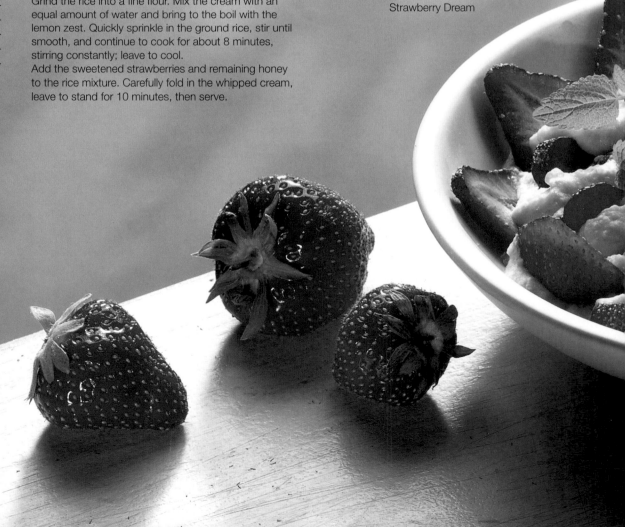

Strawberry Granita

1 vanilla bean
Honey according to taste
1 lb 2 oz (500 g) strawberries
3 Tbs lemon juice
1 bottle of Prosecco or dry sparkling wine

Slit open the vanilla bean and boil in 2¹/₂ cups (500 ml) water for 20 minutes. Take out the bean, stir in the honey and allow the honey water to cool.
Wash the strawberries and purée in a blender with the lemon juice, then add the cold honey water.
Put the mixture in a suitable bowl (stainless steel) and transfer to the freezer; every 20 minutes stir from the edge so that small ice crystals do not collect at the edge. The granita needs 3–4 hours to set.
Put 2 scoops of granita in each champagne glass and pour over the Prosecco.

Strawberry Whip
(Illustration below)

Serves 2

11 oz (300 g) strawberries
¹/₂ a banana
1¹/₄ cups (250 ml) yogurt
3 Tbs heavy cream
1 Tbs lemon juice
2 Tbs honey
¹/₂ tsp vanilla extract

Wash and halve the strawberries, then slice the banana. Purée the fruit with a little yogurt, then add the remaining yogurt and the other ingredients and purée until a foamy, creamy drink is produced. Serve well chilled.

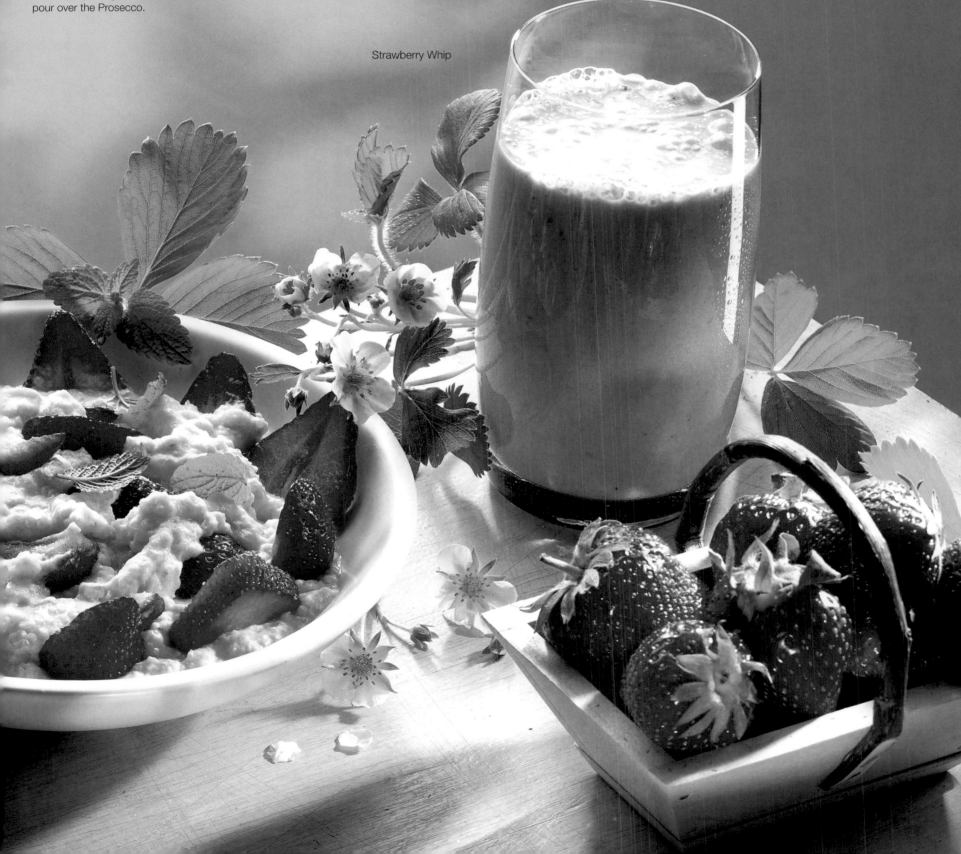

Strawberry Whip

Exotic Fruits

For a long time now many fruits that originally came from other parts of the world have been a familiar sight in our fruit and vegetable stores. Many of them have been native to Mediterranean countries for hundreds of years, many even for thousands of years, such as fig and pomegranate trees. The oldest reached Europe, like many of our indigenous varieties of fruit, via Asia Minor and the Near East. The Moors played a particularly important role here. They were famous for their highly developed horticulture and agriculture. From the 8th century they introduced several types of fruit and vegetables into Spain, which was then part of their territory. The new varieties then reached other European countries from the Iberian Peninsula.

The discovery of America gave Europe new vegetables that could be established there, but fruits native to America could not become acclimatized in Europe. The prickly pear, cherimoya, and cape gooseberry (physalis) are exceptions. Fruits such as the lulo or lucuma, the coronilla or pitahaya are still real exotic fruits even in international markets. Papayas have now become well-known. No other South American fruit can, however, match the popularity of the pineapple. Other exotic varieties have only been introduced and grown in increasing numbers during the last few decades. The kiwi fruit which began to be cultivated, at first timidly, during the 1970s in Mediterranean countries is a particular example. As it thrives best in the southern European climate, it has now become a common fruit for fruit growers there, but for a long time it has not been as profitable to produce as was once hoped.

The less subtropical regions of Europe with a suitable climate have also recently become interested in mangoes, lychees, carambolas, and other types of fruit. There are now businesses there that use ecological methods. In general the range of organically-grown exotic fruits is, however, still limited. There are several pioneering projects in African, Central and South American countries as well as Sri Lanka which encourage this type of cultivation and at the same time provide the small local farmer with a livelihood. The conventional production of tropical fruits, in particular of bananas, is often in the hands of large, Western companies who exploit the workers, expose them to pesticides and insecticides, and at the same time overexploit nature.

As a rule, organic exotic fruits are much more expensive than those produced conventionally. This is due not least to the fact that initiatives based on humanitarian, social, and environmental measures do not aim to maximize profits but to improve living conditions. The following selection is limited to exotic fruits that are grown organically or are available wild.

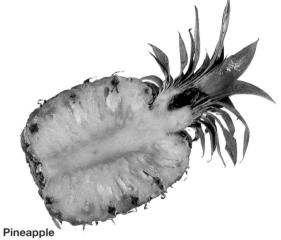

Pineapple
Native to South America; grown in many tropical countries; contains the enzyme bromeline which splits protein, helps digestion, and has medicinal properties; rich in minerals and, when ripe, vitamins, low in calories. Organic pineapples come from West African countries and Sri Lanka.

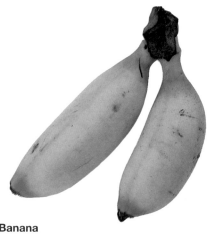

Banana
The most important fruit exported actually comes from Asia; grown in Central and South America, some countries on the west coast of Africa, as well as India; rich in vital substances. Grown organically on the Canary Islands, in Israel, the Dominican Republic, Ghana, Togo, and Burkina Faso (formerly Upper Volta).

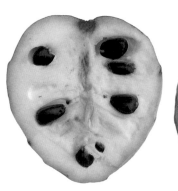

Cherimoya (Annona, Custard Apple)
Comes from the Peruvian Andes; scaly, greenish yellow fruit usually the size of an apple with an inedible skin; whitish, flavorsome, sweet flesh with a taste similar to that of a banana, with numerous brown seeds about the size of beans. Small quantities grown organically in Andalucia in southern Spain.

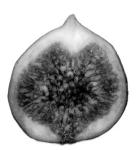

Fig
Common in the Middle and Near East, but for centuries has been cultivated around the Mediterranean; many varieties with different colored fruits from yellow to green and red to purple; when fresh rich in minerals and iron. Grown organically in Italy, France, Spain; trees often grow wild in southern countries.

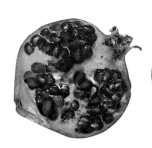

Pomegranate
A fruit which was often praised and portrayed in oriental cultures, gave Granada its name; under a tough, leathery skin, that keeps it fresh for a long time, cells contain angular seeds, enveloped by soft, juicy flesh; the seeds can be taken out, or eaten if the fruit is young; a lot of juice which can be used for many things produced organically in Spain and Italy.

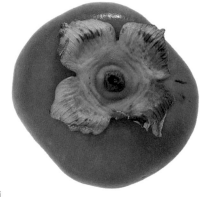

Kaki
Originates from the Far East, kaki trees grow well in the Mediterranean climate; planted in gardens there for decoration on account of its bright orange-red fruit; smooth, tomato-like skin; when fully ripe, sweet, pleasant, but not very strong taste; high carotene content; also dried. Organic from Italy and Spain.

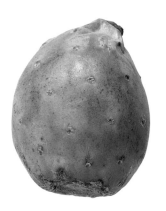

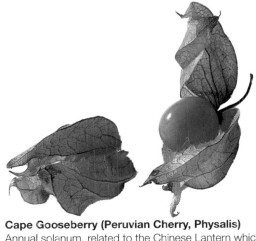

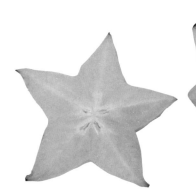

Prickly Pear (Opuntia)
Comes from Mexico and spread to the Mediterranean countries where it naturalized; often planted as an impenetrable hedge; fig-shaped fruit red when ripe with unpleasant tufts of bristles; peel with care (and gloves); vitamin-rich, sweet, discreetly aromatic fruit best spooned out. Grown organically in Sicily and southern Spain.

Cape Gooseberry (Peruvian Cherry, Physalis)
Annual solanum, related to the Chinese Lantern which adorns many gardens; first cultivated in South Africa in a big way. The vitamin-rich, yellowy fruit the size of a cherry is surrounded by a parchment-like husk; sweet-and-sour and aromatic flavor. Among other places, comes from Africa and New Zealand; also thrives in organic orchards in the Mediterranean.

Carambola (Star Fruit)
Originates from India and Malaysia; small tree, strangely enough an oxalis; yellow, vitamin-rich fruit with a smell of jasmine; when ripe, shiny amber-colored with five or six prominent ribs; cutting it across produces decorative stars; eat with the skin on. Organic carambolas come from southern Spain and West Africa.

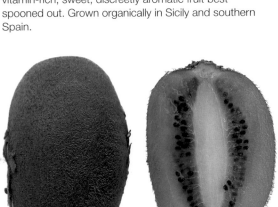

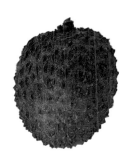

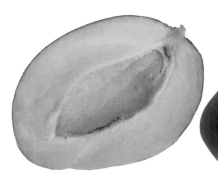

Kiwi Fruit (Chinese Gooseberry)
Spread widely from New Zealand, grows like a liana; very rich in vitamin C; under the thin, hairy, brown skin is a bright green flesh with black seeds; fresh, sweet-and-sour flavor; either cut in half and spoon out or peel; can be used in many ways. Among other places, organically grown in Italy, Spain, and France.

Lychee
Highly regarded fruit in China, its native country; tall trees growing in subtropical climates form large panicles; fruit at first has soft, red skin which dries to form a scaly, hard, protective husk; the highly aromatic, slightly soapy, pale flesh surrounds a large, brown seed. Since 1996 organic lychees have been available from the Malaga area of southern Spain.

Mango
The Indians' favorite fruit; usually an irregular shape, from green and yellow to red-colored fruit with thin, inedible skin; very juicy, rich yellow, delicious flesh that is not easy to remove from the thin, long, fibrous seed; can be used in many ways. Organically grown in Ghana, Togo, Sri Lanka, and southern Spain.

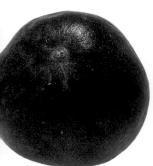

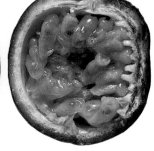

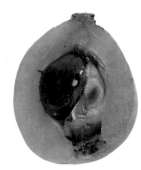

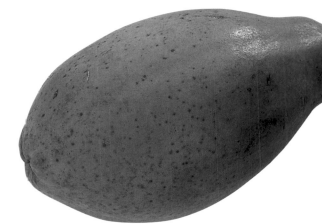

Maracuja (Passion Fruit)
Cultivated in many warm places in Europe on account of its wonderful flowers which are reminiscent of symbols of the passion. However, only in hot regions do the liana-like plants bear their round to oval-shaped fruit which is very irregular in size. Small quantities are grown organically in Africa and California to be eaten fresh by spooning out the flesh and numerous seeds.

Medlar
Pome grown in Mediterranean countries on small trees with long, decorative leaves. The orange, yet always brown-speckled, fruit rich in beta-carotene with large, shiny, brown seeds ripens in spring. Often somewhat tart, it is similar to the apricot in taste, but has a leathery skin. Grown further north, the skin is brown when it is picked, it is smaller and has a tangy taste.

Papaya
From Central America; is cultivated today in many tropical regions; oval, long, yellow fruit which, when ripe, resembles the melon in texture and flavor; grows on unbranched, hollow trees; very sweet, vitamin-rich flesh surrounding numerous small, dark, sharp seeds; papain, which is used in medicine and as a meat tenderizer, is obtained from the sap of papaya trees. Grown organically on the Canary Islands and in West Africa.

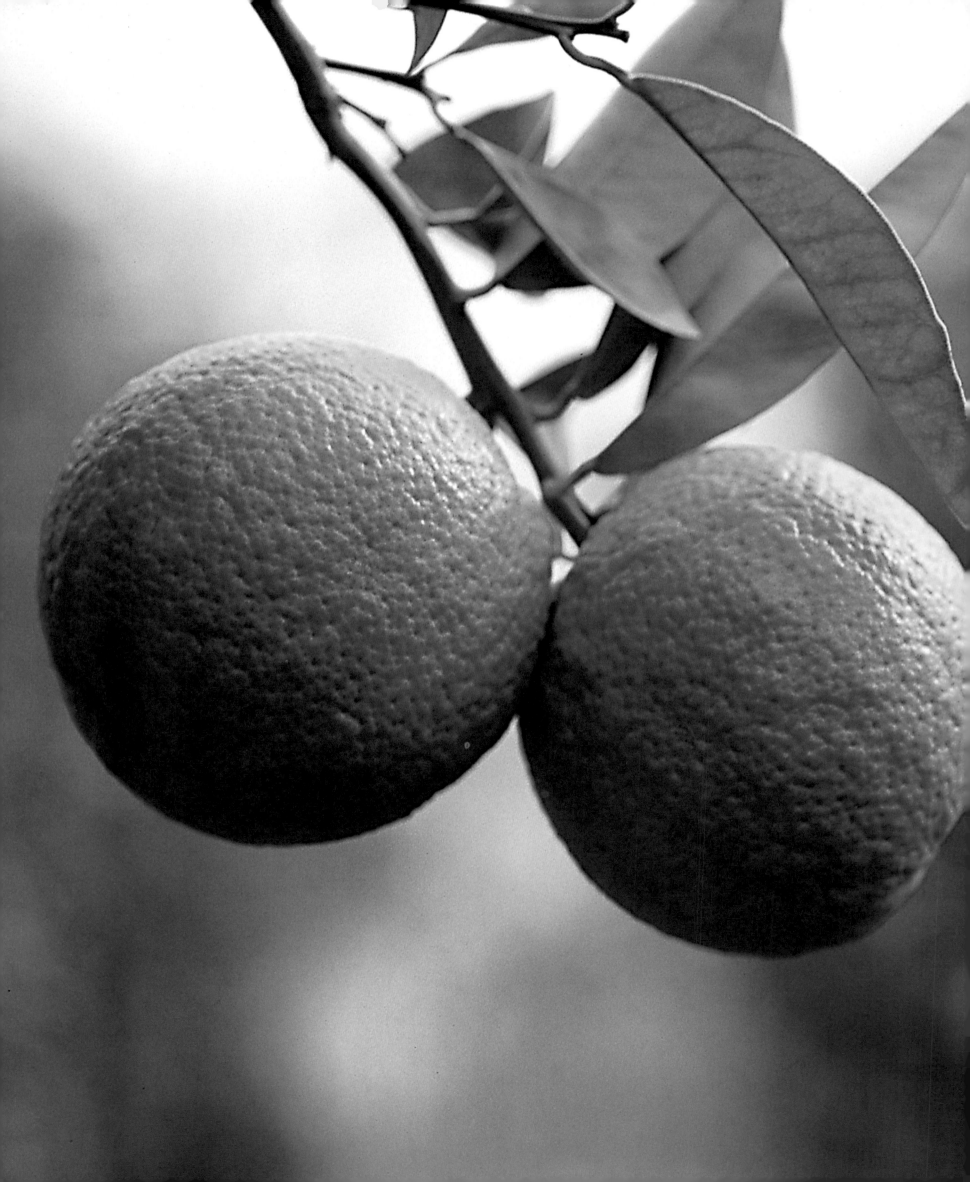

Organically Grown in Andalucia

Oranges and Lemons

Around Alora with its picturesque Moorish castle, about half way between Malaga and Cordoba, various fincas have specialized in organic cultivation. 300-year-old olive trees are an indication that this is land that has been developed and cultivated by man for a very long time. There is also a tradition of orange growing. Odd bitter orange trees with their round, reddish fruits, which have irregular, thick and rough skins, testify to this. They were once used to make English marmalade and were the first citrus fruits planted in Spain.

Citrus fruits originally came from South East Asia and *Citrus senensis*, the sweet orange, from China, while bitter oranges were introduced into Andalucia as ornamental plants by the Moors in the 11th century. Even today numerous evergreen orange trees line the streets in southern Spain. Sweet oranges only reached Spain 400 or 450 years later through Italian and Portuguese merchants. For their part the Spaniards, like the Portuguese, then laid out the first plantations in America. Oranges, however, continued to be mainly used as ornamental trees or for medicinal purposes. The first sweet orange orchard was not planted until 1781. From then on their cultivation developed at a terrific rate.

The oldest sweet orange trees in the Alora region have been there for a hundred years. They are Vernas which bear rather small, round, or pear-shaped fruits with soft, thick skins. They do not ripen until the end of winter and can be picked into the summer. As their acid is rather aggressive they are not to the discriminating taste of foreign customers and so are rarely exported but used to make juice. On the other hand, the Valencia Late variety is very popular. It is a late, robust, common variety, whose new flowers are already in the process of forming when the fruits are still ripening. Its season extends from mid-April through July. When it is fully ripe, the medium-sized, spherical, or slightly oval fruit has a pleasant, very balanced, sweet flavor, but is very sharp if it is picked too early.

The trees in these citrus groves are fully-grown. Some tower over 32 feet (ten meters) high. As orange trees produce new wood they must be pruned regularly. To do this the workers disappear under the pergola-like foliage and saw out old branches from the inside. Time seems to have stood still in these orchards, whose age can be seen in the old natural crosses between oranges, clementines, and lemons. Even the machines used to loosen the soil belong to another era. Obviously here the traditional cultivation method

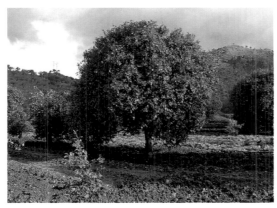

A fully-grown orange tree can reach a height of 26 to 32 feet (8 to 10 meters) and an age of over 100 years.

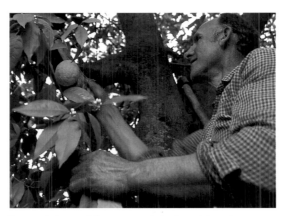

The main harvest for oranges is in the winter when citrus fruits are in great demand in northern European countries for their high vitamin C content.

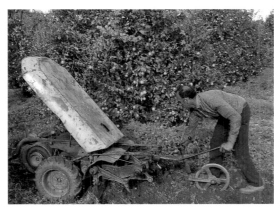

The soil is loosened under the orange trees with this manually operated motor-assisted harrow. Green manure is then spread there.

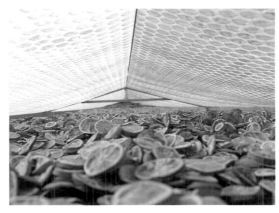

Despite organic cultivation, old varieties of orange do not sell, but sliced and dried they can be used for fruit teas.

linked to nature merges into organic farming. However, the idyll has an economic drawback: such old orchards that have been growing continuously, are no longer profitable. If such paradises are to remain then some imagination is needed in addition to a love of nature, the land, and old ruins. What can be done with an orange variety, such as the Verna, that is no longer in demand? The oranges are sliced and spread out in a – still experimental – solar tunnel dryer. Dried in this way they are excellent for tea, either alone or in fruit blends, hot or cold.

To reduce the risk involved, diversification is also practiced. Lettuce, Chinese cabbage, broccoli, zucchini, and tomatoes can thrive outdoors on the most fertile slopes. It is difficult for small and medium-sized farms to survive in the organic market with citrus fruits alone. Naturally lemon trees also grow in the hot climate. These are mainly of the old variety, also called Verna, which holds its own unchallenged. While the bright yellow fruits ripen, the spiny trees form new flowers and beautiful, young, eggplant-colored leaves. Verna is a juicy, thin-skinned lemon which rarely contains seeds. It can be picked from February through September. Then Prim(m)ofiori comes along which provides vitamin C in the winter.

In contrast to conventionally-grown lemons and oranges, whose zest is usually treated with poisonous preservatives and must, therefore, never be used in drinks, dishes, or cakes, the zest of organically-grown citrus fruits has a naturally matt surface and smells pleasantly fruity. In all the recipes in this book only organically-grown fruit, whose zest is untreated, is used.

Energy Providers with Medicinal Properties

As is well known, oranges and lemons are rich in vitamin C, but they also contain vitamins B1, B2, B6, niacin, and vitamin E as well as provitamin A, the minerals potassium, magnesium, phosphorus, calcium, and trace elements such as iron, zinc, fluorine, copper, and sulfur. They therefore stimulate energy, help to prevent cancer and are antibacterial. Lemon juice, which is also used to season dishes, has a healing effect on infections in the mouth and throat area, but thanks to its vital substances and roughage, it also ensures that arteries remain elastic, and cholesterol and uric acid levels are reduced.

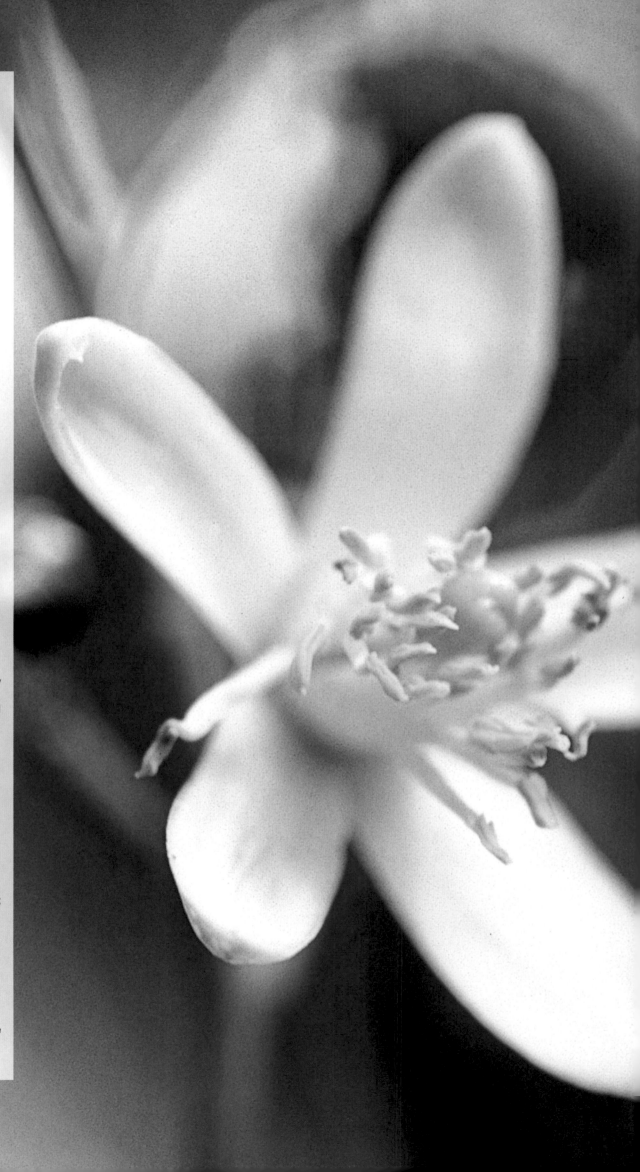

Citrus Fruits

Clementine
This reddish, often bulbous, delicious citrus fruit is a hybrid of the bitter orange and tangerine. Rather dark flesh, no seeds, sweeter than tangerines; is almost always eaten fresh. Available November through mid-March.

Grapefruit
Contrary to general belief, it is not a pummelo and grows on relatively small trees. Its slightly bitter fruits, which hang in clusters like grapes, and stimulate the appetite and digestion, are also considerably smaller. Grown in warm regions virtually worldwide, in the Mediterranean it ripens between November and April.

Kumquat
A taste for this miniature orange the size of a plum has only been acquired very gradually in Europe. Its exceptional quality is the smooth, edible, bitter sweet skin rich in essential oils. Full of flavor with a marked sharpness it is a real pleasure eaten fresh or excellent for marmalade.

Limequat
A cross between the lime, which is not very resistant to the cold, and the more robust kumquat. The result is a thorny bush producing round or plum-shaped, yellow or greenish-yellow fruit with a bitter tasting skin. Very juicy, scented, sharp, and rich in vitamin C.

Lime
No other citrus fruit is as sensitive to the cold as the lime which, therefore, only thrives in tropical climates. Its fruit is smaller than the lemon's, considerably juicier, and has a pronounced flavor. Its skin is thin, breaks easily and, when ripe, has a yellowy-green color. Distinctive fine flavor for salads, dishes, or drinks.

Tangerine
It may be sweet and full of flavor but its many seeds can spoil the enjoyment of eating it. Therefore the flat, loose-skinned fruit, which is easy to peel, is losing its popularity. Numerous new varieties are, however, based on the tangerine, and the satsuma, a practically seedless variety, is popular.

Orange
Hundreds of varieties of the 26 to 32 foot (8 to 10 meter) high trees exist wherever it is warm. A distinction is made according to color between deep red blood and pale oranges. Paler varieties, which ripen in winter, are the most popular eating oranges.

Pummelo
The giant among citrus plants can grow to double the height of an orange tree and produce fruit weighing several pounds. Yellow or pink, thick skin; slightly bitter, sweet-sour, distinctive flavor. Usually eaten fresh or drunk as juice.

Lemon
Today cultivated worldwide in the subtropics and widespread in the Mediterranean area where the often bushy tree has acclimatized well. The sharp lemons contain not only a lot of vitamin C, but a wealth of minerals and trace elements. They are antiphlogistic, strengthen tissues, and stimulate the movement of the bowels.

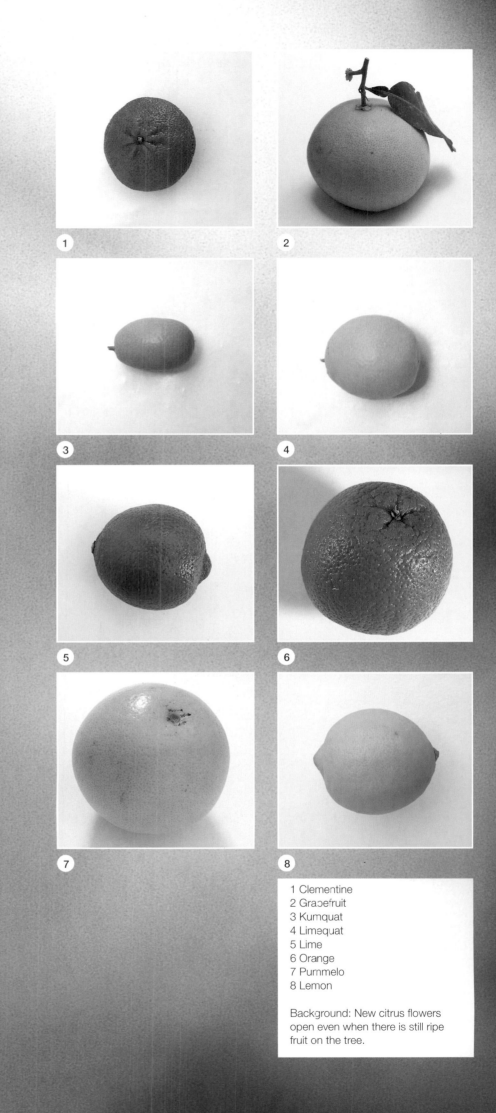

1 Clementine
2 Grapefruit
3 Kumquat
4 Limequat
5 Lime
6 Orange
7 Pummelo
8 Lemon

Background: New citrus flowers open even when there is still ripe fruit on the tree.

Recipes with Lemons and Oranges

Lemon Butter

1 cup (250 g) soft butter
Grated zest of 1 lemon
Juice of 1 lemon
$\frac{1}{2}$ tsp coarsely ground black pepper
$\frac{1}{2}$ tsp coarse salt
1 Tbs finely chopped lemon balm

Beat the butter until light and creamy, then mix in all the ingredients. Put in a container and leave in the refrigerator to go hard. Serve for spreading on bread, with fish or broiled meat.

Sicilian Lemon Salad
(Illustration below right)

6 juicy lemons
Arugula leaves
7 oz (200 g) black pitted olives
Coarse salt, black pepper
2 Tbs olive oil

Peel the lemons with a sharp knife, removing the pith, cut into segments and remove any seeds. Leave in cold water for 10 minutes; carefully take out of the water, place in a colander, and leave to stand for another 10 minutes.
Place the arugula in a serving dish, arrange the lemon segments and olives on it. Season with salt and plenty of freshly-milled black pepper, drizzle with the olive oil and serve immediately.

Sole Fillets in Lemon Sauce

2 lemons
8 sole fillets
$\frac{1}{4}$ cup (50 g) butter
Coarse salt, black pepper
Flour
1 Tbs vodka
1 carton crème fraîche

Thinly peel one lemon so that no pith is left on the zest; cut the zest into very thin strips; squeeze out the juice. Dab the sole fillets dry and sprinkle with some lemon juice.
Peel the other lemon with a sharp knife, removing the pith, cut into segments and put to one side.
Preheat the oven to 200 °F (100 °C).
Heat the butter in a very large saucepan. Season the fillets and toss in the flour. Fry for about 3 minutes on each side. Then keep warm on a plate in the oven.
Add the vodka and remaining lemon juice to the juices left in the pan and stir. Add the crème fraîche, strips of lemon zest and cook rapidly on a high heat until the sauce has reduced by half. Season with salt and pepper.
Place the sole fillets and lemon segments in the sauce and simmer for 1 minute.
Serve immediately on the warmed serving plate.
Goes well with wild rice and seasonal salad.

Chicken in Mustard and Lemon Sauce
(Illustration right)

1 small red bell pepper
2 tsp hot mustard
4 Tbs lemon juice
1 Tbs grated lemon zest
3 Tbs olive oil
1 young chicken (about 2 lb 8 oz/1.2 kg)
$\frac{1}{4}$ cup (50 g) butter
1 lemon, divided into 8 pieces
Parsley

Remove the seeds from the bell pepper and cut into rings. Mix well with the mustard, lemon juice and zest, and olive oil.
Cut the chicken into several portions and coat on all sides with the mustard and lemon mixture; marinade for at least 2 hours.
Preheat the oven to 350 °F (180 °C).
Melt the butter in an ovenproof pan. Place the chicken portions in it skin-side down and put in the oven. After 30 minutes turn the chicken portions over, add a few spoonfuls of water and cook for a further 30 minutes, until the skin has turned brown. Place on a warmed plate and decorate with the lemon wedges and parsley.

Lemon Tart
(Illustration below)

$3\frac{1}{3}$ cups (400 g) fine whole wheat flour
$1\frac{1}{2}$ tsp baking powder
1 cup (250 g) cold butter
3 Tbs honey
2 lemons
$3\frac{1}{2}$ oz (100 g) candied lemon zest
3 egg yolks
9 oz (250 g) Ricotta

Sieve the flour and baking powder into a bowl. Chop the butter into small pieces and add to the flour together with 1 tablespoon of honey. Quickly knead everything together to form shortcrust pastry, adding a little water if necessary. Put the pastry into the refrigerator for 60 minutes.
Preheat the oven to 350 °F (180 °C).
Grease a $9\frac{1}{2}$ inch (24 cm) spring clip pan.
Roll out the pastry and line the pan with it. Grate the zest of one lemon and squeeze half of it; slice the other lemon thinly. Finely chop the candied lemon zest. Whisk the egg yolks with the remaining honey until foamy, then stir in the lemon juice, grated zest, candied lemon zest, and Ricotta.
Put the mixture into the pan and cover with the lemon slices. Using your thumb press the pastry edge down all the way round until it is just above the filling.
Bake the tart in the oven for about 60 minutes.

Roast Veal with Orange

Serves 6

2 lb 3 oz (1 kg) leg of suckling calf
1 Tbs finely chopped rosemary
Coarse salt, white pepper
$\frac{1}{6}$ cup (40 g) butter
3 Tbs olive oil
3 oranges
$\frac{1}{2}$ cup (100 ml) vegetable stock
$\frac{1}{2}$ cup (100 ml) dry white wine
1 Tbs brandy
$\frac{3}{4}$ oz (20 g) cold butter

Preheat the oven to 400 °F (200 °C).
Rub rosemary, salt, and pepper into the meat. Melt 2 tablespoons (30 g) of butter and put into a roasting pan with the olive oil. Place the meat in the roasting pan and put into the oven.
Grate the zest of one orange and squeeze out the juice. After 20 minutes pour the orange juice over the meat; pour on the vegetable stock and white wine. Turn the meat over after 60 minutes, adding some water if necessary. Peel the two remaining oranges with a sharp knife, removing the pith; cut into segments and put to one side.
After 45 minutes take the roast out of the oven and allow to rest for 10 minutes.
In a saucepan heat 2 teaspoons (10 g) of butter, add the orange segments, stew them for 2 minutes and then add the brandy.
Take the roast meat out of the pan, remove the sediment from the pan, transfer into a small saucepan, reduce if necessary, and season. Thinly slice the roast, put onto a preheated plate, and arrange the orange segments around the meat. Add the orange sauce to the contents of the saucepan, bring to the boil, remove from the stove, and stir in the cold butter.
Serve the sauce separately from the meat.

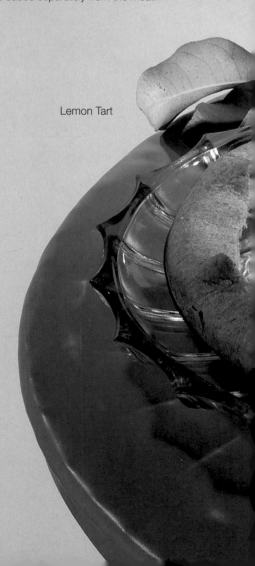

Lemon Tart

Recipes with Oranges

Fennel and Orange Salad

2 large ripe oranges
3 fennel bulbs
2 small red onions
Juice of $\frac{1}{2}$ a lemon
6–8 Tbs olive oil
Pinch of English mustard powder
Coarse salt, white pepper
3 Tbs roughly chopped walnuts

Peel the oranges with a sharp knife, removing the pith; catch any juice that comes out while doing this; cut the oranges into segments.

Thinly slice the fennel and onions, setting some of the green part of the fennel to one side. Arrange the fennel slices and orange segments in a fan shape on a large plate and arrange the onion rings on top.

Mix the orange juice you collected with the lemon juice, olive oil, mustard powder, salt, and pepper, and pour over the salad. Leave to stand for at least 30 minutes, then finely chop the green part of the fennel and sprinkle over the salad, together with the walnuts.

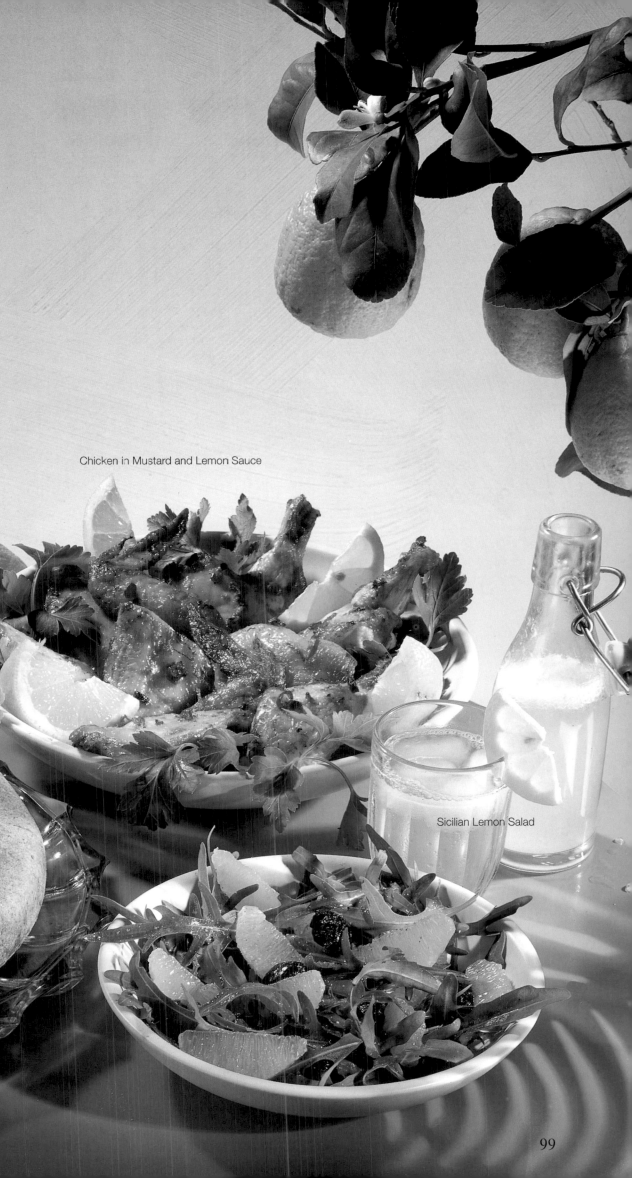

Chicken in Mustard and Lemon Sauce

Sicilian Lemon Salad

99

Juicy and Refreshing

Melons

As members of the same family as the pumpkin, the round or oval melons are actually vegetables. However, they are used and prepared almost exclusively as fruit. They like the Mediterranean climate, provided they receive enough water. As they trail, climb, and need quite a bit of space they are rarely cultivated organically in greenhouses. There are many varieties that differ in size and flavor. Basically a distinction is made between musk melons and water melons.

Musk melons include, for example, Honeydew, Ogen, and Netted melons as well as the fragrant Cantaloupes. The skin of musk melons is netted, ribbed, or grooved, and they have golden flesh which, when ripe, is highly scented, and is extremely rich in vitamin A. The seeds, which must be removed before the melon is eaten, are in a hollow in the center of the fruit. The fruit is ripe if it gives slightly when the end opposite the stem is pressed with a finger.

Water melons, which are natives of the African steppe, are now cultivated throughout the Mediterranean region. They can weigh up to 33 pounds (15 kilograms) and contain valuable minerals. The seeds are right in the flesh (which is usually red) and can be removed with a sharp knife. It is not very easy to tell if a water melon is ripe. It is best to choose fruit with a matt skin and tap it with a finger – it should sound hollow like a drum. Melons not only cleanse the kidneys, but are thirst-quenching as they contain 90 to 95 percent water. Their low calorific value makes them ideal as part of a diet.

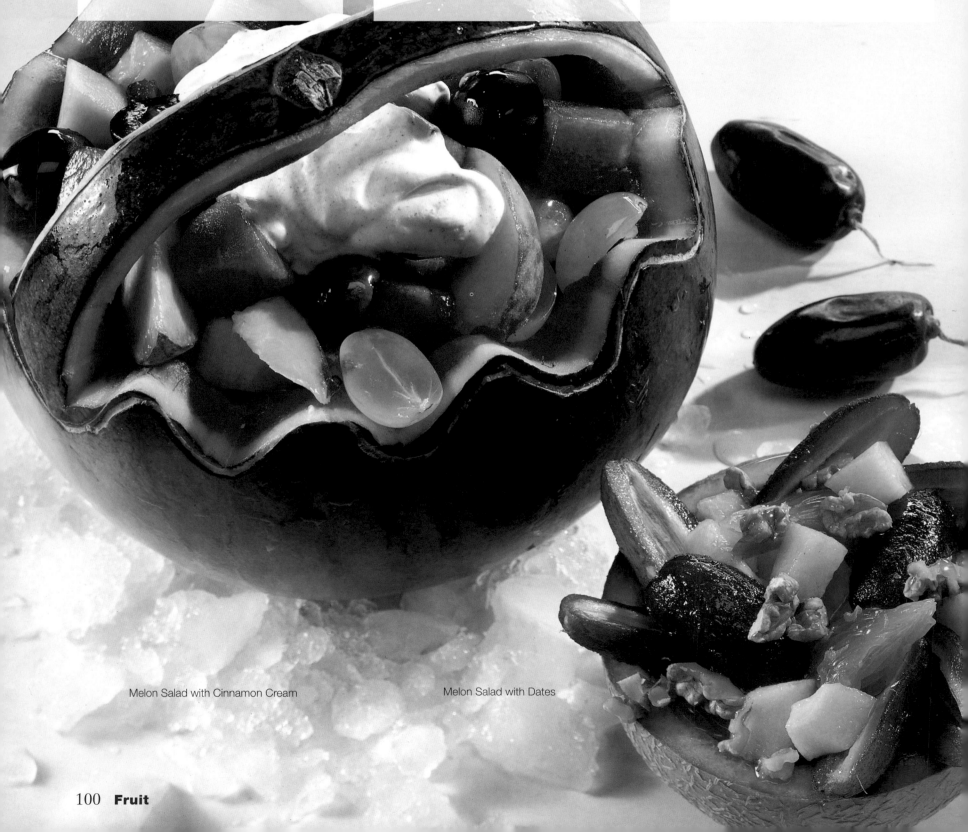

Melon Salad with Cinnamon Cream

Melon Salad with Dates

Melon Salad with Cinnamon Cream
(Illustration below left)

1 medium-sized water melon
1 small Cantaloupe
2 peaches
3¹/₂ oz (100 g) white grapes
3¹/₂ oz (100 g) black grapes
1 tsp lemon juice
3 Tbs grape juice
2 Tbs honey
1 cup (200 ml) heavy cream
Pinch of cinnamon
1 Tbs maple syrup
9 oz (250 g) farmer's cheese

Cut the top third off the water melon and hollow out the inside. De-seed the flesh, cut into cubes, and put to one side.
Straighten the base of the melon so that it stands up. Serrate the top edge with a sharp knife.
De-seed the flesh of the Cantaloupe and cut into cubes. Halve, pit, and slice the peaches. Halve the grapes and de-seed if necessary. Carefully mix the fruit together, including the cubes of water melon, and put into the hollowed out water melon.
Mix the lemon juice and grape juice with the honey and pour over the fruit. Whip the cream with the cinnamon until stiff. Mix the farmer's cheese with the maple syrup and fold in the cream.
Decorate the melon with a few spoonfuls of cream and serve the rest separately.

Melon Salad with Dates
(Illustration left)

1 Netted melon
1 pink grapefruit
7 oz (200 g) fresh dates
3¹/₂ oz (100 g) roughly chopped walnuts
2 Tbs honey
1 Tbs lemon juice
2 Tbs Cointreau

De-seed the melon flesh and cut into cubes. Peel the grapefruit with a sharp knife, removing the pith, and cut into segments. Skin, halve, and pit the dates.
Carefully mix the fruit and walnuts together. Mix the honey, lemon juice, and Cointreau to make a sauce and pour over the melon salad.
Leave to steep in the refrigerator for 60 minutes. Carefully mix once more and serve chilled.
Serve with cinnamon cream.

Melon with Ham

1 Cantaloupe
3¹/₂ oz (100 g) air-dried ham
Mint to decorate
Black pepper

De-seed the flesh of the melon and cut into small cubes.
Place a small dish upside down in the center of a large round serving plate and arrange the slices of ham over the dish. Place the melon cubes around the ham, season with freshly ground pepper and decorate with the mint.

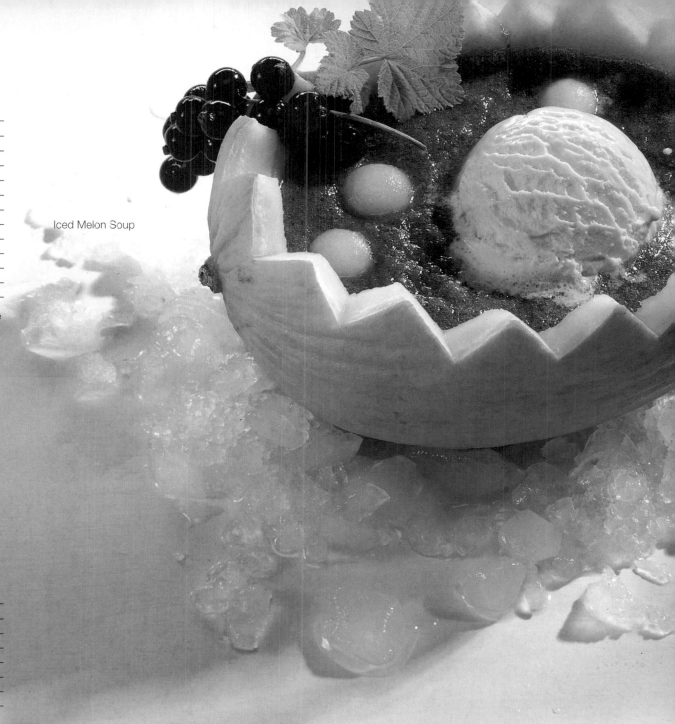

Iced Melon Soup

Iced Melon Soup
(Illustration above)

1 Honeydew melon
9 oz (250 g) red currants
1 Tbs lemon juice
1¹/₂ cups (300 ml) black currant juice
3 Tbs maple syrup
4 scoops vanilla or soft fruit ice cream

Halve and de-seed the melon. Using a melon baller scoop out 12 small balls and put to one side. Scrape out the rest of the flesh with a spoon. Take the stalks off the red currants – except for a couple of bunches – and purée in a blender with the scraped-out melon flesh, lemon juice, black currant juice, and maple syrup
Divide the fruit purée between four dishes, add three melon balls and a scoop of ice cream to each, and decorate with the red currants.

Melon with Blackberries

14 oz (400 g) blackberries
3 Tbs honey
2 Tbs sea buckthorn juice
1³/₄ oz (50 g) roughly chopped hazelnuts
2 small Ogen melons
1 cup (200 ml) whipping cream
¹/₂ tsp vanilla extract
Mint to decorate

Wash the blackberries. Mix 2 tablespoons of honey and the sea buckthorn juice, pour over the blackberries and leave to stand for 10 minutes.
Lightly dry fry the hazelnuts, add the remaining honey, allow to boil down a little, and cool. Halve and de-seed the melons. Remove the flesh with a spoon and put to one side.
For decoration, serrate the edges of the melon halves and straighten their bases so that they stand up; then put the halves onto plates.
Whip the cream with the vanilla until very stiff. Cut the flesh of the melons into cubes, mix with the marinaded blackberries, the hazelnut praline, and cream, put into the melon halves and decorate with mint.

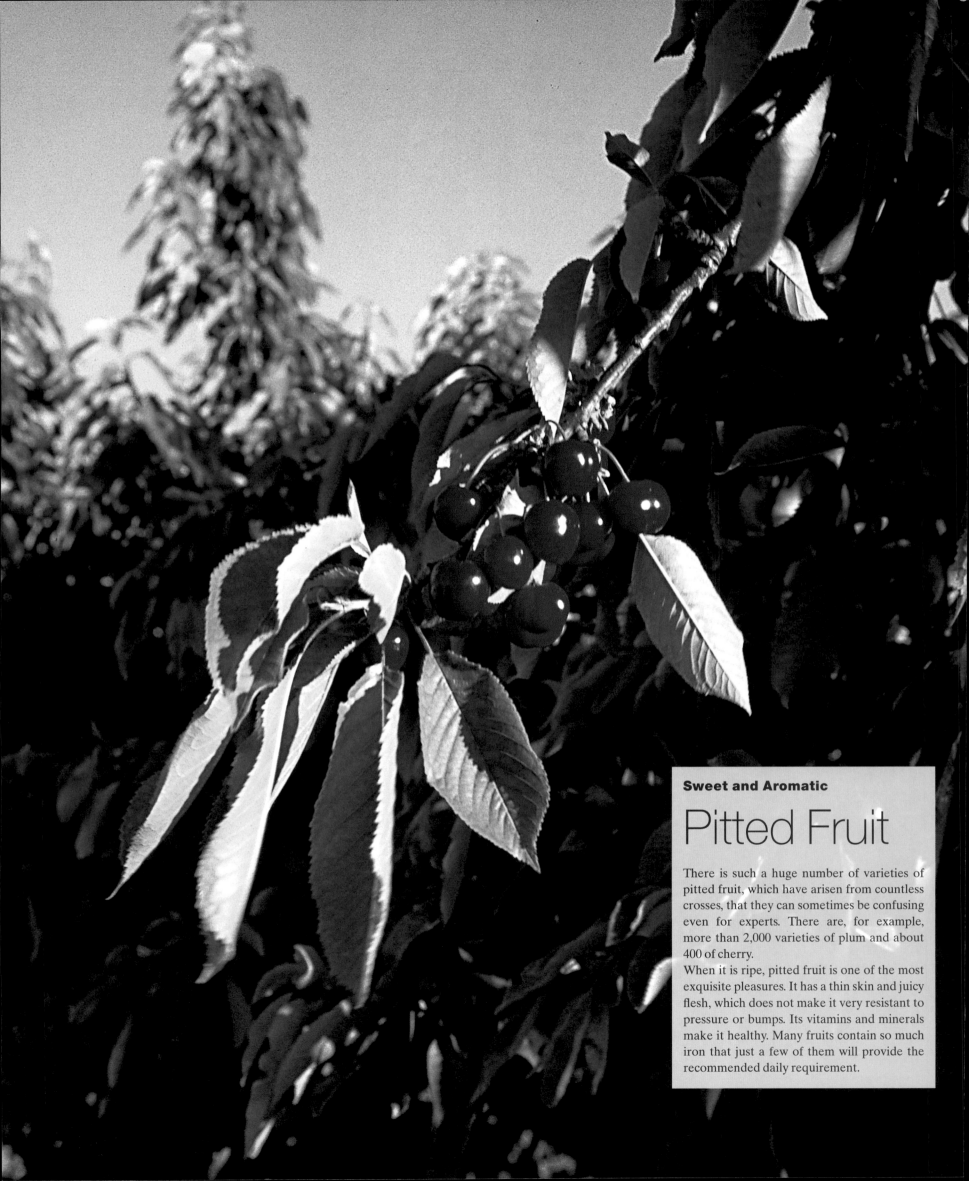

Sweet and Aromatic

Pitted Fruit

There is such a huge number of varieties of pitted fruit, which have arisen from countless crosses, that they can sometimes be confusing even for experts. There are, for example, more than 2,000 varieties of plum and about 400 of cherry.

When it is ripe, pitted fruit is one of the most exquisite pleasures. It has a thin skin and juicy flesh, which does not make it very resistant to pressure or bumps. Its vitamins and minerals make it healthy. Many fruits contain so much iron that just a few of them will provide the recommended daily requirement.

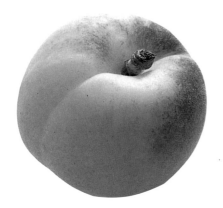

Apricot

Originally a native of Central Asia, this rose plant soon spread throughout the Near East. Easily damaged during transportation, therefore usually picked unripe and so disappointing. When ripe, the yellow to orange velvety fruits are sweet and full of flavor, high in calcium, iron, and provitamin A, and have a pleasantly refreshing sharpness. Available from May through September mainly from Greece, Italy, Spain, and France, but are also cultivated in the Balkan countries. Fresh, as dried fruit (see p. 115), and excellent as jam.

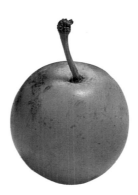

Mirabelle

Belongs to the plum family, with the epithet *syriaca*, which refers to its native country. The fruit loves warmth and will not endure much frost; acclimatized best in Lorraine, Alsace, and south west Germany; the best known variety is the late-flowering Mirabelle de Nancy; thrives well in southern Europe, but not highly regarded. Small, round, yellow fruit which ripens late in August, with slightly red cheeks. Firm, sweet to very sweet flesh which comes away from the pit easily. Often as whole fruit, compote or jam, or distilled to make delicately flavored mirabelle liquor.

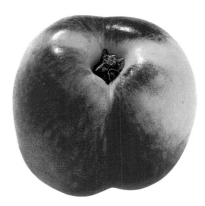

Nectarine

Related to the peach probably from a chance cross with the plum and continued to be cultivated in the last few decades. Its skin is smooth, yellow to dark red in color, the flesh is firm, and it is less susceptible to bruising, much to the delight of those involved in growing and selling it. Nevertheless usually picked when firm so it rarely attains the delicious, juicy flavor it has when fully ripe, a flavor which links it to its ancestors. It then far surpasses them in provitamin A. Cultivated in Mediterranean countries, it is available from the end of May through September.

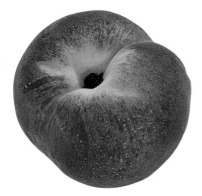

Peach

Was a highly valued fruit in its native China where it was regarded as a symbol of immortality. Today cultivated world wide, but delicate and needs warmth and humus; it places high demands on organic farmers. The main regions are the Mediterranean countries where white clingstone fruit is the first to ripen in May, also yellow varieties from June. Because they are sensitive to pressure they are usually picked green. When ripe, rich in vital substances, including vitamin E and iron, and very juicy. Only keep for a short time, store in a cool place, and throw away any fruit that is even slightly bad.

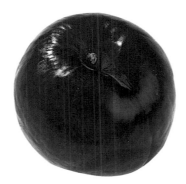

Plum

Prunus domestica is the generic term for the numerous varieties of plum, as well as mirabelles, gages, and damsons. In the narrow sense, it mainly describes frosty, reddy-blue or blue round fruit with very juicy, soft, yellow flesh which quickly cocks to a pulp. In northern countries from July through September, but early and late varieties and imports from the south extend the season. Contains a large amount of vitamin B1 and minerals. Refreshing, despite sweetness, thanks to fruit acids, and aids digestion. Can be used in cakes, for purée, compote, juices, can be dried, or distilled.

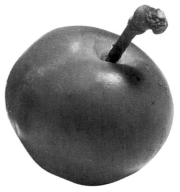

Gage

Greenish, medium-sized round fruit with a distinct cleft, but also purple varieties. The thick bloom – which occurs on all plums – consists of a natural, protective, waxy coating. Aromatic flavor, often extremely sweet and juicy. Originally from the south, because of its resilience to frost spread north where the famous Greengage variety has been found since the middle of the 17th century. Particularly rich in potassium which is very important for the heart. Fruit can be eaten fresh, but also good for preserving or for jam.

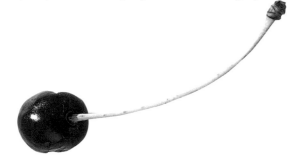

Sour Cherry

Cherries are divided into sour cherries, sweet cherries, and the less important hybrid cherries, crosses of the first two. Cultivated mainly in Europe where they thrive practically throughout except in the very far north. The sour cherries, which are highly valued in the more northerly countries, contain greater amounts of magnesium, iron and, naturally, fruit acid, which stimulates the metabolism, than the sweet varieties. Almost exclusively processed, they are used in the home for making cakes, creams, compote, jelly, and juices, but are used in many different ways in food and drinks. Harvested in July and August.

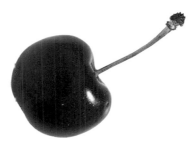

Sweet Cherry

Heralds the arrival of summer when it ripens in May in the south, considered in Asian and Roman mythology to be a gift from the gods. Italy and Germany are the main producers today. Numerous varieties divided into soft-heart cherries and firm-fleshed cherries. Colors range from light yellow to red and almost black, with the darker containing more minerals and surpassing sour cherries in potassium, calcium, and vitamin C. Overall their vital substances are considered to be hematinic and stimulate growth. Mostly eaten fresh and used, preserved and dried in many different ways. Main season June and July.

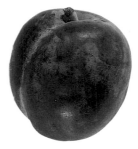

Damson

Long fruit often tapering off with flat, pointed pit which comes away easily. Red, but mostly dark blue with a lighter circlet and yellowy-brown flesh, ripening in September and October. Its main benefit is the firmness of its flesh which means it transports well, stores well, and is good for cooking or baking as it keeps its shape. Particularly popular in northern countries, above all for cakes, as, despite a pronounced sweetness, it has a succinct sharpness and a characteristic flavor. In addition to being eaten fresh, it can be preserved, frozen, dried, or distilled.

Recipes with Plums

Damson Strudel
Mechtildshausen Damson Strudel

Dough

2¹/₄ cups (270 g) fine whole wheat flour
1¹/₂ Tbs (25 g) yeast
¹/₄ cup (50 ml) milk
²/₃ cup (70 ml) light cream
1 Tbs cane sugar
1 egg
Pulp of 1 vanilla bean
Pinch of coarse salt
1 Tbs grated lemon zest

Block of butter

²/₃ cup (170 g) butter
4 tsp (20 g) whole wheat flour

Filling

1 lb 2 oz (500 g) damsons
2 Tbs honey
1 tsp cinnamon
3 Tbs breadcrumbs
1 egg yolk

For the dough, the evening before sieve the flour into a bowl, make a well, and crumble in the yeast. Gently heat the milk and cream and pour onto the yeast. Add the sugar, mix inwards with flour from the edge, cover, put in a warm place, and leave to rise for 30 minutes. Add the remaining ingredients and knead to form a fairly firm dough. Put the dough in the refrigerator and leave to rise overnight.
Take the butter out of the refrigerator.
For the block of butter, the next day mix the butter and flour. Roll the dough out thinly on a floured work surface. Then place the block of butter on the dough and wrap up, pressing the edges down well. Fold the flaky pastry again and roll out so that there are three layers.
Now roll the pastry out to form a rectangle, approximately 12 x 28 inches (30 x 70 cm).
For the filling, pit and chop the damsons, and mix with honey and cinnamon. Sprinkle the pastry with breadcrumbs and spread the damsons over it. Roll up the strudel, brush with egg, and bake in the oven at 400 °F (200 °C) for about 25 minutes, or until golden brown on top.

Damson Dumplings
(Illustration below)

2¹/₂ cups (300 g) fine spelt flour
1 tsp each cinnamon and baking powder
Pinch of coarse salt, grated zest of 1 lemon
9 oz (250 g) farmer's cheese
3 Tbs honey
¹/₂ cup (125 g) cold butter, in small pieces
30 medium-sized damsons
1 egg yolk, 1 tsp milk

Mix the flour with the cinnamon, baking powder, salt, and lemon zest. Next mix the farmer's cheese and honey with the flour then incorporate the butter. Set aside for 40 minutes. Shape the pastry into a long roll and cut this into 30 equal pieces. Form each piece into a dumpling containing a damson (not pitted), and place on a greased tray. Mix the egg yolk with the milk and brush over the dumplings. Preheat the oven to 400 °F (200 °C) and bake the dumplings for about 35 minutes.

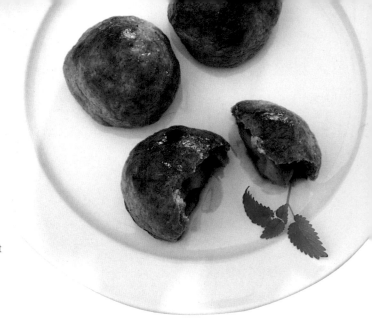

Austrian Damson Doughnuts

Austrian Damson Doughnuts
(Illustration above)

2 cups (250 g) fine rye flour
¹/₄ cup (50 g) butter
3 egg yolks, 2 Tbs honey
16 damsons, 16 almonds
1 tsp cinnamon
Oil for frying

Knead the flour, butter, egg yolks, and honey to form a smooth dough, roll out very thinly and cut out 32 circles approximately 3 inches (8 cm) in diameter.
Pit the damsons and fill each one with an almond. Place each damson on a pastry circle and cover with another circle, pressing the edges of the pastry down well right round the damson and about ³/₈ inch (1 cm) from the

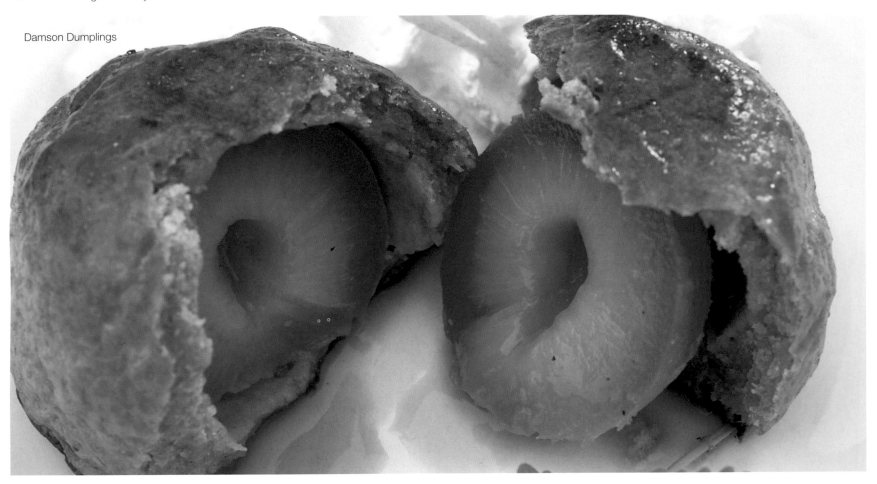

Damson Dumplings

fruit. Heat plenty of oil and deep fry the doughnuts. Drain on paper towels. Sprinkle cinnamon over and serve while still warm.

Cherry Rice Pudding

11 oz (300 g) untreated rice
Pinch of coarse salt
1 tsp cinnamon
1 tsp vanilla extract
3 eggs
1/3 cup (80 g) butter
3/4 cup (80 ml) heavy cream
4 Tbs honey
Grated zest of 1 lemon
1 lb 6 oz (600 g) cherries
3 Tbs chopped almonds

Simmer the rice with the salt and spices in 2 1/2 cups (500 ml) water for 40 minutes, then leave to soak. Separate the eggs. Beat half the butter until creamy. Add the egg yolks, cream, honey, and lemon zest to the butter and mix. Pit the cherries and, together with the butter mixture, mix into the rice. Beat the egg whites and fold into the cherry and rice mixture. Preheat the oven to 350 °F (180 °C). Grease an ovenproof dish and pour in the mixture. Lightly dry fry the almonds in a saucepan, sprinkle over the rice, and dot the remaining butter on top. Bake in the oven for 50–60 minutes.

Black Forest Gateau

Biscuit base
6 eggs
4 Tbs honey
1/2 tsp vanilla extract
Pinch of coarse salt
1/2 tsp baking powder
1 Tbs cocoa
1 1/2 cups (170 g) very fine wheat flour

Filling
1 lb 10 oz (750 g) sour cherries
1 Tbs honey
1 tsp carob powder
2 Tbs kirsch
5 cups (1 l) whipping cream, well chilled
1 Tbs cocoa
1 bar semisweet chocolate

For the biscuit base, separate the eggs. Beat the egg yolks, honey, and vanilla with 6 tablespoons of water until light. Preheat the oven to 400 °F (200 °C). Beat the egg whites with the salt until stiff. Mix the baking powder and cocoa well with the flour. Fold the egg white and flour mixture alternately into the egg yolk mixture. Grease a 10 1/4 inch (26 cm) springform pan, pour in the mixture, smooth out, and bake for 20 minutes. For the filling, pit the cherries, setting 10–12 to one side. Mix the remaining cherries in a bowl with the honey, carob powder and 2 tablespoons of water. Cut the cooled biscuit base into two horizontally and drizzle over the kirsch. Whip the cream until stiff. Spread cream thickly on the first base, arrange the cherries on it, and cover with cream. Place the second base on top. Grate the chocolate. Cover the side and top of the gateau with cream. Dot the top with cocoa, cover the side with grated chocolate. Decorate the top with piped cream and the reserved cherries.

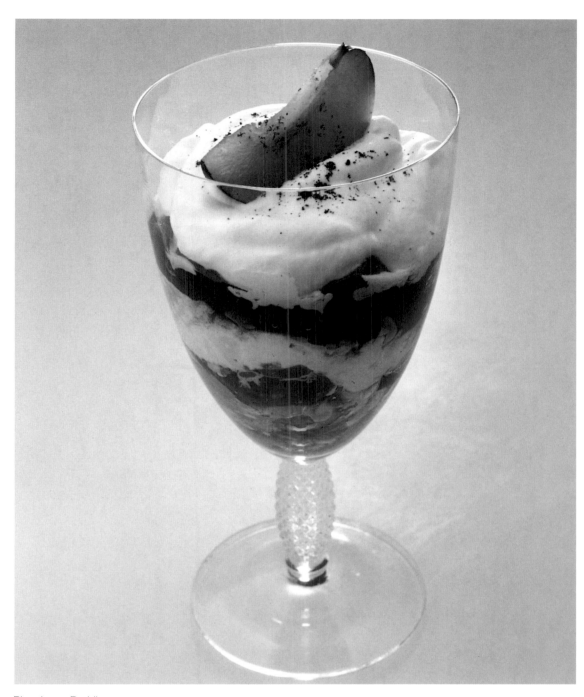

Plum Layer Pudding

Plum Layer Pudding
(Illustration above)

1 lb 2 oz (500 g) plums
1 cinnamon stick
1 Tbs honey
6 rusks
4 1/2 oz (125 g) chopped almonds
1 1/4 cups (250 ml) whipping cream
1 tsp vanilla extract

Pit and quarter the plums, and bring to the boil briefly with 4 tablespoons of water and the cinnamon stick. Sweeten with honey if necessary. Remove the cinnamon stick and leave the mixture to cool. Put the rusks in a cloth and roughly crush with a rolling pin. Lightly dry fry the almonds and mix with the rusk crumbs. Whip the cream with the vanilla until stiff. Put the cooled plums, the rusk and almond mixture, and the cream alternately into tall glass dishes. Finish with a layer of cream, and decorate with a slice of plum.

Plum Sorbet with Cinnamon

9 oz (250 g) very ripe plums
3 egg yolks
5 Tbs honey
2 Tbs rum
1 tsp cinnamon
2 cups (400 ml) whipping cream

Pit the plums and put in a saucepan and stew for 5 minutes, stirring constantly. Press through a sieve and leave to cool.
Beat the egg yolks with the honey until creamy, then gradually stir in the rum and cinnamon.
Whip the cream until very stiff and fold in the cold plum purée. Put into a stainless steel bowl and leave in the ice compartment for 4 hours to go solid.
Serve with a fresh plum sauce made by puréeing 7 ounces (200 g) pitted plums with 4 tablespoons plum wine in a blender.

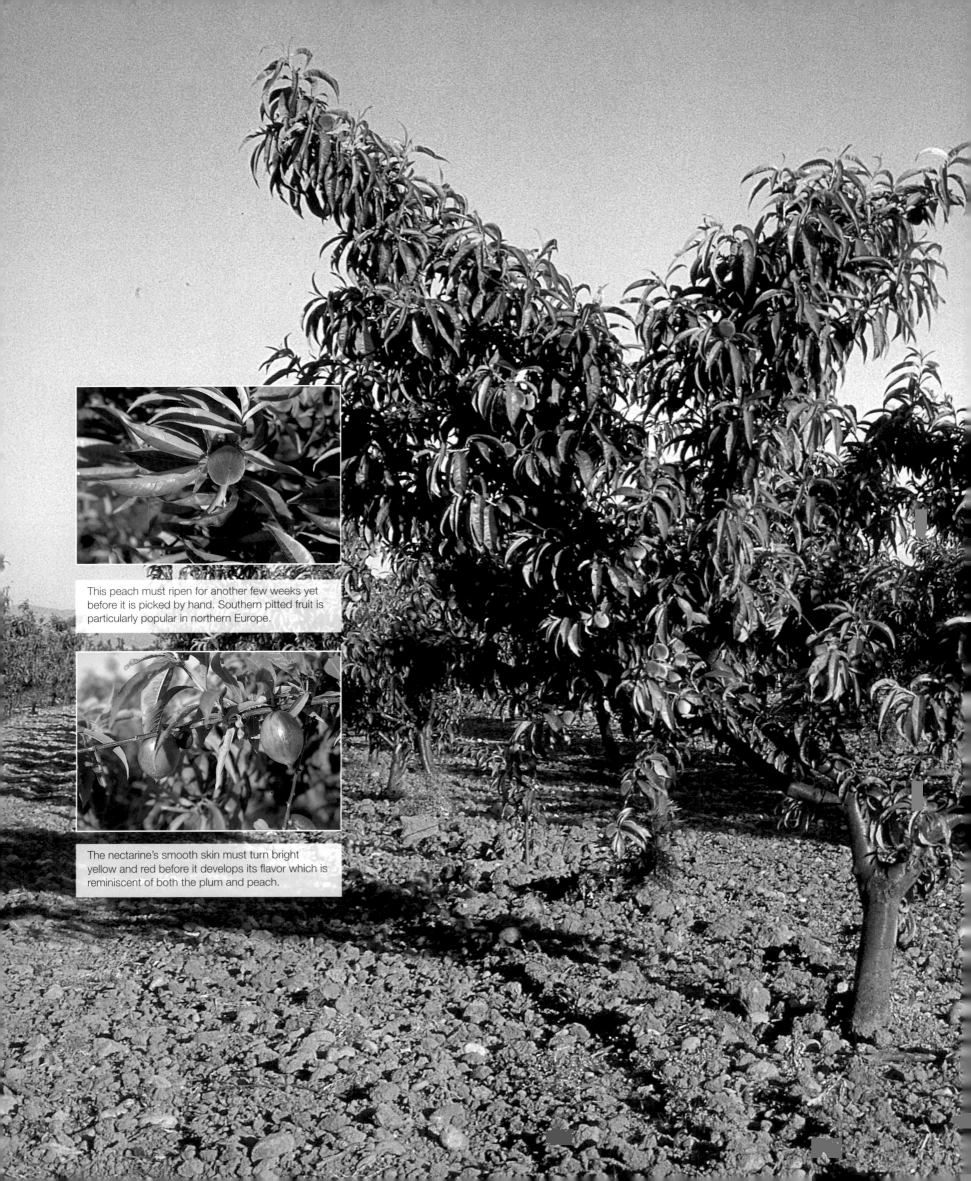

This peach must ripen for another few weeks yet before it is picked by hand. Southern pitted fruit is particularly popular in northern Europe.

The nectarine's smooth skin must turn bright yellow and red before it develops its flavor which is reminiscent of both the plum and peach.

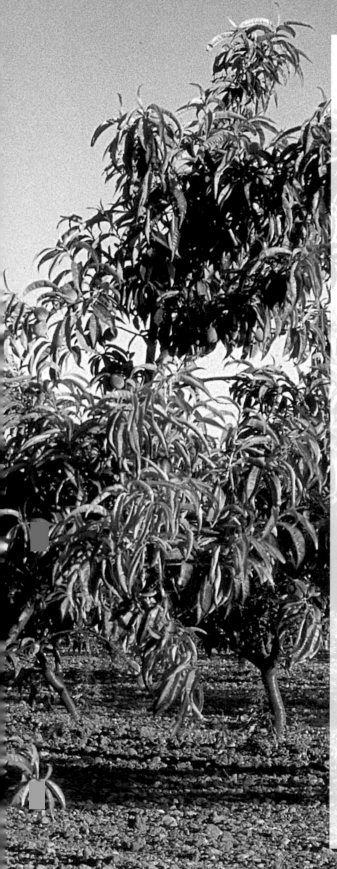

Seductive Summer Pleasures

Southern Pitted Fruit

Apricots, peaches, and nectarines rank among the greatest of summer pleasures. The latter have only arrived in the last decade but with their smooth skins, white or yellow flesh, mild juice, and a taste similar to that of a plum they are winning more and more fans and are holding their own in third place in the league of southern pitted fruit.

Apricots and peaches go back much further. Both fruits made quite an impression on Alexander the Great, with the former being discovered in the Armenian Caucasus, the latter in Persia. Consequently they were given the names of *Prunus armeniaca* and *Prunus persica*, Armenian and Persian plums – wrongly, as apricots and peaches originally come from China and probably reached the Near East via the silk route.

The seductive fruits found great favor with the Arabs, and it was the Moors that introduced them into Spain. It was not long, though, before Arabic doctors took exception to peaches which, they said, were bad for the stomach. It is proven today that they have a dehydrating and slightly laxative effect as well as being extremely beneficial for kidney diseases. Apricots, however, were held in high regard by doctors in the East. Although their qualities are similar to those of the peach they are considerably richer in provitamin A which has a positive effect on growth, the eyes, liver, and skin.

The Moors brought apricots to Roussillon as early as the 10th century. They became acclimatized in the east Pyrenees region of France, which enjoys a Mediterranean climate, five hundred years before they were planted in the Rhône valley. Even today the red-cheeked Rouge du Roussillon is one of the most famous varieties. However, it only started to be cultivated commercially at the foot of the almost 9,200 foot (2,800 meter) high Canigou in 1820. The crisis in the wine-growing industry at the beginning of the 20th century caused many winegrowers in the hot plateaux around Perpignan to switch from traditional winegrowing to the cultivation of apricots.

The warm Roussillon region is not only one of the most important regions for growing apricots but also peaches, which were enthusiastically received and grown in France from the 15th century. This is also the case for fruit cultivated organically. They are some of the most delicate of fruits. In conventional fruit growing apricots and peaches are generally planted on sterilized soil which makes them even more delicate. It is usual to spray them with fungicides and pesticides two dozen times. As both types of fruit are easily damaged during transportation there has been a move towards more robust varieties, more often than not at the expense of flavor. In addition, they are often picked unripe and never achieve the exquisiteness of fruit which has ripened on the trees.

In organic cultivation apricots and peaches place great demands on the fruit farmers, who provide the trees, which are preferably grown on chalky soil, with compost and green manure that is particularly suited to their needs. The farmers then try to increase the trees' resistance by spraying them several times with herbal brews and organic preparations. Once the harvest period arrives, which lasts from the end of May through the end of September, it is a matter of getting the fruit to the customer within two days. There is, though, nothing to compare with the flavor of those bought at markets in the region or direct from the producers: ripened on the tree and freshly picked.

Background: This healthy peach grove in the northern Rhône valley is an example of the high standard of organic fruit growing, as peaches are one of the most delicate of fruits.

Recipes with Apricots, Peaches, and Nectarines

Apricot Chutney

1 lb 2 oz (500 g) apricots
9 oz (250 g) onions
9 oz (250 g) rhubarb
2 oz (50 g) ginger
Juice of 1 lemon
Juice of 1 orange
$^1/_3$ cup (80 g) raisins
$1^1/_2$ cups (300 ml) fruit vinegar
1 tsp mustard seeds
Pinch of cayenne pepper
Pinch of saffron powder
2 Tbs honey

Pit and roughly chop the apricots. Thinly slice the onions and chop the rhubarb into $^3/_8$ inch (1 cm) thick pieces. Finely grate the ginger.
Boil the fruit and vegetables with the lemon and orange juice and the remaining ingredients for about 60 minutes until they are a soft consistency; season to taste.
Pour the chutney into jars and seal tightly. Store in a cool, dark place and allow to mature for several weeks for the taste to develop fully.
Can be kept for about 6 months unopened; after opening keep in the refrigerator.

Peaches in Marsala

4 large yellow peaches
2 Tbs butter
2 Tbs honey
$^3/_4$ cup (150 ml) dry Marsala

Blanch the peaches in boiling water, remove the skins, halve and pit them.
Preheat the oven to 400 °F (200 °C).
Grease an ovenproof baking pan and place the peaches in it cut side down. Mix the honey with the Marsala and pour over the fruit.
Bake in the oven for 25 minutes.

Nectarines in Lemon Marinade

(Illustration below left)

1 lb 10 oz (750 g) ripe nectarines
4 Tbs honey
Juice of 1 lemon

Halve and pit the nectarines, and slice thinly using a sharp knife. Arrange side by side on a plate.
Mix the honey with the lemon juice and pour over the nectarines. Leave to marinade in the refrigerator for 60 minutes and serve chilled.

Peach Cream

(Illustration below)

5 peaches
2 Tbs lemon juice
7 oz (200 g) farmer's cheese
$1^1/_4$ cups (250 ml) heavy cream
1 Tbs honey
Lemon balm

Immerse 4 peaches briefly in boiling water, peel, halve, and pit; purée with the lemon juice. Mix the farmer's cheese with half the cream and the honey, stir in the peach purée and chill.
Whip the remaining cream until stiff and fold into the mixture; pour into individual serving dishes.
Slice the remaining peach, arrange around the peach cream and decorate with a few leaves of lemon balm.

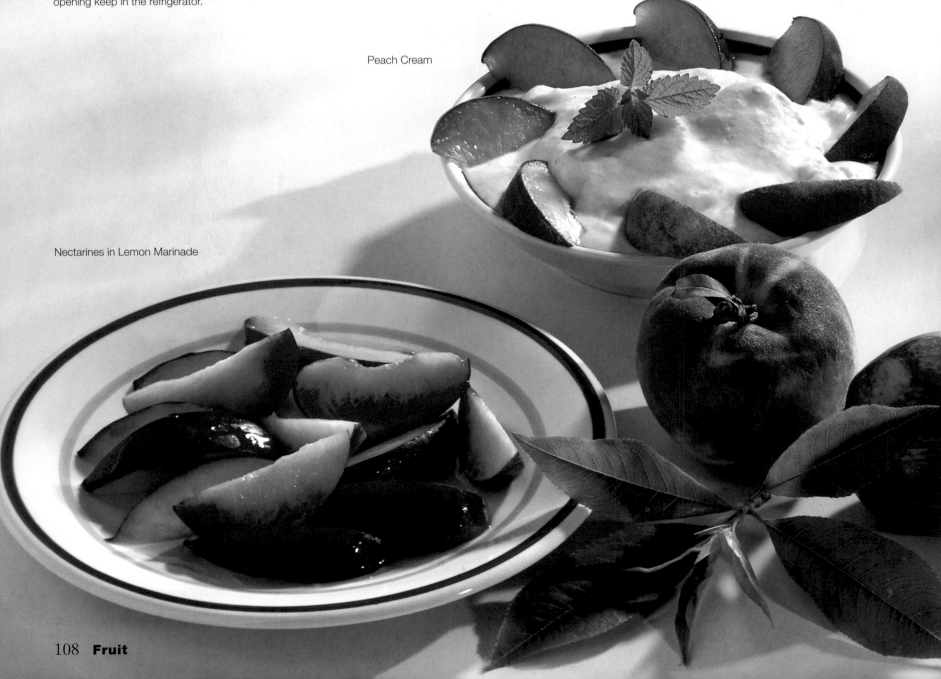

Peach Cream

Nectarines in Lemon Marinade

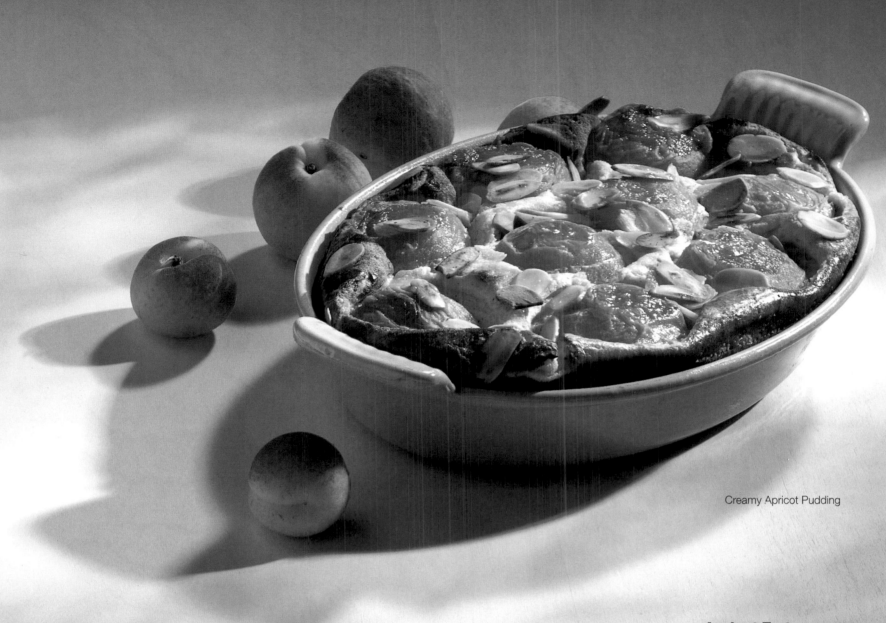

Creamy Apricot Pudding

Apricot Tart

2 cups (250 g) whole wheat flour
1 tsp baking powder
1/2 cup (125 g) cold butter, in small pieces
1 Tbs cane sugar
Grated zest of 1 lemon
Pinch of coarse salt
1 egg
1 lb 10 oz (750 g) apricots
1/5 cup (40 ml) apricot brandy
2 Tbs honey
2 Tbs apricot jam
3 1/2 oz (100 g) slivered almonds

Sieve the flour and mix with the baking powder. Add the butter, sugar, lemon zest, salt, and egg and knead into a smooth shortcrust pastry; if necessary, add 1–2 tablespoons of cold water. Cover and leave the pastry in the refrigerator for 60 minutes.
Blanch, peel, and halve the apricots. Heat 2 tablespoons of water, apricot brandy, honey, and apricot jam in a large saucepan. Add the fruit and simmer for 5 minutes.
Remove the apricots using a ladle and leave to cool. Boil the juice that is left to form a syrup.
Preheat the oven to 400 °F (200 °C).
Grease a springform pan and line with the pastry, prick the bottom with a fork. Cover the pastry with the apricots and press the pastry edge over the fruit slightly. Pour over the syrup and sprinkle with the almonds.
Bake the tart for 40 minutes.

Creamy Apricot Pudding
(Illustration above)

1 lb 2 oz (500 g) apricots
2 eggs
1/2 cup (100 g) butter
1 lb 2 oz (500 g) farmer's cheese
3 Tbs heavy cream
2 Tbs fine spelt flour
1 Tbs cornstarch
1 Tbs honey
1/2 tsp vanilla extract
1 Tbs breadcrumbs
3 Tbs slivered almonds

Halve and pit the apricots and stew them briefly in a little water. Separate the eggs. Mix together the egg yolks, 1/3 cup (80 g) butter, farmer's cheese, cream, flour, cornstarch, honey, and vanilla. Beat the egg whites until stiff and fold into the cream mixture.
Preheat the oven to 350 °F (180 °C).
Grease an ovenproof dish, sprinkle in the breadcrumbs and 1 tablespoon of almonds, pour in the mixture, place the apricots on top and sprinkle over the remaining almonds. Dot the remaining butter on the top of the pudding. Bake in the oven for about 45 minutes.

Apricots with Golden Rivesaltes

12 ripe apricots
2 Tbs finely chopped almonds
3 Tbs honey
3 Tbs lemon juice
1/2 bottle Rivesaltes doré or ambré

Halve and pit the apricots. Arrange in a dish cut side up and sprinkle with the almonds.
Mix together the honey, lemon juice, and wine and pour over the fruit. Chill for 60 minutes.
Note: A Rivesaltes made from white grapes, a naturally sweet wine from Roussillon, often develops an apricot flavor after a few years, when it is referred to as *doré* or *ambré*.

109

Pear Cake

Yeast Dough

1²/₃ cups (200 g) whole wheat flour
1 Tbs (15 g) yeast
Milk
1 oz (25 g) lard
1 egg
Pinch of coarse salt

Filling

8–10 medium-sized aromatic pears
14 oz (400 g) farmer's cheese
2 eggs
¹/₂ cup (100 g) cane sugar
1 Tbs whole wheat flour

Crumble Topping

2 cups (250 g) whole wheat flour
¹/₂ cup (125 g) butter
¹/₃ cup (90 g) cane sugar

For the dough, sieve the flour into a bowl, make a well and crumble in the yeast, pour in some lukewarm milk and mix with a little flour. Cover and leave to rise for 30 minutes.

Add the lard, egg, salt, and a small amount of milk. Knead well together and gradually add enough milk to give a soft dough. Cover and leave to rise in a warm place for a further 30 minutes.

For the filling, wash and peel the pears leaving some of the peel on. Then halve the fruit, and remove the core and stem.

Mix the farmer's cheese with the eggs, sugar, and flour until creamy.

For the crumble, mix together the flour, butter, and sugar. Preheat the oven to 375 °F (190 °C). Put the risen yeast dough into a 10¹/₄ inch (26 cm) springform pan and press flat.

Cover the dough base with a thin layer of the cheese mixture. Place the pear halves close together on the mixture cut side down. Put the remaining mixture on top and smooth out the surface. Then spread the crumble topping over evenly and gently press down. Bake the cake in the oven for about 50 minutes.

Note: The recipe for this pear cake has been passed down through many generations and comes from eastern Europe where pears are used in a variety of ways.

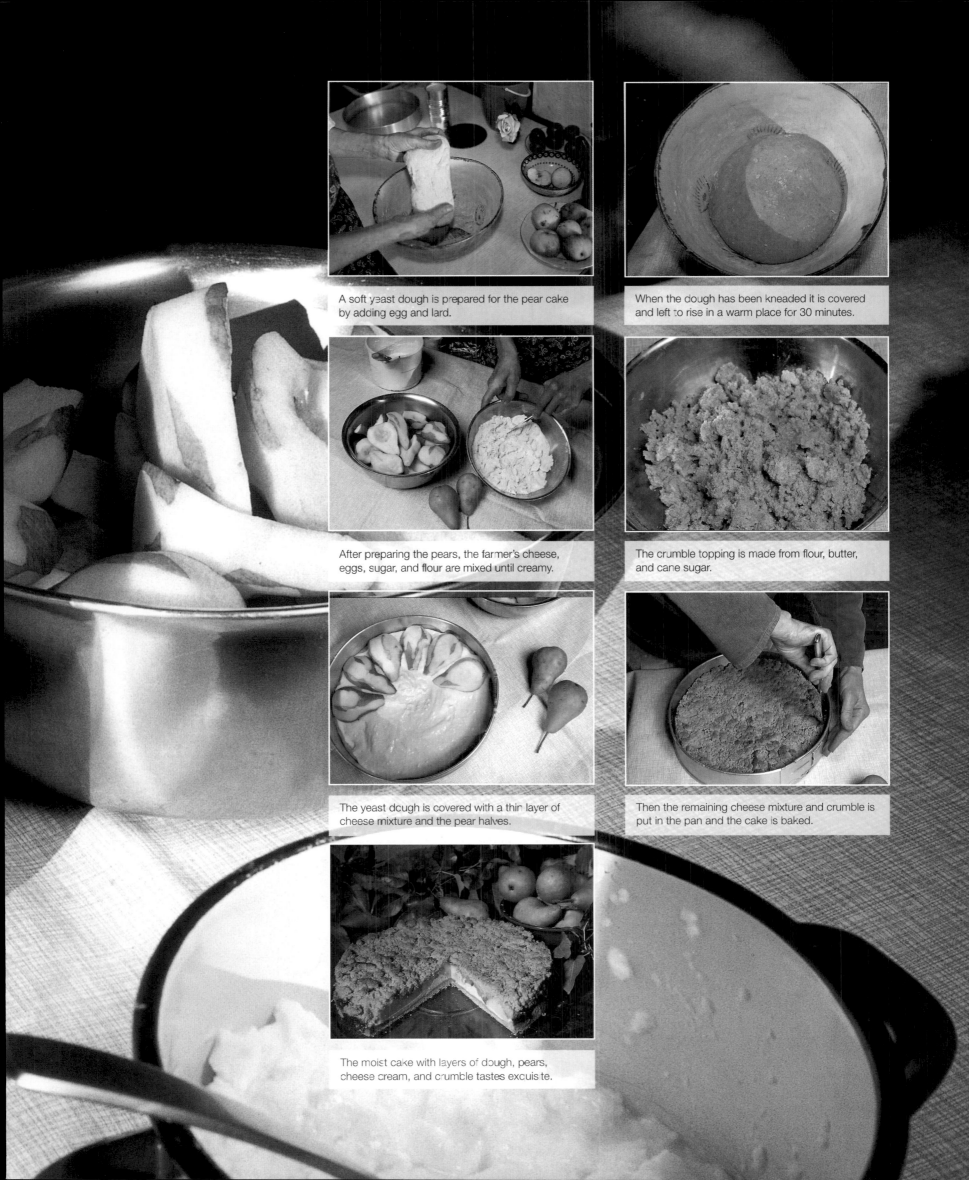

A soft yeast dough is prepared for the pear cake by adding egg and lard.

When the dough has been kneaded it is covered and left to rise in a warm place for 30 minutes.

After preparing the pears, the farmer's cheese, eggs, sugar, and flour are mixed until creamy.

The crumble topping is made from flour, butter, and cane sugar.

The yeast dough is covered with a thin layer of cheese mixture and the pear halves.

Then the remaining cheese mixture and crumble is put in the pan and the cake is baked.

The moist cake with layers of dough, pears, cheese cream, and crumble tastes excuisite.

Jam

Even if sugar is viewed critically, with justification, in wholefood, you do not need to give up sweet spreads or delicious fruit coulis completely. The best method is simply to purée fresh fruit, add spices according to your taste, and sweeten if necessary with honey, cane sugar, or fructose according to taste. Then the ingredients are mixed thoroughly, the purée is put in a screw top jar and kept in the refrigerator.

This quick method produces excellent jam in which the fruit's vital substances are preserved, as are those of the honey. It will keep longer if it is put in small screw top jars. Because it will only keep for a limited length of time it is not suitable for storing or for preserving large quantities of fruit. However, as it can also be made from frozen fruit, homemade jam can be enjoyed outside of the fruit season. It tastes delicious not only on bread, but is excellent as compote, fruit sauce with desserts, and in cakes.

Cherry Jam

7 oz (200 g) pitted sweet cherries
2 Tbs honey
$\frac{1}{2}$ tsp vanilla extract
1 Tbs fruit liquor (Maraschino)

Purée the cherries and mix with the other ingredients. Put into screw top jars which have been rinsed out with hot water, close tightly, and put in the refrigerator immediately. Use within 10 days.

Strawberry Jam

14 oz (400 g) strawberries
1 tsp finely chopped peppermint
1 Tbs lemon juice
2 Tbs cane sugar

Halve the strawberries and purée with the other ingredients. Put into screw top jars which have been rinsed out with hot water, and close tightly. Use within 10 days.

Gooseberry Jam

11 oz (300 g) gooseberries
Pinch of finely chopped thyme
4 Tbs honey
1 tsp cornstarch

Chop up the gooseberries and gently heat with the other ingredients, stirring constantly. Put into screw top jars which have been rinsed out with hot water, close tightly, refrigerate, and use within 2–3 weeks.

Raspberry Jam

14 oz (400 g) raspberries
1 tsp very finely chopped balm
Pinch of ground coriander
1 tsp lemon juice
3 Tbs honey

Purée the raspberries and press through a very fine sieve. Add the other ingredients and mix with the fruit purée. Put into screw top jars which have been rinsed out with hot water, close tightly, and put in the refrigerator immediately. Use within 10 days.

Rhubarb Jam
(Illustrations below)

1 lb 2 oz (500 g) rhubarb
9 oz (250 g) bananas
9 oz (250 g) dried apricots
Pectin-based organic gelling agent
9 oz (250 g) honey

Chop the rhubarb, bananas, and apricots into small pieces and put into a large saucepan. Add the gelling agent, heat and mix into a homogenous mixture using a beater. Remove from the stove and allow to cool a little, then stir in the honey. Put the jam into screw top jars which have been rinsed out with hot water, and close tightly. Store in a cool, dark place. Use within 4 weeks.

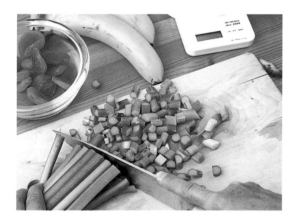

With its distinctive flavor, rhubarb is a popular and easy-to-use ingredient for jams, fruit sauces, and desserts.

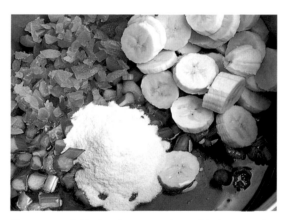

Bananas and dried apricots are often added to round off the taste. The other ingredients are honey and a pectin-rich gelling agent.

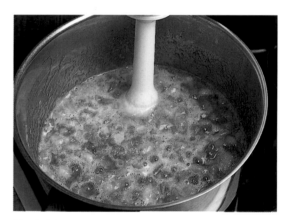

The fruit is heated with the gelling agent and then puréed with a beater. When the purée has cooled a little, the honey is added.

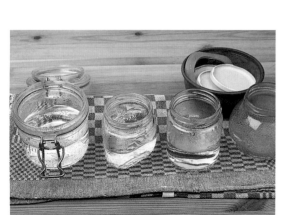

The jars must be washed thoroughly and rinsed out with hot water to sterilize them.

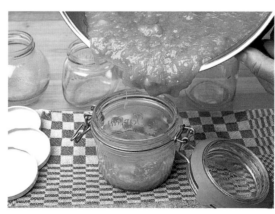

The hot jam is put into preserving jars or jars with screw-on lids which are closed tightly.

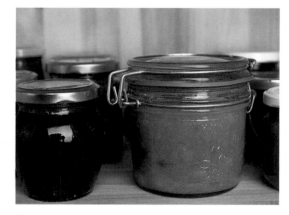

Gently prepared jams only keep for a short time and must be stored in a cool, dark place.

Apricot Jam with Vin Santo

9 oz (250 g) dried apricots
$1/2$ cup (100 ml) Vin Santo
1 lb 2 oz (500 g) fresh apricots
1 Tbs lemon juice
7 oz (200 g) honey

Chop the dried apricots into small pieces, put into a shallow bowl, pour over the Vin Santo, and leave to stand for 6 hours.
Pit and chop the fresh apricots. Drain the soaked apricots and purée with the fresh apricots and lemon juice. Then add the honey.
Put the jam into screw top jars which have been rinsed out with hot water, close tightly, and put in the refrigerator immediately. Use within 10–14 days.

Pruneaux d'Agen and Armagnac Jam

9 oz (250 g) Pruneaux d'Agen (see p. 134)
2 Tbs finely chopped walnuts
$1/2$ tsp cinnamon
Pinch of ground cloves
Pinch of nutmeg
1 Tbs Armagnac
1–2 Tbs lemon juice
1–2 Tbs honey

Pit the prunes and chop into small pieces. Purée with the walnuts, spices, Armagnac, and some lemon juice; add lemon juice and honey to taste.
Put into screw top jars which have been rinsed out with hot water, and close tightly. Use within 4 weeks.

Apple and Carrot Jam

1 lb 2 oz (500 g) carrots
2 tart apples (Cox's Orange Pippins)
Juice of 2 lemons
$1/2$ tsp cinnamon
9 oz (250 g) honey

Finely dice the carrots and simmer in $1^{1}/_{4}$ cups (250 ml) water for 15 minutes, then purée.
Coarsely grate the apples and add to the carrots along with the lemon juice and cinnamon. Cook for 2 minutes, then leave to cool. When the ingredients are hand-hot stir in the honey.
Put the jam into jars which have been rinsed out with hot water, and close. Store in a cool, dark place. Use immediately.

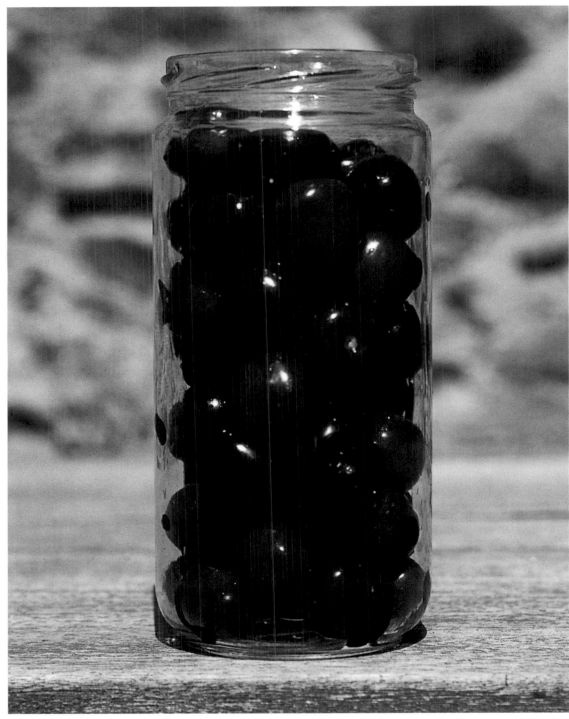

Not all cherries can always be eaten fresh. If they are put into jars with some cane sugar and water, and the fruits preserved, they are a reminder of early summer days, in the middle of winter.

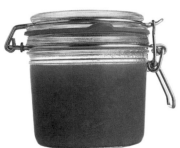

Apricot Jam
Vin Santo gives it that extra something

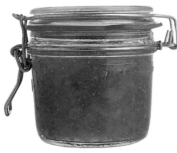

Gooseberry Jam
Thyme gives it a taste of the Mediterranean

Raspberry Jam
Mixed cold and delicately spiced

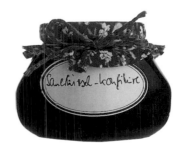

Cherry Jam
Deliciously fresh and with a dash of liquor

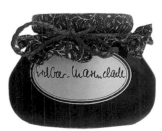

Strawberry Jam
Flavored with peppermint

Dried Fruit

Drying is the oldest and simplest method of preserving fruit. In more northerly parts of the world fruit such as apples or pears was cut into pieces, and hung on string in an airy place or over a stove. This method produced rather unappetizing looking but, due to the sugar concentration, delicious nibbles for the family's own consumption. They lasted significantly longer than stored fruit and could be used soaked as compote or for cakes.

In contrast to fruit that is dried at very high temperatures, often over 200 °F (100 °C), during which most vital substances are lost, gentler methods can be used, of which the most natural is sundrying. In southern and eastern countries dried fruit is an important part of the storecupboard and is used in numerous recipes. It used to be an indispensable element of a nomad's diet and was regarded as an ideal food to take on journeys. In general, figs and dates were two of the most important basic foodstuffs in many eastern countries.

Fresh fruit usually consists of 80 to 90 percent water. As a rule, drying reduces this amount to approximately 25 percent. This leads to a carbohydrate concentration which often increases four to sixfold in relation to weight. The natural increase in the energy value linked to this is almost as great. Less spectacular, but still considerable is the rise in protein, fat, and roughage content. The concentration of minerals and trace elements is also significant with the amounts of potassium, phosphorus, calcium, and iron in particular increasing. While drying clearly reduces the vitamin C content, a larger amount of vitamins B1, B2, B6, niacin, and quite often vitamin E, results from gentle drying methods. Dried fruit can, therefore, be used as an energy food, as well as candy for children, and can add vital substances to many dishes, particularly when uncooked. In addition it is an alternative way of sweetening desserts, cakes, and sauces.

Conventional dried fruit is, however, treated with considerable amounts of sulfur dioxide to prevent discoloring and to combat pest infestation. This, though, destroys the vitamin B1 and can lead to a number of unpleasant symptoms such as headaches and indigestion. For the same reason the fruit is gassed with methyl bromide, a nerve gas, which does evaporate quickly but not without leaving a residue.

Sulfur and chemical poisons must not be used on dried fruit grown organically. Instead quickfreezing is often used today to destroy the eggs of unpleasant pests. The cold is generally the best way of protecting fruit once it has been dried. This also applies in the domestic household. The range

of gently-dried, organic fruit has increased considerably in the past few years with most of it coming from Mediterranean countries. Although quality is much better thanks to modern processes, you should check each packet carefully, something that the regulation transparent packets make possible.

If dried fruit is not simply eaten raw or in granola or fruit salads, it is advisable to soak the fruit overnight in fruit juice or alcohol, depending on what it is to be used for. Then it is perfect for puréeing or cooking. A whole range of dried exotic fruit is now available as snacks. The first ones on the market were treated with sugar, sulfur, and oil, but there are now pineapples, banana slices, kiwi fruits, lychees, mangoes, and papayas from organic plantations.

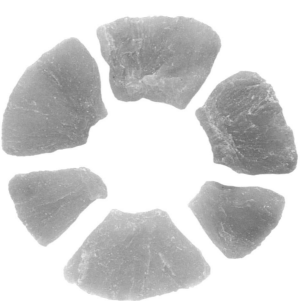

Pineapple
Also grown organically, then cubed and sun-dried; there is thus a concentration of the fruit's sweetness and flavor; an alternative to candy.

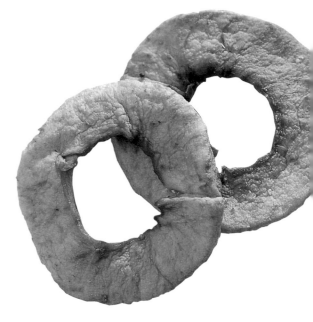

Apple
Mainly available in rings; of a soft consistency, but slightly tough; chopped up small in granola, better still soaked in apple juice, good in compote.

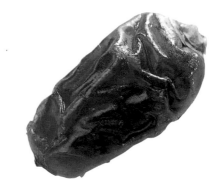

Date
Delicious fruit from the enormous palm of the same name; enhances not only fruit salads, but also avocado salads for example; can be stuffed with nuts or cheese.

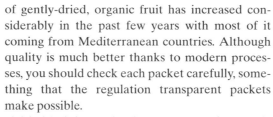

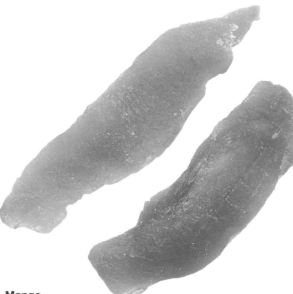

Mango
They are sundried in slices on plantations in several African countries where they are cultivated organically; best used for granola and fruit salad, but also with aperitifs.

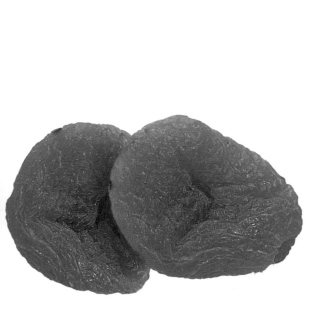

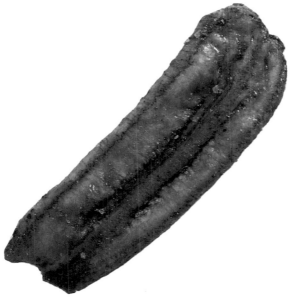

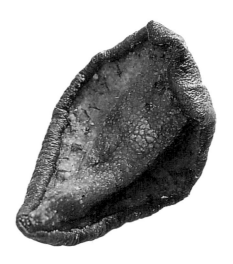

Apricot
Available in halves or as whole pitted fruit, are darker and have more flavor when sun-dried; excellent in creams or jam when soaked, then puréed.

Banana
Dried in various ways, as slices or whole; very intense flavor and particularly kind to the stomach.

Pear
Often dried as halves with distinctive flavor; chopped up raw and added to granola or cakes; soaked and cooked as compote or in desserts.

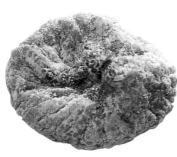

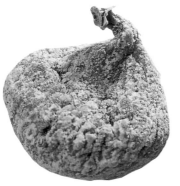

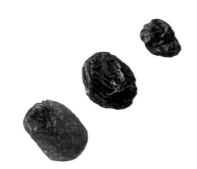

Currant
Originally from Greek Corinth; dried fruit from small, seedless red grapes; not sulfurized even in conventional methods; excellent for baking and cooking.

Raisin
Often generic term for all dried grapes; from various types of vine and for all uses; particularly large and sweet varieties are produced in California.

Sultana
Once only larger, fleshier, Turkish relations of the currant from white, seedless grapes; raw in granola or fruit salad, but above all for baking.

Fig
At its best and most tasty when dried whole and not pressed; can be used in cakes, salads, and for compote.

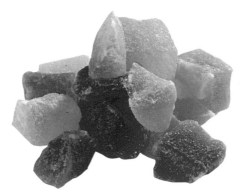

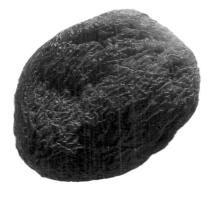

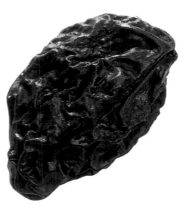

Papaya
Chopped up small and dried, the yellow pieces enhance granola and fruit salad, with the fruit maintaining its ability to stimulate digestion.

Peach
Dried as halves, browny orange, rather tough, and much less aromatic than, for example, apricots; more enjoyable when soaked; in desserts or compote.

Prune
With or without pit, whole or halved; sour-sweet or very sweet – always an intense flavor; a pleasure raw; exquisite soaked and served with meat, in desserts, or ice cream.

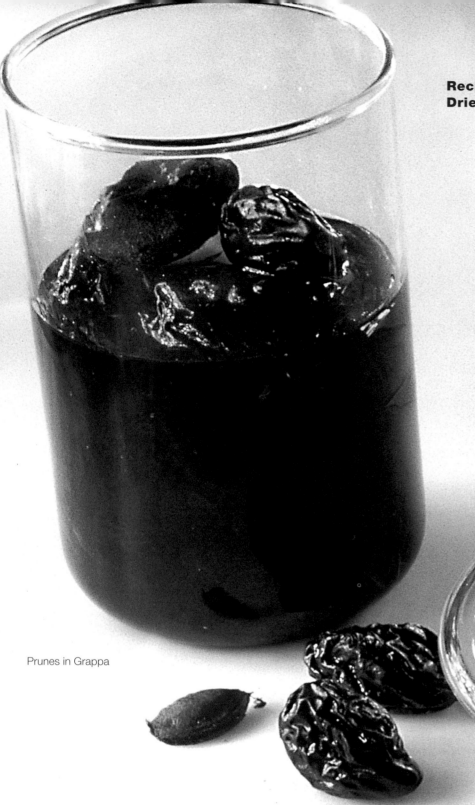

Prunes in Grappa

Recipes with Dried Fruit

Apricot Yogurt Mousse

9 oz (250 g) dried apricots
1^1/$_2$ cups (300 ml) white wine
1 Tbs peach liqueur
3 pots yogurt
Pectin-based organic gelling agent
2 Tbs honey
1 cup (200 ml) whipping cream
1 tsp butter
2 oz (50 g) almonds

Soak the apricots in the white wine for 6 hours; then squeeze out well, collecting the juice. Mix the fruit with the peach liqueur, purée and add the yogurt. Bring to the boil the liquid in which the fruit has been soaked and reduce down to about ^{1}/$_2$ cup (100 ml). Add the gelling agent and boil for 2 minutes, stirring constantly. Mix in the honey and leave the mixture to cool, stirring occasionally; then add to the apricot-yogurt mixture. Whip the cream until very stiff and fold into the mixture. Pour into champagne glasses and chill for 60 minutes.
In the meantime melt the butter and toast the almonds in it; leave to cool. Sprinkle the almonds over the mousse and serve.

Dried Fruit Compote
(Illustration above right)

Serves 2–3

3 dried figs
3 prunes
3 dried apple rings
3 dried pear rings
3 dried apricots
3^1/$_2$ cups (700 ml) apple juice
1 Tbs honey
^{1}/$_2$ tsp vanilla extract
Pinch of cardamom

Soak the dried fruit overnight in the apple juice. The next day, bring to the boil briefly. Add the honey, vanilla, and cardamom.
Serve hot or cold.

Prunes in Grappa
(Illustration above left)

3^1/$_2$ oz (100 g) prunes, with pits
3^3/$_4$ cups (750 ml) Grappa or pomace

Wash and drain the prunes, put into a wide-necked container, large enough to hold 5 cups (1 liter) of liquid, fill up with Grappa and put in a dark place.
After 2 days the prunes will have soaked up the liquor and given it their flavor. The longer the prunes are left, the more intense the flavor will be.

Potato and Oat Dumplings with a Dried Fruit Sauce
(Illustration below)

Dried Fruit Sauce
2 oz (50 g) dried pear slices and apple rings
2 Tbs raisins
1¼ cups (250 ml) apple juice
½ cinnamon stick
1 Tbs arrowroot

Dumplings
1 lb 2 oz (800 g) cooled, cooked potatoes
1½ cups (180 g) medium-coarse oatmeal
1–2 eggs
Bunch of finely chopped parsley
½ tsp herb salt
Pinch of nutmeg
Coarse salt

For the fruit sauce, soak the dried fruit overnight in the apple juice and the same amount of water. Bring the fruit to the boil in the liquid in which it has been soaking, adding the cinnamon. Blend the arrowroot with some water, add to the fruit, and bring to the boil.

For the dumplings, peel and finely grate the potatoes. Add the oatmeal, eggs, herbs, and spices to the potatoes and knead into a dough.

Form the mixture into dumplings and put into boiling salted water. When they rise to the surface simmer for a further 3 minutes. Then remove from the water and drain well.

Pour the fruit sauce onto the plates, arrange the dumplings on top, and serve immediately.

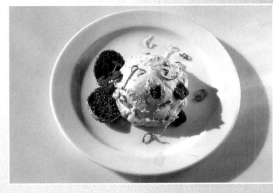

Orange and Fig Cream

6 dried figs
Juice of 2 oranges
1 orange
7 oz (200 g) Mascarpone
1 Tbs honey
½ cup (100 ml) whipping cream
½ tsp vanilla extract
Pinch of aniseed
Pinch of cardamom
1 Tbs grated orange zest
1 tsp grated lemon zest

Chop the figs into strips and leave to soak in the orange juice for 4 hours.

Peel the orange – put the zest to one side – cut it into segments, and chop into small pieces.

Mix the Mascarpone and honey well. Whip the cream until stiff and fold into the Mascarpone mixture.

Add the spices and lemon and orange zest. Finally, mix the figs with the orange juice and orange pieces.

Using a tablespoon put two scoops onto plates. Cut thin strips from the orange zest using a zester and use to decorate the cream.

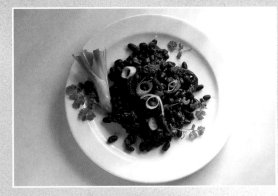

Adzuki Bean and Dried Apricot Salad

8 dried apricots
¾ cup (150 ml) apple juice
5 oz (150 g) adzuki beans
3 Tbs red wine vinegar
2 Tbs safflower oil
1 Tbs honey
1 tsp herb salt
Black pepper
1 Tbs finely chopped thyme
1 leek
2 red onions
Bunch of chervil, finely chopped
Bunch of parsley, finely chopped

Chop the apricots up small and soak in the apple juice overnight. Soak the beans in water overnight.

Drain the beans and cook in fresh water, then drain again. Make a marinade with the vinegar, oil, honey, salt, pepper, and thyme and leave the beans to cool in it. Add the apricots and apple juice and marinade well.

Chop the onions and leek into rings and add to the apricot and bean mixture, along with the herbs. Mix the ingredients together well and season to taste before serving.

Dried Fruit
Compote

Potato and Oat Dumplings with a Dried Fruit Sauce

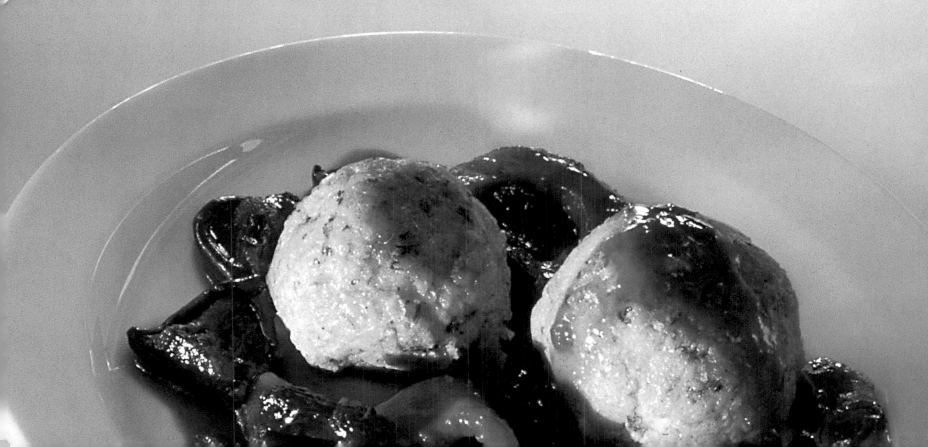

A French Specialty

Pruneaux d'Agen

After California, south west France is the main producer of prunes, the very famous Pruneaux d'Agen. Today only one variety is cultivated, the Prune d'Ente, which is excellent for drying and so has replaced all other varieties down the centuries. It was probably the Crusaders who brought them with them from Syria in the Middle Ages, and monks who were responsible for spreading them in the area north of Agen. This town on the banks of the Garonne gave them their name although they are mainly grown in the Département of Lot-et-Garonne, extending up to Bergerac.

The Prune d'Ente has a frosty purple skin, with a partly reddish, partly pink tinge, and is oval-shaped. Its special quality becomes clear when it is dried. It then has a shiny black appearance and soft consistency, it melts in the mouth, its inside is a rich yellow to amber color and full of flavor. Being a southern plant, it loves sunny slopes, cannot tolerate late frosts, and is sensitive to wind. It likes deep clayey and chalky soils, but not ones that are too moist or sandy. It therefore survives long periods of rain as badly as it does droughts. The trees, which when fully-grown reach a height of 13 to 16 feet (4 to 5 meters), are planted usually 23 by 23 feet (7 by 7 meters) apart in soil which has been well prepared with decomposed manure and compost. Green manure is often used. It is very important that the trees are trained, allowing them a 3.6 foot (1.10 meter) high trunk. Up until the sixth year, when the trees start to produce fruit, the plum grower carefully prunes the tree so its branches form a pyramid shape with the twigs arranged in a herringbone pattern. Pruning it means that the crown of the tree receives plenty of air, and the tree is healthy and the fruit of good quality. The balance of the organic fertilizer and irrigation also increases the tree's natural resistance.

The optimum ripeness of the fruit is an important factor in producing prunes. This requires the foliage to be healthy and plentiful, and the yield to have been controlled, through early thinning out. There are several indicators as to when the fruit is ripe:

- an accumulation of sugar in the flesh,
- a decrease in the acid content,
- a deeper skin coloring,
- a softening of the flesh,
- the fruit dropping without its stem.

Harvesting starts in the second half of August and continues through to the beginning of October. While large concerns use special machines to

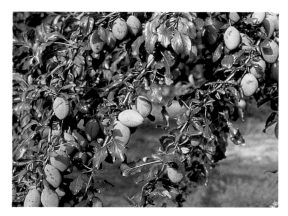

Prunes d'Ente shortly before they are ripe enough for picking.

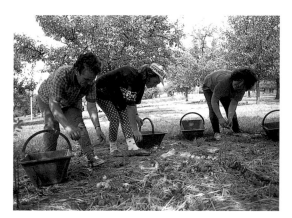

The plums which have fallen are picked up immediately and put into small baskets.

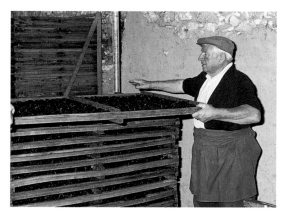

The plums are spread out on frames, which are stacked on trolleys, and wheeled into the huge drying ovens.

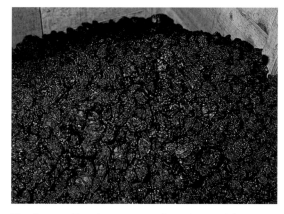

The famous French prunes can be eaten straight away, without having to be soaked.

shake the trees, organic fruit farmers mainly work by hand. But in this case the fruit is not picked. Keeping to the traditional way, experienced harvesters knock sticks against the individual branches. As the ripe plums fall off easily, and what is important, without their stems, this process does not damage the trees. Furthermore, unripe fruit remains on the tree, which helps improve its quality. The fruit is then picked up off the ground. Using this method one person collects between 770 and 1,100 pounds (350 and 500 kilograms) of plums per eight hour working day. Three to five days are needed to harvest 200 trees which normally cover an area of 2.5 acres (one hectare).

The plums are spread out in a single layer on frames, between which air can circulate. In the past they were dried in the sun or bread ovens. Today the frames, which are stacked on trolleys, are wheeled into large drying chambers or tunnels. Hot air is blown into these and moist air sucked out. There is a total of 18 to 24 hours between the pre-drying phase, which occurs at 117 °F (60 °C), and the *finition* (finishing process), which takes place at 150 °F (75 °C). The aim is to reduce the plums' moisture content to 21 to 23 percent, and at the same time preserve and increase their flavor through an initial cooking stage. On the other hand, caramelization has to be prevented as it spoils the flavor and gives the plums an undesirable brown color. The temperature inside the fruit must, therefore, not exceed 150 °F (75 °C).

The plums are dried as soon as they are harvested. They are then stored in large wooden boxes at a temperature of 14 to 20 °F (7 to 10 °C) in a dark room with 70 percent humidity, to prevent them from going bad. Before they are sold, the Pruneaux d'Agen undergo a brief, hot water bath so that their moisture content increases by about 10 percent. This gives them an attractive shine and exquisitely soft consistency, and means that the consumer can eat them straight away.

2.5 to 3.5 pounds of fresh fruit is needed to make one pound of prunes, depending on degree of ripeness and size. Because of their high roughage content they are marvelous for the digestion. They are rich in provitamin A, as well as B vitamins, potassium, phosphorus, magnesium, and iron, and, with their carbohydrate content, are a healthy, nerve-strengthening, and effective source of energy.

Right-hand page: Knocks from a stick start the branches of the plum trees swinging so that the ripe plums fall down.

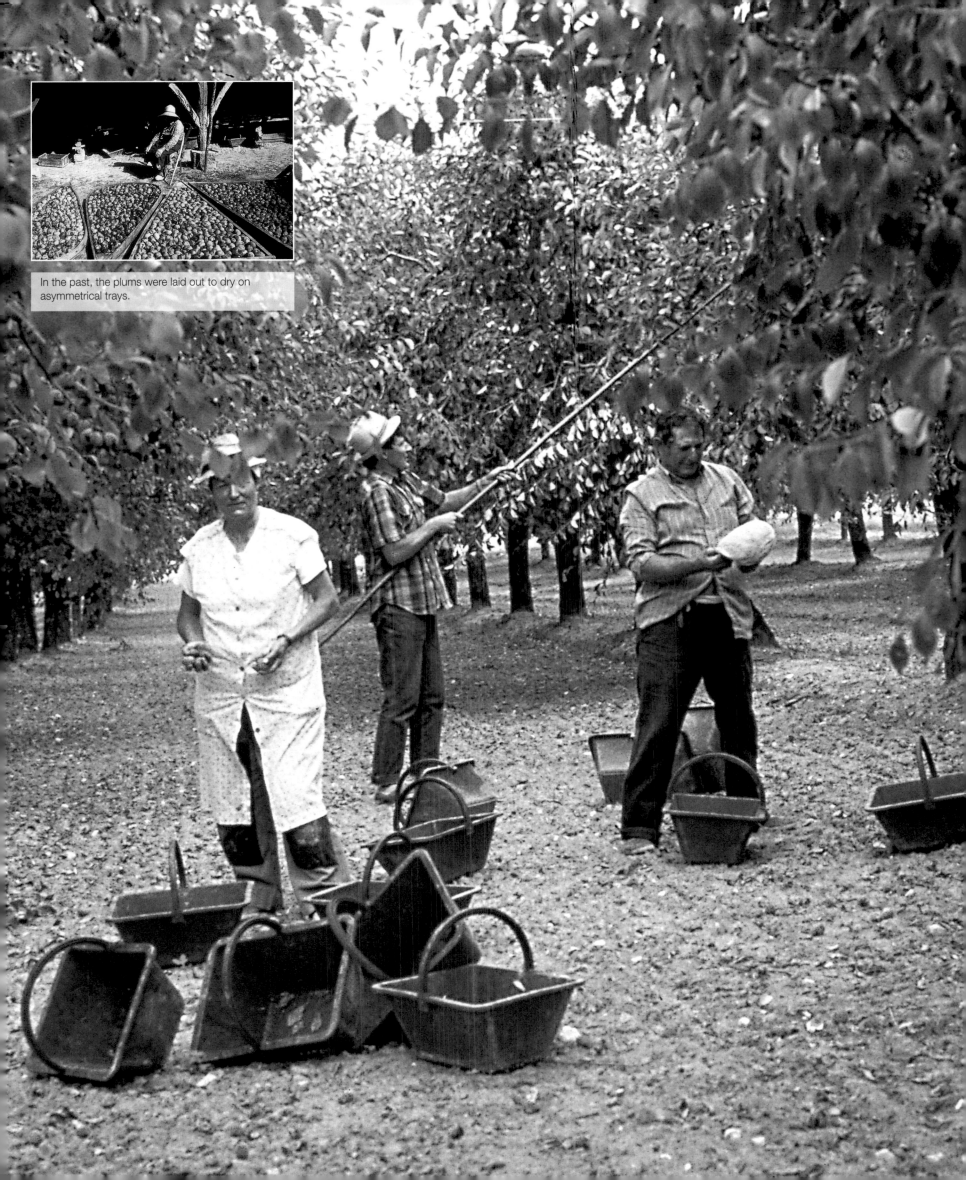

In the past, the plums were laid out to dry on asymmetrical trays.

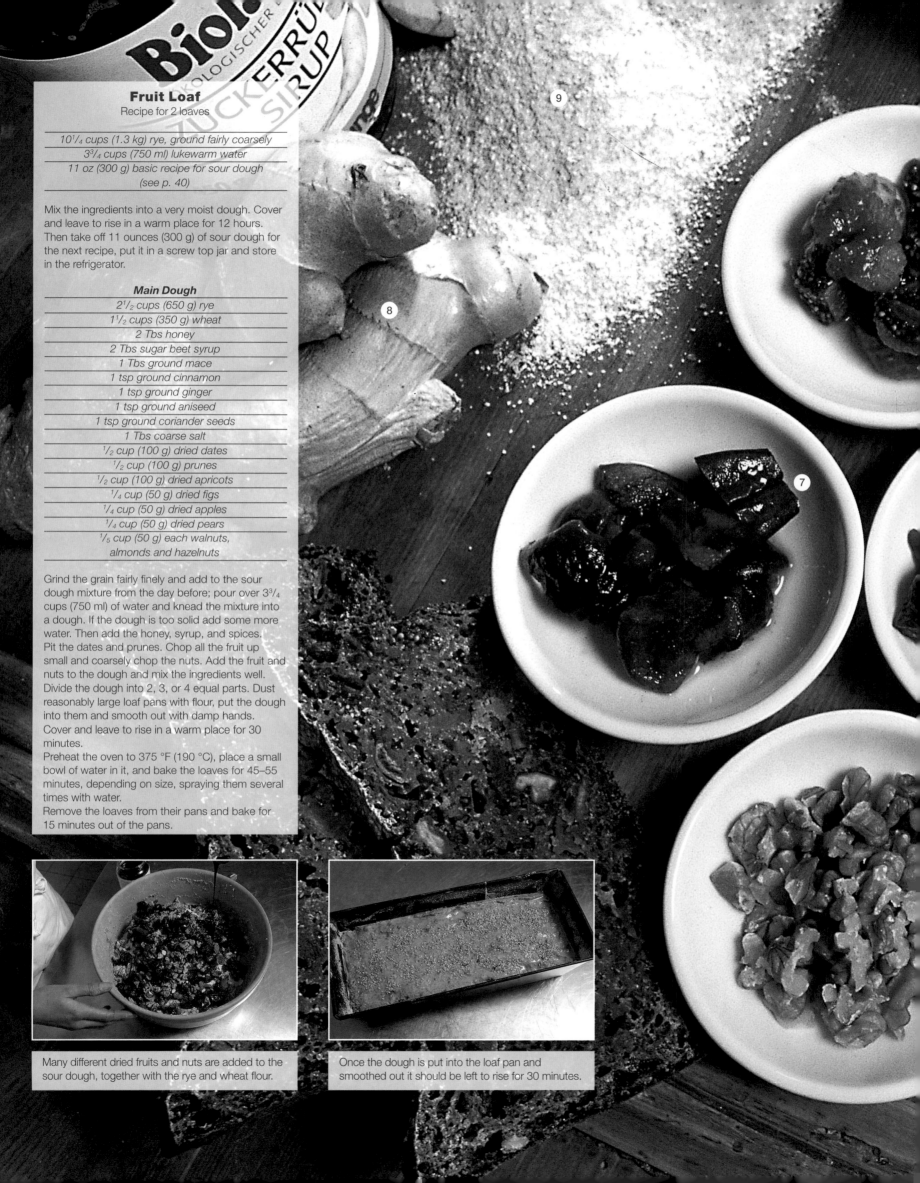

Fruit Loaf
Recipe for 2 loaves

10¼ cups (1.3 kg) rye, ground fairly coarsely
3¾ cups (750 ml) lukewarm water
11 oz (300 g) basic recipe for sour dough
(see p. 40)

Mix the ingredients into a very moist dough. Cover
and leave to rise in a warm place for 12 hours.
Then take off 11 ounces (300 g) of sour dough for
the next recipe, put it in a screw top jar and store
in the refrigerator.

Main Dough
2½ cups (650 g) rye
1½ cups (350 g) wheat
2 Tbs honey
2 Tbs sugar beet syrup
1 Tbs ground mace
1 tsp ground cinnamon
1 tsp ground ginger
1 tsp ground aniseed
1 tsp ground coriander seeds
1 Tbs coarse salt
½ cup (100 g) dried dates
½ cup (100 g) prunes
½ cup (100 g) dried apricots
¼ cup (50 g) dried figs
¼ cup (50 g) dried apples
¼ cup (50 g) dried pears
⅕ cup (50 g) each walnuts,
almonds and hazelnuts

Grind the grain fairly finely and add to the sour
dough mixture from the day before; pour over 3¾
cups (750 ml) of water and knead the mixture into
a dough. If the dough is too solid add some more
water. Then add the honey, syrup, and spices.
Pit the dates and prunes. Chop all the fruit up
small and coarsely chop the nuts. Add the fruit and
nuts to the dough and mix the ingredients well.
Divide the dough into 2, 3, or 4 equal parts. Dust
reasonably large loaf pans with flour, put the dough
into them and smooth out with damp hands.
Cover and leave to rise in a warm place for 30
minutes.
Preheat the oven to 375 °F (190 °C), place a small
bowl of water in it, and bake the loaves for 45–55
minutes, depending on size, spraying them several
times with water.
Remove the loaves from their pans and bake for
15 minutes out of the pans.

Many different dried fruits and nuts are added to the
sour dough, together with the rye and wheat flour.

Once the dough is put into the loaf pan and
smoothed out it should be left to rise for 30 minutes.

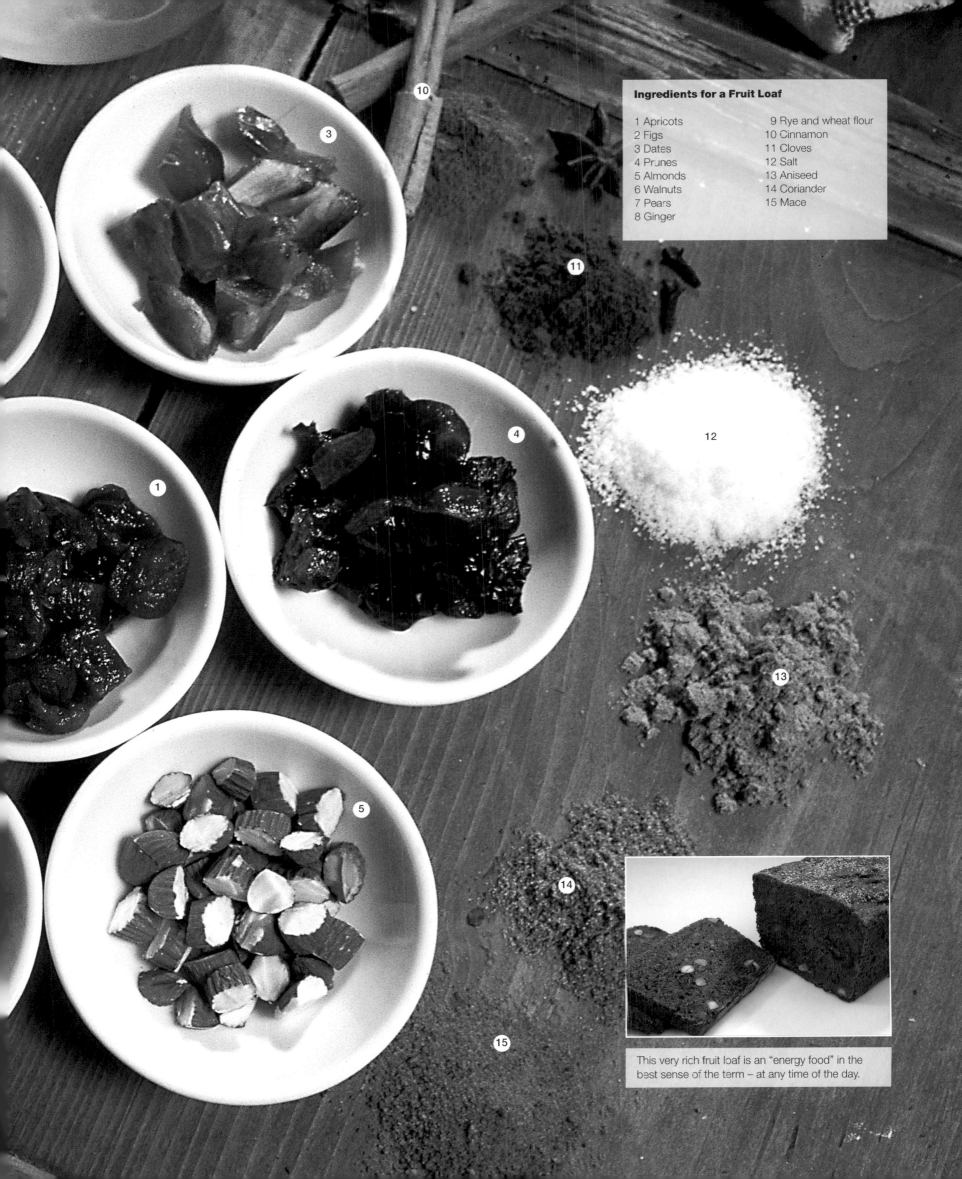

This very rich fruit loaf is an "energy food" in the best sense of the term – at any time of the day.

Nutritious and Filling

Nuts

Nuts are historically considered to be one of man's first foods. One of their main advantages is that they can be stored. In America many Indian tribes stocked up predominantly with nuts for the winter and were supposed to have lived exclusively off them often for weeks at a time.

Under the term nuts, a distinction can be made between, on the one hand, the edible seeds of fruits, and, on the other hand, the fruits themselves. They are extremely nutritious and a valuable foodstuff. Walnuts and Brazil nuts have over 700 calories per 3.5 ounces (100 grams). It is, though, not only because of their energy values that nuts put most fruit in the shade. Apart from pulses, they have the highest protein content in the vegetable kingdom by about 15 to 25 percent. They even compare favorably with meat and fish with their protein being more digestible. With the exception of coconut and chestnuts, they are rich in unsaturated fats, particularly linoleic acid (see pp. 20–21), which is why they are beneficial for heart and vascular problems. Nuts do, though, have the disadvantage of going rancid quickly as they can be made up of over 60 percent oil. This is particularly the case when they are shelled.

Their health value is increased by the abundance of vital substances. They are rich in vitamins and mostly contain many B vitamins, especially B1, B2, and B6, which stimulate growth, the nervous system, and brain functions, as well as astonishing amounts of vitamin E, which not only prevents the nut oil from oxidizing too quickly, but also helps to protect cells in the human body. With comparatively high concentrations of calcium, potassium, phosphorus, and magnesium, nuts provide the body with important mineral constituents for growth and metabolism.

Because of these concentrated, positive properties, nuts make excellent provisions and provide an energy boost when one is needed. They are highly valued ingredients in wholefood cookery precisely because they increase the protein content, provide essential fatty acids, and supply important vitamins. Their natural shells not only keep these substances in an optimum condition, but they also guarantee that they have not been denatured with salt, inferior fats, and additives.

A Nut Glossary

Cashew
The kidney-shaped nut, which grows at the end of an apple-like, edible fleshy stalk, originally comes from the West Indies. Its hard shell contains a corrosive toxin used in industry. Today it is cultivated in Africa and India as well as South America, and is only sold shelled. The whole white nuts, which are also available roasted and salted, taste best.

Peanut
It is the outsider of the pulse family. The plant is an annual shrub which pushes its fruit into the earth where it matures a few inches below the surface. The pods dry there and are then lifted. Peanuts, which are grown in nearly all hot countries, are an important foodstuff. They are very rich in protein and oil. When raw they taste a bit like beans, when roasted they have a nutty flavor.

Sweet Chestnut
It grows wild in Mediterranean countries, but has spread to southern Germany and England. Prime specimens reach heights of over 65 feet (20 meters). Its edible seeds are enclosed in thorny hulls, which burst open when they are ripe. The somewhat smaller maroons are better tasting. Before the introduction of potatoes they were an important foodstuff. They were served with vegetables and meat, and used as flour in bread and cake mixtures.

Hazelnut
Common throughout Europe a long time ago, hazelnuts, which are nutritious and keep well, were one of man's first foods. Today the shrubs are cultivated mainly in Turkey and the other Mediterranean countries. The numerous varieties are divided into more round, and long shapes. Hazelnuts, with their beautiful hard husks, usually come from Germany or France and are generally sold shelled.

Coconut
The fruit of a palm which grows to a height of 100 feet (30 meters) and thrives in tropical regions. The nuts are surrounded by a thick fibrous layer which is used for rope, mats, sacks, etc. If the coconut is fresh it will contain liquid which you can hear if you shake it. Avoid any that are mildewy at the eyes. Its fat, with predominantly saturated fatty acids, does not play a part in wholefood.

Macadamia
A particularly delicious, fine nut native to Australia and discovered by the explorer McAdam in 1857. Today the small, evergreen trees are also grown in Africa, America, and Spain. The round nuts, which are somewhat larger than hazelnuts, are surrounded by a thin, semisolid shell that can be cut open with a knife. Unfortunately they are almost always sold shelled, often roasted in oil and then salted.

Almond
Almond trees grow around the Mediterranean, but are also cultivated in the Near East, California, and elsewhere. The drupe fruit which is related to the peach is surrounded by a furry, rough outer shell which splits when ripe and releases the hard, light brown nutshell. If you cannot buy sweet almonds in their shells, you should if possible choose ones with thin, brown skins and not the blanched or ground sort.

Brazil Nut
It comes from a tropical tree which reaches a height of over 165 feet (50 meters), but is rarely cultivated. The nuts are gathered. They are found, often two or three dozen together, in spherical capsules about the size of a head which fall to the ground in late fall. The actual nuts have a thin, but very hard, three-sided shell. They are usually sold in this shell. Be careful that it is not bad inside.

Pecan
Native to the southern United States, the nuts, which resemble acorns, were important winter supplies for Indian tribes. Today the largest plantations of these trees which often reach a height of 130 feet (40 meters) are in the southern states. They are now also grown in other countries and continents, and are related to the walnut tree. Pecan nuts are available shelled and unshelled, but the thin shells are easy to crack.

Pine Nut
Umbrella Pines, which add charm to Mediterranean coasts, form cones the size of a fist. The long seeds are on the hard segments of the cones. If the protective brown skin is removed small ivory-colored spindles appear. Their contents are similar to nuts. A valuable ingredient in Iberian, Italian, and oriental cookery, they are always sold shelled and sometimes roasted.

Pistachio
The evergreen tree has been cultivated for many thousands of years in the Near East where its small kernel can be eaten raw or is used in dishes for its greenish color. When ripe the pale shells split open by themselves and release the uneven kernel which is surrounded by a darker skin. Often available roasted and salted with or without shells.

Walnut
The imposing, sweeping tree, a native of the Far East, is common in all milder regions today. The main producer is California, in Europe it is France and Italy. On the tree the nuts are encased in a green leathery hull which splits open when the nut is ripe. The inside of its two halves forms a subdivided shell containing the kernels. They are also available without shells, but are more popular as whole nuts.

Right-hand page:	4	Hazelnut	10	Walnut
1 Cashew nuts	5	Coconut		
2 Peanuts	6	Almonds		
3 Sweet chestnut	7	Brazil nut		Background: A sweet chestnut tree in blossom.
	8	Pine nut		
	9	Pistachio		

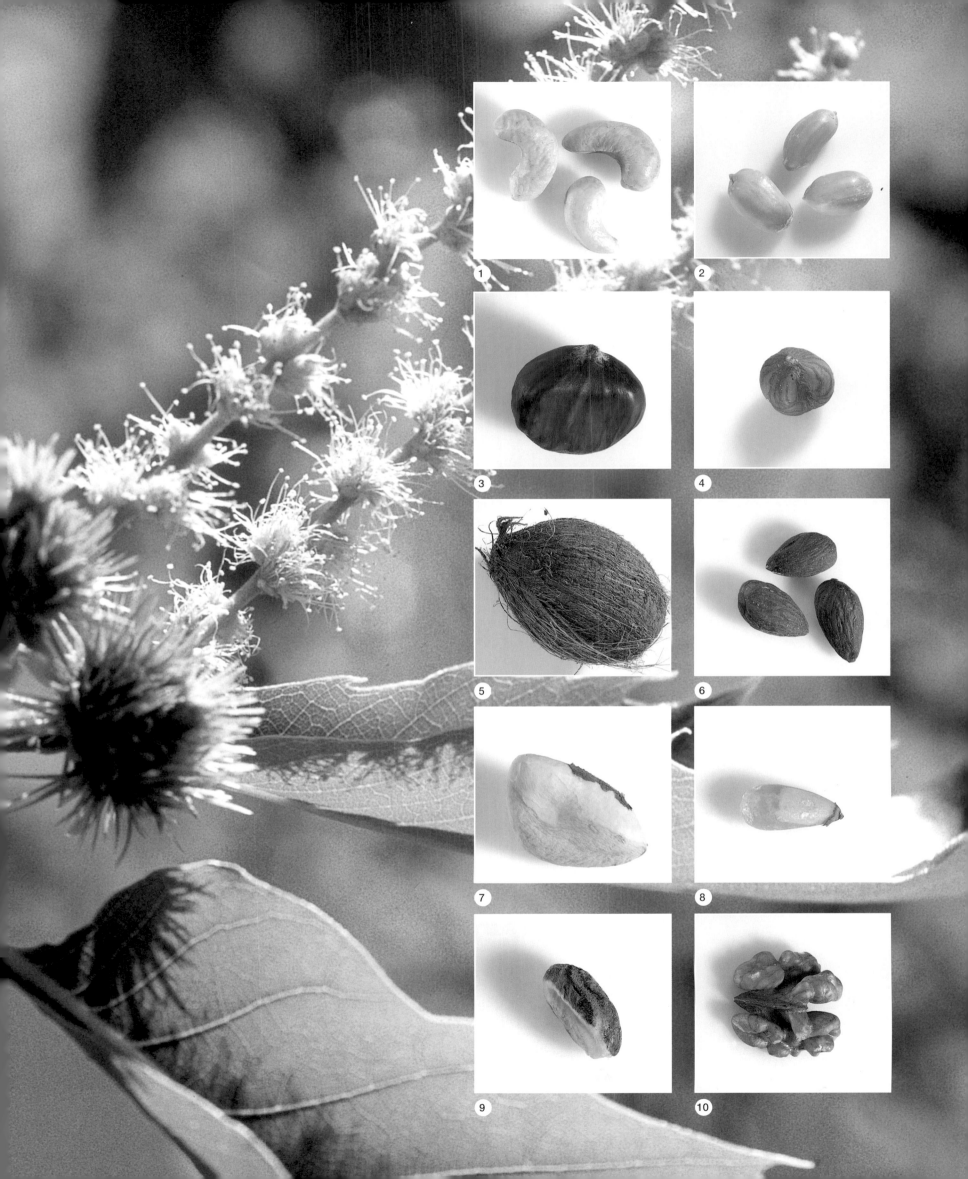

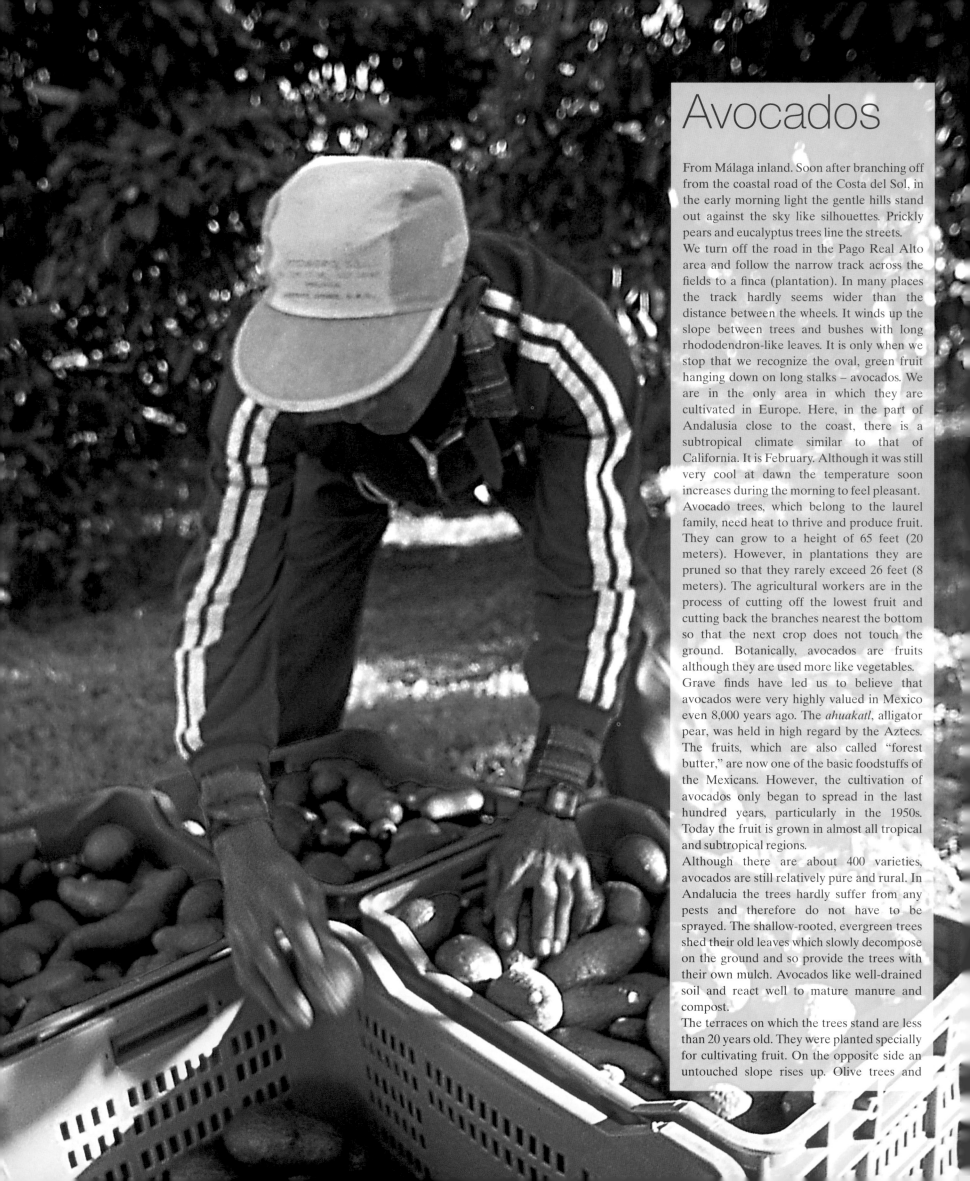

Avocados

From Málaga inland. Soon after branching off from the coastal road of the Costa del Sol, in the early morning light the gentle hills stand out against the sky like silhouettes. Prickly pears and eucalyptus trees line the streets.

We turn off the road in the Pago Real Alto area and follow the narrow track across the fields to a finca (plantation). In many places the track hardly seems wider than the distance between the wheels. It winds up the slope between trees and bushes with long rhododendron-like leaves. It is only when we stop that we recognize the oval, green fruit hanging down on long stalks – avocados. We are in the only area in which they are cultivated in Europe. Here, in the part of Andalusia close to the coast, there is a subtropical climate similar to that of California. It is February. Although it was still very cool at dawn the temperature soon increases during the morning to feel pleasant. Avocado trees, which belong to the laurel family, need heat to thrive and produce fruit. They can grow to a height of 65 feet (20 meters). However, in plantations they are pruned so that they rarely exceed 26 feet (8 meters). The agricultural workers are in the process of cutting off the lowest fruit and cutting back the branches nearest the bottom so that the next crop does not touch the ground. Botanically, avocados are fruits although they are used more like vegetables.

Grave finds have led us to believe that avocados were very highly valued in Mexico even 8,000 years ago. The *ahuakatl*, alligator pear, was held in high regard by the Aztecs. The fruits, which are also called "forest butter," are now one of the basic foodstuffs of the Mexicans. However, the cultivation of avocados only began to spread in the last hundred years, particularly in the 1950s. Today the fruit is grown in almost all tropical and subtropical regions.

Although there are about 400 varieties, avocados are still relatively pure and rural. In Andalucia the trees hardly suffer from any pests and therefore do not have to be sprayed. The shallow-rooted, evergreen trees shed their old leaves which slowly decompose on the ground and so provide the trees with their own mulch. Avocados like well-drained soil and react well to mature manure and compost.

The terraces on which the trees stand are less than 20 years old. They were planted specially for cultivating fruit. On the opposite side an untouched slope rises up. Olive trees and some holm oaks are growing in the distance. A small, whitewashed, but deserted Finca stands on the top of the hill. For centuries cattle were kept and olives harvested on the hills. Then progress brought water pipes. The slopes were taken over by fruit growing while vegetables were now grown intensively in the valley.

The organic cultivation of avocados in Europe is due to the initiative of two Germans. Under the name of "Campiña Verde" (green fields) and starting from Córdoba, they began to convince Andalucian farmers about organic methods, advise them about switching over and cultivation, and look after the marketing of their organic products throughout Europe. The hardy avocado trees were particularly suited to organic cultivation, something in which the first Finca in the Entre Rios municipality specialized in the mid-1980s. Now a good 120 acres (50 hectares) of magnificent trees extend over gentle slopes. In order to be able to harvest the pitted fruit, the workers move between the high rows of trees with elevating platforms. It is particularly important that the avocados are cut off individually to guarantee top quality. In this way the stalk remains on the fruit and so the latter can ripen to its optimum condition and is protected against rot at its most delicate point. The freshly picked avocados are taken in small crates to the nearby producers' association and are packed according to size ready for transporting. According to the regulations, for size 12 there are to be 12 fruits in the boxes which hold 8.8 pounds (4 kilograms), for size 28 there are to be 28.

Several Fincas now specialize in the organic cultivation of avocados. By planting several varieties they are able to supply avocados nine months a year; only from July through September no avocados are available. Of the five varieties Bacon, Fuerte, Pinkerton, Hass, and Reed, Hass has the best flavor. Rudolf Hass, a German mailman who emigrated to America, discovered the rough-skinned variety in his garden in California at the beginning of the 1930s. He propagated the variety which had developed from a natural cross. Its special feature is its skin which turns a dark color as it ripens, making the Hass the only variety of avocado that gives the consumer a visual indication of when it is ready to be eaten. Because of its nutty flavor the Hass is the preferred fruit of all avocado lovers.

In order to be able to supply high quality fruit, the ripening time is established as precisely as possible in organic cultivation. This is not at all

Left-hand page: Avocados are always harvested when they are "tree ripe." They are still hard and inedible then. They only become ripe enough to eat after storage. Because of their hardiness, avocado trees are particularly suited to organic cultivation.

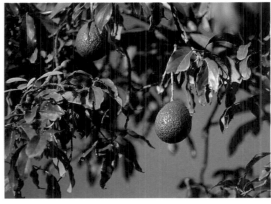

Avocados are the fruits of very hardy, evergreen trees which hardly suffer from disease or insects.

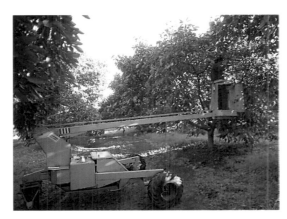

The laurel plants, which love the subtropical climate, reach a height of 65 feet (20 meters). Special elevating platforms are needed for harvesting.

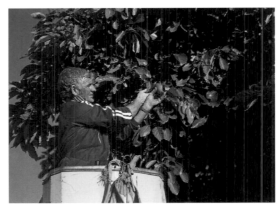

The self-propelled platforms lift the workers up to the tops of the trees where the fruit is cut by hand. In this way the stalk remains on the fruit.

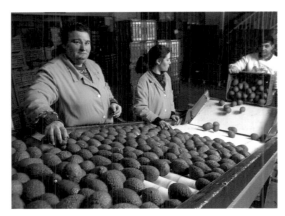

The freshly picked fruit is prepared for the market by the cooperative.

Preparing for the Market

- The fruit is first put on a moving belt and all those that are damaged or too small are taken out.
- After going through a blower, the fruit passes over brushes which clean any dirt off it.
- Then there is another, even stricter selection, and sorting according to weight.
- The grading line then shakes each fruit to the appropriate area for its weight, currently to the nearest 0.35 ounce (10 grams), soon, however, to the nearest 0.07 ounce (2 grams).
- The avocados are packed by hand according to size in normal commercial boxes which hold 8.8 pounds (4 kilograms).

easy as the fruit does not give any clues externally. Avocados never ripen on the tree; they only achieve so-called "tree ripeness," and it is not until they have been picked that they become ripe enough to eat. Tree ripeness is determined by establishing the oil content which must exceed a high minimum. Then a test is carried out to determine how near to being ready for eating the fruit is before it is harvested.

Like all fruit, avocados only develop their abundance of vital substances when they are ripe. They are amazing things as, apart from olives and nuts, they are the only fruit that contains any amount of fat. It is not rare for the fat content to be over 20 percent. This is made up of extremely healthy, polyunsaturated fats, in particular linoleic acid which the human body needs to be able to form vital tissue hormones. These fatty acids also have the function of absorbing vitamins which accounts for the avocado's amazingly high vitamin E content. Above and beyond this, the fruit contains all the essential amino acids as well as potassium and iron in particular. This combination of substances, which is extremely rare for plants, makes the avocado an exceptionally healthy and energy-giving food.

How to Handle Avocados

- Buy firm – and therefore undamaged – fruit and let it ripen at home.
- Only buy soft, ripe fruit, which often has bruises, in exceptional cases.
- Choose fruit with stalks, which shows that the fruit was cut from the tree; the stalk also protects against rot.
- Avocados ripen quicker if they are kept at room temperature with other fruit.
- The fruit keeps longer if it is stored between 8–20 °F (4–10 °C).
- They cannot tolerate temperatures that are too low or even frost, as the flesh turns a dark color without ripening.
- The fruit is ready to eat if it gives when pressed with a finger.
- Only the Hass variety becomes visibly darker or black as it ripens.
- If possible choose the Hass variety, as it has the best flavor.
- Once it is cut open, the flesh oxidizes quickly. Therefore only cut it open shortly before using it or brush with lemon juice or vinegar.
- An avocado half will keep in the refrigerator for 1–2 days if the pit is not removed, the flesh is brushed with lemon juice, and it is wrapped well in plastic wrap.
- Avocados will only keep in the freezer if mashed and mixed with lemon juice; defrost in the refrigerator.

Avocados – Delicious and Versatile

- On their own, especially the Hass and Pinkerton varieties
- Just with some coarse salt sprinkled over
- With vinaigrette or salad dressing according to taste
- In any salad as a delicate and decorative addition
- Mashed, seasoned with lemon juice and coarse salt, as a delicious spread or exquisite sauce
- Puréed as a refreshing shake or in fruit juice cocktails
- As a mild, delicious, easily digestible food for children, rich in vital substances
- Puréed with some cream to accompany vegetables or whisked into hot stock

Nutritious Content of the Avocado

With its fat content of almost 24 percent – principally consisting of highly nutritious polyunsaturated fats – the avocado is the fruit that is richest in fat. But it has other valuable nutrients. These are: 2 g protein – 4 g carbohydrate, of which 3.3 g fiber – 503 mg potassium – 10 mg calcium – 29 mg magnesium; as well as 13 mg vitamin C. All in all: 223 kcal/932 kJ per 100 grams.
Note: 1 g = 0.0353 oz; 1 mg = 0.001 g

Varieties of Avocado

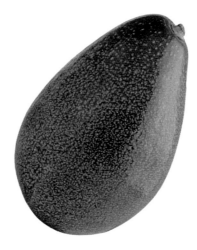
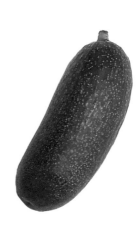
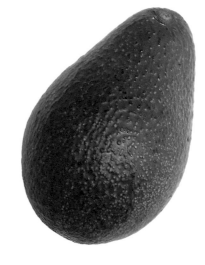

Bacon
Smooth, yellow speckled, dark green, soft thin skin, oval-shaped. October through end of December

Cocktail Avocado
From Fuerte trees; rare, thumb-sized, unpollinated, pitless, mild tasting fruit

Fuerte
Very common, a lightly speckled green, leathery skin, long pear-shaped; full of flavor. November through end of March

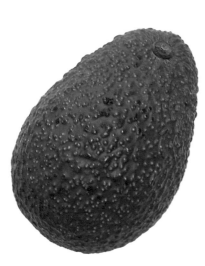
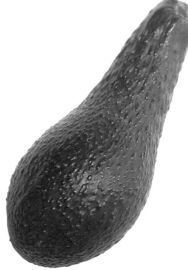
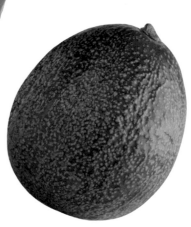

Hass
Green at first, dark purple to black as it ripens, rough grained, thick, hard skin; excellent nutty flavor; small fruits provide proportionally more flesh. January through mid-June

Pinkerton
Dark green, narrow, long shape with rough grained skin; high in fat, keeps well. November through end of February

Reed
Round, very large, shiny green fruit with slightly rough, medium-thick skin; mild flavor. April through end of July

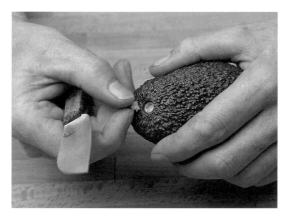
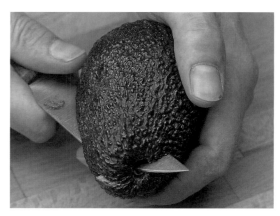

The stalk shows that the fruit was cut from the tree. It protects it against rot and decay.

Hold the avocado and, using a knife, cut it open lengthways around the pit in the middle.

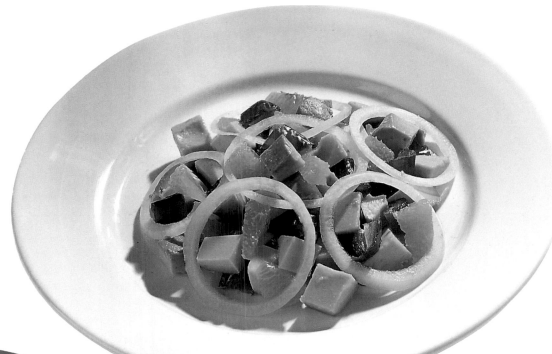

Avocado Salad with Dates and Oranges

Guacamole

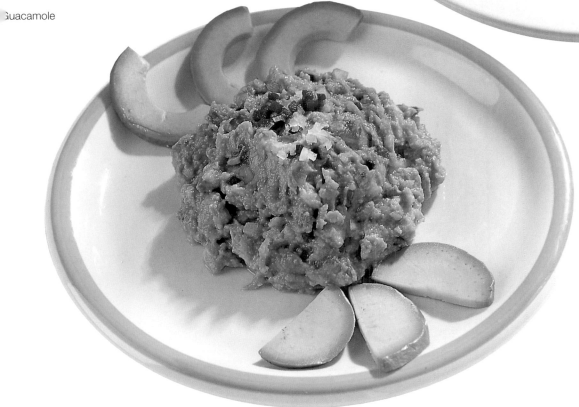

Avocado Salad with Dates and Oranges
(Illustration above)

5 oz (150 g) dates
1 orange
1 onion
2 avocados
²/₃ cup (125 ml) vinaigrette

Pit the dates and chop into small pieces.
Peel and dice the orange.
Chop the onion into rings.
Cut the avocado flesh into cubes.
Mix all the ingredients in a salad bowl and pour over the vinaigrette – made from vinegar, oil, salt, and pepper; mix well.

Guacamole
(Illustration above left)

1 tomato
¹/₂ small onion
2 medium-sized avocados
1 Tbs lemon juice
Coarse salt, black pepper

Skin, de-seed, and dice the tomato.
Finely chop the onion.
Take out and mash the avocado flesh. Mix with the lemon juice, salt, and pepper, then fold in the tomato and onion.
Serve with toast as an appetizer.
Also delicious as a dip, for example with seafood, or with salad. A truly vegetarian alternative to mayonnaise.

Note: Guacamole is a Mexican specialty which was originally made with hot chilis and garlic.

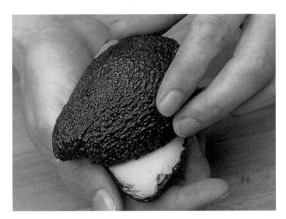

Then turn the two halves against one another so that the top comes away from the large pit, and carefully take it apart.

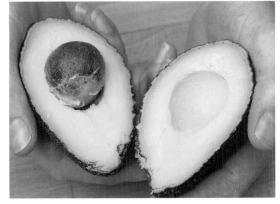

Fully ripe avocados have light yellow flesh. The pit is removed by using a knife to carefully lever it out.

127

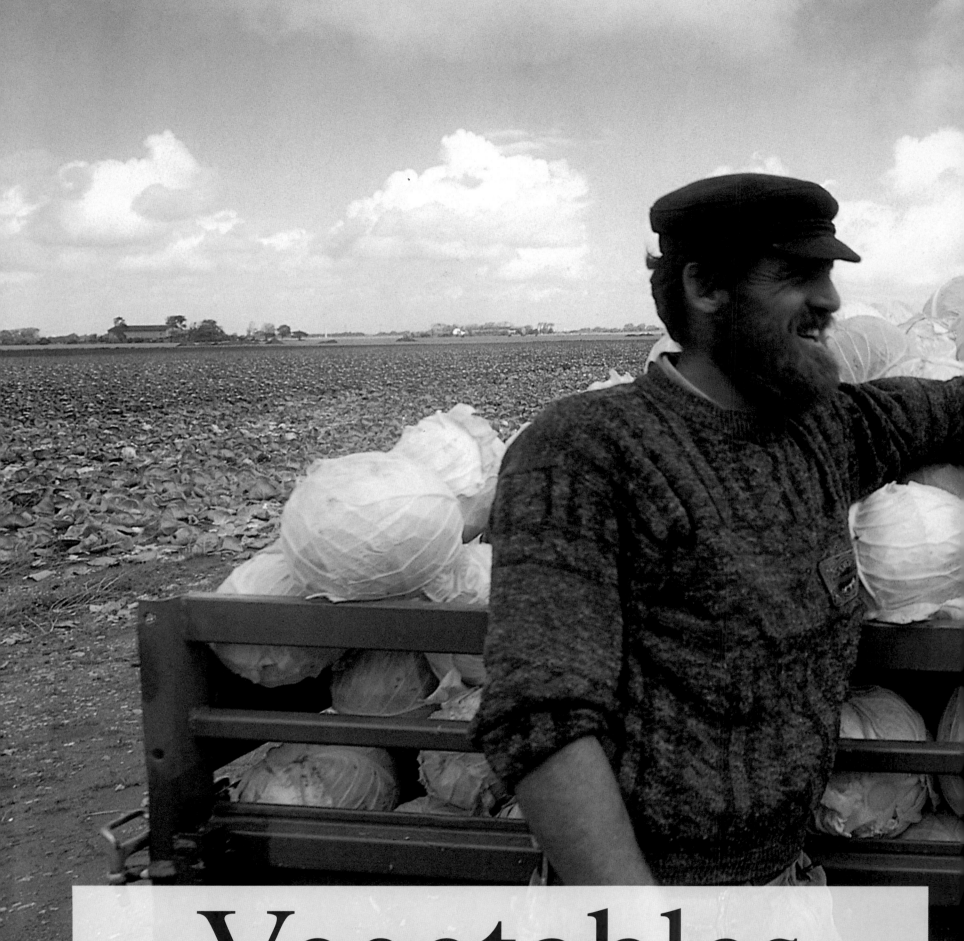

Vegetables

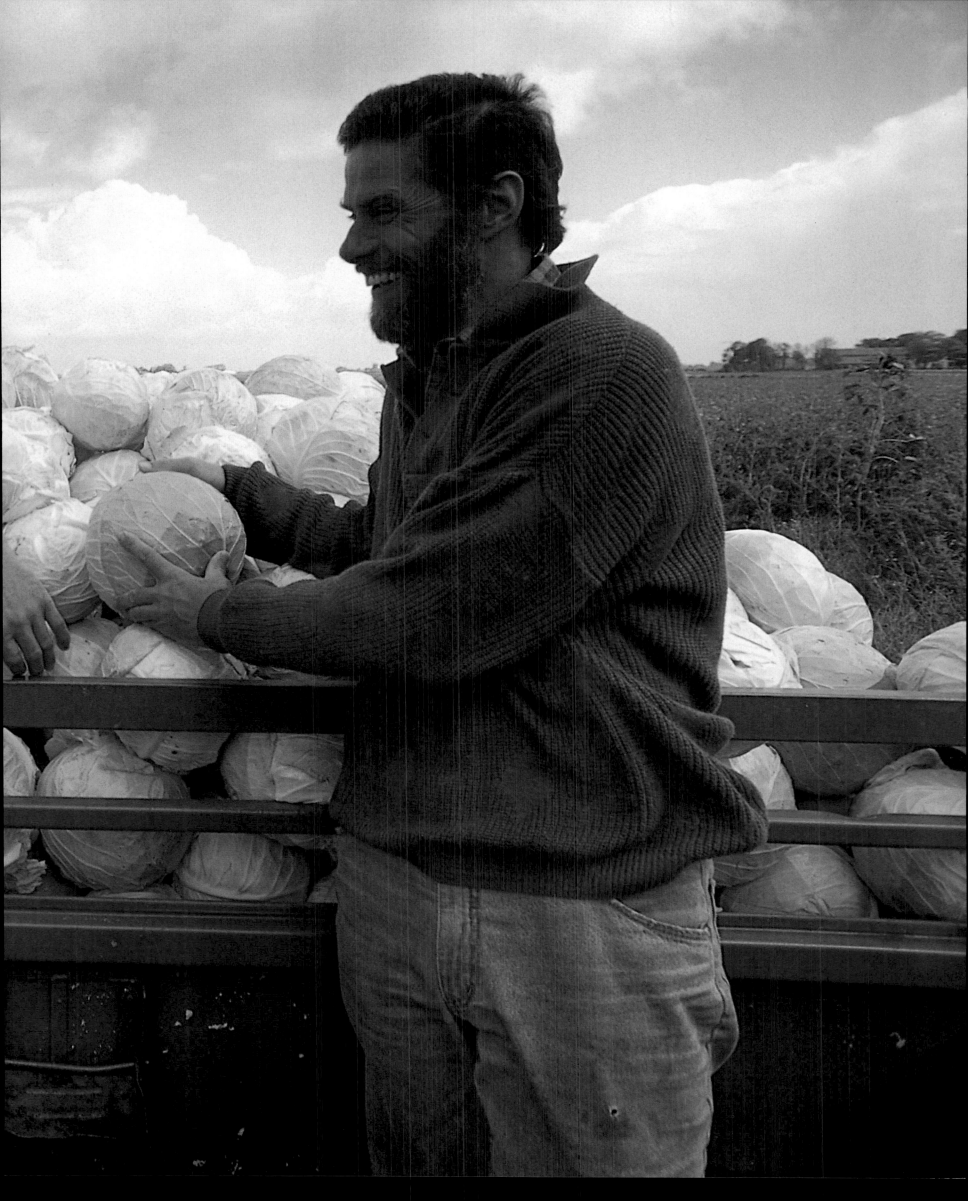

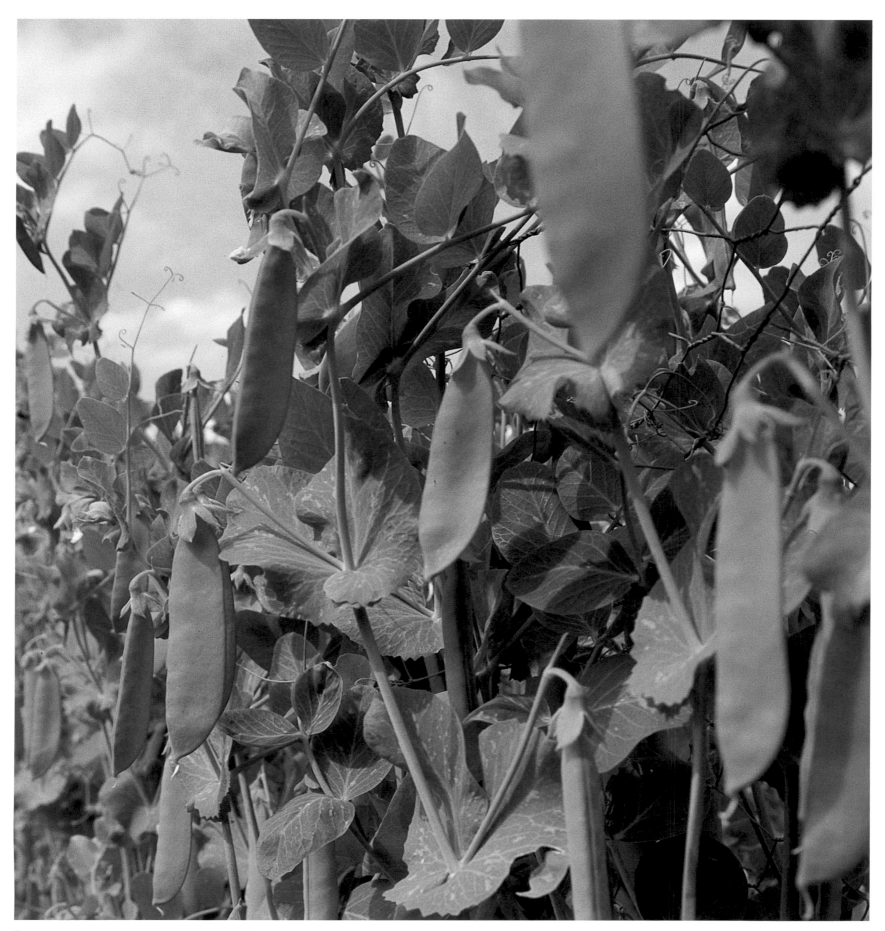

Peas enrich the ground naturally with nitrogen. This means that they play a very important part in organic farming.

Previous double page: White cabbage is healthy, rich in vitamins and (when organically grown) very easy to digest.

Whatever we choose to eat, there is no other foodstuff so rich in nutrients as vegetables. They have a wealth of vitamins, minerals, and fiber together with enzymes and hormones – all essential for health, immunity to disease and well-being, yet they contain comparatively few calories. This means that we can feast on vegetables to our hearts' content without piling on the pounds.

These riches within vegetables do have one drawback – namely that they disappear with great speed. Vitamins are affected by exposure to light, air, and heat; minerals are water-soluble. This makes it important to learn the correct way to handle vegetables. Ripe vegetables are at their nutritional peak at the moment that they are harvested. After 24 hours they will have lost between a quarter and a third of their vitamin content, rising to a half after three days.

Standard growing techniques depend heavily on the use of synthetic fertilizers and chemicals, and the environment in which the produce is grown is usually deprived of natural sunlight. Worse still, the environment may be an energy-guzzling greenhouse. The time and distance between harvest and consumer can be kept as short as possible by buying locally grown vegetables that are in season. Organically grown produce from other countries is always useful to provide vegetables that are out of season, and to extend the range of produce available to the customer. Vegetables offer a huge variety of roots, tubers, leaves, stalks, flowers, fruits, and seeds – guaranteed to whet the appetite. However, their nutrients have to overcome the hurdle of preparation. The nutrients will only remain intact as long as the vegetable is served raw. Mediterranean cookery is particularly healthy, because salad and raw vegetables form a part of every meal. If vegetables have to be cooked, then they should be exposed to heat as quickly and gently as possible, preferably in a little butter or oil and/or in very little water. This method of cooking not only preserves all the nutrients, but also creates an excellent consistency, color, and taste sensation.

Gourmet and Garden Vegetables

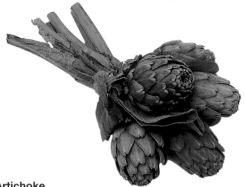

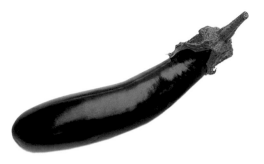

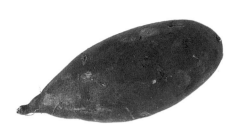

Artichoke
This giant thistle is very popular in Mediterranean countries. The finest part is the "heart" that is best served cooked. It can be eaten raw, but only if young and tender. In its raw state it can be finely chopped and added to salads.

Eggplant
Originating from India, this delicate, fleshy vegetable should never be eaten raw because of its high Solanin content (Solanin is a poisonous alkaloid). It has a bland flavor and is excellent when steamed, baked, or fried.

Sweet Potato
Sweet potato originates from South America but is also very popular in China; botanically, it is a type of convolvulus, which often produces spindle-shaped tubers. Sweet and floury, it tastes best fried.

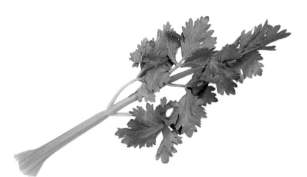

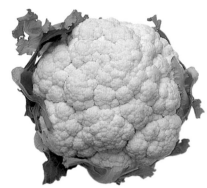

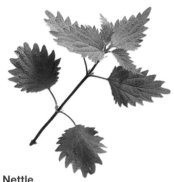

Celery
Related to celeriac, celery no longer needs to be wrapped in paper or "earthed up" but is self-blanching. It retains its piquant flavor whether eaten raw, or cooked. The leaves can be used for seasoning.

Cauliflower
Cauliflower, a cabbage with a flower-like appearance, is very indigestible when grown with artificial fertilizers, but organic cauliflowers taste extremely good. Delicious raw, and if cooked should be boiled, or fried until "al dente."

Stinging Nettle
Its use as a vegetable is not widely known, but it is very healthy and has a purifying effect on the blood; very beneficial in cases of rheumatism or gout. Use the youngest leaves, and blanch them to remove the sting.

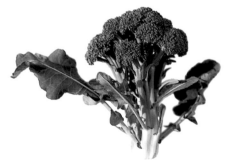

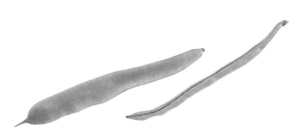

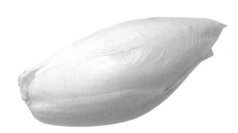

Broccoli
Richer in vitamins than its close relative the cauliflower, this sprouting cabbage is entirely edible – the stalks and leaves are delicious. A very versatile vegetable, which should always be eaten cooked.

Dwarf and String Beans
A gift from Central and South America, these vegetables are rich in carbohydrates and nutrients, but contain Phasin – a poison – that can only be removed by long, slow, steaming.

Belgian Endive
Produces only roots in the first year of growth, and in the second year, light-colored, bitter-sweet, spindle-shaped vegetables. Mass produced in hydroculture, they taste good steamed, and in salads.

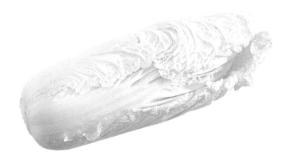

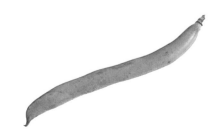

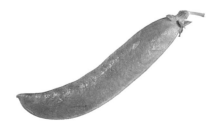

Chinese Leaf
A fast-growing, fall harvest crop that is a distant member of the cabbage family. Good in salads, or lightly steamed. Very digestible and rich in minerals, it has a subtle flavor.

Fava Beans
An Asiatic legume, they grow in a thickly lined pod. Fava (or broad) beans are particularly flavorsome when first picked; do not store and always cook them thoroughly. Delicious in salads and purées.

Peas
Grown all around the world, but rarely eaten fresh from the pod. They are delicious when lightly cooked, make excellent additions to salads, and add a delicate sweetness to mixed vegetable dishes.

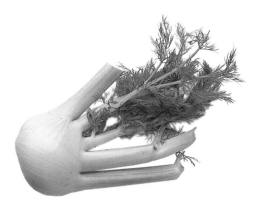

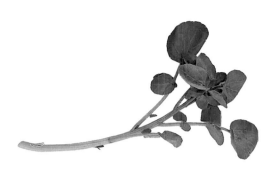

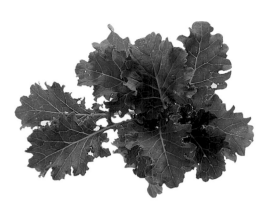

Fennel
This aromatic Mediterranean vegetable is at its most plentiful during the winter months. A delicate and fresh addition to salads, it is also good steamed or baked.

Mountain Spinach
A wild vegetable that is occasionally grown in the garden, a member of the spinach family with triangular, dusty looking leaves. It needs to be washed carefully, can be boiled, steamed, or used in salads.

Green Cabbage
Particularly favored in northern Europe, this popular leaf cabbage has a very high nutritional value, being rich in vitamin C and provitamin A. It is especially tender and tasty after the season's first frost. Best when just lightly steamed.

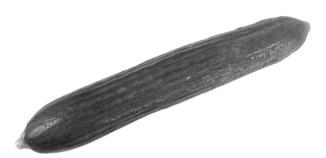

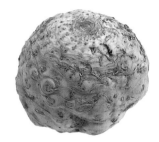

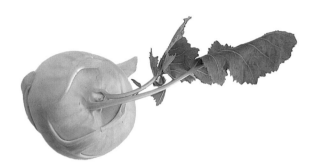

Cucumber
A climbing plant with many varieties, the most popular being the pickling cucumber. The skin should only be eaten if the cucumber is organically grown. Add salt just before serving. A good stewing vegetable.

Celeriac
An aromatic vegetable, rich in vitamin B and essential oils, celeriac has a diuretic effect, purifies the blood, and helps calm the nerves. It is commonly eaten raw, but is also good in salads and stews.

Kohlrabi
An unusual shaped, rough-skinned, sprouting tuber, kohlrabi can be eaten boiled, or grated in its raw state into salads. The leaves are good in salads or cooked like spinach.

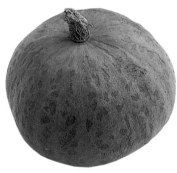

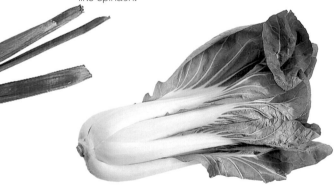

Squash
Widely grown in Italy, their seeds are used for oil in Eastern Europe. Available from fall for use in creamy soups, chutneys, and pickles, or to serve as a simple side vegetable.

Leeks
A type of lily, with pale sprouting roots. Only organic leeks are easy to digest. They have a delicate, distinctive flavor and stimulate the kidneys, liver, and gallbladder.

Swiss Chard
Very popular in Switzerland and the Mediterranean countries, Swiss chard should be prepared in the same way as spinach. Regular chard should be cooked like asparagus.

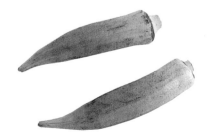

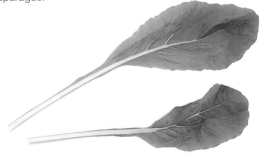

Carrots
Rounded or long, these root vegetables are popular all over the world. They are rich in betacarotene (provitamin A) and are delicious raw or cooked and eaten with young leaves.

Okra
Common in the eastern Mediterranean, these long green vegetables are very useful in stews and mixed vegetable dishes. Before use, blanch in vinegar and water. Do not refrigerate.

Pak Choi
Closely related to Chinese leaf and Swiss chard, this grows best in a temperate climate. Subtly flavored, it should be lightly steamed and the stalks prepared like asparagus. It is also good in salads.

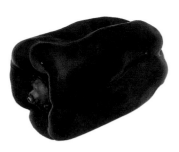

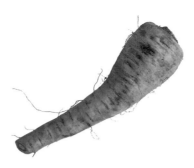

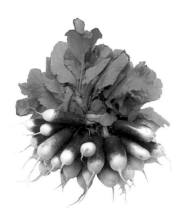

Bell Peppers
Originally from South America, this sun-loving vegetable has a very high vitamin C content. May be eaten raw in salads, or can be broiled, braised, stuffed, or pickled.

Parsnip
A large, flavorsome vegetable that keeps well. It is rich in vitamins and high in fiber. Very popular in England and Scandinavia and used for purées and stews. The leaves can be used for seasoning.

Pink Radishes
Very popular as nibbles, and good for the gallbladder, liver, stomach, and bowels. Radishes are normally eaten raw in salads, or used as a garnish. The small leaves can be used in soups.

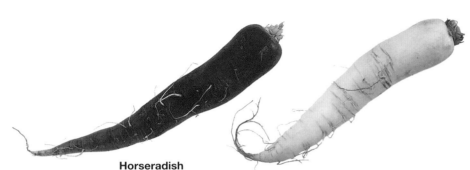

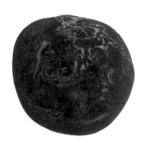

Horseradish
Eternally popular, long, root vegetable with healing qualities (due to its mustard oil content), it is often eaten raw. The peppery taste can be lessened by salting the radish before eating it.

Scorzonera
The black skin conceals creamy-white flesh that is particularly rich in vitamins and minerals. A fall and winter vegetable.

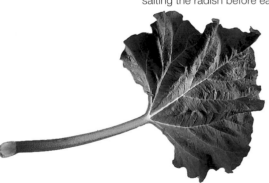

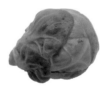

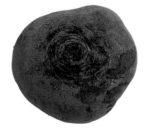

Rhubarb
Although it looks like a vegetable (since it is a rhizome), its stalks are used like a fruit. The leaves are poisonous and the stalks should always be cooked. It can be stewed, put into pies, and made into jam.

Brussels Sprouts
Buds resembling small cabbages are formed on the stalk of the plant. Full of goodness, sprouts should be eaten as soon after picking as possible. Serve boiled as a side vegetable, in a gratin, or in a warm salad.

Beet
A specialty of northern and central Europe, beet has a high vitamin and mineral content and is a good source of protein. As long as it is organically grown, it is extremely healthy and can be eaten raw or cooked.

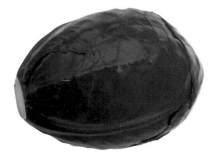

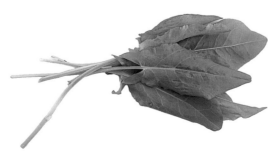

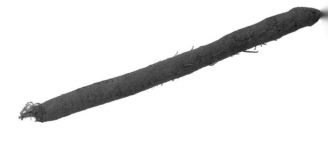

Red Cabbage
A cabbage with a firm dark red head that is available from early summer, but has its main crop in winter. Whilst early red cabbage is very good in salads, the later crop is better boiled or steamed. It combines well with apples or chestnuts.

Sorrel
The garden variety can be used as a vegetable or an herb. Always use the youngest, freshest leaves. Wonderful for fish sauces, cream soups, or as a piquant side vegetable.

Salsify
Relatively unknown and difficult to prepare, gloves should always be worn when preparing this vegetable. Salsify helps cell growth and repair. It has a similar flavor to asparagus.

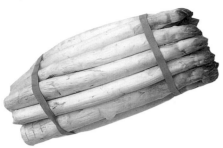

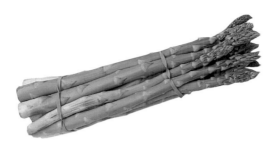

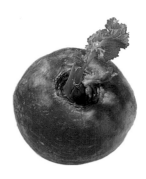

Asparagus
Long-lasting stalks with delicious tips, the above-ground variety is green and the underground variety is white. Green asparagus is richer in nutrients and can be cooked without having to be peeled.

Rutabaga
This definition includes swedes and English turnips. They should always be boiled, and are often mashed. A very fine root vegetable.

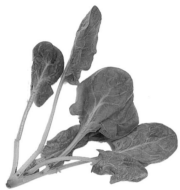

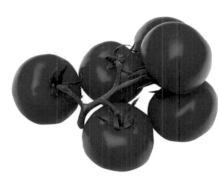

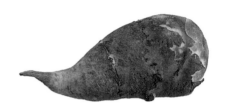

Spinach
A vitamin-rich leaf that is full of iron and good for the stomach. Young leaves can be used raw in salads or lightly steamed. Can be added to soups, flans, and vegetable bakes. Has a short shelf life.

Tomatoes
A vegetable superstar that comes in all shapes and sizes – round, oval, tiny, and heavy. Eat raw, steamed or boiled. Use for sauces and juices. Unbeatable.

Jerusalem Artichoke
A sweet-tasting tuber used by the North American Indians, that tastes equally good raw, sliced and steamed, or puréed.

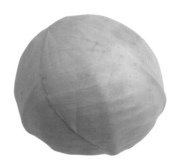

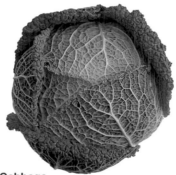

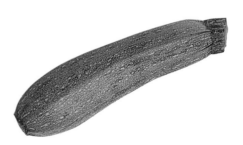

White Cabbage
A cabbage variety that is popular all around the world. Available with a round, or pointed, head, early cabbages can be eaten raw in salads, later ones should be steamed. Use in soups, vegetable bakes and to make sauerkraut.

Savoy Cabbage
Very popular in northern Europe and Russia, this cabbage has distinctive leaves. The summer harvest tastes mildly piquant, and the flavor becomes stronger in the winter crop. Eat cooked, and use in stews.

Zucchini
A non-proliferating variety of squash, with long, angular fruits. Small zucchini can be eaten raw in salads, while larger ones should be lightly steamed or stuffed. The flowers are delicious fried.

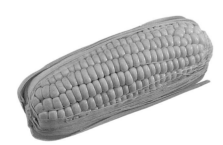

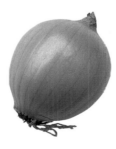

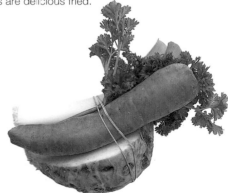

Corn
A sweet variety of maize, with tender kernels. Boil in unsalted water or broil. Eat on the cob, in salads or in mixed vegetable dishes.

Onions
The most popular ingredient, used in every kitchen in the world, onions are also valued for their healing properties. There are numerous varieties available. Cut just before use. A very versatile vegetable.

Vegetables for Stock
Carrots, celeriac, leeks, and parsley give vegetable stock its typical flavor.

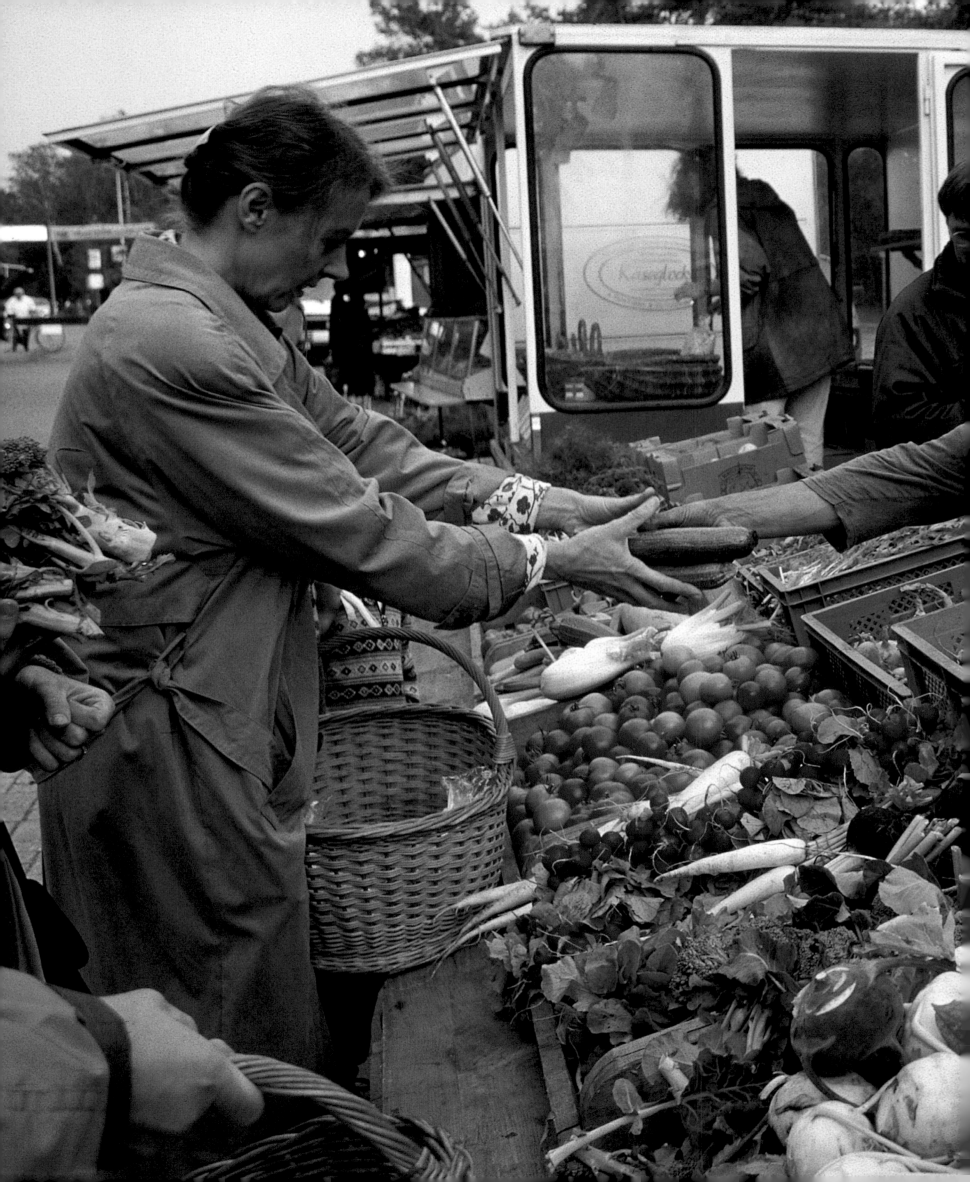

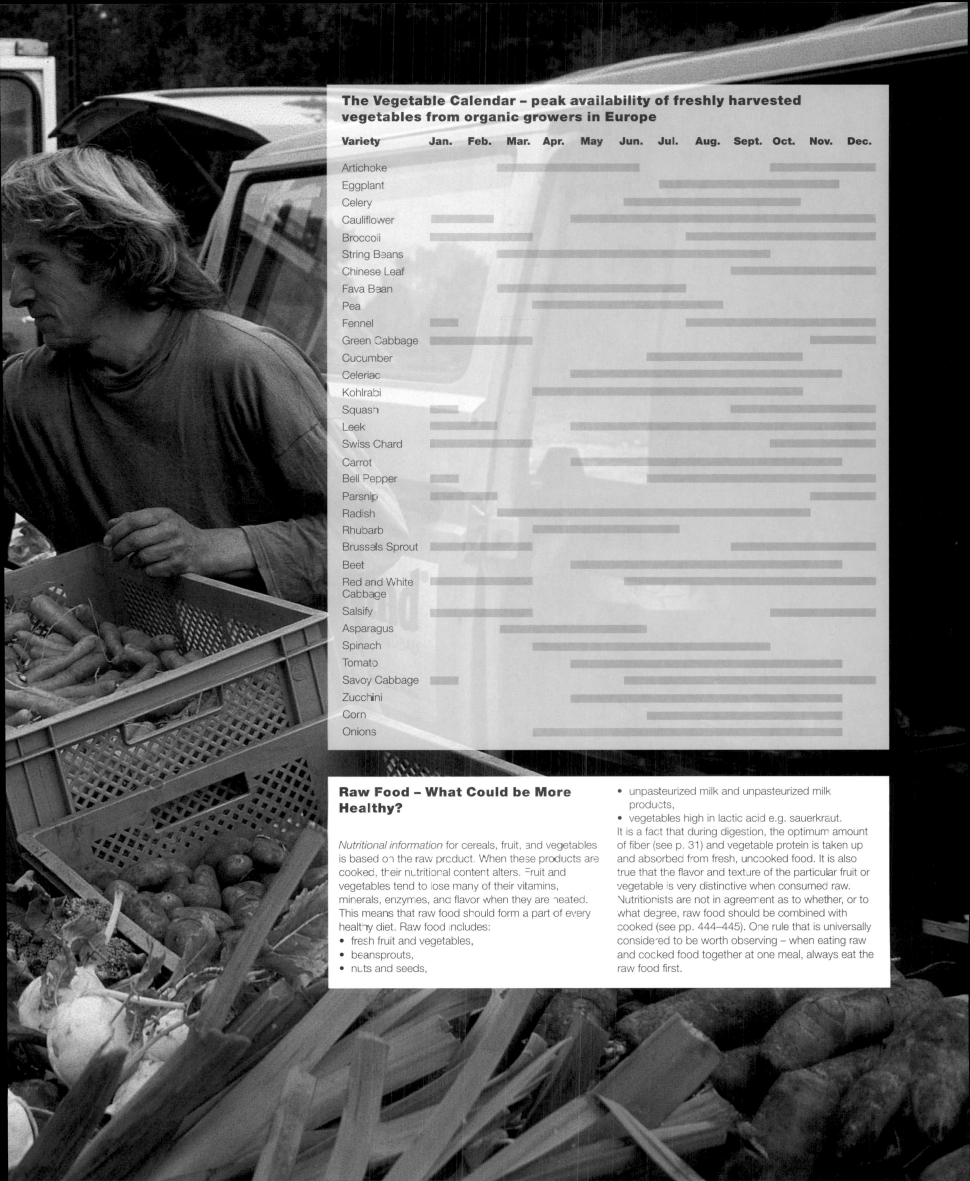

The Vegetable Calendar – peak availability of freshly harvested vegetables from organic growers in Europe

Variety	Jan.	Feb.	Mar.	Apr.	May	Jun.	Jul.	Aug.	Sept.	Oct.	Nov.	Dec.
Artichoke												
Eggplant												
Celery												
Cauliflower												
Broccoli												
String Beans												
Chinese Leaf												
Fava Bean												
Pea												
Fennel												
Green Cabbage												
Cucumber												
Celeriac												
Kohlrabi												
Squash												
Leek												
Swiss Chard												
Carrot												
Bell Pepper												
Parsnip												
Radish												
Rhubarb												
Brussels Sprout												
Beet												
Red and White Cabbage												
Salsify												
Asparagus												
Spinach												
Tomato												
Savoy Cabbage												
Zucchini												
Corn												
Onions												

Raw Food – What Could be More Healthy?

Nutritional information for cereals, fruit, and vegetables is based on the raw product. When these products are cooked, their nutritional content alters. Fruit and vegetables tend to lose many of their vitamins, minerals, enzymes, and flavor when they are heated. This means that raw food should form a part of every healthy diet. Raw food includes:

- fresh fruit and vegetables,
- beansprouts,
- nuts and seeds,
- unpasteurized milk and unpasteurized milk products,
- vegetables high in lactic acid e.g. sauerkraut.

It is a fact that during digestion, the optimum amount of fiber (see p. 31) and vegetable protein is taken up and absorbed from fresh, uncooked food. It is also true that the flavor and texture of the particular fruit or vegetable is very distinctive when consumed raw. Nutritionists are not in agreement as to whether, or to what degree, raw food should be combined with cooked (see pp. 444–445). One rule that is universally considered to be worth observing – when eating raw and cooked food together at one meal, always eat the raw food first.

Vegetable Soup

This easy vegetable soup is made from the magnificent variety of vegetables that can be found in the garden. It adapts to each season and reflects the time of year that it is made. Fresh herbs should be used when available. Onions, potatoes, and parsley form the basis of the soup.

1 medium onion, 2 leeks
5$\frac{1}{2}$ lbs (2.5 kg) seasonal vegetables (e.g. carrots, green beans, kohlrabi, white cabbage, celeriac, tomatoes)
1 lb 2 oz (500 g) potatoes
2 Tbs sunflower oil
3 Tbs finely chopped herbs (e.g. basil, hyssop, oregano, marjoram, lovage, sage)
Coarse salt
9 oz (250 g) brussels sprouts
2 Tbs finely chopped parsley

Finely chop the onion. Slice the remaining vegetables into rings or cubes and dice the potatoes. Heat the oil in a large saucepan, add the onions and fry gently until they are transparent. Add the leeks and cook gently. Then add the remaining vegetables with the herbs. Pour boiling water over the ingredients until the pan is full, add the salt, and simmer until the vegetables are just cooked through. Cook the brussels sprouts in a separate pan until they are tender. Just before serving, add the sprouts to the soup, and sprinkle liberally with parsley.

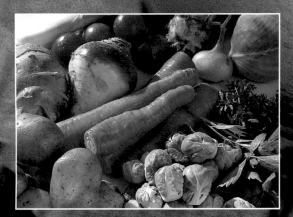

The ingredients for vegetable soup vary according to the season.

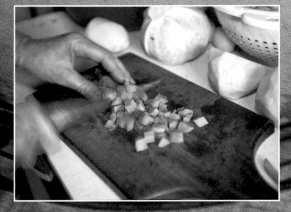

Easy to make, but requires a lot of preparation, as all the vegetables are cut into small pieces.

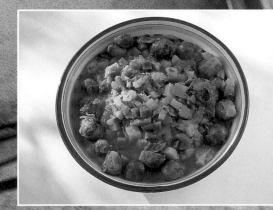

The superb range of vegetables available turns this simple soup into a delicious treat.

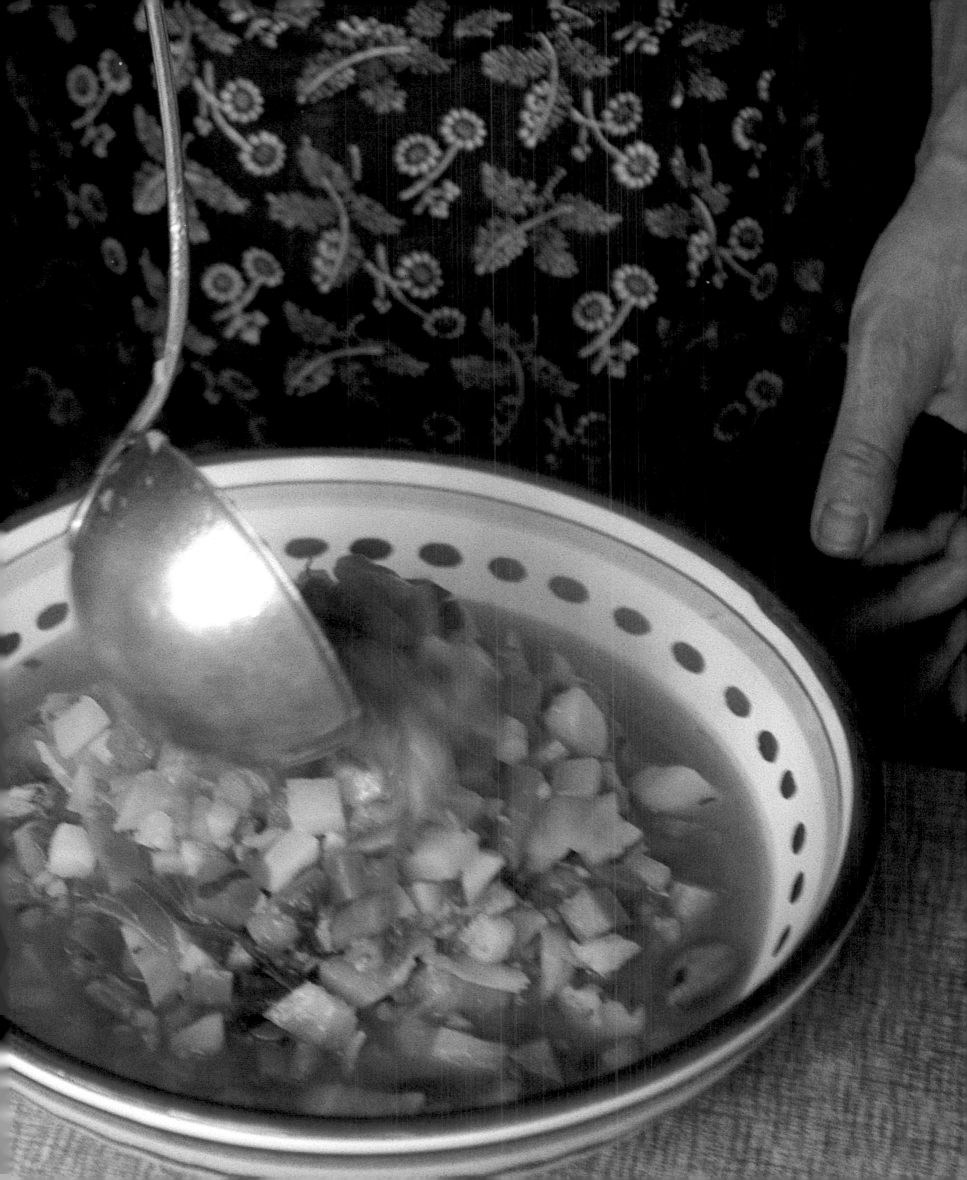

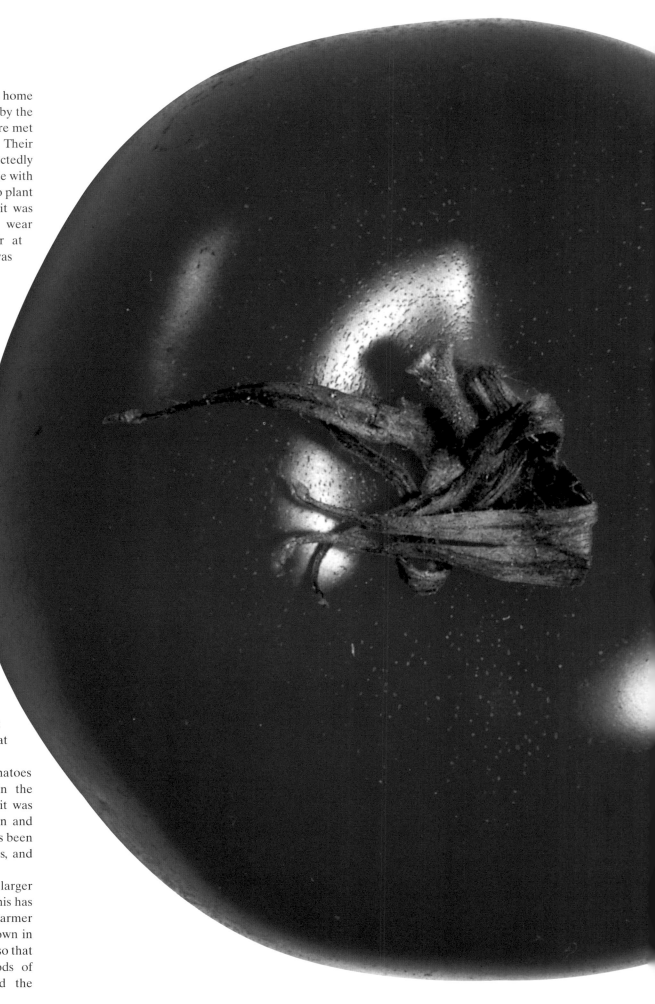

Love or Paradise Apples

Tomatoes

When Columbus first brought tomato plants home from America (where they were cultivated by the Aztecs, who called them "tomatl") they were met with deep suspicion by the Europeans. Their unique, intense scent, and their unexpectedly aromatic flavor filled the 16th century people with scepticism. Later, the upper classes began to plant tomato plants in their flower gardens, as it was very fashionable for society women to wear garlands of tomato flowers in their hair at parties. The fruit of the tomato plant was simply thought to be a colorful curiosity.

There were a few daring tomato-eaters, and very soon, rumors were spreading about the aphrodisiac effect of these Solana (members of the "nightshade" family). This led to tomatoes being known as "love apples" or "paradise apples." It was not until the 18th century that they found popularity in southern Europe.

The first champion of the tomato was none other than the forebear of all gastronomic literature, Grimod de la Reynière (1758–1838), who was in the process of publishing his "Gourmands' Almanac" between 1803 and 1813. He claimed in his book that the tomato was first brought to Paris shortly after the revolution, already having been cultivated in Provence and other parts of southern France. Before then, it was completely unknown. By 1807 there was a reasonable supply of tomatoes available in Paris.

Grimod refers to the fruit both as "tomato" and "love apple" and praises its suitability for sauces. He shares his own recipe for stuffed tomatoes, and claims that this was the only recipe in existence (at that time) to use tomatoes as an ingredient.

Even so, it took another century before tomatoes were grown in the gardens and used in the kitchens of northern Europe. Until then, it was thought that tomatoes needed a lot of sun and were sensitive to frost. Tomatoes had always been grown in sheltered corners, or greenhouses, and were treated like annual plants.

In the last 50 years, tomatoes have formed a larger proportion of the vegetables that we use. This has led to their cultivation in large fields (in warmer regions) or under glass, where they are grown in artificial conditions and fed with chemicals, so that they ripen in record time. These methods of cultivation destroy both the flavor, and the nutrients of the tomato.

When compared with tomatoes grown under these conditions, organic, sun-ripened tomatoes have a marvelous scent and are full of vitamins, minerals, anti oxidants, and essential oils. Organic farms in northern Europe take great care to make their cloches as close to the natural environment as possible. The results are consistently amazing. The amount of extra time that it takes to grow tomatoes is a small matter when compared to the time it takes to grow other vegetables.

It is definitely worth growing these low-calorie fruits because of the beneficial effect they have on our health. They stimulate the whole body, protect against disease, stimulate secretions and, because of their wealth of vitamins, they can give protection against cancer.

There are a huge number of tomato varieties available, ranging from tiny cherry tomatoes (also known as cocktail tomatoes) to plum tomatoes and large, slicing tomatoes. Tomatoes even vary in color, and yellow to almost black tomatoes can be bought from specialist stores.

In more southern countries, pale, greenish tomatoes are favored for salads. However, care should be taken with green tomatoes, as the green indicates the presence of Solanin (which exists in plants of the nightshade family.) The green parts should always be removed before eating, or cooking with the fruit. Moldy, or half rotten tomatoes should always be discarded. as mold may indicate the presence of carcinogens.

It is generally recommended that tomatoes are skinned before being used in recipes. This is done by pouring boiling water over the tomatoes and then the skins can be easily removed. For more sophisticated recipes, the seeds too may need to be removed; however, it is advisable to leave the seeds in for ordinary family meals, as the seeds are very high in fiber.

Baked Tomatoes

4 large slicing tomatoes
4 garlic cloves
1 bunch flat-leafed parsley
4 canned anchovy fillets
4 Tbs (60 g) whole wheat breadcrumbs
2 egg yolks
3 Tbs olive oil
1 tsp oregano
White pepper
Coarse salt

Preheat the oven to 460 °F (250 °C). Cut the tomatoes in half and scoop out the seeds and flesh with a teaspoon. Set aside. Mince the garlic and chop the parsley and anchovies. Mix together with the breadcrumbs, egg yolk, oregano, pepper and 2 tablespoons of the oil, until it forms a smooth paste, then season to taste with salt.
Fill the hollowed out tomatoes with this mixture. Grease an oven proof dish using the remaining oil, place the tomatoes in the dish, and bake for 10–15 minutes.
Serve at once.

Tomato Pizza

Dough

1 lb 2 oz (500 g) whole wheat flour
1 1/4 oz (42 g) yeast
1 pinch cane sugar
Coarse salt
2 Tbs olive oil

Sauce

1 lb 11 oz (750 g) vine ripened tomatoes
1 bunch basil
3 garlic cloves
1 Tbs olive oil
Coarse salt, white pepper
1 pack buffalo Mozzarella
2 oz (50 g) freshly grated Pecorino

To make the dough: sift 14 ounces (400 g) of the flour into a large bowl and make a well in the center. Dissolve the yeast and the sugar in 1 1/2 cups (300 ml) of lukewarm water and pour this into the well in the flour. Cover and leave for 20 minutes.
Add about 1/2 a teaspoon of salt and the oil to the flour mixture, and mix until it forms a smooth dough. If the mixture seems sticky, add a little more flour.
Knead the dough thoroughly for at least 5 minutes and shape into a ball. Place in a large bowl, dust with flour, cover, and leave to rise for 2 hours.
Plunge the tomatoes into boiling water, skin, and deseed. Chop the tomato flesh into cubes.
Chop the basil finely, keeping a few leaves for a garnish. Mince the garlic, and fry with the basil in the olive oil. Add the tomatoes, bring briefly to the boil, then lower the heat and simmer gently, for about 30 minutes. Season to taste with salt and pepper. Leave to cool.
When the dough has risen, place on a floured work surface and stretch it with your hands. Form it into a large round, and using your thumbs, make a rim around the edge. The pizza should be about 1/4 inch (1/2 cm) thick and at least 12 inches (30 cm) in diameter. The crust should be slightly thicker than the rest of the pizza. Preheat the oven to 460 °F (250 °C).
Place the dough onto a greased baking sheet or pizza plate, and leave to rise for a further 30 minutes. Slice the Mozzarella. Spread the sauce on the pizza, sprinkle with the grated Pecorino, and top with the Mozzarella. Bake for about 15 minutes, or until the crust is browned.
Remove from the oven, leave to stand for about 2 minutes, garnish with the remaining basil leaves, and serve.

Tomato and Bread Salad

1 lb 2 oz (500 g) dried, sliced, whole wheat bread
4 Tbs red wine vinegar
1 garlic clove (peeled)
1 lb 2 oz (500g) firm slicing tomatoes
2 red onions
A few basil leaves
2 Tbs olive oil
Coarse salt, white pepper
Black olives

Place the bread in a bowl, dilute the vinegar with 1 1/2 cups (300 ml) of water, and pour over the bread. Leave it to stand for 10 minutes, remove the bread, and squeeze it to remove excess liquid.
Rub the inside of a salad bowl with the garlic clove and place the bread in the bowl. Slice the onions and tomatoes and place on the bread. Tear the basil leaves into pieces, and add to the salad, together with the oil. Garnish with olives and serve.

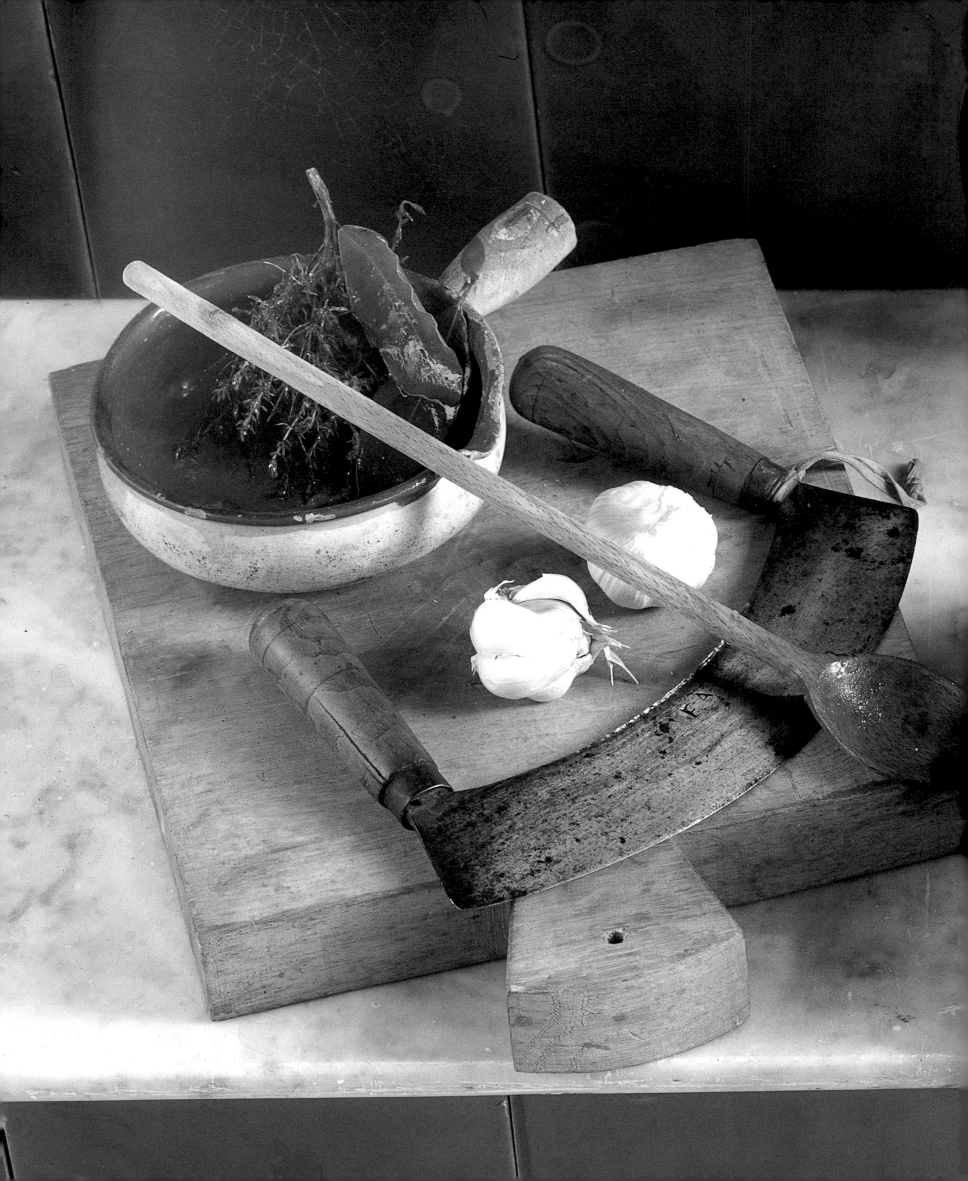

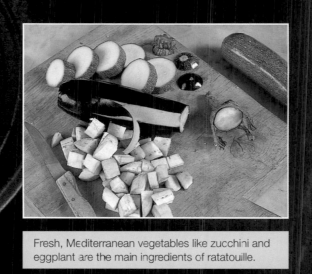

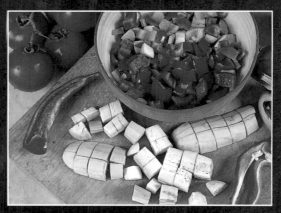

Fresh, Mediterranean vegetables like zucchini and eggplant are the main ingredients of ratatouille.

Pieces of halved and deseeded red and green bell peppers add color to the dish.

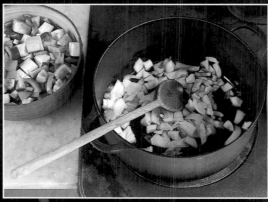

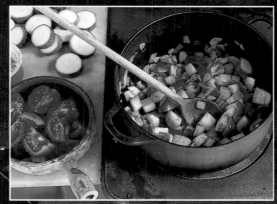

Olive oil is an especially important flavor carrier as are onions, which should be only lightly browned.

Eggplant and bell pepper both taste better when they have been braised for a short time.

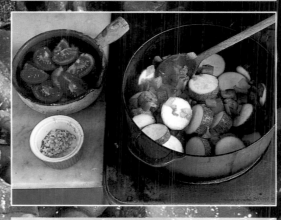

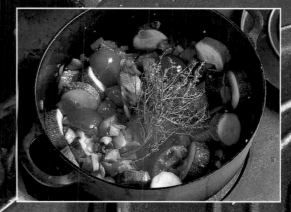

After putting the zucchini in the stew, add the tomatoes. They should be as ripe as possible

The stew gets its aromatic flavor from garlic and herbs – particularly thyme.

Ratatouille
Provençal Vegetable Stew

4 small zucchini
2 eggplants
2 red and 2 green bell peppers
4 large ripe tomatoes
2 onions
3 garlic cloves
8 Tbs olive oil
Coarse salt, black pepper
1 bouquet garni

Slice the zucchini into ½ inch (1 cm) rounds and dice the egg plant. Halve and deseed the peppers, then slice them. Plunge the tomatoes into boiling water, skin and quarter. Finely chop the onion and mince the garlic. Preheat the oven to 350 °F (180 °C)

Heat the olive oil in a large casserole, add the onions and fry until lightly browned. Then add the eggplant and peppers and braise briefly. Next add the zucchini and tomatoes. Season with salt and pepper, and sprinkle with garlic.

Stir the stew thoroughly, then place the bouquet garni – made of parsley, rosemary, marjoram, thyme, tarragon, and savory – on top of the vegetables. Cover the casserole.

Place in the oven and leave to cook for 60 minutes. Alternatively, simmer on the hob, over a low heat for 50–60 minutes. Remove the bouquet garni and serve.

Mediterranean Vegetable Recipes with Eggplants and Bell Peppers

Eggplant Rolls with Mozzarella Filling
(Illustration below center)

2 eggplants
Coarse salt
2 packets buffalo Mozzarella
Corn oil
Whole wheat flour
1 bunch large-leafed basil
White pepper
4 ripe tomatoes

Cut the eggplants lengthways into slices approximately ½ inch (1 cm) thick. Sprinkle with salt and set aside for 30 minutes to remove their bitter juices. Rinse, squeeze out any excess liquid, and pat dry with paper towels. Slice the Mozzarella. Pour plenty of oil into a skillet. Coat the eggplant slices in flour, and pan fry in the oil. Leave to drain on paper towels.
Preheat the oven to 400 °F (200 °C).
Place a slice of Mozzarella onto each slice of eggplant and season well with pepper. Roll them up together and secure with a cocktail stick.
Skin, deseed, and dice the tomatoes. Place the tomatoes in an ovenproof dish, season well, sprinkle with the basil leaves, and place the eggplant rolls on the top.
Bake for about 15 minutes.

Bell Peppers with Tomatoes

11 oz (300 g) onions
2 Tbs olive oil
2 lbs 3 oz (1 kg) red and green bell peppers
2 garlic cloves
1 lb 11 oz (750 g) ripe tomatoes
Coarse salt
White pepper

Roughly chop the onions. Heat the oil in a large saucepan, add the onions and cook until transparent. Halve the bell peppers, remove the seeds and cut into strips lengthways. Crush the garlic and add to the pan, together with the peppers.
Skin and quarter the tomatoes and add to the pan. Cook over a medium heat, stirring frequently, adding a little more liquid if the stew is getting dry. Season to taste with salt and pepper. Serve warm or cold.

Stuffed Bell Peppers

1 medium eggplant
Coarse salt
1 onion
2 garlic cloves
3 Tbs olive oil
4½ oz (125 g) ground lamb
1 bunch flat-leafed parsley
1 egg
3½ oz (100 g) freshly grated hard cheese
Whole wheat breadcrumbs
Black pepper
1 lb 2 oz (500 g) red, green, and yellow bell peppers
½ cup (100 ml) vegetable stock

Cut the eggplant into small cubes, sprinkle with salt and set aside for 60 minutes to remove the bitter juices. Rinse, and dry well.
Finely chop the onion and the garlic and pan fry gently in 2 tablespoons (30 ml) of olive oil. Add the eggplant and ground lamb, brown thoroughly, and leave to cool.
Finely chop the parsley and add to the lamb, together with the egg and cheese. Sprinkle enough breadcrumbs into the mixture, so that it just binds together, but is not too stiff. Season to taste with salt and pepper.
Preheat the oven to 350 °F (180 °C).
Cut a lid out of each of the bell peppers, carefully remove all the seeds and stuff with the lamb mixture; replace the lids on the peppers.
Using the remaining oil, grease an ovenproof dish and place the bell peppers in the dish. Pour the stock around the peppers and bake for 30 minutes in the oven until they are cooked through.

Eggplant Balls

Eggplant Balls
(Illustration below left)

Coarse salt
1 lb 6 oz (600 g) eggplant
2 Tbs (30 g) chopped basil
2 garlic cloves
3½ oz (100 g) freshly grated Pecorino
1 egg
Whole wheat breadcrumbs
Corn oil

Bring a large saucepan of salted water to the boil. Remove the stalks from the eggplants and place the eggplants in the boiling water; allow to boil vigorously for 5 minutes. Drain off the water and leave to cool. Squeeze any excess liquid from the eggplants and chop finely. Place in a bowl, add the basil, crushed garlic, Pecorino, egg and a large pinch of salt, and mix thoroughly. Add enough breadcrumbs to hold the mixture together.
Form the mixture into walnut-sized balls and coat in breadcrumbs.
Heat plenty of corn oil in a deep pan. Fry the eggplant balls in batches, so that they have enough room to move about in the oil. They should be golden-brown after about 5 minutes.
Leave to dry on paper towels.
Eggplant balls are delicious hot or cold.

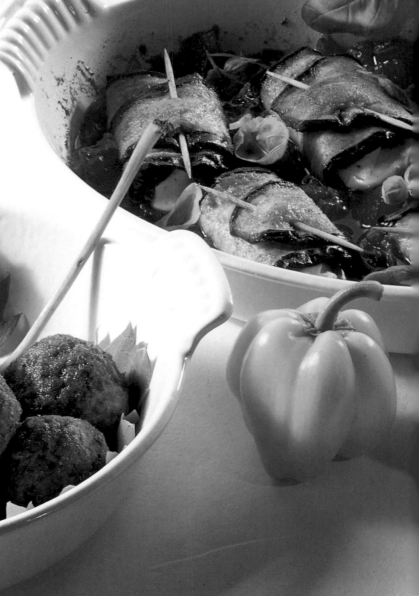

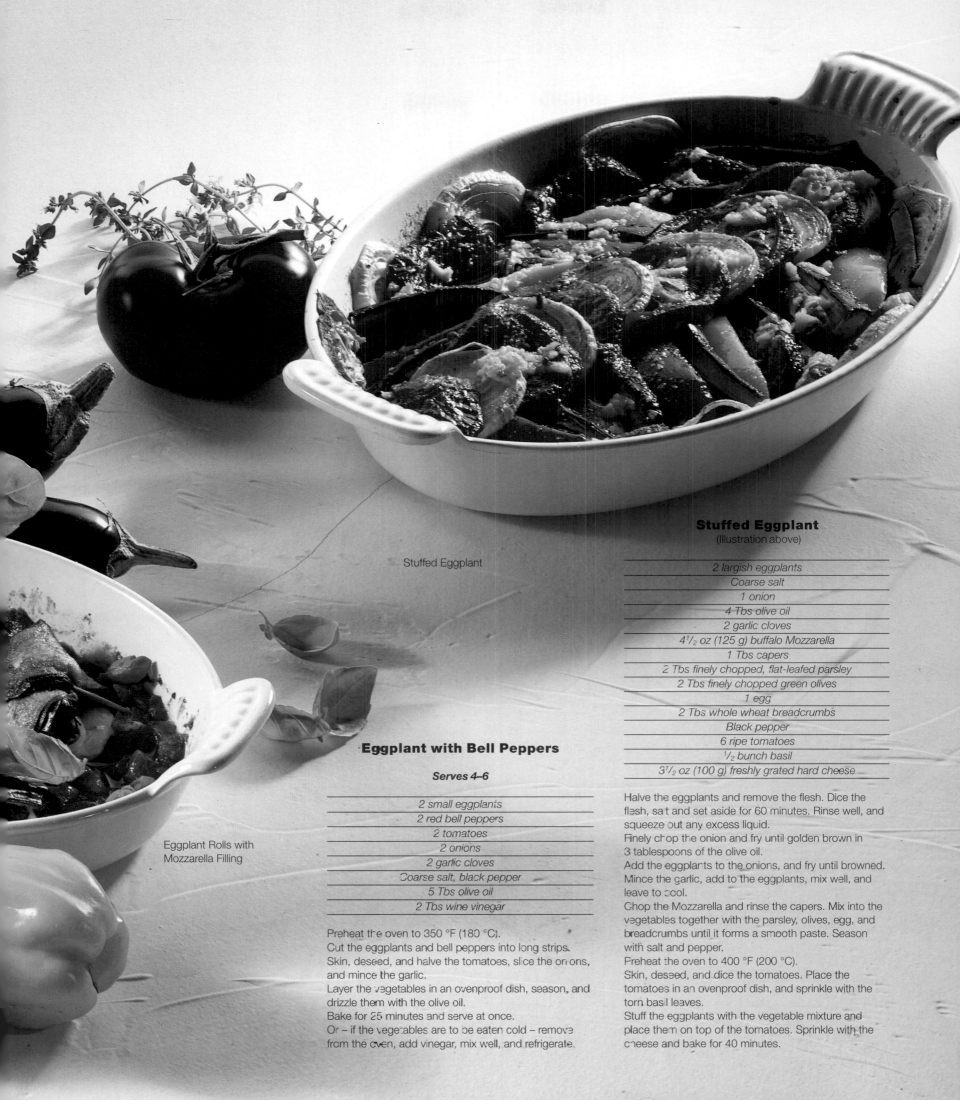

Stuffed Eggplant

Eggplant Rolls with
Mozzarella Filling

Stuffed Eggplant

(Illustration above)

2 largish eggplants	
Coarse salt	
1 onion	
4 Tbs olive oil	
2 garlic cloves	
4¹/₂ oz (125 g) buffalo Mozzarella	
1 Tbs capers	
2 Tbs finely chopped, flat-leafed parsley	
2 Tbs finely chopped green olives	
1 egg	
2 Tbs whole wheat breadcrumbs	
Black pepper	
6 ripe tomatoes	
¹/₂ bunch basil	
3¹/₂ oz (100 g) freshly grated hard cheese	

Halve the eggplants and remove the flesh. Dice the
flesh, salt and set aside for 60 minutes. Rinse well, and
squeeze out any excess liquid.
Finely chop the onion and fry until golden brown in
3 tablespoons of the olive oil.
Add the eggplants to the onions, and fry until browned.
Mince the garlic, add to the eggplants, mix well, and
leave to cool.
Chop the Mozzarella and rinse the capers. Mix into the
vegetables together with the parsley, olives, egg, and
breadcrumbs until it forms a smooth paste. Season
with salt and pepper.
Preheat the oven to 400 °F (200 °C).
Skin, deseed, and dice the tomatoes. Place the
tomatoes in an ovenproof dish, and sprinkle with the
torn basil leaves.
Stuff the eggplants with the vegetable mixture and
place them on top of the tomatoes. Sprinkle with the
cheese and bake for 40 minutes.

Eggplant with Bell Peppers

Serves 4–6

2 small eggplants	
2 red bell peppers	
2 tomatoes	
2 onions	
2 garlic cloves	
Coarse salt, black pepper	
5 Tbs olive oil	
2 Tbs wine vinegar	

Preheat the oven to 350 °F (180 °C).
Cut the eggplants and bell peppers into long strips.
Skin, deseed, and halve the tomatoes, slice the onions,
and mince the garlic.
Layer the vegetables in an ovenproof dish, season, and
drizzle them with the olive oil.
Bake for 25 minutes and serve at once.
Or – if the vegetables are to be eaten cold – remove
from the oven, add vinegar, mix well, and refrigerate.

145

Artichokes

Cynara was an outstanding beauty with long, blonde hair who caught Jupiter's eye. However, she rejected his advances. This enraged the king of the gods, so he turned her into a spiny plant – the *Cynara scolymus*. This is the story of the artichoke. Artichokes are perennial plants that yield a good crop for 4–5 years. After this time, they become weaker and should be replaced by new plants. In southern countries, the main crop can be harvested from December through May but, depending on the variety of plant, artichokes can be harvested all year round. Further north they are a specialty of organic greenhouse agriculture.

Each plant must be well fertilized, and then it will yield seven to eight flowerheads that grow after one another. These flowerheads are cut just before they bloom and then they can be eaten.

There are many different types of artichoke. The small, long and violet-colored varieties are particularly good to eat raw. Artichokes must always be very young and fresh so they do not form any coarse fibers (known as the "choke").

The heart should be cut away from the leaves and then sliced into slender strips (a delicious salad ingredient). Larger, rounder artichokes are usually cooked, and only the heart and the fleshy lower parts of the leaves are eaten. Their slightly bitter, nutty flavor makes artichokes a great delicacy. We have the artichoke to thank for Cynarine, a chemical that purifies the liver and gallbladder, strengthens the bladder and kidneys, and soothes the symptoms of rheumatism. This is obtained from the stalk and the leaves, where it can be found in a concentrated form, and is used for medicinal purposes.

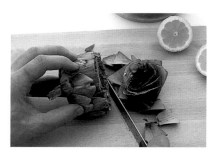

To obtain the heart and base, cut a large section off the top of the artichoke.

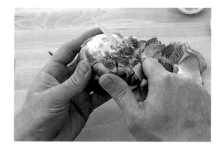

Using a sharp knife, remove the coarse, outer leaves from the base of the artichoke.

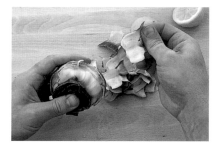

With your fingers, pull the tender, inner leaves away from the heart.

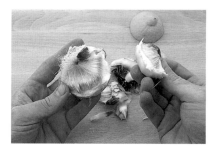

Remove the inedible "choke" by scraping it away from the heart with a teaspoon.

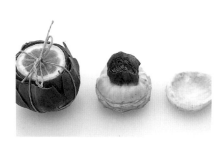

Three ways of eating an artichoke: trimmed and lightly boiled, the tender heart, and the delicate base.

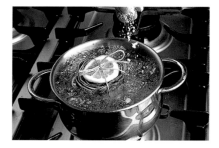

The use of a lemon slice tied onto the artichoke removes the need to add vinegar to the water during cooking.

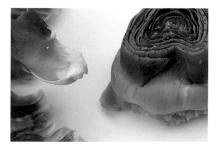

All good things take a little time, and artichokes need to be cooked for at least 35 minutes.

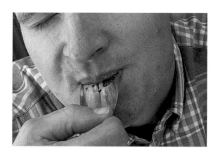

The French way: dip the bases of the leaves into a sauce, and scrape off the bottom part with your teeth.

How to Prepare Artichokes

• 1. The easiest way to cook an artichoke is the "French way," where a large artichoke is eaten whole. Break off the stalk and discard – or keep for use in another recipe – and bring a pan of salted water to the boil. Add a dash of vinegar or lemon juice, then place the artichoke in the pan and cook for about 45 minutes, or until tender. Remove with a ladle, leave to drain upside-down until cool enough to handle. Allow one artichoke per person and serve with a choice of sauces.

• 2. True gourmets accept that often only a quarter, or even a fifth of the artichoke is actually edible. If the artichoke is not properly trimmed, then the texture is spoiled by the presence of tough, coarse fibers.

• 3. When preparing small or violet-colored artichokes, break off the stalk, remove the tough, outer leaves, and trim the pointed tips of the remaining leaves until they are $3/4$–$1^1/2$ inches (2–4 cm) long (this varies according to the age and freshness of the artichoke). Using a knife or a pointed spoon, part the central leaves and scrape out the "choke." Place the artichoke directly into water with vinegar or lemon juice, to avoid discoloration. Cook in boiling, salted water for 30–40 minutes (according to size). These varieties can also be steamed or simmered in a sauce.

• 4. Artichokes – like so many other vegetables – taste best when cooked until "al dente." It is very difficult to judge the exact cooking time since they vary in length, thickness, and weight.

• 5. The stalks can be as delicious as the artichoke bases. This is why smaller artichokes are sold with such long stalks. Remove any leaves from the stalk and then peel. Cut into bite-sized pieces and cook with the artichoke heads.

• 6. There are two ways of preparing the base of a large artichoke. To obtain the base without any leaves attached, break off the stem and remove the leaves. These can now be cooked and served separately with a dipping sauce. Then scrape away the choke and remove any small leaves from the base. Alternatively, trim all the leaves (leaving about $1^1/4$ inches (3 cm) of each leaf attached), then remove the "choke" and any coarse leaves from the base. Either method of preparation requires the artichokes to be soaked in water with a dash of vinegar or lemon juice as soon as they have been cut, to avoid discoloration. Finally, cook in boiling, salted water for 25 minutes, or steam with other vegetables.

• 7. To stuff a large artichoke, break off the stalk, remove the outer leaves, and trim the points of the remaining leaves.

Then simmer for 40 minutes in salted water with a dash of lemon juice or vinegar, and leave to drain. Press the leaves apart and remove the choke. Now the artichoke can be stuffed.

• 8. Artichokes should never be cooked in aluminum pans, as aluminum causes artichokes to turn an unpleasant, dirty color.

• 9. Fresh artichokes have a firm stalk, which gives slightly when pressed with a fingernail. Soft stalks, opened flowerheads, and brown or dry leaf tips are all signs that the vegetable is past its best.

• 10. Cooked artichokes should be eaten within 24 hours. If they are left longer they lose their consistency and flavor and become indigestible.

Artichokes – French Style

4 large Roman artichokes
¹/₂ tsp coarse salt

French Dressing

4 hard cooked eggs
2 raw egg yolks
4 Tbs olive oil
4 Tbs white wine vinegar
1 tsp hot mustard
Coarse salt, white pepper
1 Tbs finely chopped chervil
1 Tbs finely chopped chives
1 Tbs finely chopped parsley
1 Tbs capers

Following the instructions on the previous page, prepare and cook the artichokes (see opposite page under 1).
Peel the hard cooked eggs and remove the yolks. Chop the egg whites finely and set aside.
Mix the hard cooked egg yolks with the fresh egg yolks, then add in the oil, vinegar, and mustard. Season to taste with salt and pepper. Finally, mix in the herbs, capers, and chopped egg whites.
Place the warm artichokes onto plates, and pour over plenty of French dressing. Eat the artichokes by pulling off individual leaves, dipping the fleshy end into the dressing, and then using the teeth to scrape the flesh away from the leaf.

Artichokes – Venetian Style

8 baby artichokes
3 Tbs finely chopped flat-leafed parsley
4 minced garlic cloves
2 oz (50 g) butter
2 Tbs olive oil
Coarse salt, white pepper

Prepare the artichokes as described on the opposite page (under 3).
Place in a pan that is large enough to take all the artichokes (right way up) next to each other. Peel the stalks and place on top of the artichokes. Add water until three quarters of the contents are covered, bring to the boil, cover, and cook on a high heat for 15 minutes.
Add the parsley, garlic, butter, and olive oil, then season well. When the butter causes the water to foam, cook uncovered for a further 5 minutes, then replace the lid.
After 30 minutes turn the artichokes so that the pointed side is down, then boil, uncovered, until all the water has evaporated.
To see if an artichoke is cooked, pull out a leaf: if it comes away from the heart easily and can be bitten through, then the artichoke is ready. If it does not, then the artichoke needs longer cooking. Add a little more water and boil until tender.
This dish is best served with rustic bread.

All leaves must be removed from the flower head to obtain the uniquely delicious "heart" – the best part of the artichoke.

Background: A field of artichokes. Artichokes are perennial plants, members of the thistle family, and have large, ragged leaves.

A High-Class Foodstuff

Potatoes

Wild potatoes have always grown in the Andes of South America. It is thought that the Incas cultivated them as long as 3,000 years ago. One of the Conquistadors, following in the footsteps of Pizarro, brought them back to Spain in the 16th century. At first, their culinary uses were not known, but it was believed that they had a healing effect. In 1565, King Philip II of Spain had them presented to Pope Pius IV as a cure for rheumatism.

The Flemish botanist Charles de Lescluse played an important part in the cultivation of potatoes across central and northern Europe, where they were known by the Latin name *Clusius*. In 1588 he took them to Austria, and when he visited Frankfurt in 1589 he campaigned for their widespread cultivation. Potatoes were soon growing in the gardens of the well-to-do as ornamental plants, and Lescluse managed to convince the Lord of Hessen-Kassel, William IV, that they had wide-ranging culinary uses.

It took another 150 years before the potato became a staple foodstuff, and it was a very popular vegetable in Ireland. Back in the 16th century, Sir Walter Raleigh, one of Elizabeth I's admirals, had brought the potato to England after one of his voyages to America. The climate in Ireland was perfect for the cultivation of potatoes, as it was mild and damp, and potatoes could be grown in the poorest soil. The Irish cooked potatoes in their skins, so that they were not only filling, but also retained all their vitamins and minerals. This helped to keep the population healthy. The potato blight of 1845 ruined that year's crop, and caused the next few harvests to fail. This was the greatest catastrophe ever to hit Ireland: the population was reduced to half its previous size because of deaths from famine and mass emigration. This disaster is still remembered by the people of Ireland today.

In the 18th century, several rulers realized that potatoes could help to relieve the famine that was sweeping the world. The King of Prussia, Frederick the Great, ordered the widespread planting of potatoes in 1756. To trick the farmers into planting the vegetable, the king had potato fields sown and had his grenadiers pretend to guard them. The farmers suspected that something precious was in the fields and stole the tubers under cover of darkness (the grenadiers duly looked away, of course). The trick had the desired effect and potatoes were grown all over Prussia.

During the Seven Years War (1756–63), the French chemist Parmentier was being held in prison in Prussia. This is where he first made the acquaintance of the potato. When he returned to

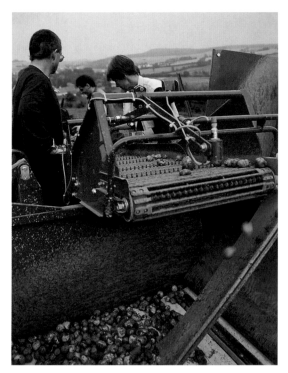

Potatoes are the most important crop for many organic farmers. The potato harvest is a high point of the farming year.

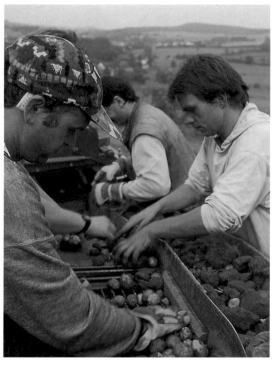

The potatoes are sorted as soon as they are harvested. Any damaged potatoes are used to make animal fodder (see illustration on the right).

France, he spent the next decade encouraging the cultivation of the potato throughout France. He had his own potato plantation in Neuilly, just outside Paris. During the reign of Louis XVI (1774–92), he managed to convince the court to eat potatoes. It was not until the 19th century that the potato was cultivated in all the countries of Europe. Today about 470 varieties of potato can be found in Europe alone.

The cultivation of potatoes has dwindled in the last 20 or 30 years. This is partly because of the large range of vegetables available. Some people believe potatoes to be fattening, because they are so filling. However, it has been known for a long time now that boiled potatoes have the same calorific value as whole milk, sole, or plums, and fewer calories than the same quantity of bread, pasta, rice, or meat.

Indeed, potatoes are a particularly valuable food source, since they contain all 8 essential amino acids, vitamins A, B1, B2, and B6, and folic acid, pantothenic acid, niacin, and vitamin C. They provide the body with trace elements, and all minerals. Potatoes are high in carbohydrates in the easily-digestible form of starch. There are few foods that provide such a balanced and nutritious contribution to our diets as the potato.

This does not apply to potato products, and potatoes that have not been organically grown. When fields have been treated with artificial fertilizers, liquid manure, pesticide, herbicide, and fungicide, then tubers that are grown in those fields absorb nitrates, traces of metal, and other poisonous substances. Their flavor is also spoiled by the chemicals in the soil.

For many organic farms in central and northern Europe, potatoes have become the most important crop. With the possible exception of carrots, there is no other vegetable where the difference in flavor between organic and non organic varieties is so marked. Organic methods of potato cultivation require a lot of work to prepare the soil for the crop. First the ground is planted with cereals or legumes – peas, beans, sweet peas, or buckwheat. In the fall, the field is fertilized with manure, in winter it is plowed, and in the new year the seedlings are prepared. Organic potatoes are planted a little later than conventionally grown potatoes, placed in rows at least 30 inches (75 centimeters) apart, and are covered with earth.

Whilst the leaves and stems above ground are unfolding and growing, below ground tubers that hold nutritional reserves for the plant are growing. It is important to keep the fields free of weeds so that the tubers can absorb as many nutrients as possible from the soil. The field is hoed and weeded frequently and the plants are checked to make sure that they are covered with enough earth. Gravel is sprinkled on the ground to deter enemies to the potato – like the Colorado Beetle. The greatest danger to a potato crop is Phytophtora – a disease that rots plants and tubers. There is no organic method of controlling this disease, which can destroy up to forty percent of the crop. This risk of disease, and the amount of preparation required to produce a potato crop accounts for the high price of organic potatoes. However, organic potatoes represent good value for money because of their superior flavor, and high nutritional value.

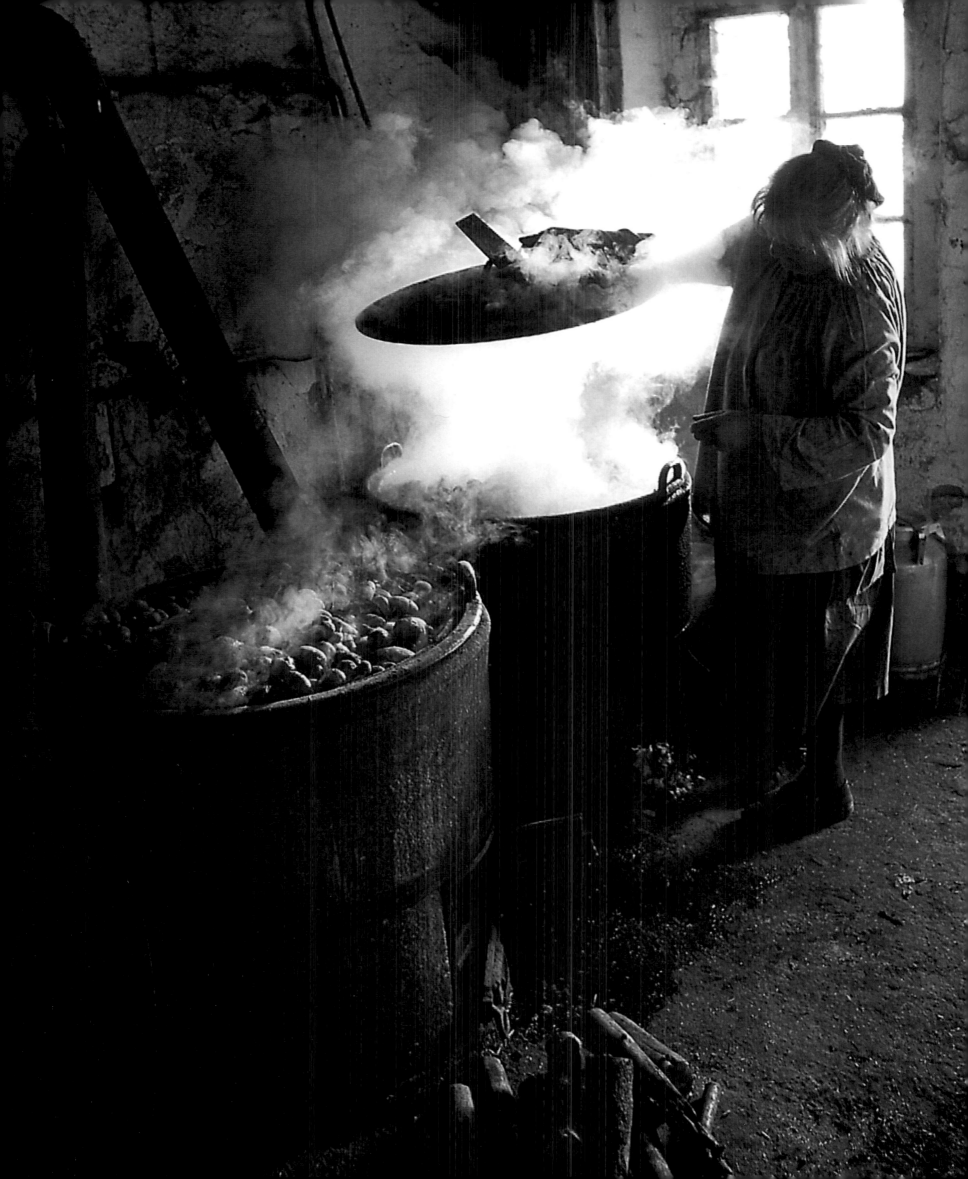

Common Varieties of Organic Potatoes

(See p. 152 for cooking characteristics of these varieties).

Agria
Mid-season, generally firm, yellow-fleshed potato whose color does not darken after cooking. Large, oval tubers; good flavor, versatile; high vitamin C content; keeps well.

Arnika
Early, generally firm, dark yellow, round to oval tubers; pleasantly moist, mild flavor; very good crop for northern regions; color darkens after January.

Cilena
Early, firm tubers with deep yellow, clear flesh; long in shape; mild, pleasant boiling and salad potato; high quality, good yield.

Cinja
Early, generally firm, dark yellow; long to oval tubers; good cooking consistency; good quality; keeps well in winter.

Exquisa
Mid-season, firm, yellowish tubers with a long, oval, pointed shape; delicate flavor, firm flesh, very good quality, but low yield; susceptible to disease.

Gloria
Very early seedlings, generally firm, pure yellow tubers with an oval to long shape; very good for all cooking purposes; medium quality, good yield.

Granola
Mid-season, generally firm, yellow, slightly rough-skinned tubers with a round to oval shape; pleasant flavor, medium quality, good yield, very robust, keeps very well.

Leyla
Very early seedlings, generally firm tubers with a dark yellow color that does not darken after cooking. Oval to long shape; very pleasant flavor, medium quality, satisfactory yield.

Linda
Mid-season, firm potato with a yellow color that does not change after cooking; relatively small, longish, tubers; very good flavor; low yield; does not keep as well as other varieties.

Nicola
Mid-season, firm potato with a yellow color that does not change after cooking. Attractive, long, oval shape; mild flavor; delicate consistency, low quality, limited keeping time.

Renate
Early, firm, yellow-fleshed potato that is oval in shape. It is important to keep the tubers covered with earth; medium yield; keeps well.

Rosella
Mid-season to late potato, generally firm, with a yellow or dark yellow color. Red skin and oval in shape, it has a distinctive flavor. Difficult to peel. It is resistant to disease, has a high yield and keeps very well.

Santé
Mid-season, floury potato with light yellow skin and flesh. Large, oval tubers; fairly good flavor, good resistance to disease, very high yield. Keeps fairly well.

Sieglinde
Early, firm yellow variety with smooth skin. Pleasant flavor and oval shape; a good consistency, particularly suitable for salads; an old variety with a medium yield.

Solara
Mid-season, firm, clear colored variety that does not deepen in color after cooking. Oval in shape with a neutral flavor, this potato cooks quickly and is extremely good quality. It has a good resistance to disease and a high yield.

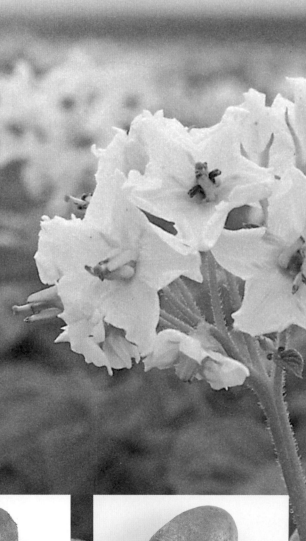

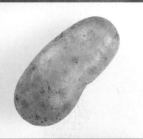

1

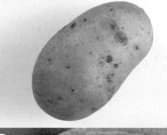

2

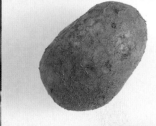

3

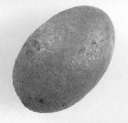

4

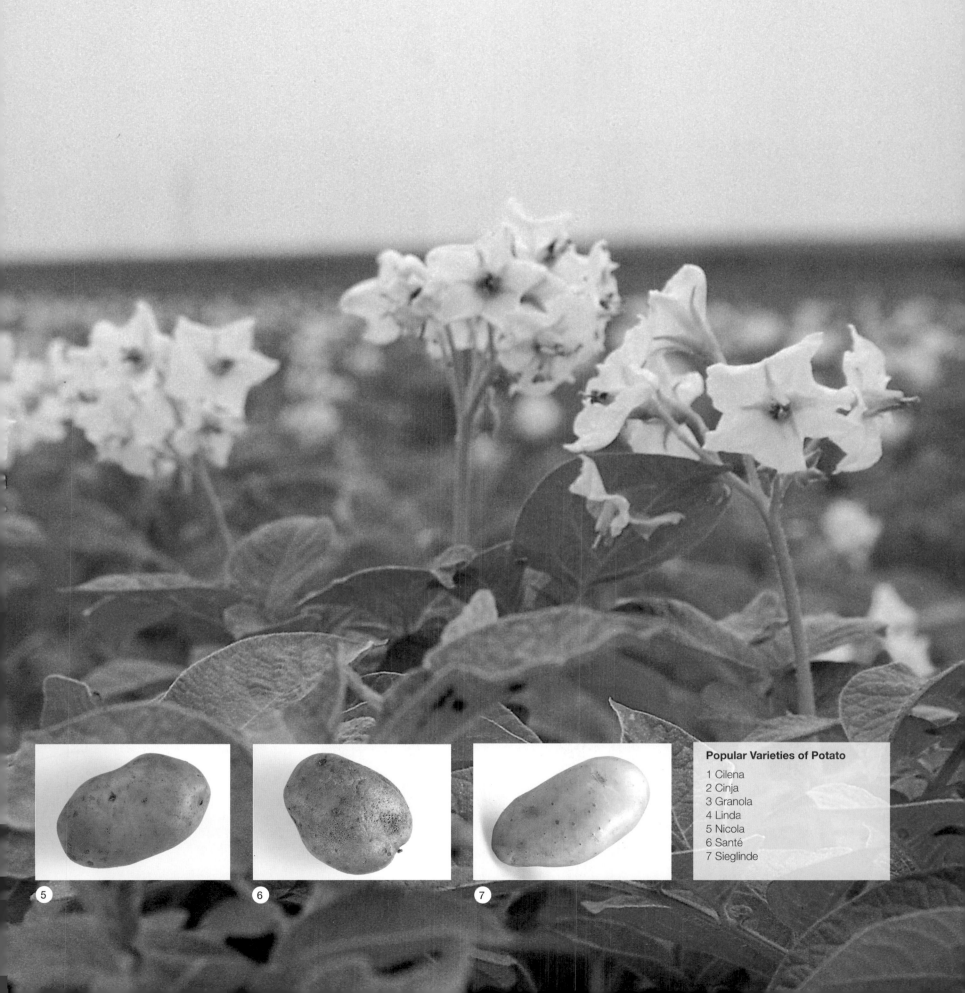

Popular Varieties of Potato

1 Cilena
2 Cinja
3 Granola
4 Linda
5 Nicola
6 Santé
7 Sieglinde

Cooking Characteristics of Potatoes

Firm These potatoes have less starch than other varieties. As a rule, their skin does not come away from the flesh during cooking. In northern Europe they are also known as "salad potatoes" because they are often used in salads. Their firm, even consistency also makes them a good choice for boiling, frying, and potato gratin.

Fairly firm These contain more starch than firm potatoes. Their skin comes away from the flesh during cooking. They can be used for every type of potato dish, but are mostly used for boiling as they absorb gravy and sauces very well. They are good boiled in their skins, but can also be used for baking,

frying, and making into french fries.

Floury, or firm, floury potatoes These potatoes have a very high starch content, and their skins come away from the flesh completely during cooking. Very good for purées or mixing into pastry. Can also be used to thicken soups.

How to tell the starch content of a potato Cut the potato in half down the middle, and rub the two halves together. The more the two halves stick together, the higher the starch content of the potato and the flourier they will be. If they do not stick together, then they are firm potatoes. Firm, floury potatoes have a medium starch content.

How to Prepare Potatoes

- Potatoes are best boiled in their skins. This ensures that no nutrients are lost. Always place potatoes into boiling water.
- Prepare and eat early potatoes as quickly as possible. After 10–14 days they begin to spoil. It is advisable to steam new potatoes since they have very tender skins.
- Always keep potatoes in a dark place or they will develop green patches, which indicates the presence of the poison Solanin, that must be removed before cooking.
- If potatoes are going to be stored for long then it is important to have a dark, dry, airy cellar that is cool, but not frosty.

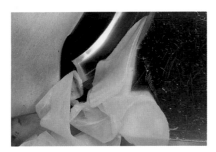

Floury potatoes are used for potato ravioli and are cut into very thin slices.

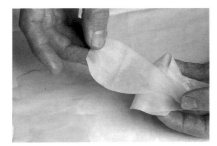

The potato slices are arranged carefully onto clean paper towels.

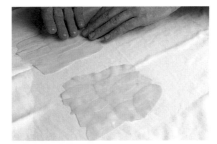

Then the slices of potato are placed so that they overlap and form squares about 5 inches (12 cm) in size.

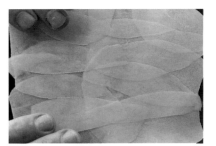

These squares made from potato slices form the basis for potato ravioli. Now they need to be set together.

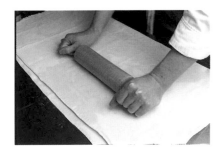

The squares are covered with another layer of paper towel, which is then dampened slightly, and pressed over with a rolling pin.

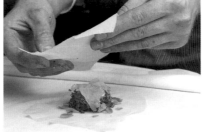

The filling is placed on top of each square – blood sausage, escarole and marjoram – and then it is covered by another square.

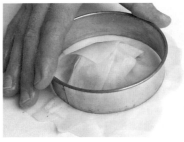

Using a pastry cutter 4 inches (10 cm) in diameter, the ravioli are cut out from the squares.

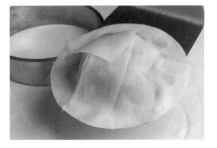

Finally the ravioli are quickly fried in oil until lightly browned, and then seasoned.

Potato Ravioli with Blood Sausage

(Illustration above and right)

5 1/2 oz (125 g) Puy lentils (see page 185)
2 Tbs Balsamic vinegar
4 floury potatoes
2 Tbs finely chopped marjoram
Escarole
4 slices blood sausage
5 Tbs olive oil
Coarse salt, black pepper
1 finely chopped shallot
3 strands saffron
1 pinch ground cumin

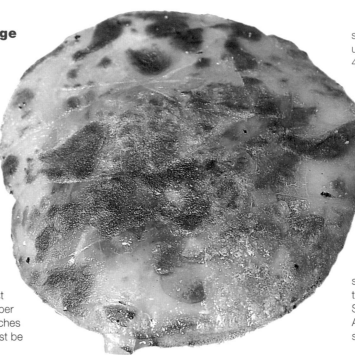

Place the lentils in water, add 1 tablespoon of vinegar, and bring to the boil. Cook for about 40 minutes, then drain, and set aside.

Cut the raw potatoes into very thin slices – it is best to use a machine for this – and lay them out on paper towels, so that they form 8 squares with sides 5 inches (12 cm) long. The size of the squares of potato must be

slightly more than the diameter of the cutter that will be used to make the ravioli – a cutter with diameter of 4 inches (10 cm) was used for the ravioli in the picture – a good size to handle.

Place one layer of paper towels on top of the potato squares, dampen the towel slightly, and run a rolling pin quickly and carefully over the towel so that the potatoes bind together. Remove the top layer of paper towel.

Onto each of 4 squares place 1/2 teaspoon of marjoram, a little sliced escarole, and 1 slice of blood sausage. Cover with a potato square, press the sides to seal, and cut out each ravioli using a round cutter.

Heat 3 tablespoons of oil in a skillet, and fry the ravioli until they begin to turn brown: season both sides with salt and pepper.

Fry the shallot in the remaining olive oil, add the saffron and cook briefly. Add the cumin and vinegar, then the lentils and mix all the ingredients thoroughly. Season to taste with salt and pepper.

Arrange the ravioli on plates with a portion of lentils and serve.

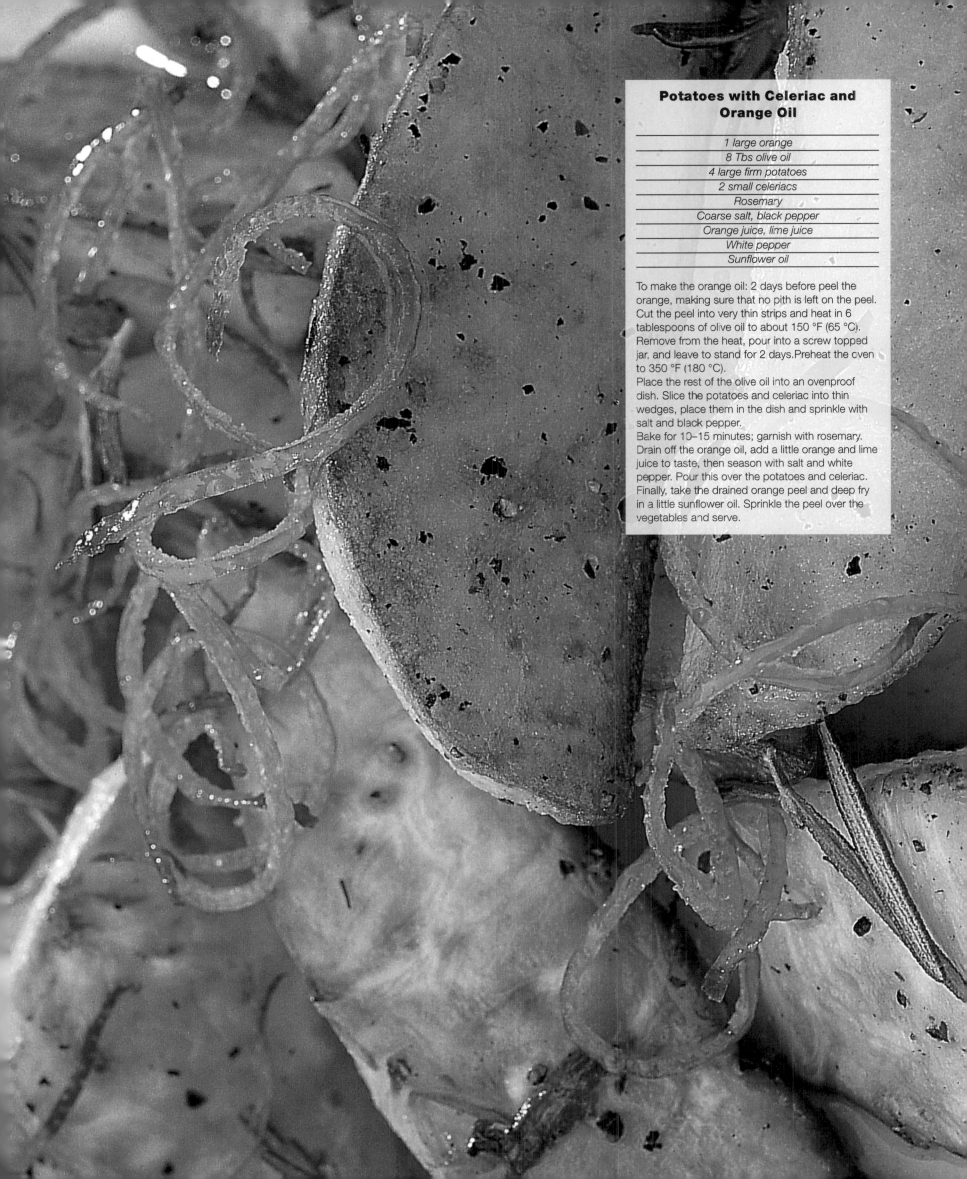

Potatoes with Celeriac and Orange Oil

1 large orange
8 Tbs olive oil
4 large firm potatoes
2 small celeriacs
Rosemary
Coarse salt, black pepper
Orange juice, lime juice
White pepper
Sunflower oil

To make the orange oil: 2 days before peel the orange, making sure that no pith is left on the peel. Cut the peel into very thin strips and heat in 6 tablespoons of olive oil to about 150 °F (65 °C). Remove from the heat, pour into a screw topped jar, and leave to stand for 2 days. Preheat the oven to 350 °F (180 °C).

Place the rest of the olive oil into an ovenproof dish. Slice the potatoes and celeriac into thin wedges, place them in the dish and sprinkle with salt and black pepper.

Bake for 10–15 minutes; garnish with rosemary. Drain off the orange oil, add a little orange and lime juice to taste, then season with salt and white pepper. Pour this over the potatoes and celeriac. Finally, take the drained orange peel and deep fry in a little sunflower oil. Sprinkle the peel over the vegetables and serve.

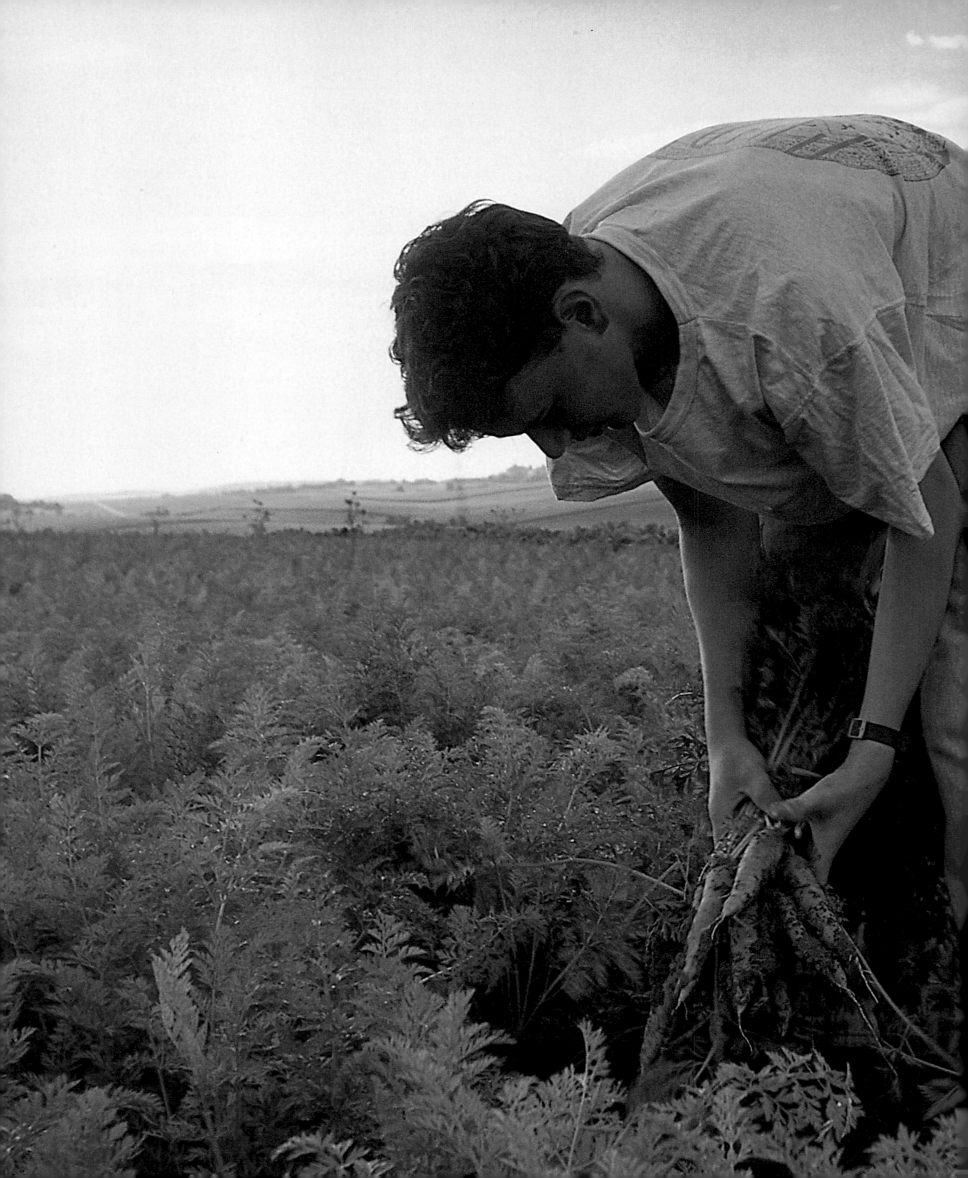

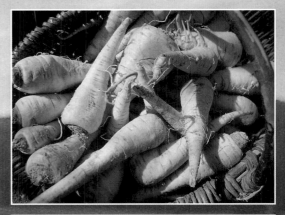

Beet
The first beets of the year can be bought in May.

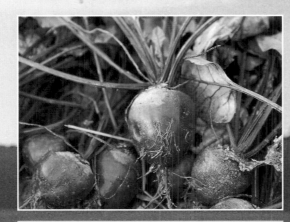

Parsnips
Young parsnips are firm, crunchy, and delicious eaten raw. They store and keep well.

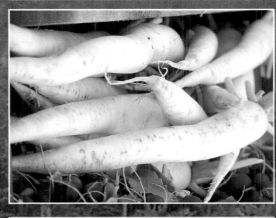

Radishes
These long, white radishes are very refreshing eaten raw – particularly in summer.

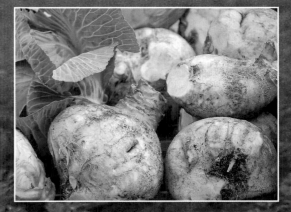

Rutabaga
Rutabaga is a spring vegetable with a green top, that can also be cooked and eaten.

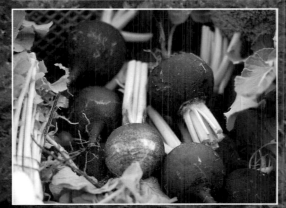

Scorzonera
These roots darken as the year goes by; they can be eaten raw, but are nicest peeled and cooked.

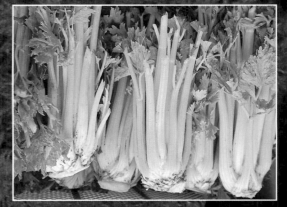

Celery
Celery makes a delicious addition to any salad, and flourishes in the fields during the summer.

Roots and Tubers

Although they belong to different families, plants that form large roots and tubers have one thing in common: they store supplies under the soil that provide energy, and are good for the health. These supplies are actually designed to see the plant through the winter and help it to form seeds in the new year. Roots and tubers generally come from biennial plants.

The most important member of the root and tuber group of vegetables has to be the carrot, although this group also includes beet, salsify, all types of radishes, kohlrabis, and even the exotic Jerusalem artichoke. There is virtually no place on earth where carrots are not grown. Wild carrots have grown in both Asia and Europe for as long as anyone can remember. Carrot seeds have been found in Neolithic dwellings. It is likely that carrots underwent a great change in appearance and flavor during the time of the Roman Empire, when they were crossed with another root *Daucus Maximus*. Since this time, carrots owe their popularity to their shape, delicate flavor, and widespread cultivation.

Carrots get their beautiful coloring from betacarotene, a substance that is bright yellow in its purest form. Carrots are a very important part of vegetarian nutrition, because they have the highest betacarotene content of any vegetable. This provitamin shows itself in human or animal bodies as vitamin A. The effect of vitamin A on the human body has not been very deeply researched, but it is thought that it plays an important part in cell growth. This is why carrots are a favorite baby food. When preparing carrots, it is important to remember that betacarotene can only be absorbed by the body if it is eaten with fat. Raw carrots are a good source of fiber and other nutrients but the betacarotene cannot be used by the body. To obtain the full nutritional benefits of carrots, they should be braised in butter – oil is high in polyunsaturated fats, which prevent betacarotene from being absorbed. Carrots are thought to help prevent cancer, because of their beneficial effect on cells. Vitamin A also helps us to see in the dark, or in poor light. A deficiency in vitamin A manifests itself as night blindness.

Carrots require certain conditions in which to grow. The ideal environment for carrots is deep, well drained, airy, slightly sandy soil, containing a high level of humus. Carrots like soil to be rich and well manured, but the manure should be old. Fresh manure may contain carrot fly, which can cause great damage to the crop.

Carrot seeds are tiny, and about five million seeds are needed to sow an acre of land. Organic farmers use special machines for sowing the seeds to save themselves the laborious work of sowing the carrots by hand.

Many farms grow carrots for babyfood. The main crop ripens over summer and fall; then these nutritious vegetables are harvested and carried off in large trucks.

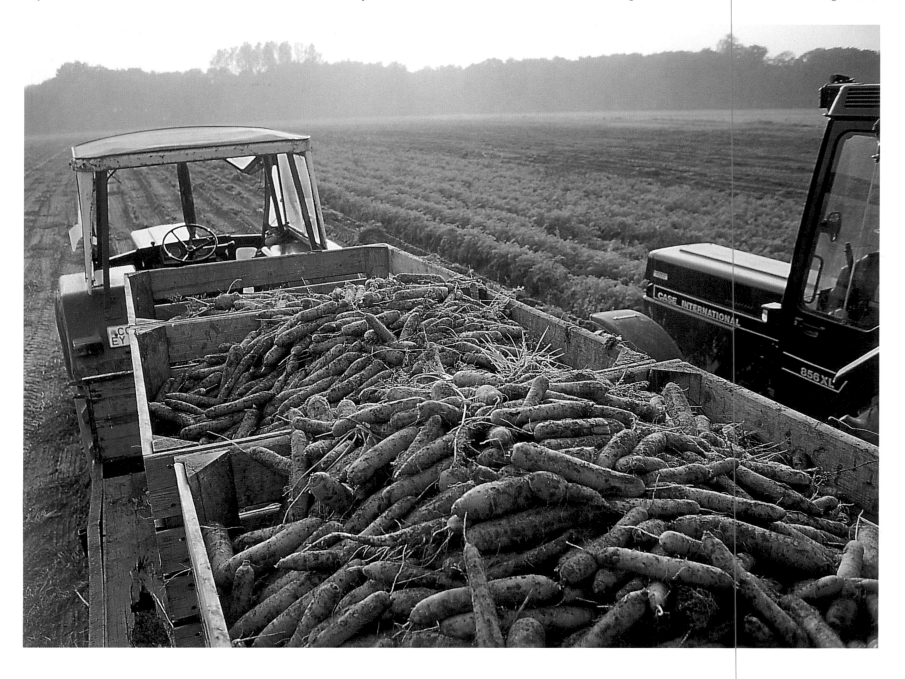

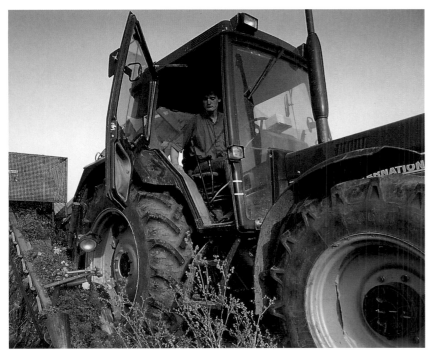

The machine grabs the carrots by the tops and pulls them out of the ground.

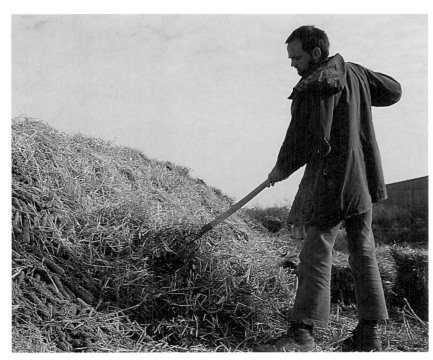

Carrots can be stored in a stack, and will last until the new year.

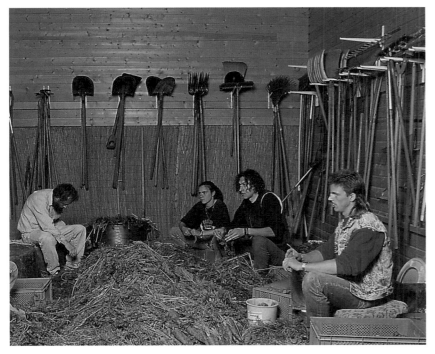

Here, the carrot tops are being removed by hand. The green tops make very good animal fodder.

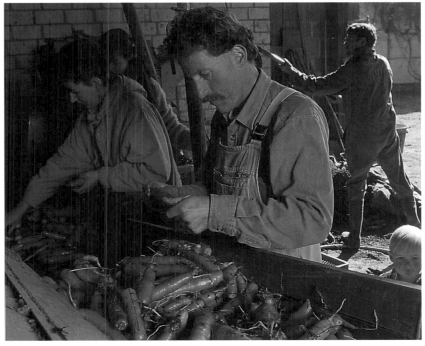

The carrots are picked over carefully, to ensure that the quality is consistently good.

The plants grow on banks that are prepared eight days before the seeds are sown. About 120 carrots grow per yard (1 meter). The banks are dug 2½ feet (75 cm) apart. Just before the carrot tops appear through the soil – usually about a week after planting – any weeds that have appeared are burnt away using a special tool. This allows the carrots to grow unchallenged for 3 to 4 weeks until they are picked. The first fresh carrots of the year can be harvested as early as mid-May in northern Europe although the main crop is from July through November. A carrot harvesting machine pulls the carrots out by the green tops, then the tops are chopped off, and the carrots are collected in a large truck. They are then taken back for storage but are not washed. Early carrots should be eaten as soon as possible as they do not keep for more than a week. To keep them for this long, it is necessary to remove the green tops and store them in the refrigerator. The fall crop (which tends to produce thicker carrots) is far better suited to long term storage. They ripen in the ground for much longer than the earlier varieties, and should not be harvested until their tops discolor.

The green tops of early carrots can be cooked and eaten with the carrots. They are delicious and full of nutrients.

Recipes with Roots and Tubers

Cream of Celeriac Soup with Sparkling White Wine
(Illustration below)

1 medium-sized celeriac
1 small onion
1 Tbs butter
1 Tbs vegetable stock granules
Coarse salt, white pepper
1 tsp lemon juice
$^3/_4$ cup (125 ml) sparkling white wine
$^3/_4$ cup (125 ml) heavy cream

Cut the celeriac into bite-sized pieces.
Dice the onion finely and sweat in the butter until transparent.
Add the celeriac and pour in 3$^3/_4$ cups (750 ml) water. Simmer the vegetables until just tender, then liquidize. Stir in the stock granules and season to taste with salt and pepper. Add the lemon juice and sparkling wine. Beat the cream until slightly thickened, add to the soup and allow to come to the boil briefly. Season again and serve at once.

Celeriac and Carrot Salad with Watercress

1 small celeriac
11 oz (300 g) young carrots
10 small radishes
1 bunch watercress
2 oz (50 g) roughly chopped walnuts

Dressing
2 Tbs sherry vinegar
2 Tbs cider vinegar
2 Tbs vegetable stock granules
1 tsp honey
1 tsp mustard
4 Tbs sunflower oil
1 finely chopped shallot
1 Tbs finely chopped parsley

Slice the celeriac, carrots, and radishes into medium-sized strips.
To make the dressing: place all the ingredients in a screw top jar and shake vigorously. Remove 2 tablespoons of dressing and set aside.
Mix the rest of the dressing with the vegetables and leave to marinate for 10 minutes.
Mix the watercress with the reserved dressing and arrange a bed of watercress on a large platter. Place the vegetables on top of the watercress, sprinkle with the walnuts and serve at once.

Jerusalem Artichoke Salad

12 medium Jerusalem artichokes
2 oz (50 g) pine nuts
1 lemon
2 Tbs olive oil
Coarse salt, white pepper
1 bunch finely chopped parsley

Cook the Jerusalem artichokes in water until tender, then peel and dice.
Dry fry the pine nuts in a skillet until evenly browned.
Halve the lemon, squeeze the juice from one half and cut the other into thin slices.
Mix the lemon juice, oil, salt, pepper, and parsley together and pour the marinade over the diced Jerusalem artichokes.
Sprinkle with pine nuts and garnish with the slices of lemon. Serve whilst still warm

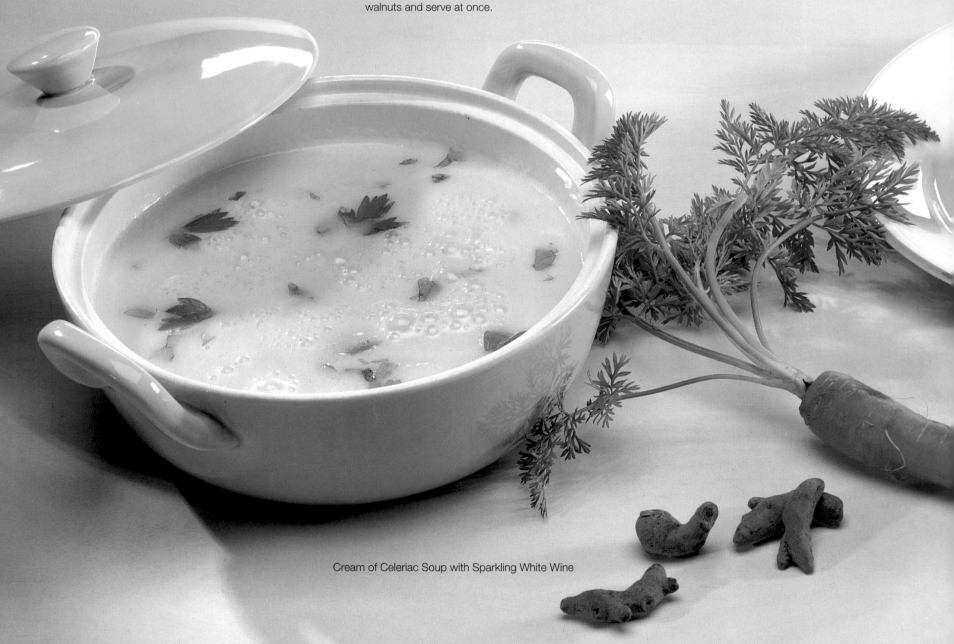

Cream of Celeriac Soup with Sparkling White Wine

Beet, Apple, and Nut Salad
(Illustration below right)

3 medium beets
1 apple
1 onion
3 Tbs white wine vinegar
4 Tbs safflower oil
1 Tbs honey
Coarse salt, black pepper
1 tsp ground cumin
Chopped hazelnuts

Grate the beets, chop the apple into small pieces, and finely chop the onion. Beat together the oil, vinegar, honey, salt, pepper, and cumin until it forms a frothy vinaigrette.
Mix together the beets, apple, onion, and hazelnuts and pour the dressing over them. Stir well, season to taste and wait 15 minutes before serving, so that the flavors can develop.

Caramelized Root Vegetables
(Illustration below center)

4 medium carrots
1 parsnip
2 Tbs olive oil
1 tsp turmeric
2 Tbs honey
4 Tbs white wine vinegar
1/2 tsp herb salt
1 pinch paprika
1 pinch ground cinnamon
1 pinch ground cloves
1 pinch cayenne pepper
Coarse salt

Cut the carrots and parsnip into long strips, heat half the olive oil and braise the carrots in the oil. Then add half a teaspoon of turmeric and 1 tablespoon of the honey to the pan. Allow to caramelize slightly, then add 2 tablespoons of vinegar to the pan together with the other spices.
Braise the parsnips in the remaining oil. Add the remaining turmeric and honey. When the parsnips have caramelized, add the other two tablespoons of vinegar, and season with salt to taste.
Arrange the parsnip and carrots attractively on the serving plates and serve as a starter.

Salsify with Ham

2 lbs (800 g) salsify
4 Tbs lemon juice
5 cups (1 l) vegetable stock
1 slice cured ham – about 2 oz (50 g) in weight
1 small onion
1 bunch flat-leafed parsley
1 Tbs olive oil
1 oz (30 g) butter
Coarse salt, white pepper

Peel the salsify either wearing rubber gloves, or rub vinegar into your hands first. Cut the salsify into 2 inch (5 cm) pieces and put into water immediately. Add 2 tablespoons of the lemon juice to the water, so that the salsify does not discolor. Bring the vegetable stock, together with 1 tablespoon of the lemon juice, to the boil. Add the salsify, simmer for 10 minutes, then drain. Finely chop the ham, onion, and parsley and brown in the oil. Add the salsify and cook, stirring frequently for about 15 minutes, until the salsify is "al dente." Stir in the butter, add the remaining lemon juice and season to taste with salt and pepper.

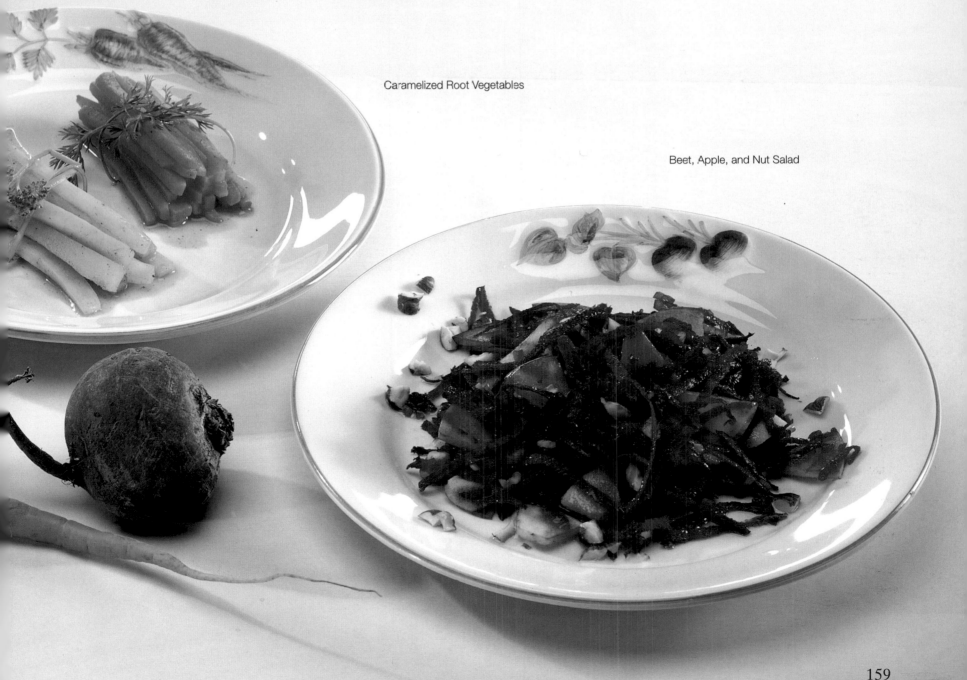

Caramelized Root Vegetables

Beet, Apple, and Nut Salad

Long Forgotten and Unappreciated

Parsnips

In earlier times, parsnips were sweet-tasting, whitish yellow root vegetables, that could grow up to 8 inches (about 40 centimeters) long. They were a type of parsley, distantly related to the carrot and were a very important part of our diet. However, the arrival of the potato reduced the parsnip's popularity. Parsnips are as nutritious as potatoes, having almost the same level of carbohydrates, a little less protein, and a little more fat. They have the same potassium and magnesium content as potatoes and are richer in phosphorus, calcium, and vitamin C.

One of the factors that contributed to the decline of the parsnip in the 18th century (when it was even more popular than the carrot) was the problem of cultivating them. They are one of the earlier crops, but need to grow for seven months before they can be harvested. Germination of parsnips is a slow and irregular process, and can take up to four weeks. The best way to tell when parsnips are ready to plant out, is by sowing radishes along with the parsnips. When the radishes are ready to be eaten, then the parsnips are ready to be planted out.

The plus points of the parsnip is its simplicity to grow and its hardiness. Parsnips can be grown in practically any soil, although they prefer to be in well-prepared, airy, deep fields or vegetable beds, where the soil is rich in humus. Like carrots, parsnips should not be fertilized by fresh manure. This is not because the carrot fly might spoil the crop, but rather that they will make deformed and not spindle-shaped tubers. Parsnips are extremely hardy, and are not at risk to any disease.

Parsnips can be harvested from October onwards and if kept covered, then they can be harvested in winter. They are available at a time of year when there are few fresh vegetables on the market. Parsnips keep very well if they are unwashed and stored in a cool place. In these conditions they will keep until spring.

In English speaking, and Scandinavian countries, parsnips are eaten as purées, or roasted in the oven. In other countries, they are only used as cow fodder or as bulk in pre-packaged foods. Parsnips are very popular in England, and are used in French and Austrian cuisine for salads and stews.

The renewed popularity of the parsnip is due to their increased cultivation in organic farming. Parsnips are both healthy and delicious, they are piquant, and have a wealth of essential oils that stimulate the digestion. Their sweet smell and unusual flavor – somewhere between a carrot and celery – makes them ideal accompaniments for salty and smoked foods. They have a nutty flavor when eaten raw. Parsnips can be used in cooking in a variety of ways: grated raw, they are delicious in salads, they can be steamed or fried, eaten alone or with other vegetables, they can be included in soups or stews. However they are served, they always provide an interesting, hearty culinary experience.

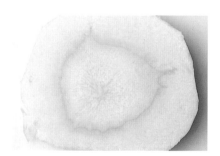
Unwashed parsnips will keep until the new year. They should be scrubbed thoroughly before use.

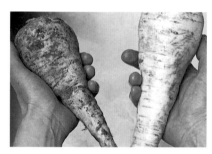
These long root vegetables were very popular as a staple food until the arrival of the potato.

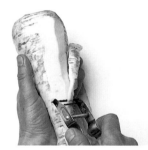
Parsnips should be peeled before use, even when they have been scrubbed.

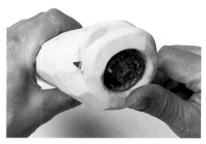
Often the top of the parsnip (where the leaves were attached) is dark brown. It is advisable to cut this out before cooking.

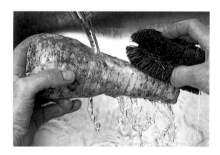
The center of a parsnip is woody, and its cortex very rich in nutrients.

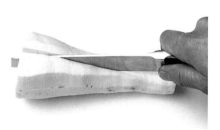
Parsnips have to be chopped, because they are so large. They should be halved lengthways before chopping.

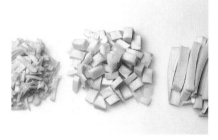
Parsnips are easiest to work with when they are chopped. They can be diced, finely chopped, or cut into strips.

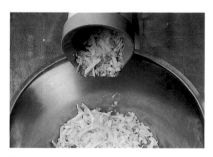
For salads, rissoles, or purées, parsnips should be grated.

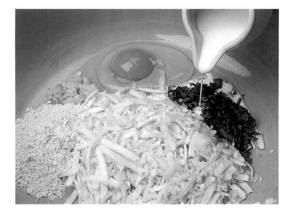
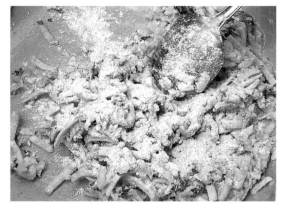
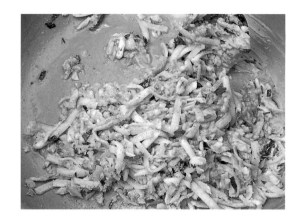

Parsnip Rissoles

2 medium parsnips
1 small onion
1 bunch flat-leafed parsley
1/2 tsp herb salt
White pepper
2 Tbs spelt flour
1 egg
1 Tbs light cream

Coarsely grate the parsnips. Finely chop the onion and the parsley and mix all the ingredients together thoroughly.
Heat plenty of oil in a skillet. Place tablespoons of the parsnip mixture into the fat and pan fry for about 7 minutes on each side.

Parsnip and Spinach Gratin

2 large parsnips
1 lb 2 oz (500 g) leaf spinach
1 medium onion
1 garlic clove
1 Tbs olive oil
Herb salt, black pepper
1/2 cup (125 ml) light cream
2 Tbs Mascarpone
1 egg
3 1/2 oz (100 g) freshly grated Emmental
Coarse salt

Cut the parsnips into 6–8 inch (15–20 cm) long, fairly wide strips and steam in a colander over a saucepan of boiling water for 3–4 minutes.
Tear the spinach into large pieces.
Finely chop the onion and garlic and brown lightly in the olive oil. Add the spinach, cover and simmer. Season with herb salt and pepper to taste.
Preheat the oven to 425 °F (220 °C).
Mix together the cream, Mascarpone, egg, and grated Emmental. Add a little coarse salt to taste.
Grease a gratin dish and place half the spinach into the dish. Cover with the parsnips and top with the remaining spinach.
Pour the cream and cheese mixture over the vegetables and bake in the oven for 15 minutes.

Parsnips in a Cream Sauce

3 medium parsnips
1 1/4 cups (250 ml) light cream
1/2 tsp herb salt
2 tsp arrowroot
1 bunch burnet saxifrage (optional)
A dash of lemon juice
Coarse salt, white pepper

Cut the parsnips into strips 1/2 inch (1 cm) wide, 1/2 inch (1 cm) thick, and about 6 inches (15 cm) long. Steam in a colander for about 5–7 minutes, then drain.
Meanwhile, bring the cream mixed with just under 3/4 cup (125 ml) water to the boil. Dissolve the arrowroot in 2 tablespoons of cold water and add to the cream. Finely chop the herb, add to the cream sauce and season to taste with lemon juice, salt, and pepper.
Arrange the parsnips on a warmed plate, and cover with the sauce.

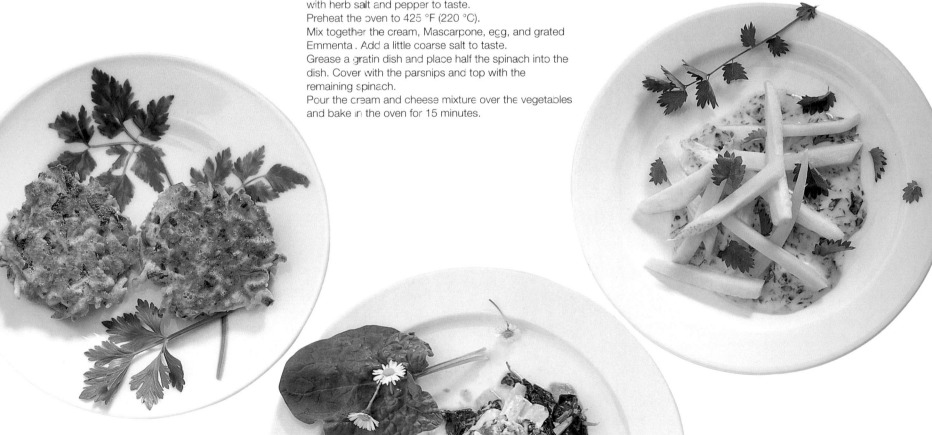

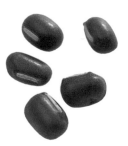

Adzuki Beans
Originally from Japan, these beans are now grown in Italy; popular in soups and rice dishes, but also used in desserts because of their sweet flavor.

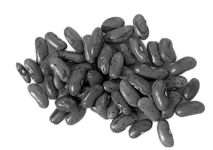

Black Eyed Peas
A variety of the green asparagus bean, with a distinctive dark spot. Very common in South America and Asia; quick-cooking with a pleasant, nutty flavor.

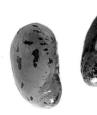

Borlotti Beans
Very popular in Italy, a brownish-red, speckled bean that turns green when cooked. Very good in salads, soups, and sauces.

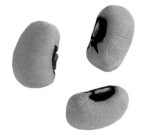

Fava Beans
Also known as broad beans, these are delicious when freshly picked and cooked. They become brown when they are dried. They should be peeled after cooking.

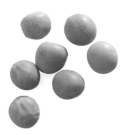

Dried Peas
A variety that ripens in the pod. They do not require peeling and should be soaked overnight before use. Very good in soups, stews, and purées.

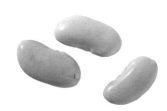

Flageolet Beans
Small, light-green, French variety with enormous versatility, and a delicious flavor, usually served as a side vegetable.

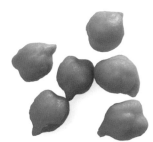

Garbanzo Beans
An annual bush with short pods; its beans are light-beige, yellow, and occasionally black. Used in Africa, Spain, and India to make flour, purées, stews, and vegetable accompaniments.

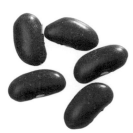

Kidney Beans
Red color and kidney shape makes these beans distinctive as does their fine aroma; very popular in South America, they are firm when cooked but have a floury consistency. Very high in fiber and good for salads, stews, and ragouts.

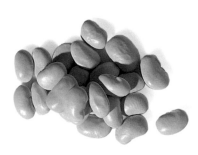

Lima Beans
An off-white bean that comes from Peru, Lima Beans are round and large with an intensive flavor. Cooking water should be changed frequently because Lima Beans have a slight prussic acid content.

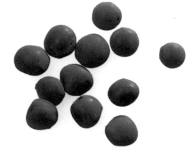

Lentils
Sorted by diameter: more than $1/4$ inch (7 mm) are "large," $1/6$–$1/4$ inch (6–7 mm) are "medium," and $1/8$–$1/6$ inch (4–6 mm) are small. They can be green or brown and the smaller the lentil, the more intense the flavor.

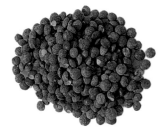

Puy Lentils
Cultivated in France, these small gray-green to blue-green lentils have a thin skin. They cook quickly and have a delicious flavor.

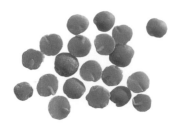

Red Lentils
Small, reddish-brown variety which are peeled and split; quick-cooking, easy to purée, use for soups, purées, and spreads.

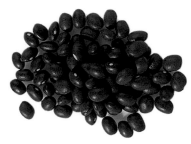

Black Beans
Kidney shaped with a shiny skin and a white center; widely grown in South America; they form the basis of black bean sauce.

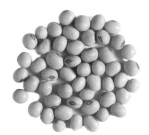

Soybeans
Grown world wide and the most important legume; used in a wide range of products; very high in protein; can be eaten cooked or sprouted in salads (see p. 170).

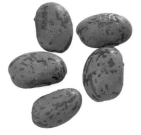

Pinto Beans
Red-brown, with attractive speckled skin that looks like quail's eggs. Pleasant flavor; good for stews, organically grown in the USA.

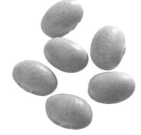

White Beans
Perhaps the best known of the legume family; becomes very soft when overcooked. Standard ingredient in many soups and stews; hearty flavor.

A Virtually Limitless Shelf Life

Dried Legumes

Legumes filled the store cupboards of people in the Dark Ages. When beans, peas, and lentils are ripened and dried, they will keep for years. Their simplicity accounts for their use in early cooking. The *Papilionaceae* family has many different varieties of plants – over 12,000 are known – and they can be grown in any soil, even dry and barren soil. These plants enrich the ground for the next crop by aerating the soil and obtain nitrogen from the air using their tubercles. Leguminous plants form a very important part of organic farming, because they help to fertilize the soil. Not only do they obtain nitrogen from the air, but also use the nitrogen to create protein. Legumes are the most important source of protein in the plant kingdom. They do not contain all the necessary amino acids but, as our ancestors discovered, if they are eaten with cereals, they provide complete proteins. Many traditional recipes in Asia, America, Africa, and Europe are based on legumes. The increased use of chemical fertilizers in modern agriculture, and the fact that legumes are often used as cow fodder, has meant that legumes do not play such an important part in our nutrition as they ought to. However, now that there is greater awareness in the world about nutritional requirements, legumes are becoming more popular, and their high protein content has led to their wide-ranging culinary uses being rediscovered.

Pea Soup, Silesian Style

1 lb 2 oz (500 g) dried whole green peas
1/4 celeriac
1 carrot
4 potatoes
1 leek
1 Tbs finely chopped lovage
4 vegetable stock cubes
4 cured or smoked sausages
3 1/2 oz (100 g) bacon
4 slices stale whole wheat bread
2 Tbs butter

Soak the peas overnight. The following day, drain the peas and place in 1 1/2 pints (2 l) fresh water and bring to the boil.
Dice the celeriac, carrots, and potatoes, slice the leeks into rings. After 20 minutes add the vegetables, lovage, and stock cubes to the peas. Cover and cook for about 60 minutes, adding a little more water if necessary.
Prick the sausages with a fork, add to the soup and cook for about 30 minutes. Finely dice the bacon, and add to the soup just before serving. Cut the bread into small squares, fry in the butter until golden brown, and pass around with the soup.

Durum Wheat Rigatoni with Red Lentils and Red Bell Pepper

1 onion
1 garlic clove
1 Tbs olive oil
5 oz (150 g) red lentils
1 tsp vegetable stock granules
1/2 red bell pepper
1 Tbs tomato paste
Coarse salt, herb salt
Pinch cayenne pepper
Pinch ground paprika
2 Tbs finely chopped flat-leafed parsley
7 oz (200 g) durum wheat rigatoni
1/2 cup (100 ml) vegetable stock

Chop the onion, mince the garlic and pan fry in the oil. Add the lentils and sweat briefly. Pour in 1 1/2 cups (250 ml) water, add the stock granules and cook the lentils for about 20 minutes. Finely dice the bell pepper, add to the lentils and cook together. Stir in the tomato paste, and season to taste with the spices. Then add the parsley. While the lentils are cooking, cook the pasta in the vegetable stock until they are "al dente," and leave to drain. Arrange on plates, pour over the lentil and bell pepper sauce, and serve.

Arugula Salad with Borlotti Beans

7 oz (200 g) dried borlotti or pinto beans
Coarse salt
5 oz (150 g) arugula
4 vine tomatoes
2 Tbs olive oil
2 Tbs balsamic vinegar
2 Tbs vegetable stock
1/2 tsp mustard
White pepper

Soak the beans overnight.
The following day, drain the beans, place in plenty of fresh water, bring to the boil and cook for 60–90 minutes depending on the age of the beans.
When the beans are cooked, add the salt and leave the beans to cool in their cooking water, then drain.
Divide the arugula among the serving plates, arrange the beans on top, and garnish with the tomato cut into eighths. Make a sauce from the remaining ingredients and pour over the beans.
Serve with oven baked polenta.

Protein and Fiber Content of Dried Legumes

Per 3 1/2 ounces (100 g)

	Protein	Fiber
Dried peas, in their skins	c. 3/4 oz (23 g)	c. 1/2 oz (16.8 g)
Garbanzo beans	c. 2/3 oz (20 g)	c. 1/3 oz (9.5 g)
White beans	c. 3/4 oz (22 g)	c. 2/3 oz (19.2 g)
Kidney beans	c. 2/3 oz (21 g)	c. 1/3 oz (8.3 g)
Soybeans	c. 1 1/4 oz (37 g)	c. 1/2 oz (12.0 g)
Lentils	c. 3/4 oz (24 g)	c. 1/3 oz (10.5 g)

In comparison: fresh legumes and vegetables each contain about 1/11–1/6 ounce (2–6 g) protein and fiber.

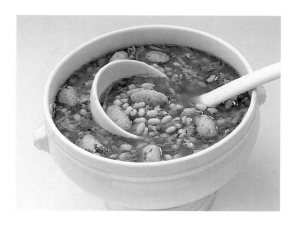

White Bean Soup with Semolina Dumplings

Soup

5 oz (150 g) dried white beans
1 tsp dried lovage
1 tsp dried savory
1 tsp dried basil
1 tsp dried marjoram
1 large pinch caraway seeds
1 bay leaf
1 lb 2 oz (500 g) fresh vegetables
3 Tbs olive oil
1–2 Tbs vegetable stock granules
1 pinch nutmeg
1 tsp coarse salt
3 Tbs finely chopped parsley
2 Tbs lemon juice

Dumplings

2 Tbs butter
2 tsp vegetable stock granules
5 Tbs corn or wheat semolina
1/2 tsp dried oregano
1/2 tsp dried basil
1 pinch nutmeg
1 Tbs farmer's cheese

To make the soup: soak the beans overnight in a saucepan filled with 1 1/4 pints (750 ml) water. The following day, add the herbs to the water and cook the beans until they are tender.
Take a selection of mixed vegetables – celeriac, kohlrabi, carrot, leek, parsnip, or Jerusalem artichoke – and chop or slice them into small pieces. Braise the vegetables briefly in the oil and add to the beans. Then add the vegetable stock, herbs, spices, and parsley, simmer over a low heat for about 10–15 minutes; add a little lemon juice to taste just before serving.
To make the dumplings: place the butter, together with 5 tablespoons (75 ml) of water in a large saucepan. Stir in the semolina, and bring to the boil. Reduce the heat, and leave the semolina to swell, then stir in the farmer's cheese.
Make dumplings out of the mixture either using your hands or 2 teaspoons. Place the dumplings into a pan of boiling, salted water. When they rise to the surface of the water cook them for a further 2–3 minutes. Remove them with a slotted spoon, leave to drain for a few moments, then add to the soup.

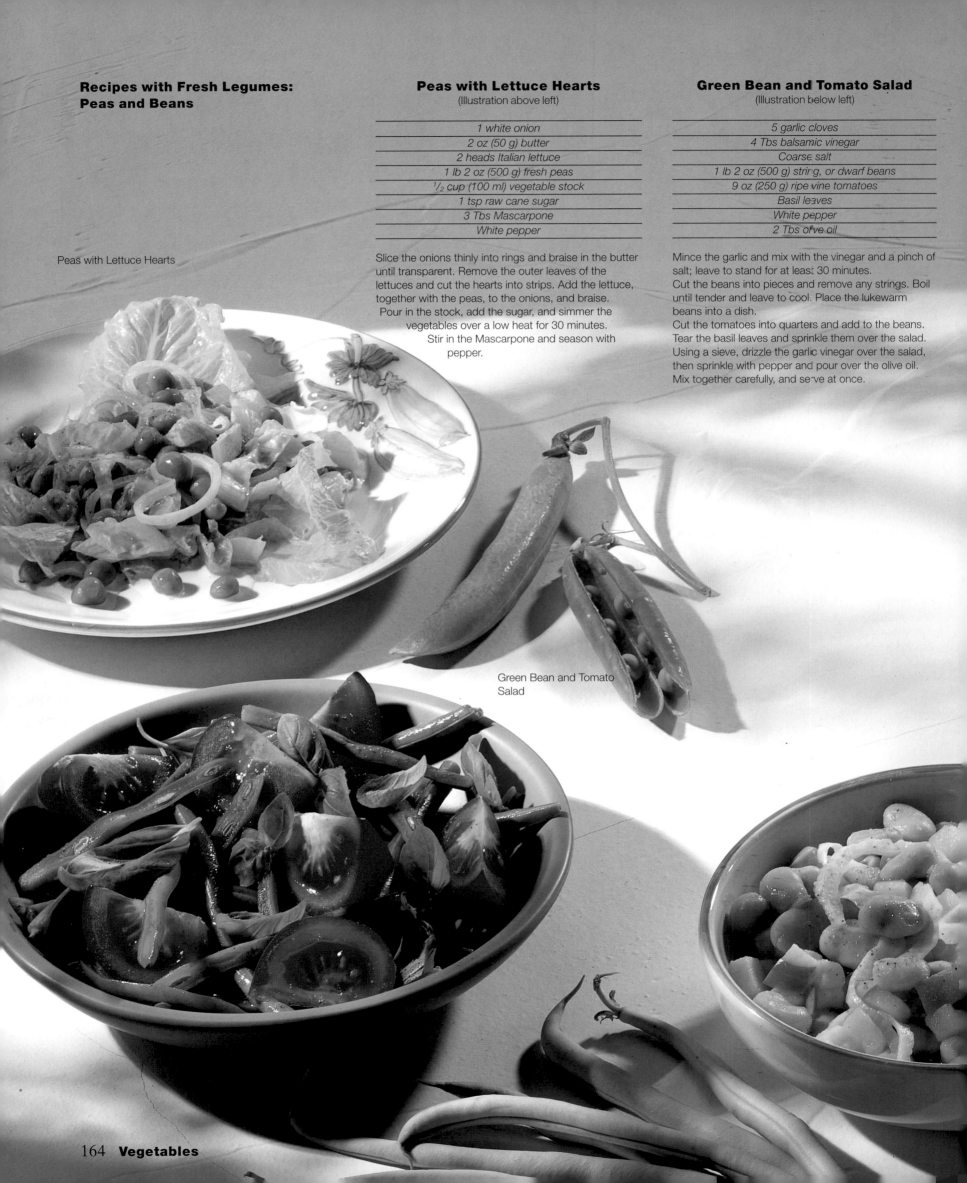

Recipes with Fresh Legumes: Peas and Beans

Peas with Lettuce Hearts
(Illustration above left)

1 white onion
2 oz (50 g) butter
2 heads Italian lettuce
1 lb 2 oz (500 g) fresh peas
1/2 cup (100 ml) vegetable stock
1 tsp raw cane sugar
3 Tbs Mascarpone
White pepper

Slice the onions thinly into rings and braise in the butter until transparent. Remove the outer leaves of the lettuces and cut the hearts into strips. Add the lettuce, together with the peas, to the onions, and braise. Pour in the stock, add the sugar, and simmer the vegetables over a low heat for 30 minutes. Stir in the Mascarpone and season with pepper.

Green Bean and Tomato Salad
(Illustration below left)

5 garlic cloves
4 Tbs balsamic vinegar
Coarse salt
1 lb 2 oz (500 g) string, or dwarf beans
9 oz (250 g) ripe vine tomatoes
Basil leaves
White pepper
2 Tbs olive oil

Mince the garlic and mix with the vinegar and a pinch of salt; leave to stand for at least 30 minutes.
Cut the beans into pieces and remove any strings. Boil until tender and leave to cool. Place the lukewarm beans into a dish.
Cut the tomatoes into quarters and add to the beans. Tear the basil leaves and sprinkle them over the salad. Using a sieve, drizzle the garlic vinegar over the salad, then sprinkle with pepper and pour over the olive oil. Mix together carefully, and serve at once.

Peas with Lettuce Hearts

Green Bean and Tomato Salad

Pasta with Sugar Snap Peas and Smoked Salmon

1 lb 2 oz (500 g) whole wheat pasta
1 shallot
1 oz (30 g) butter
9 oz (250 g) sugar snap peas
9 oz (250 g) Mascarpone
2 oz (50 g) freshly grated hard cheese
Coarse salt, white pepper
3 1/2 oz (100 g) wild smoked salmon

Cook the pasta in boiling, salted water until "al dente."
Finely chop the shallot.
Melt the butter in a large skillet and braise the shallot in the butter until transparent.
Blanch the peas in boiling, salted water for 5 minutes, drain, and rinse in cold water.
Add the Mascarpone to the skillet of shallots, allow it to melt, add the peas and leave to simmer for 5 minutes.
Stir in the cheese and season the mixture with salt and pepper. Add the pasta.
Serve on warmed plates and sprinkle strips of smoked salmon over the pasta.

Green Beans in Mint Sauce

1 lb 9 oz (700 g) green beans
2 Tbs olive oil
1 garlic clove
1 Tbs vinegar
2 Tbs chopped mint
Coarse salt

Cook the beans in boiling, salted water until they are just tender. Drain, place in a bowl, and keep warm.
Heat the oil in a skillet and add the garlic, stirring well.
Add the vinegar, mint, and salt, and mix together well.
Heat the sauce, pour over the beans and serve at once.

Fava Beans with Fennel and Apple

(Illustration below left)

2 Tbs butter
1 lb 9 oz (700 g) fava beans
1 fennel bulb
1 apple
Coarse salt, white pepper

Melt the butter in a skillet over a low heat.
Add the beans with a little water and simmer for 15–20 minutes.
Cut the fennel into fine strips, core and dice the apple.
Add the fennel and apple to the beans, cover and cook for a further 6 minutes. Remove the lid and cook until almost all the liquid has evaporated. Season to taste with salt and pepper.
Serve with Ricotta or cottage cheese, and bread.

String Beans with Tomatoes

2 Tbs olive oil
1 small onion
1 lb 2 oz (500 g) tomatoes
1 garlic clove
2 lbs 3 oz (1 kg) string or dwarf beans
1 cup (200 ml) vegetable stock
1 tsp oregano
Coarse salt, white pepper

Heat the oil in a casserole, finely chop the onions and braise in the oil until transparent.
Skin and quarter the tomatoes. Mince the garlic and add to the onion. Braise for 2 minutes then add the tomatoes. Remove any strings from the beans, break the beans into pieces and add to the tomatoes.
Stir the mixture well and pour in the stock. Sprinkle the oregano over the top, cover and simmer for 30 minutes.
Remove the lid, and cook until all the liquid has evaporated and the beans are cooked. Season with salt and pepper.

Fava Bean and Pecorino Sauce

9 oz fava beans
1 bunch peppermint
1 garlic clove
4 Tbs grated Pecorino
2 Tbs olive oil
Coarse salt, white pepper

Blanch the beans in boiling water for 2 minutes. If the beans are very large, they should be peeled.
Roughly chop the mint and liquidize with the remaining ingredients. If the sauce seems too thick, add a little olive oil to make it thinner. Season with salt and pepper to taste.
Serve with pasta or meat. The sauce should not be kept, as it loses its freshness very quickly.

Braised Fava Beans

7 oz (200 g) white onions
2 Tbs olive oil
2 tomatoes
14 oz (400 g) fava beans
2 tsp vegetable stock granules
Coarse salt, white pepper
2 Tbs finely chopped parsley

Chop the onions. Place the oil in a casserole, add the onions, and braise until transparent.
Skin, deseed, and chop the tomatoes. Add the tomatoes, beans, and stock granules to the onions.
Cover and cook for about 30 minutes. Add more water if it looks dry. Season with salt and pepper, garnish with parsley, and serve.

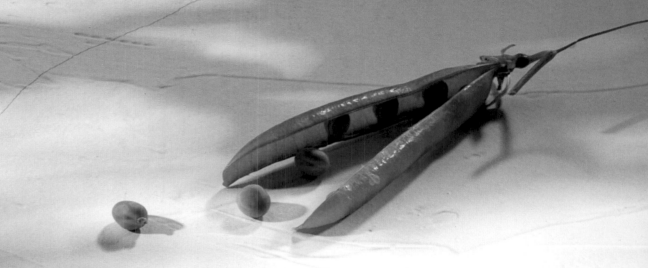

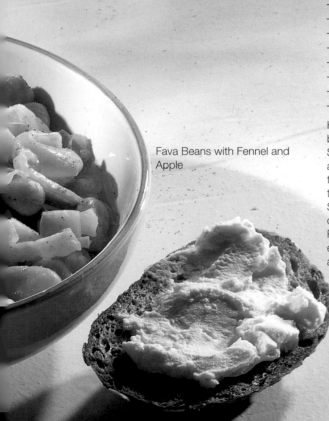

Fava Beans with Fennel and Apple

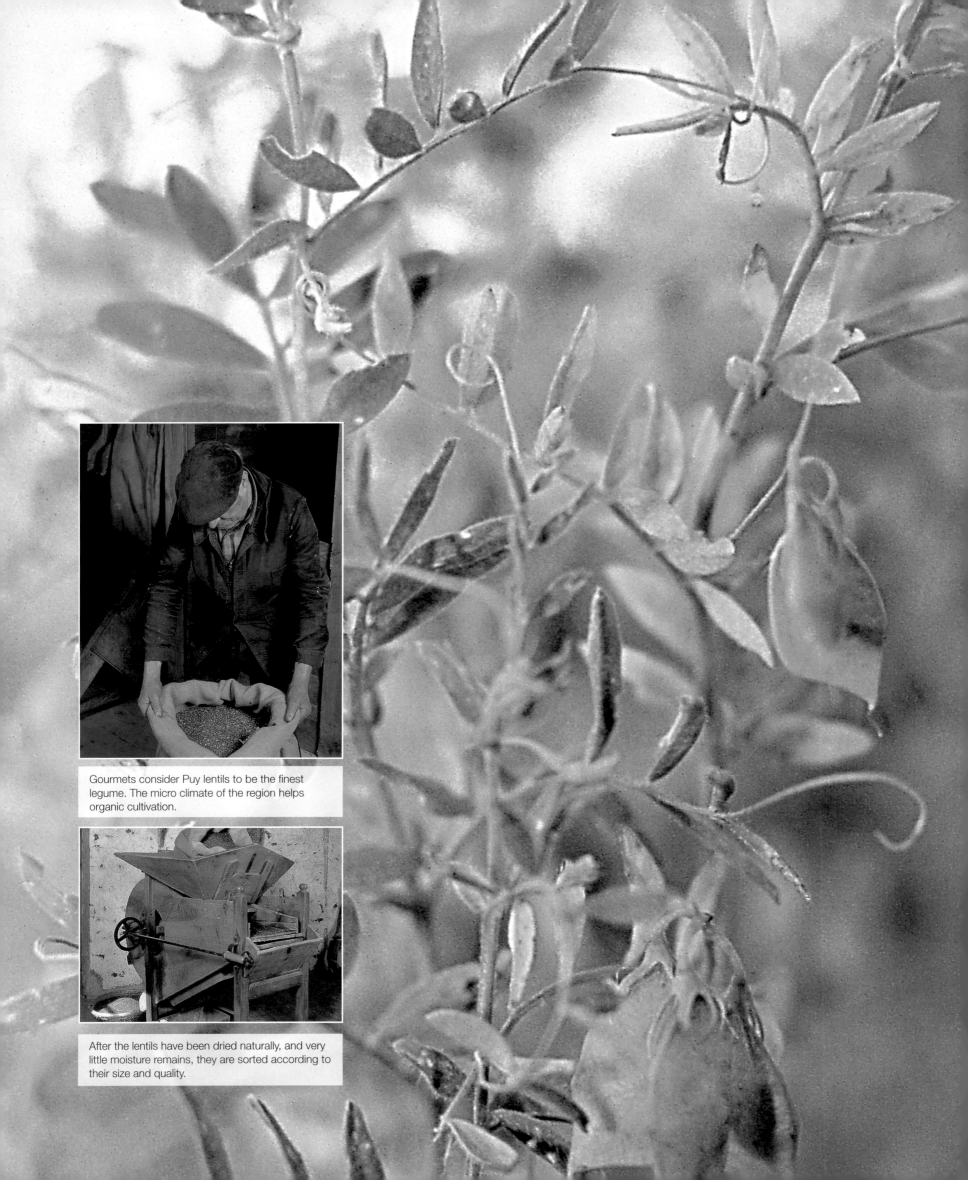

Gourmets consider Puy lentils to be the finest legume. The micro climate of the region helps organic cultivation.

After the lentils have been dried naturally, and very little moisture remains, they are sorted according to their size and quality.

Europe's Most Famous Lentils

The Green Lentils of Puy

Europe's most famous lentils come from the Auvergne, the volcanic region in the center of France. To be more precise, they come from Velay, whose main town Puy is overlooked by three volcanoes. Excavations from the time of Roman Gaul show that these lentils have been cultivated for nearly 2,000 years. Their green color is provided by the blue pigment Anthozyan, which creates a blue-green color when it covers the yellow kernel. Sometimes the lentils have a deep blue marbled color, which happens if the pigment is not evenly distributed. This pigment – which can also be found in blueberries and black grapes – has a beneficial effect on the arteries.

Puy lentils are an especially small variety, being only $^1/_6$–$^1/_5$ inch (4–5 millimeters) in diameter and only $^1/_{12}$–$^1/_{10}$ inch (2–2.5 millimeters) wide. The skin forms a greater proportion of the lentil and is especially aromatic. Puy lentils retain more minerals than other varieties, and have a particularly high iron and magnesium content. These minerals are contained in the kernel of the lentil.

It is not only the high nutritional value of Puy lentils that accounts for their popularity, they also have a thinner skin than other lentils and are less starchy. These factors mean that Puy lentils require a short cooking time and have a firm consistency when cooked. They turn an attractive brown color when cooked and keep extremely well.

There are about 700 farmers in Velay, who sow a total of 6,000 acres (about 2,500 hectares) with lentils. They plant a very old variety called "Anicia." The time to sow the lentils is in March and April when the temperature of the soil rises above 41 °F (5 °C). There is a tradition of observing the phases of the moon – lentils should be sown when the moon is waning, in the last quarter – and they need to be placed 1 inch (2–3 centimeters) below ground, to germinate properly. The distance between rows of lentils is 6–8 inches (15–20 centimeters). This means that there are about 350 seeds per square yard (square meter) and about 220 pounds (100 kilograms) seed per hectare.

The fields are at an altitude of 1,800 to 3,600 feet (600–1,200 meters) and are not fertilized. Since Puy lentils are for the most part grown on volcanic soil, which is extremely fertile, the lentils obtain their nitrogen from the air. It is now known that it is not only the volcanic soil that gives Puy lentils their distinctive characteristics, as they have been grown in other types of soil with a reasonable amount of success. A more important factor in the cultivation of Puy lentils is the micro climate. No matter what the season, Le Puy enjoys warm weather. The Cantal and the Margeride mountains in the south west together with Vivarais in the south east form a protective barrier and often produce the Mistral. The geographic surroundings result in long hours of sunshine and warm, dry, winds.

If the plants have to endure lower temperatures when they are germinating, then the weather has usually picked up by the time that they are ripening and provides the warm conditions in which they flourish. The intense heat of the region has a debilitating effect on the lentils and prevents them from reaching their optimum starch levels and makes their skins paler. These factors account for their unusual culinary qualities. The harvest takes place from the end July through the beginning September. By this time the lentils have ripened naturally and have a moisture content of only 14–16 percent, or even less. Then they are sorted by size and quality and packaged. They are ideal for organic cultivation because they do not require fertilizers and enrich the ground with nitrogen. This makes lentils an ideal intercrop.

Puy Lentils "Au Naturel"

1 stick celery
1–2 carrots
2 onions
2 oz (50 g) bacon
2 Tbs olive oil
1 cup (200 ml) white wine
1 lb 2 oz (500 g) Puy lentils
1 Tbs vegetable stock granules
1 sprig thyme
2 bay leaves
1 tsp butter
Coarse salt, black pepper

Dice the vegetables and cut the bacon into strips. Braise in the oil. Add the white wine and reduce the liquid by a half.
Pick over the lentils and add to the vegetables. Add three times the volume of water together with the stock granules, thyme, and bay leaves. Simmer for 25–30 minutes depending on how firm or soft you want the lentils to be.
Drain the lentils, keeping the cooking liquid. Cook 3 tablespoons (45 g) of the lentils in the cooking water until they are very soft. Liquidize them and add to the other lentils. Mix thoroughly add the butter, season with salt and pepper, and serve.

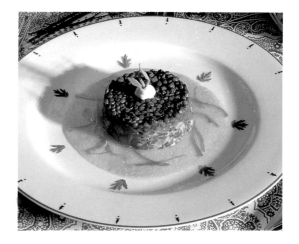

Salmon Tartare with Puy Lentils
(Illustration above)

2 onions
5 oz (150 g) Puy lentils
1 bouquet garni
2 tsp vegetable stock granules
3 Tbs olive oil
2 Tbs white wine vinegar
1 Tbs mustard
Coarse salt, black pepper
11 oz (300 g) salmon
3 shallots
3 small gherkins
1 hard-cooked egg
1 Tbs finely chopped parsley
1 Tbs finely chopped tarragon
Lemon juice
$^1/_2$ orange
2 Tbs orange juice

Chop the onions, and pick over the lentils. Place them both in a pan, add three times the volume of water, the stock granules, and the bouquet garni.
Simmer for 20–25 minutes, then drain the lentils.
Make a vinaigrette from the 2 tablespoons (30 ml) of oil, vinegar, mustard, salt, and pepper. Add a third of this to the warm lentils.
Cut the salmon into small pieces. Finely chop the shallots, gherkins, and egg. Add to the salmon together with the rest of the vinaigrette, the parsley, and the tarragon; mix well, season to taste with lemon juice and salt. Refrigerate and leave for 30 minutes. Fill a small flan dish – about 4 inches (10 cm) in diameter – two thirds full with the salmon tartare and press down well. Place a layer of lentils on top and press, so that the mixture holds together.
Peel the orange making sure that there is no white pith in the peel, then cut into very fine strips. Make a dressing from the remaining oil, orange juice, salt, and pepper and add the peel to the dressing. Arrange the salmon tartare on plates and pour a little orange dressing around each salmon tart.

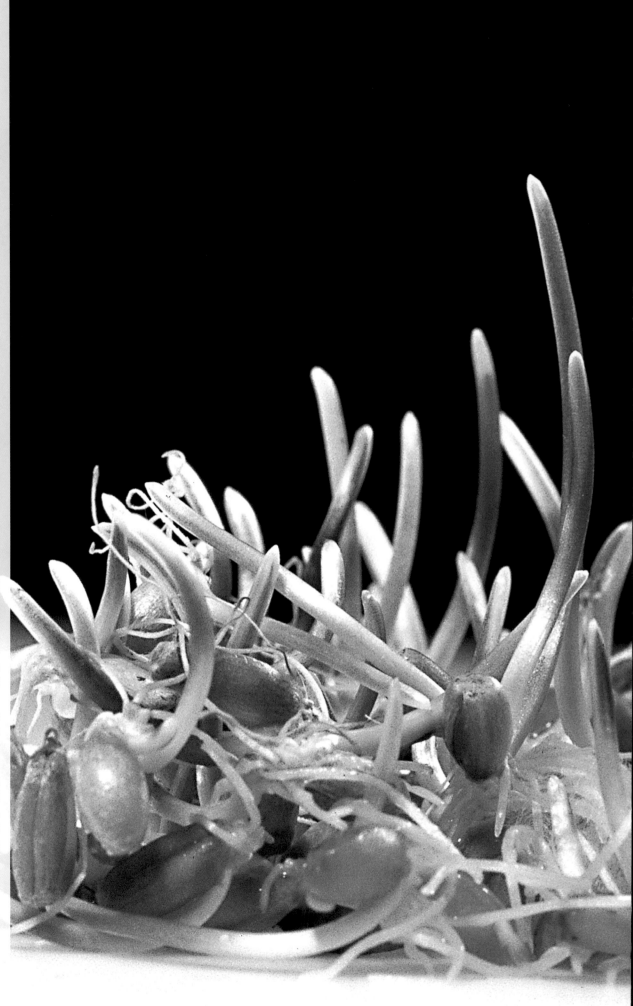

Seeds and Sprouts

Since the seed of a plant contains everything that the potential plant requires, it is not surprising that it releases a lot of energy when it begins to sprout. It has a concentrated supply of nutrients so that it can survive the first stages of germination, until it grows roots and is able to obtain nutrition from the soil. A seed – whether from a cereal, a legume, an oil-producing plant, or a nut – contains a large amount of carbohydrate, protein, and other nutrients. This accounts for the miracle that unfolds when the seed begins to sprout. Germination requires water, warmth, oxygen, and light.

Water is the catalyst in the germination process. It dampens the skin that has protected the seed so well for so long – in some types of seeds the potential for germination can remain for years, decades, or even centuries. As soon as the water touches the inside of the seed, the germination process can begin, as long as the surroundings are warm. If the environment is too cold or too hot then germination will not take place, or it will stop and the seed will be spoiled. Most types of seeds require a temperature of between 66 and 73 °F (19 and 23 °C). Rice needs a little more warmth and time, and will start to sprout after a few days at 86 °F (30 °C). The right temperature, combined with water, creates an atmosphere that activates the enzymes. Enzymes consist mostly of protein and an activating substance – often a vitamin or metallic element. Active substances cause a change in the molecular structure of the seed, awakening it from its dormant state and creating a chemical reaction.

This reaction develops further. After the water has entered the skin of the seed, then oxygen, the fundamental element of all life, can force its way in. This wakes the seed and starts the process of growth. Everything inside the seed works to provide it with all the nutrients and energy that it requires. Amazing chemical changes take place and hormones play an important part in these changes. Inside the seed, molecules bind

Background: This rather eerie picture shows some well germinated rye sprouts.

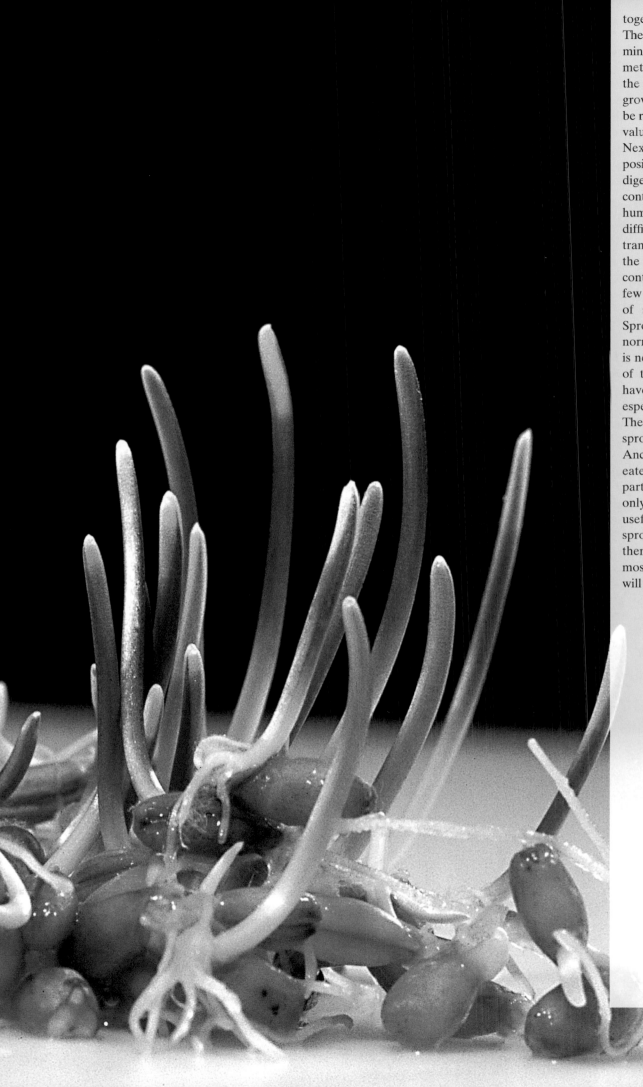

together, grow and change their structure. The quantity of essential amino acids and vitamins increases, and starch is retained for metabolism. While the seed – also through the presence of light – is visibly beginning to grow, and in the few days that it takes for it to be ready to eat, it has increased its nutritional value four fold.

Next come the enzymes, which have a positive effect on human metabolism and digestion. In comparison to seeds, the mineral content of sprouts is much easier for the human organism to use. The starch, which is difficult to digest, has for the most part, been transformed into glucose – much easier for the human body to absorb. The vitamin content of sprouts is quite astonishing. In the few days of germination, the vitamin content of sprouts can increase by 100 percent. Sprouts also contain vitamin B12 which is normally only found in animal products. B12 is necessary for cell growth and maintenance of the nervous system. American scientists have proven that B12 is present in sprouts, especially legume sprouts.

The discovery of the incredible vitality of sprouts took place thousands of years ago. Ancient sources have shown that sprouts were eaten, especially in Asia, where they formed a part of daily nutrition. However, they are only just being recognized in Europe as a useful source of nutrients. It is not difficult to sprout seeds at home, and to incorporate them into daily meals. In this way, even at the most inconvenient times, a fresh, healthy food will be at your disposal.

The Seeds Best Suited for Germination

In principle, any seed which comes from a plant that grows something edible can be used for sprouting (as long as it has not been chemically treated). However, there are seeds available that are specially intended for sprouting and these are the best ones to use.

These are generally cereals, legumes, and oil seeds.

• Cereals: there is a difference between the so-called "pseudo cereals," with amaranth, buckwheat, and quinoa on one side and spelt, barley, oats, millet, rye, and wheat on the other. Amaranth and quinoa require a relatively high temperature, 77 °F (25 °C), to germinate and should not be pre-soaked, whereas buckwheat should be soaked for 12 hours. These "pseudo-cereals" are edible after 3–4 days. "Proper" cereals need to be soaked for 9–15 hours, but can be eaten after only 2–3 days, when the seed swells. Spelt and wild rice are not suitable for sprouting because they have been dried.

• Legumes: The best legumes for sprouting are adzuki beans, peas, garbanzo beans, lentils, mung beans, and soybeans. They should be soaked for 6–15 hours depending on their size and they can be eaten 3 days later. Soybeans take a week to sprout and have to be kept in very damp conditions. Their sprouts are about 1 inch (3 centimeters) long. Soybeans should be washed thoroughly in very hot water before eating.

• Oil and other types of seeds: Alfalfa (Lucerne), clover, linseed, cress, pumpkin seed, red and white radishes, mustard seed, and sunflower seeds. The amount of soaking required varies for each type of seed. Alfalfa, linseed, and cress need little or no soaking, while the other types of seed require between 4 and 8 hours before germination can take place. All these seeds need about 4–6 days to produce sprouts and they make very good salad ingredients.

How to Grow Seedlings and Sprouts

Equipment The most simple container to use is a preserving jar covered with a piece of gauze or muslin. The cloth can be held in place by a rubber band. Sprouting equipment is becoming easier to obtain; it is often made of pottery or plastic and the jars themselves are divided into levels, so that more than one type of seed can be sprouted at one time.

Amount For a standard bowl in sprouting equipment (which usually has a diameter of 7 inches (18 centimeters) about 2 tablespoons (30 grams) of seeds should be used. This ensures that the seeds have enough room to sprout. Allow 1/2–1 tablespoon of seeds per person for salads, or 1–2 tablespoons of seeds if the sprouts are for a stir-fry.

Preparation It is advisable to pick the seeds over before you start. Unless very small seeds are to be sprouted, allow sufficient time for water to permeate the skins. The amount of soaking time will depend on the size of the seeds and the thickness of their skins, cereals and legumes taking more time than oil seeds. It is advisable as well as practical to soak the seeds overnight.

Germination The seeds need moisture and warmth for germination to take place. The best place to start off the germination process is a dark cupboard. The temperature should be around 68–69 °F (20–21 °C) (see left hand column). If the seeds become too damp they will spoil. This is why proper sprouting boxes have layers, so that air can circulate around the seeds. If you are using a jar to sprout the seeds, simply rinse them, shake off any excess water and

leave them to grow. From the second day the seeds need a little light, but should not be placed in direct sunlight. They should be rinsed frequently, preferably twice daily, so that they do not become moldy. Cress, and some types of cereals do produce fine hairs or a slimy substance that should not be confused with mold. Seeds that require a longer germination time should be kept scrupulously clean.

Before Use When the seeds or sprouts have grown to the desired length, they should be washed before use in fresh water and then drained. It is also a good idea to sort through them and remove any that have not sprouted. Legumes, particularly, can be as hard as stones and are a danger to the teeth. To make sure that the legumes are free of indigestible substances, the sprouts should be washed in hot water if they are to be eaten raw. Blanching the sprouts before using them in dishes is generally recommended.

Serving Suggestions Seedlings and sprouts add a distinctive flavor to salads. They range from tasting nutty, to tasting peppery. They should only be added to dishes just before serving, or they lose their flavor. The hotter seeds can be used as seasoning. Sprouts combine well with cereals, small sprouts make very good additions to dips and sauces.

Storage Seedlings and sprouts should be eaten immediately, no matter what variety they are. Because a cold environment stops them from growing, they can be kept in a sealed container in the refrigerator for 48 hours.

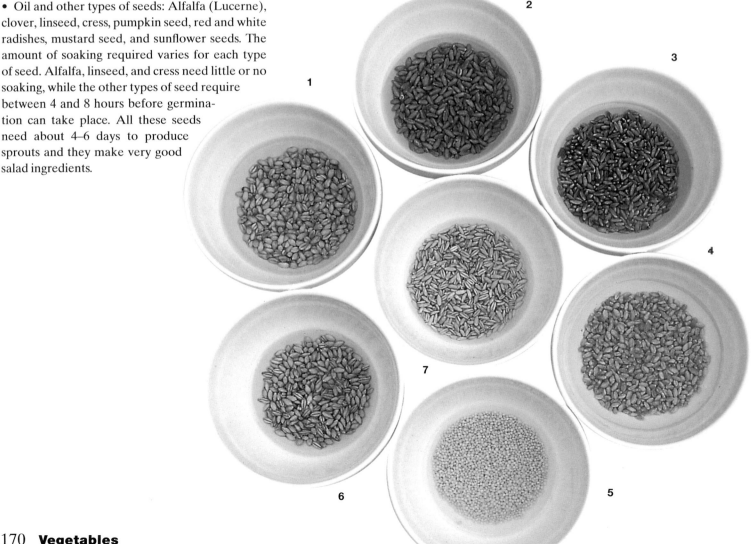

1 Wheat
2 Spelt
3 Rye
4 Wheat
5 Millet
6 Naked barley
7 Naked oats

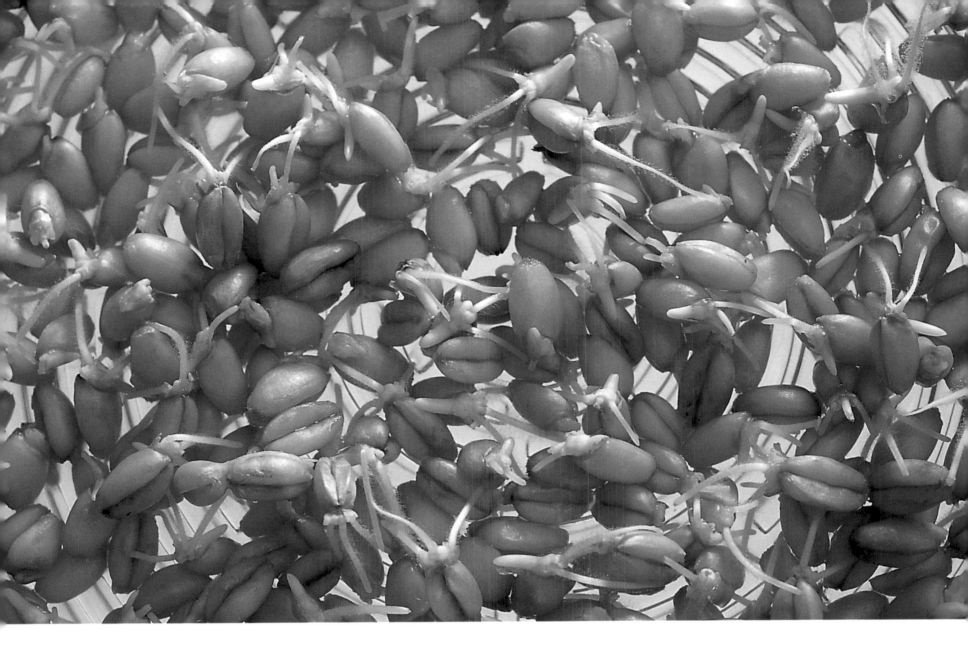

Above: Cereals, legumes, and oilseeds are all suitable for sprouting. After 2–3 days when they have reached the stage shown, they are ready to eat.

Sprouting Salad

¹/₄ cup (45 g) each of spelt, barley, and rye
1 Tbs (15 g) alfalfa
1 green, 1 red, and 1 yellow bell pepper
1 garlic clove
1 shallot
1 bunch arugula
2 Tbs red wine vinegar
3 Tbs olive oil
1 Tbs honey
2 Tbs finely chopped chervil
1 pinch cayenne pepper
1 pinch herb salt
Coarse salt, black pepper

Sprout the seeds 3 days before serving the salad. Deseed and dice the bell peppers. Mince the garlic and shallot, finely chop the arugula, leaving a few whole for garnish.
Mix the vegetables and sprouts together.
Make a dressing using the remaining ingredients, and season to taste. Dress the salad, toss it carefully, allow the flavors to develop, and serve.

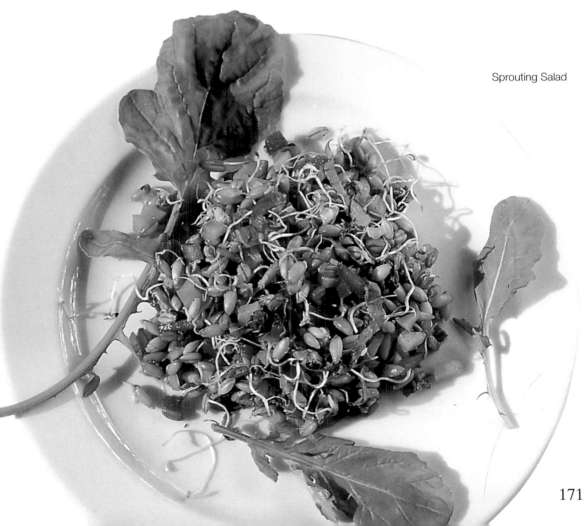

Sprouting Salad

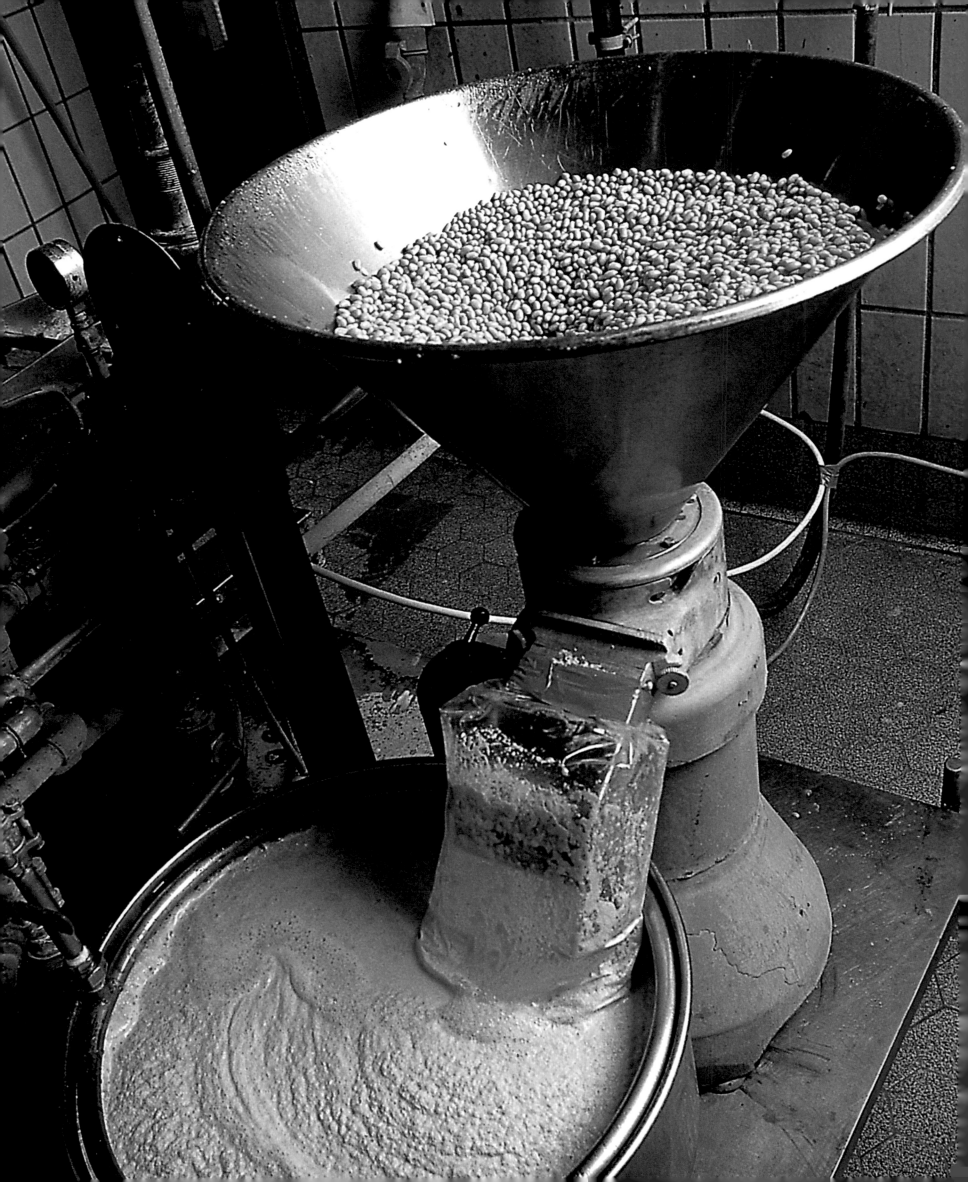

The Protein Miracle

Soybeans and Tofu

Soybeans, which belong to the *Glycine* family, have become the best known legume of the 20th century. They have been grown in China for thousands of years and are a staple part of the Chinese diet. *Sou* is revered along with rice, wheat, barley, and millet as one of the five holy grains.

The annual soy plants resemble dwarf bean plants and are about three feet (one meter) high. They

Soybeans have a higher protein content than all other types of food, including meat, fish, and poultry. The soy protein is especially valuable to us because it contains all eight amino acids and contains large enough quantities of seven of these amino acids to satisfy human nutritional requirements. Soy is 40 percent protein but contains only 18 percent fat, which is made up of unsaturated fatty acids including linogen, which is essential for the metabolism. It also has a large quantity of lecithin, a substance that plays an important part in the nervous system. In addition, soy has a high mineral content, a very high vitamin E content, and is rich in vitamins B1 and B2.

Soy was brought to Japan 1,000 years ago by Buddhist monks and has formed a part of the daily diet in Japan, and other countries in the Far East. It

fodder, as they have lost most of the valuable vitamins and oils. This creates a vicious circle for the developing countries. They increase their soy cultivation and ruin their fields using western chemicals and fertilizers, to make products that are used to increase the western meat industry. As world hunger increases, this high protein food – which could be used directly to feed people – is being fed to animals. Only 6 percent of soy is consumed direct by human beings while the rest is wasted on animals.

The soy industry makes other products – the best known being TVP (textured vegetable protein). The high protein content of soy makes it ideal for all types of production, and it is used to make artificial fibers, varnish, and even plywood. Soy has become a raw material with a wealth of uses.

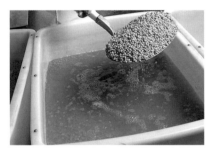
To make tofu, the soybeans must be thoroughly rinsed and soaked.

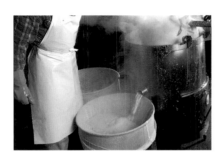
The soy milk is boiled and poured through a sieve, to remove any pieces of bean.

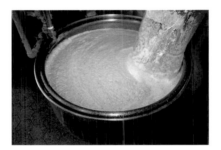
A separating agent like Nigari is added to the soy milk to separate curds and whey.

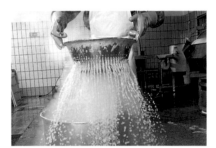
The mixture is shaken so that the whey drains off.

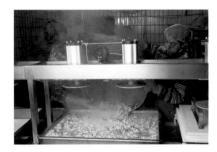
The proteinous mixture that remains still contains a lot of moisture, so it is put in a press.

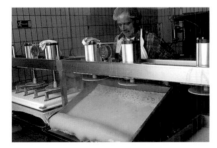
The tofu is pressed into a large block, which is later divided into portions.

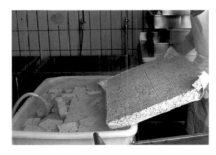
The warm tofu blocks are placed in large tubs of cold water to cool.

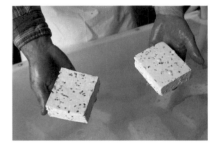
Tofu is sold in small blocks. It can also have added spices, nuts, or vegetables and is available smoked.

have an unusual feature – they are hairy. The leaves, stems, and beans are all, to some degree, covered in hair. Soy plants have many buds, which are tiny, off-white or even violet in color. These buds form the legume pods, which contain up to five seeds, all varying in size and color. These seeds grow to be $^1/_5$–$^1/_2$ inch (5–12 millimeters) in diameter and range from white through red and green through black in color. The most popular types – there are about 300 – are pale yellow. The unripened seeds can be cooked fresh and served as a side vegetable but they are generally used when dried.

Left hand page: Tofu begins life as soy milk which is made by liquidizing soybeans.

was first brought to Europe in the 18th century and did not reach the USA until the 19th century. Even after its arrival, it did not achieve great culinary popularity. Nowadays the thinking towards this "wonder bean" has changed dramatically; in the United States the production of soy has escalated in the last ten years. Over 62 million acres (25 million hectares) are used to grow soybeans and this makes America the highest producer, with Brazil coming second. Argentina and other developing countries are also considering increasing their cultivation of the wonder bean.

This boom in cultivation it not linked to the discovery of the health benefits of soy, but is purely because of its high protein content and its oil. Soybeans are used to make concentrated food, and also soy oil and margarine. The by-products of the margarine production are used for animal

Quite apart from the effect of soy on world hunger, and its ecological consequences which can be debated at great length, soy is extremely versatile and has an unusual quality, first discovered by the resourceful Chinese. Apart from beansprouts, which are an important ingredient for Chinese cooking, they divided soy products into two groups: fermented and unfermented.

The most important member of the first group is soy milk. It is obtained by soaking yellow soybeans for 12 hours. The beans are then liquidized and stirred into eight to ten times their volume of water. The whole mixture is boiled for fifteen minutes, then it is filtered. Manufacturers use a centrifuge system, heat treat the milk then homogenize and pasteurize it. This destroys the distinctive flavor of the milk; organic production does not use these techniques. Soy milk is officially described as a "drink" because of trade description regulations. It replaces animal milk in many East Asian countries, and is similar to cow's milk, although it has a higher protein content. It can be used in the same way as cow's milk and makes milk shakes, buttermilk, yogurt, and tofu. Tofu is made from soy milk and can be made at home. *To* stands for bean, and *fu* stands for coagulated. The coagulate – calcium or magnesium sulfate, or more commonly the Japanese sea salt Nigari – is stirred into warm soy milk. Coagulation takes place quickly and in just a few minutes the protein separates itself from the whey. The whey is then drained off and the solid matter is put into containers and pressed. Depending on the amount of pressure applied (this should be for 20–30 minutes) the tofu will have a soft or firm consistency. It is then cut, chilled, packaged, and possibly flavored with vegetables, nuts, spices, or it can be smoked.

Tofu is 12–14 percent protein and contains all eight amino acids in well balanced quantities.

Tofu is more nutritious than meat, fish, and milk. It is only 4–5 percent fat and this fat is mostly unsaturated fatty acids. The B vitamins and minerals of the soybean remain undamaged by the tofu-making process. Tofu is only lacking in one respect – it has no flavor, but this should not be seen as a disadvantage. On the contrary, it adds to the versatility of this soy cheese. Tofu can absorb the flavors of any ingredients. Tofu was discovered in China about 2,000 years ago, and became a very important ingredient. It was even more important in Japan. Tofu did not reach Europe until the 1970s, when it was made by a few small manufacturers in Belgium and Holland. There were a few tofu pioneers in other countries but it was not until the beginning of the 1980s that tofu production increased. Since then, research into the nutritional benefits of tofu have increased its popularity, together with the growing trend to eat less meat. There are over 300 organically produced tofu products on the market, which are increasingly available in supermarkets.

Different Types of Tofu
- 1 Natural tofu: This has no added flavors; it can be marinated, fried, broiled, boiled, and prepared in a variety of different ways.
- 2 Tofu with mung bean sprouts, sesame, coarse salt, parsley, and other herbs; for salads.
- 3 Smoked tofu: marinated n spicy soysauce then smoked over birchwood; use in stir fries or on bread.
- 4 Tofu with hazelnuts; especially rich in fatty acids and protein; eat cold on bread, with fruits, or in salad.
- 5 Vegetable tofu: with finely diced vegetables and herbs, very versatile, an especially colorful addition to soups.
- 6 Tofu with mushrooms, onions, and coarse salt: a specialty that can be eaten cold, but tastes delicious when fried.

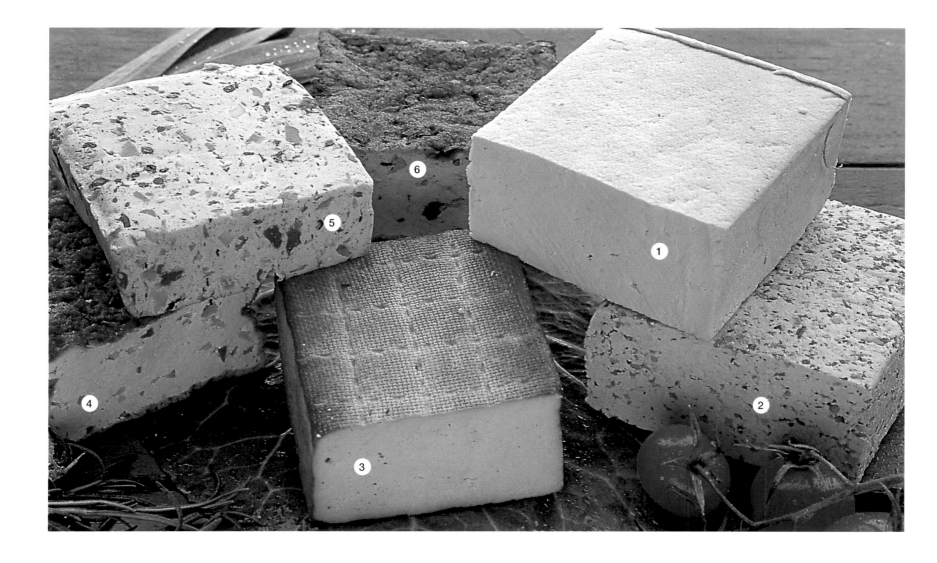

Soybean Glossary

Chiang
A Chinese spicy paste made from soybeans and rice that can be made into a sauce

Ketjap
Soysauce made from black, fermented soybeans

Kinako
Powder made from roasted soybeans

Kori-tofu
Dried tofu, soaked to form silken tofu and sold as silken tofu

Miso
This Japanese spice mixture made from soy and rice comes in many different forms and is usually used as stock for a soup

Natto
Whole, cooked soybeans that are fermented and turn dark brown; served in Japan as a side dish

Nigari
A Japanese salt that contains magnesium sulfate; a natural coagulate used to make tofu

Okara
Soy bran that is left after the soy milk has been filtered; used dried to make noodles

Silken Tofu or Kinugoshi
Very soft tofu that is made without pressing the soy milk solids; use for sauces and purées

Seitan
Made from wheat protein, but flavored with soysauce which increases the content of Lysine

Soy Meat
TVP (textured vegetable protein); manufactured industrially and using non ecological methods it is a meat substitute that is 50 percent protein

Soy Flakes
Made from cooked, whole soybeans; use like cereal flakes

Soy Granules
Made from granulated, pre roasted, and cooked beans. An alternative to soy meat

Soy Flour
Available in two different varieties; as fat free flour – made as a by-product of oil extraction – or from whole, ground beans; added to cereal flours and cereal products

Soy Milk
Used as a substitute for cow's milk in many countries. It is made from puréed soybeans that are liquidized with water; used to make soy cheese, tofu, and other "dairy" products

Soy Oil
Normally obtained by chemical processes; a denatured oil

Soysauce
This sauce, made from fermented soy and wheat, is available in two different varieties; dark, strong Koikuchi, and light mild Usukuchi

Tamari
Actually called Tamari shoyu, a pure Chinese soysauce with a low wheat content

Tempeh
A soy product made from an enzyme process that creates a white fibrous mass which is very nutritious, especially if it is made from whole soybeans

Tofu
Rather like a soft cheese and varying in consistency; can be used for frying, boiling, purées, and sauces

Yuba
The skin that forms during the soy milk process and considered a delicacy when eaten fresh; normally available sliced and dried

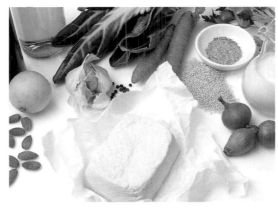

Tofu, millet, almonds, Swiss chard, carrots, and onions contribute to this delicious wholefood recipe (see right).

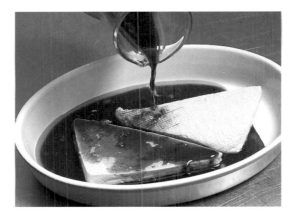

Natural tofu has no flavor. This marinade made from olive oil, soysauce, garlic, and lemon juice gives it extra taste.

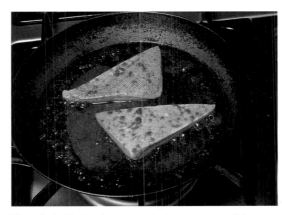

The tofu is fried in the marinade, turns an appetizing brown color and has a slightly smoky flavor.

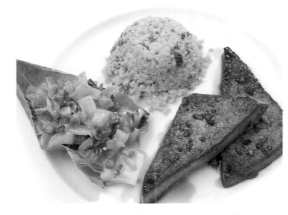

Tofu, Swiss chard, and millet complement the flavor of the tofu perfectly and add extra nutrients to the meal.

Marinated Tofu with Almond Millet and Swiss Chard
(Illustrations left)

7 oz (200 g) plain tofu
3 Tbs olive oil
4 Tbs soysauce or tamari
Juice of $^1/_2$ lemon
$^1/_2$ tsp herb salt
2 garlic cloves
$^3/_4$ cup (125 g) millet
1$^1/_4$ cups (250 ml) vegetable stock
Coarse salt, black pepper
3 Tbs finely chopped almonds
2 Tbs finely chopped parsley
1 lb 2 oz (500 g) Swiss chard
$^1/_2$ onion
1 Tbs butter
$^1/_2$ tsp vegetable stock granules
$^1/_2$ cup (100 ml) heavy cream
1 small carrot
1 tsp arrowroot
1 pinch nutmeg

Cut the tofu into triangles. Make a marinade out of oil, soysauce, lemon juice, and herb salt. Add one clove of minced garlic and leave the tofu in the marinade. Rinse the millet under hot then cold water. Dry fry it briefly, then add the vegetable stock and simmer for 8 minutes. Season to taste with salt and pepper and simmer for a further 20 minutes. Mix in the parsley and almonds just before serving.

Meanwhile, prepare the Swiss chard by removing the stalks. Chop the stalks, cut the leaves into strips. Finely chop the onion and the rest of the garlic, and braise in the butter until it is transparent. Add the chard stalks and braise. Dissolve the stock granules in 5 tablespoons of boiling water. Pour into the onion mixture and add the chard leaves. Braise until the leaves wilt.

Dice the carrots and add to the chard.

Mix the cream with the same volume of water and add to the chard and carrot mixture. Add the arrowroot, dissolved in a little water and use to thicken the vegetable sauce. Season with salt, pepper, and nutmeg.

Fry the tofu in the marinade. Serve with the millet and Swiss chard and serve at once.

Tempeh Salad with Raisins and Walnuts

Tofu mayonnaise
5 oz (150 g) soft tofu
1$^1/_2$ Tbs apple vinegar
1 finely chopped gherkin
1 Tbs sesame oil, 1 Tbs soysauce
$^1/_2$ chopped garlic clove
1 pinch cayenne pepper
1 pinch sweet paprika
1 tsp mustard
1 finely chopped onion

Salad
5 oz (150 g) tempeh (see Soya Glossary on left)
Groundnut oil for deep frying
1 peeled, finely diced apple
3 Tbs (45 g) raisins
4$^1/_2$ oz (125 g) chopped walnuts

For the tofu mayonnaise, mix all ingredients together. To make the salad, deep fry the tempeh, dice and stir into the mayonnaise with the remaining ingredients.

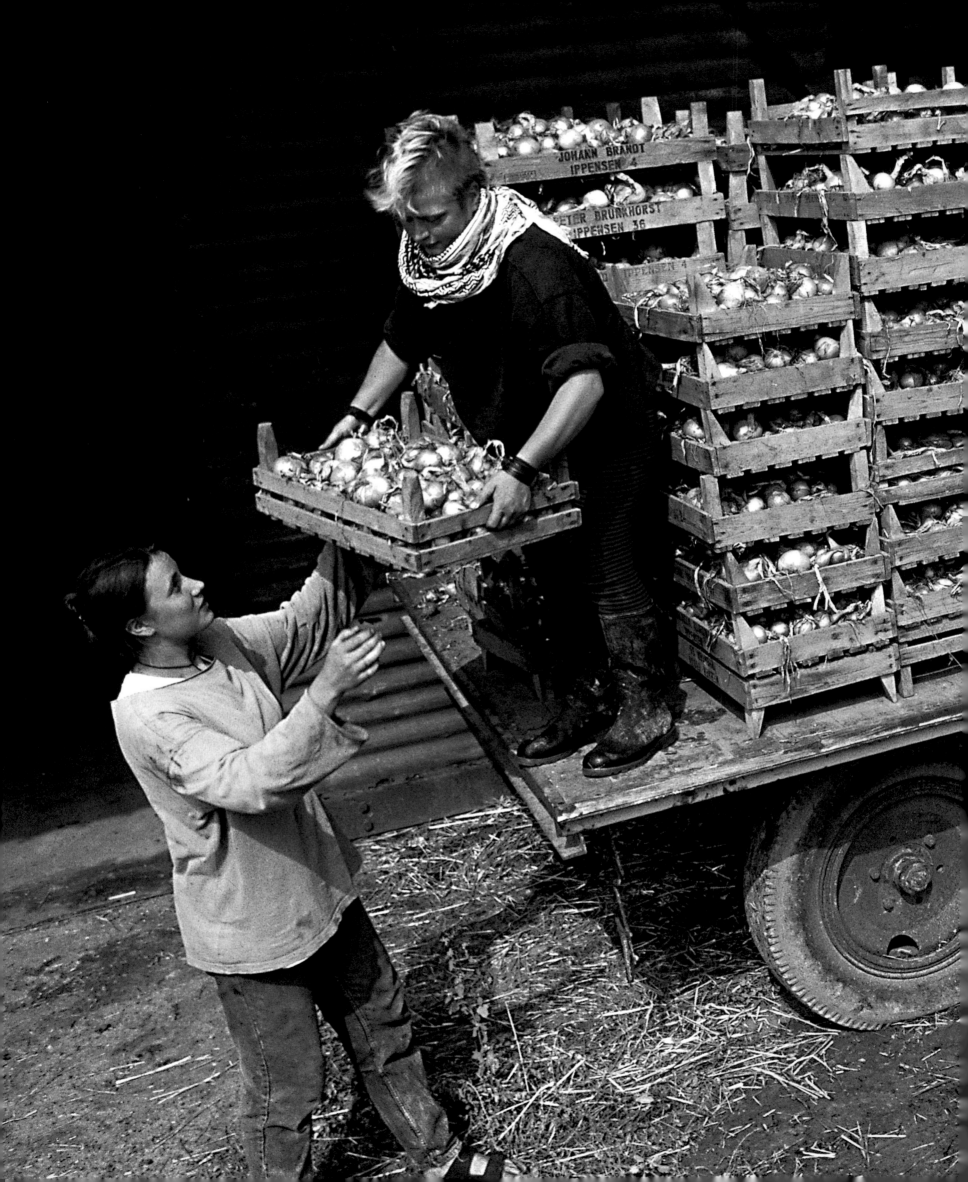

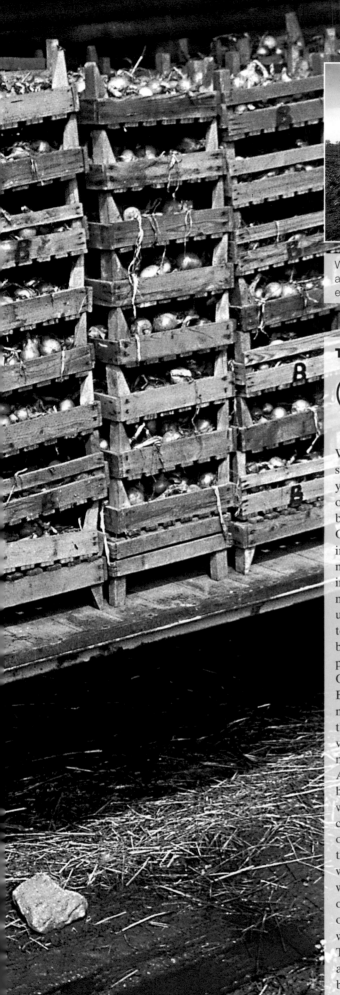

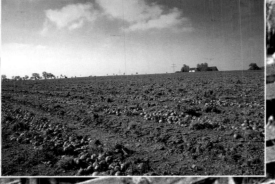

When the weather allows, onions can be dug up and left to dry in the fields. This helps them keep especially well.

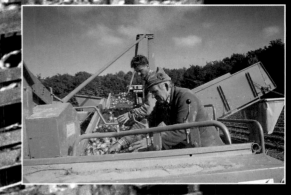

When the onions are brought in, they are sorted before they are packed so that only good quality onions reach the shops.

The Vegetable Antibiotic

Onions

What would cooking be without onions? The smell of onions frying in butter or olive oil fills your senses and arouses the appetite. Raw onion juice is less appetizing, being rather bitter and peppery, but it is extremely healthy. Onions – and to some degree leeks – have incredible medicinal properties and act as a natural antibiotic. They fight infection, inflammation, and fungal infection. In folk medicine, when mixed with honey, they were used to treat worms, and they were also used to treat coughs, colds, and even asthma. Their beneficial effects have been scientifically proven – particularly against arteriosclerosis. Onions are rich in B vitamins, and vitamins C, E, and A and contain trace elements and minerals. They can help prevent cancer. It is the essential oils in onions that are really valuable; these sulfurous oils stimulate the membranes of the digestive organs.

Asia and southern Europe came across the healing powers of the onion many years ago when they discovered its versatility as a cooking ingredient. In Ancient Egypt the onion was a staple foodstuff. The building of the pyramids would not have been possible without the onion, which helped keep the workforce healthy. Nowadays onions are one of the most popular vegetables and are grown on all continents, particularly in those with warm climates.

There are different methods of cultivation, and different types of onions. Gardeners like bulb onions, baby onions that have been grown from seed and are very easy to grow into large onions. They do not keep as well as onions that have been grown from seed, but bulb onions can be harvested more quickly.

Here are some varieties of seed onions.

• Scallions: sown in August and harvested the following spring when they have formed small white onions. Their peppery stalk is also edible.

• Spanish onions: this mild bulb needs a warm climate which is why this variety is often grown in Mediterranean countries.

• Salad onions: these are stalks that widen at the base. The green part is eaten.

• Pickling onions: these are the size of hazelnuts and are harvested in summer. They are rarely used fresh, but rather for making pickles.

• Red onions: very popular in southern Europe, reddish, violet colored onions that have a pleasant, aromatic flavor. Ideal for salads.

• Shallots: these differ from the other varieties of onion because the stalk of the plant grows more than one bulb. There are dozens of tiny oval onion bulbs on each plant stalk. Shallots have a delicate taste and are used for flavoring dishes.

• Cooking onions: these come in two varieties, the sowing onions (seed) and the bulb onions. Bulb onions ripen more quickly, and grow larger than seed onions. These can be used in all recipes and are available all through the winter.

Background: When the onions are packed without their leaves and are stored in crates they will keep for a long time. They should be stored in cool and airy conditions and will keep until the beginning of the following year.

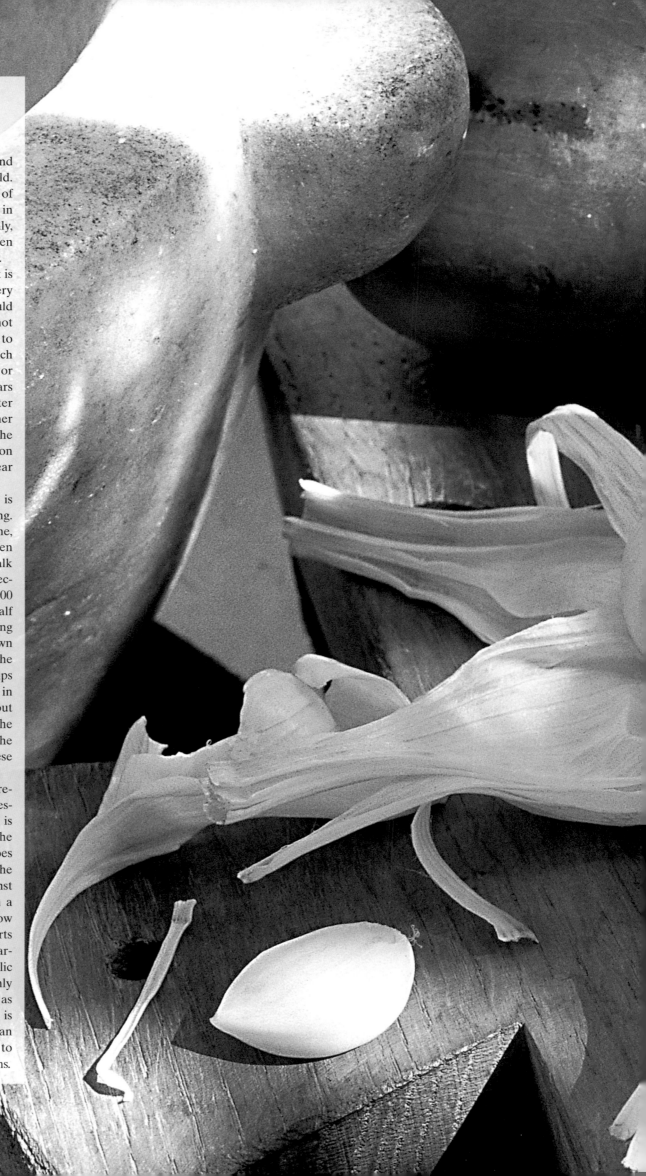

Garlic

Garlic is grown on thousands of acres of land in all the warm countries of the world. Organic farmers do not use large amounts of land for garlic cultivation, producing it in relatively small fields. In Spain and Italy, organic farmers who grow garlic on five to ten acres (2 to 4 hectares) are the big producers. Garlic likes a warm, sunny environment. It is a member of the lily family and requires very little attention. The ideal soil for garlic would be fertile, light, chalky, or limy. It should not be over watered as this will cause the bulb to rot. There is a special rotation of crops which begins with four years of lucerne. Then one or two crops of garlic are planted after two years of cereal crops like wheat or barley. After this, a third cereal crop is planted or another garlic crop, depending on the fertility of the soil. This is followed by thorough fertilization of the ground with manure and the ten year cycle ends with a last garlic crop.

At the end of the summer, the ground is prepared – with deep plowing and harrowing. Before the garlic can be planted by machine, the bulbs have to be divided into cloves. Then the cloves are soaked in a mixture of chalk and copper to protect them from fungal infection. About 1,800 to 2,200 pounds (800–1,000 kilograms) are required to sow two and a half acres (1 hectare) of land. These planting cloves are mass-produced, and are grown from seed by some larger farms who grow the cloves from their own seed supply. This helps to stop viruses – which appear regularly in organic agriculture – spreading throughout organic farms. Most planting is done in the fall, and the most popular varieties are the white or violet white types of garlic. These varieties have a lower yield, but keep well.

Weeding is carried out mechanically, when required although occasionally it is also necessary to weed by hand. Organic manure is spread on the field in the spring and the farmer has to be vigilant that the crop does not become damaged by mildew or rust. The farmer can take certain precautions against these dangers by sprinkling the field with a sulfur solution. The first signs of rust show themselves on cereals and grass. Garlic starts to ripen at the end of June and is then harvested by machine. In earlier years, the garlic was left to ripen in the fields, protected only by its leaves. This is no longer possible, as garlic is a protected crop, so now drying is carried out in the farmyard. Garlic bulbs can be sold half dried almost immediately, but to dry garlic completely takes about eight months.

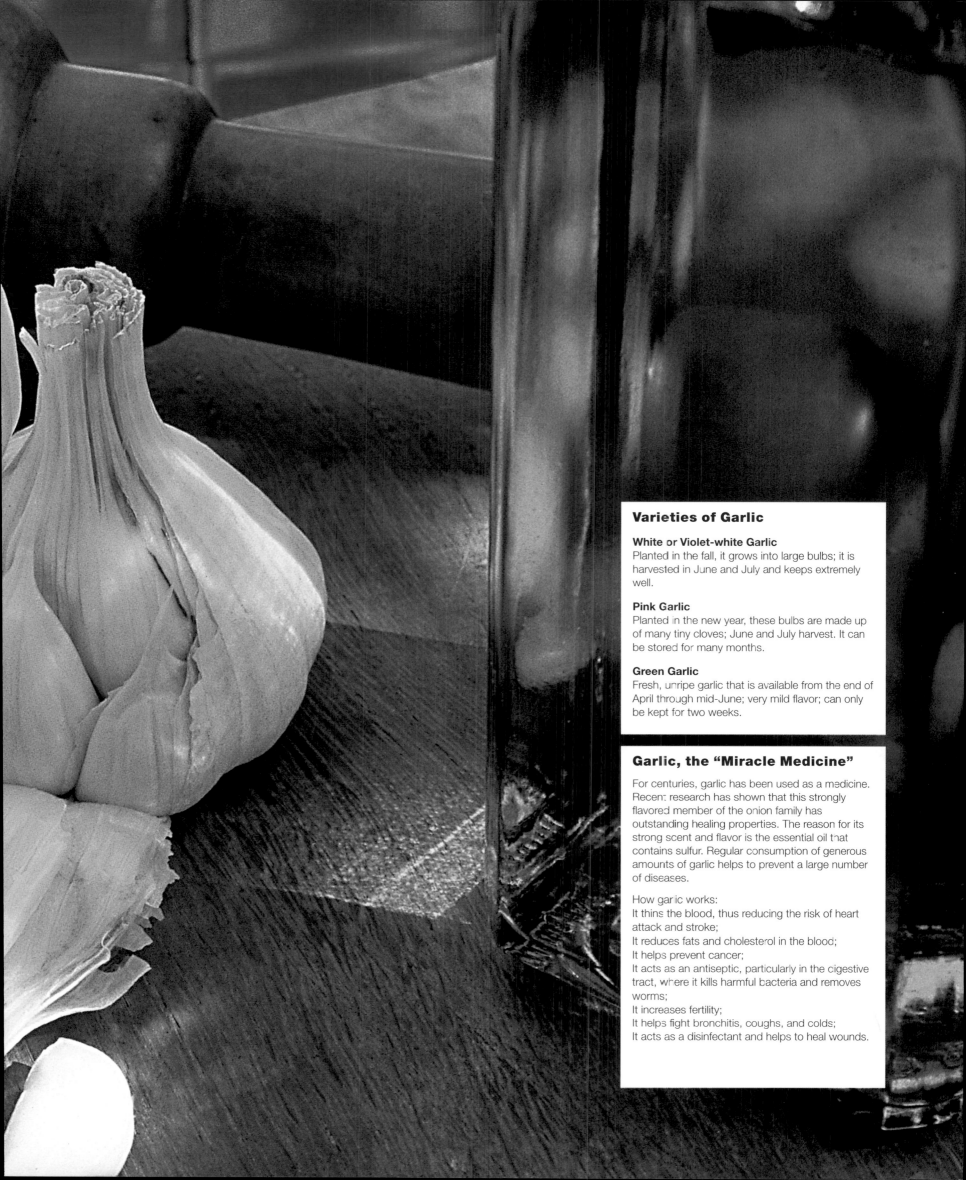

Varieties of Garlic

White or Violet-white Garlic
Planted in the fall, it grows into large bulbs; it is harvested in June and July and keeps extremely well.

Pink Garlic
Planted in the new year, these bulbs are made up of many tiny cloves; June and July harvest. It can be stored for many months.

Green Garlic
Fresh, unripe garlic that is available from the end of April through mid-June; very mild flavor; can only be kept for two weeks.

Garlic, the "Miracle Medicine"

For centuries, garlic has been used as a medicine. Recent research has shown that this strongly flavored member of the onion family has outstanding healing properties. The reason for its strong scent and flavor is the essential oil that contains sulfur. Regular consumption of generous amounts of garlic helps to prevent a large number of diseases.

How garlic works:
It thins the blood, thus reducing the risk of heart attack and stroke;
It reduces fats and cholesterol in the blood;
It helps prevent cancer;
It acts as an antiseptic, particularly in the digestive tract, where it kills harmful bacteria and removes worms;
It increases fertility;
It helps fight bronchitis, coughs, and colds;
It acts as a disinfectant and helps to heal wounds.

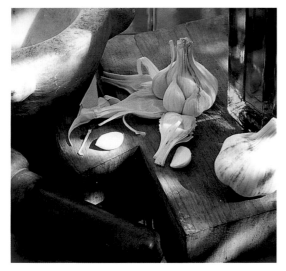

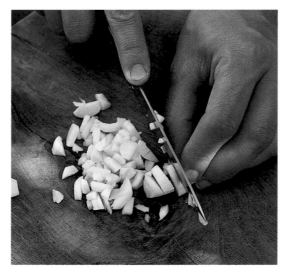

Aïoli

1 garlic bulb
1¼–1½ cups (250–300 ml) olive oil

Divide the garlic into cloves, peel and chop the flesh. Either pound the garlic using a pestle and mortar, or reduce to a pulp in a liquidizer.
Add the olive oil drop by drop to the garlic mixture. When the sauce becomes too thick, add the oil a little more slowly until the mixture becomes a paste.
Add a little salt, if desired, and a few drops of lemon juice.
Aïoli makes a good accompaniment to grilled or broiled fish, dried cod, and lamb and can also be served with broiled vegetables and boiled potatoes. It tastes even better served the next day.

It was probably the Romans who first made a paste from garlic and olive oil and discovered aïoli. The quality of aïoli depends on the garlic, which should be as young and plump as possible.

Inhabitants of Provence, Catalonia, and Castile dispute the origin of aïoli. The first step in its preparation is to separate the garlic bulb into cloves, which are then chopped and peeled.

Garlic Mayonnaise

10 garlic cloves
¼ tsp coarse salt
3 egg yolks
1¼ cups (250 ml) olive oil
2 tsp lemon juice
Black pepper

This is a milder version of Aïoli. It is important that all the ingredients are at room temperature.
Pound the garlic with the salt and mix together thoroughly with the egg yolks.
Keep beating the mixture and slowly add the olive oil in a steady stream. Once half the oil has been mixed in, the mixture is emulsified and the rest of the oil can be added a little more quickly.
Finally, stir in the lemon juice and season the mayonnaise with pepper.

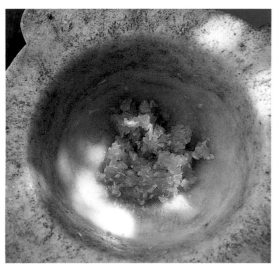

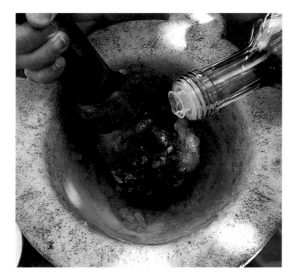

To make traditional aïoli, it is important to use old-fashioned utensils – if possible a stone mortar and a pestle made out of fine olive wood.

When the garlic has been thoroughly crushed with a pestle, another ingredient is added – olive oil, which should be cold-pressed. It should be poured into the garlic drop by drop at first, then in a steady stream.

Rouille

2 ripe red bell peppers
1 large floury potato
6 garlic cloves
1 small red chili pepper
1 pinch saffron strands
1 tsp coarse salt
1 cup (200 ml) olive oil

Roast the bell peppers whole in the oven: skin, deseed, and cut into pieces. At the same time, boil the potato in its skin, rinse in cold water, and peel. Pound together the garlic, chili, saffron, and salt in the mortar.
Stirring the paste, gradually add the olive oil until the mixture has the consistency of a creamy purée.
This hot garlic and pepper paste is delicious spread on toast and served with fish soups. It also makes a good accompaniment to broiled or poached fish.

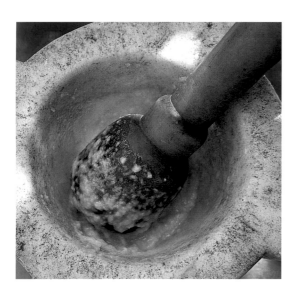

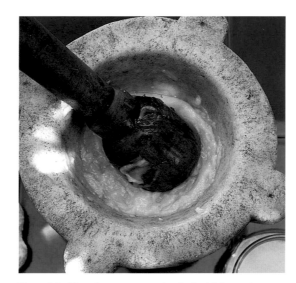

Making a stiff paste from garlic and olive oil using only a pestle is a real art. The pestle must rotate very quickly.

True aïoli differs from mayonnaise in that it has a less firm consistency and a paler color. It is also extremely peppery.

Previous double page: Garlic is an extremely healthy and versatile seasoning ingredient – it can be pickled, pounded, minced, pressed, or simmered as a whole clove.

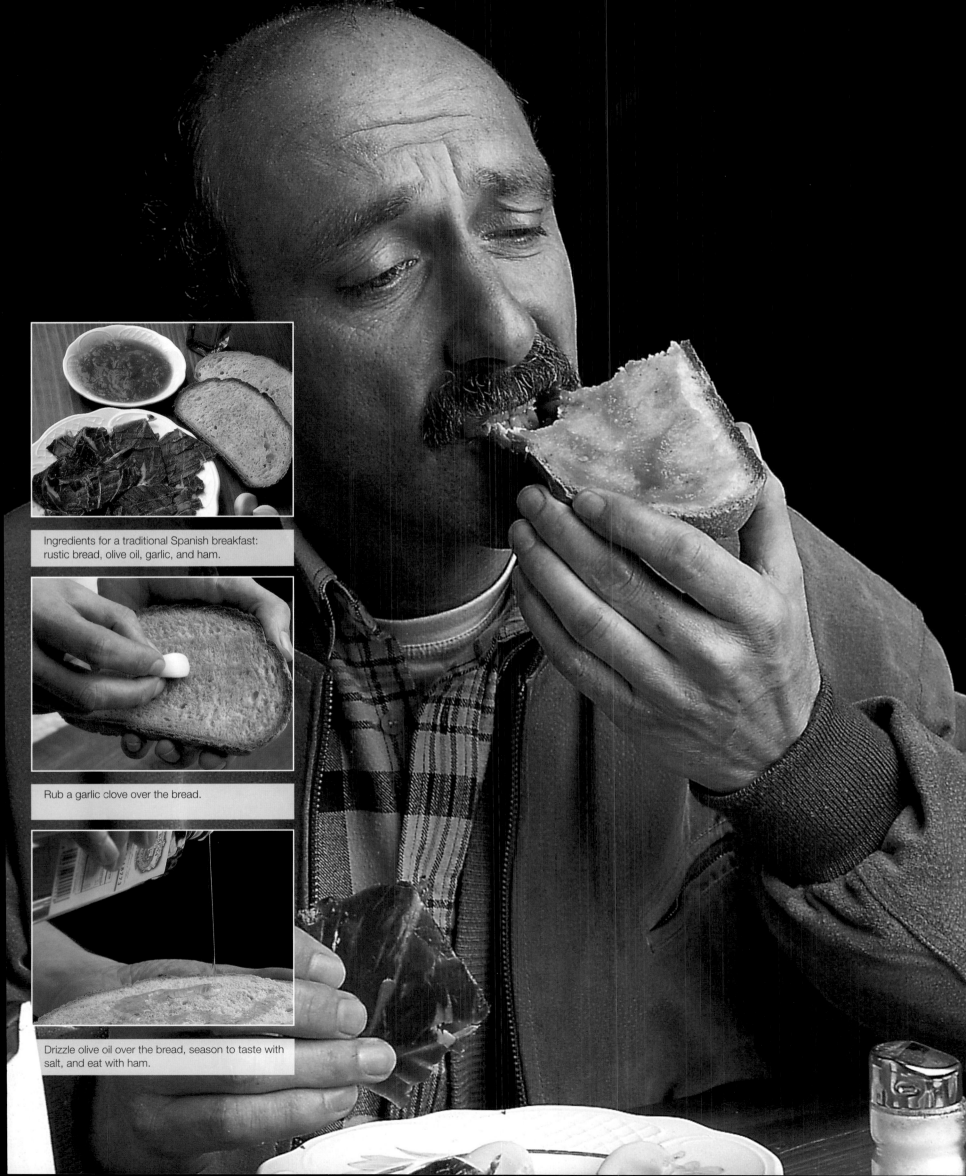

Ingredients for a traditional Spanish breakfast: rustic bread, olive oil, garlic, and ham.

Rub a garlic clove over the bread.

Drizzle olive oil over the bread, season to taste with salt, and eat with ham.

Recipes with Garlic

Romesco Sauce
(Illustration below right)

2 oz (50 g) almonds
3 garlic cloves
1 tomato
Coarse salt, black pepper
1 tsp paprika
5 Tbs olive oil
1 Tbs white wine vinegar

Peel and roast the almonds. Using a pestle and mortar, pound the almonds and the garlic.
Skin and deseed the tomatoes and add to the garlic and almond mixture. Mix together until it forms a smooth paste; season to taste with salt and pepper.
Add the olive oil, paprika, and vinegar.
Romesco Sauce is a good accompaniment to broiled or baked fish, and fried or baked vegetables.

Garlic Purée

12 large garlic cloves
1/2 cup (100 ml) vegetable stock
1/4 cup (50 g) butter
1/4 cup (30 g) whole wheat flour
3/4 cup (150 ml) milk

Halve the garlic cloves, simmer for about 10 minutes in the vegetable stock then purée.
Melt the butter, stir in the flour and add the milk, stirring well.
Then add the garlic purée and simmer for 5 minutes.
Garlic purée makes a good accompaniment to broiled lamb.

Baked Garlic
(Illustration below left)

4 fresh garlic bulbs
(each about 7 oz – 200 g – in weight)
Black pepper
Coarse salt
8 slices whole wheat toasting bread
1/3 cup (80 g) butter

Preheat the oven to 460 °F (250 °C).
Place the garlic bulbs on a baking sheet lined with parchment paper, and bake in the oven until the skins have darkened.
Peel the individual cloves and mash with a fork; add pepper and salt.
Toast the bread, and spread with butter and the baked garlic. Baked garlic is a good accompaniment to Mediterranean vegetables.

Garlic Marinated in Olive Oil

2–3 red bell peppers
1 lb 2 oz (500 g) garlic cloves
Olive oil

Mince the peppers and layer alternately with the garlic in a sterilized jar. Pour over enough olive oil so that there is at least 1/3 inch (1 cm) oil above the vegetables.
Fasten the jar securely, put in a dark place and leave to marinate for at least 4 weeks.
The preserved garlic and the garlic oil are ideal for use in meat dishes and salad dressings.

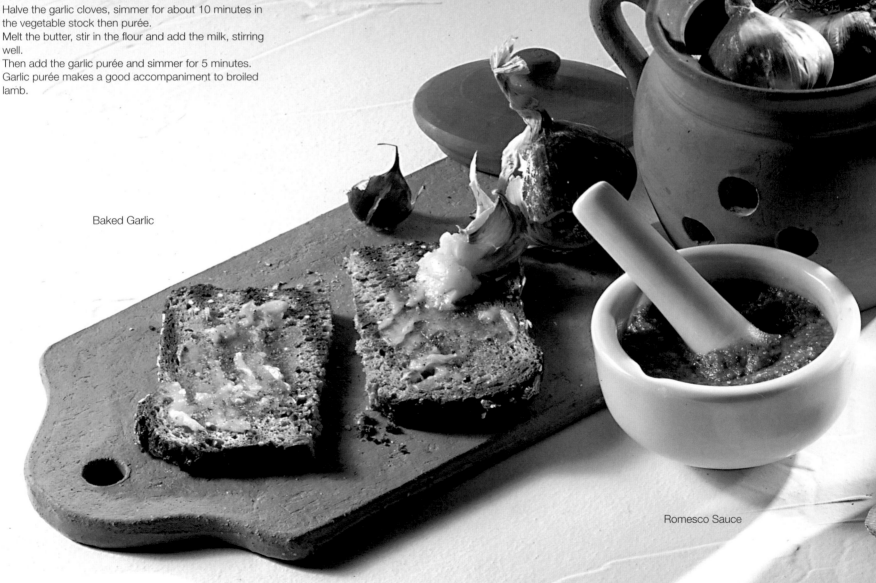

Baked Garlic

Romesco Sauce

Balkan Style Pickled Garlic
(Illustration below)

1 cup (200 ml) white wine
1 cup (200 ml) white wine vinegar
2 Tbs honey
4 red chili peppers
2 sprigs thyme
1 tsp coarse salt
1 lb 2 oz (500 g) garlic cloves
Olive oil

Bring the wine, vinegar, honey, chili, thyme, and salt to the boil together with a cup (200 ml) of water.
Add the garlic and leave for 24 hours so that the flavors can combine. Bring to the boil again, and simmer for 5 minutes.
Pour into sterilized screw top jars, and cover with a layer of olive oil to prevent air reaching the pickle. Leave in a cool, dark place for at least 3 weeks.
The marinade can be used as a garlic vinegar.

Balkan Style Pickled Garlic

Marinated Mozzarella with Garlic
(Illustration below)

4 packets Mozzarella
A few leaves radicchio lettuce
2 small red onions
1 red chili pepper
8 garlic cloves
$1/4$ tsp coarse salt
1 bunch flat-leafed parsley
1 bunch basil leaves
2 Tbs lemon juice
$1/2$ cup (120 ml) olive oil

Slice the Mozzarella and arrange on a bed of radicchio. Slice the onions and chili into fine rings and scatter over the Mozzarella.
Pound the garlic and salt until it forms a smooth paste. Finely chop the basil and parsley and add the remaining ingredients to make a dressing; pour over the Mozzarella.
Leave for at least 1 hour.
Serve with warm garlic bread.

Marinated Mozzarella with Garlic

Dried Cod in Hot and Spicy Garlic Sauce

$1^1/2$ lbs (700 g) dried cod
1 garlic clove
1 dried red chili pepper
3 Tbs olive oil
Black pepper

Soak the cod in cold water for at least 24 hours, changing the water frequently. Cut the fish into small pieces, rinse well, and leave to drain.
Finely chop the garlic and break the chili into pieces. Gently pan fry the garlic and chili in the oil, then remove the pieces of chili.
Place the pieces of fish in the skillet with the garlic, making sure that the fish is skin side down. Sweat in the oil for 20 minutes, stirring frequently. The stirring ensures that the garlic, oil, and gelatine in the fish skin combine to make a sauce with the consistency of mayonnaise. Season to taste with pepper. This dish is delicious served with boiled potatoes.

Garlic Soup with Muscatel Grapes

11 oz (300 g) rustic white bread (crusts removed)
4 garlic cloves
Coarse salt
4 Tbs olive oil
2 Tbs sherry vinegar
5 oz (150 g) ground almonds
$3^3/4$ cups (750 ml) ice cold water
7 oz (200 g) muscatel grapes

Slice the bread and soak in water for 5 minutes. Squeeze out the excess water and tear into pieces. Liquidize the bread, garlic, $1/4$ tsp coarse salt, oil, and vinegar. Then add the almonds and stir in the water until it forms a creamy soup. Chill for 3 hours. Halve the grapes and remove the pits.
Season the cold soup with salt, pour into bowls, and garnish with the grapes.

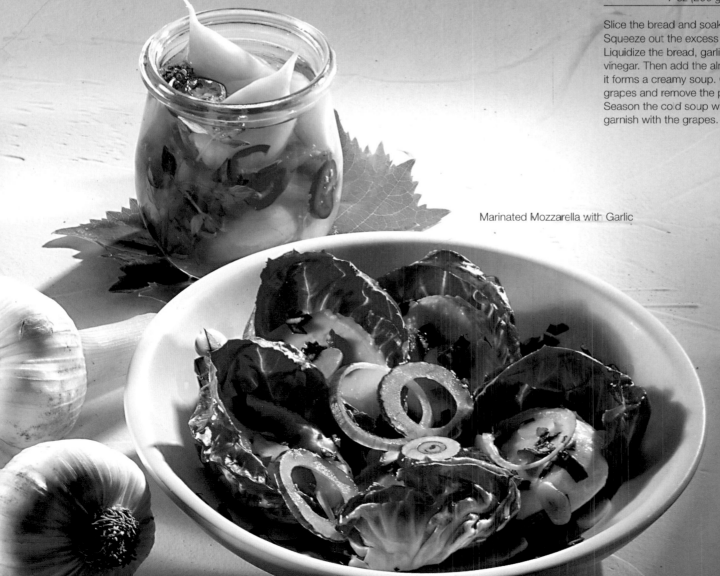

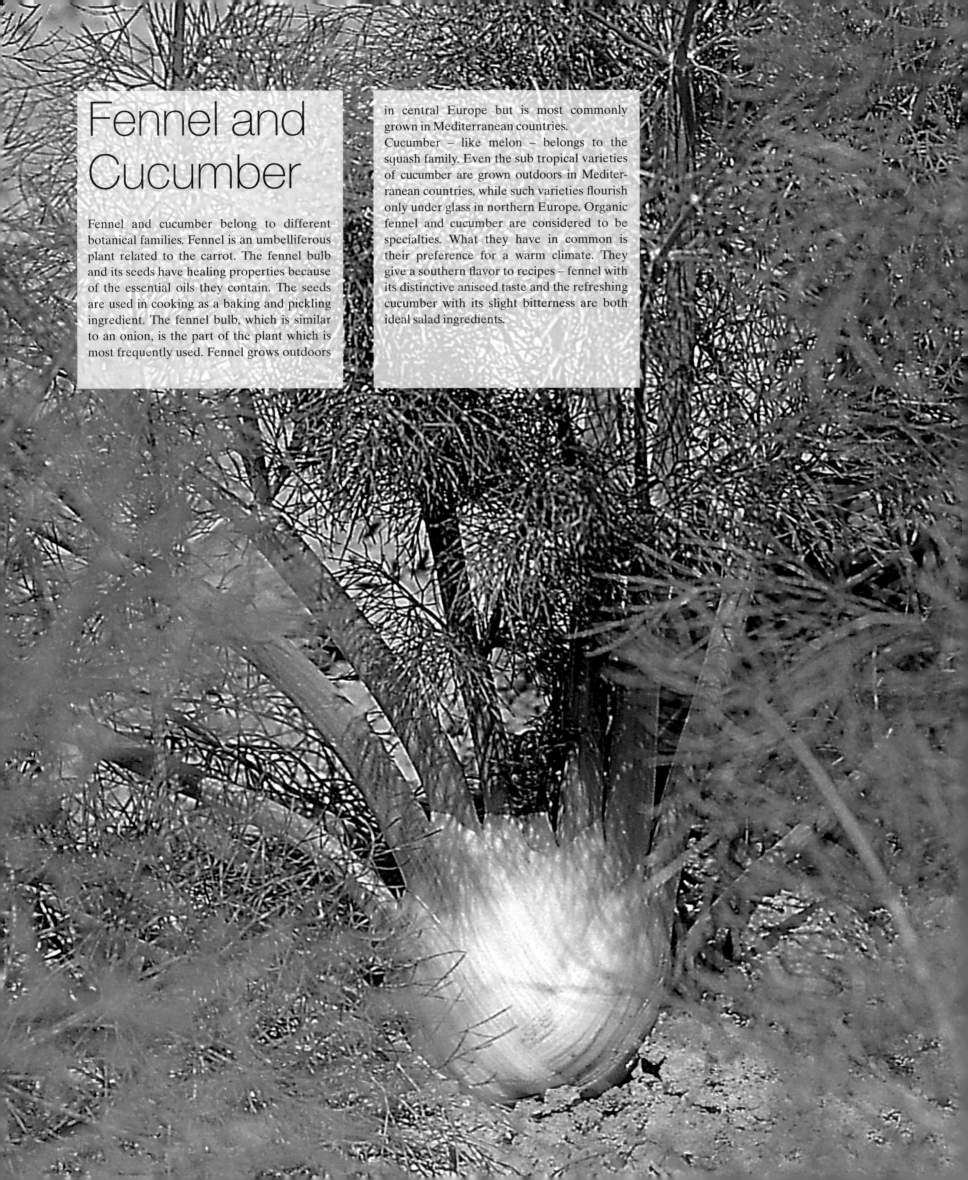

Fennel and Cucumber

Fennel and cucumber belong to different botanical families. Fennel is an umbelliferous plant related to the carrot. The fennel bulb and its seeds have healing properties because of the essential oils they contain. The seeds are used in cooking as a baking and pickling ingredient. The fennel bulb, which is similar to an onion, is the part of the plant which is most frequently used. Fennel grows outdoors in central Europe but is most commonly grown in Mediterranean countries.

Cucumber – like melon – belongs to the squash family. Even the sub tropical varieties of cucumber are grown outdoors in Mediterranean countries, while such varieties flourish only under glass in northern Europe. Organic fennel and cucumber are considered to be specialties. What they have in common is their preference for a warm climate. They give a southern flavor to recipes – fennel with its distinctive aniseed taste and the refreshing cucumber with its slight bitterness are both ideal salad ingredients.

Fennel Gratin

2 lbs 3 oz (1 kg) fennel
$1/2$ tsp coarse salt
$3^1/_2$ oz (100 g) Swiss cheese
5 oz (150 g) Roquefort
1 cup (200 ml) sour cream
$1/2$ tsp fennel seeds
Black pepper

Remove the green parts of the fennel and set aside.
Cut the fennel bulb into narrow strips and remove the stalk.
Cook in boiling, salted water for about 5 minutes until it is "al dente." Drain and set aside.
Preheat the oven to 400 °F (200 °C).
Grease a baking pan and spread the fennel out in it.
Grate the Swiss cheese, crumble the Roquefort and mix the two cheeses with the sour cream.
Add the fennel seeds and season the cheese mixture with pepper.
Pour the cream and cheese mixture over the fennel and bake in the oven for 15 minutes.
Chop the green fennel leaves and sprinkle over the dish just before serving.

Marinated Fennel

1 lb 2 oz (500 g) fennel
2 shallots
$3/_4$ cup (125 ml) sherry
2 Tbs balsamic vinegar
1 Tbs honey
1 Tbs fennel seeds
Coarse salt, black pepper

Remove the green parts of the fennel and set aside.
Halve the fennel bulbs, remove the stalk and cut the vegetables lengthways into strips. Cook in boiling, salted water for about 5 minutes until it is "al dente." Drain and set aside.
Finely dice the shallots and mix together with the sherry, vinegar, honey, fennel seeds, salt, and pepper to make a marinade.
Place the fennel into the marinade while it is still warm and leave for 3 hours. Just before serving, finely chop the green parts of the fennel and sprinkle over the dish.

Chilled Cucumber Soup

1 medium salad cucumber
11 oz (300 g) yogurt
1 cup (200 ml) buttermilk or kefir
1–2 garlic cloves
Coarse salt, black pepper
6 mint leaves

Peel, deseed, and chop the cucumber and purée with the buttermilk and yogurt.
Mince the garlic and stir the garlic juice into the cucumber soup.
Finely chop 2 mint leaves and add to the soup.
Season to taste with salt and pepper.
Chill for 2 hours. Just before serving, garnish with the remaining mint leaves.

Fennel and Orange Salad

2 oranges
1 lemon
4 small fennel bulbs
4 Tbs olive oil
$1/_2$ tsp coarse salt
Black pepper
10 black olives
2 Tbs raspberry vinegar

Peel the lemon and one of the oranges. Separate the fruit into segments and retain the juice. Squeeze the second orange.
Remove the stalk and greenery from the fennel, setting the green parts aside.
Cut the fennel lengthways into narrow strips. Warm the orange and lemon juice in a skillet with 2 tablespoons of the olive oil. Add the fennel and season with salt and pepper.
Add the lemon and orange segments and cook briefly.
Remove the fennel and the fruit from the skillet, pour the juice from the skillet into a container and mix with the raspberry vinegar.
Finely chop the green parts of the fennel, add half to the liquids with the remaining olive oil and stir well.
Arrange the slices of fennel with the fruits on plates and pour the sauce over the top. Stone the olives and use, together with the remaining green parts of the fennel, to garnish the dish.

Cucumber in Cream Sauce

1 salad cucumber
1 shallot
2 Tbs butter
$1/_2$ cup (100 ml) white wine
1 tsp vegetable stock granules
1 bunch dill
1 container crème fraîche
White pepper

Halve and deseed the cucumber, then chop into pieces 1 inch (2.5 cm) thick.
Finely chop the shallots and braise in the butter until transparent.
Add the wine and the stock and cook over a high heat for 5 minutes.
Roughly chop the dill and add to the cucumber with the crème fraîche; season with pepper.
Cucumbers in cream are an excellent accompaniment to fish dishes.

Cucumber and Fennel Salad with Gorgonzola Dressing

1 garlic clove
1 salad cucumber
1 fennel bulb
Juice of 1–2 lemons
$3^1/_2$ oz (100 g) Gorgonzola
1 tsp mustard
4 Tbs olive oil
Coarse salt, white pepper

Peel the garlic and rub it around the inside of a salad bowl.
Slice the cucumber and the fennel and set aside the green parts of the fennel.
Place the vegetables in the salad bowl and sprinkle with a little lemon juice.
Mix the Gorgonzola with 2 tablespoons of lemon juice, the mustard, and a little olive oil until it forms a thick cream; season to taste with salt and pepper.
Mix the remaining olive oil and lemon juice together, pour over the salad and toss the salad thoroughly.
Arrange the salad on individual plates.
Pour the cheese dressing over the salad and decorate each plate with a sprig of fennel greenery.

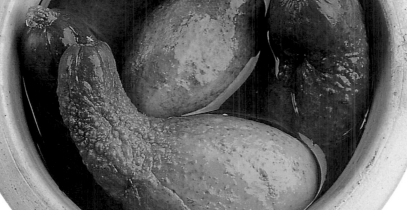

Pickled cucumbers: in lightly salted water with a little dill and garlic

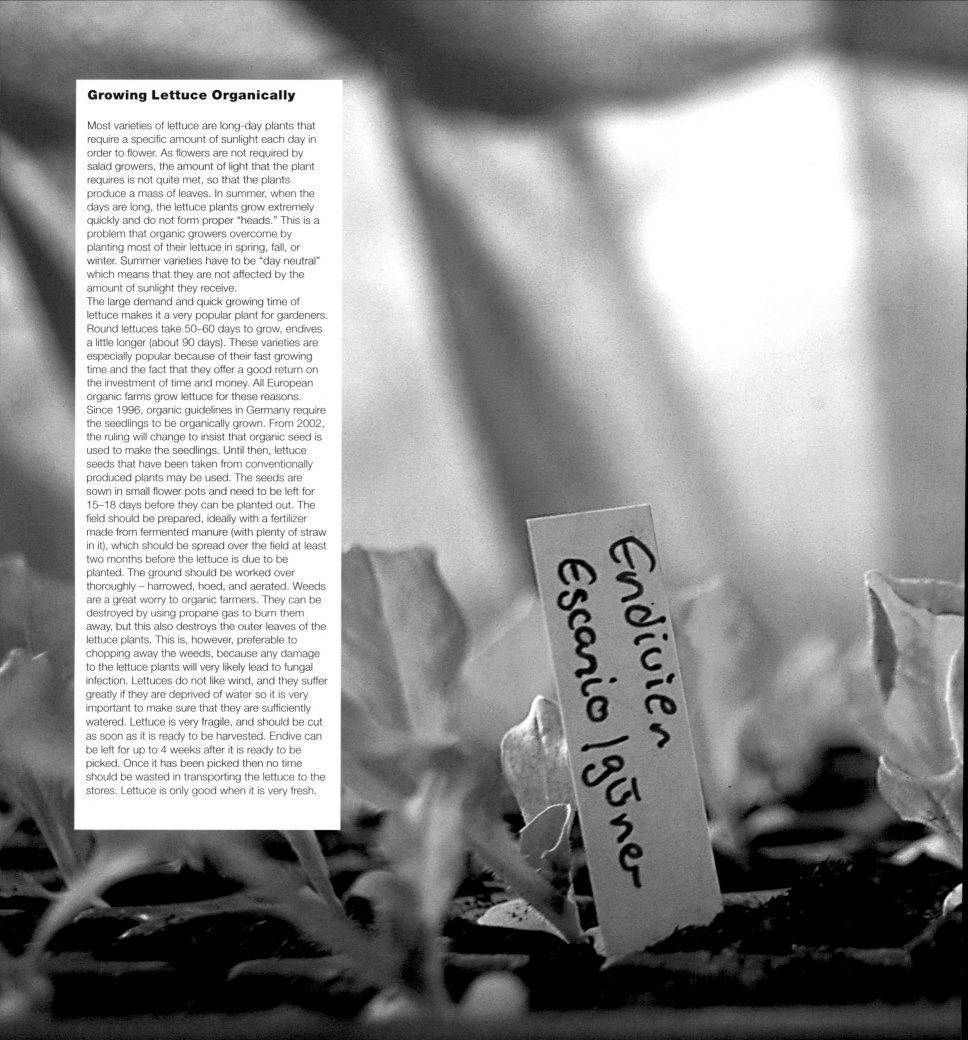

Growing Lettuce Organically

Most varieties of lettuce are long-day plants that require a specific amount of sunlight each day in order to flower. As flowers are not required by salad growers, the amount of light that the plant requires is not quite met, so that the plants produce a mass of leaves. In summer, when the days are long, the lettuce plants grow extremely quickly and do not form proper "heads." This is a problem that organic growers overcome by planting most of their lettuce in spring, fall, or winter. Summer varieties have to be "day neutral" which means that they are not affected by the amount of sunlight they receive.

The large demand and quick growing time of lettuce makes it a very popular plant for gardeners. Round lettuces take 50–60 days to grow, endives a little longer (about 90 days). These varieties are especially popular because of their fast growing time and the fact that they offer a good return on the investment of time and money. All European organic farms grow lettuce for these reasons. Since 1996, organic guidelines in Germany require the seedlings to be organically grown. From 2002, the ruling will change to insist that organic seed is used to make the seedlings. Until then, lettuce seeds that have been taken from conventionally produced plants may be used. The seeds are sown in small flower pots and need to be left for 15–18 days before they can be planted out. The field should be prepared, ideally with a fertilizer made from fermented manure (with plenty of straw in it), which should be spread over the field at least two months before the lettuce is due to be planted. The ground should be worked over thoroughly – harrowed, hoed, and aerated. Weeds are a great worry to organic farmers. They can be destroyed by using propane gas to burn them away, but this also destroys the outer leaves of the lettuce plants. This is, however, preferable to chopping away the weeds, because any damage to the lettuce plants will very likely lead to fungal infection. Lettuces do not like wind, and they suffer greatly if they are deprived of water so it is very important to make sure that they are sufficiently watered. Lettuce is very fragile, and should be cut as soon as it is ready to be harvested. Endive can be left for up to 4 weeks after it is ready to be picked. Once it has been picked then no time should be wasted in transporting the lettuce to the stores. Lettuce is only good when it is very fresh.

Lettuce

There is no other member of the vegetable kingdom that offers as much freshness and delicacy as lettuce. Salad forms a part of every meal in southern Europe, and its popularity is increasing every year in the rest of Europe. However, no other vegetable suffers so much from conventional growing techniques. Lettuce absorbs all poisons, particularly nitrates. If lettuce is grown in a greenhouse it can contain twice as much nitrate as organic salad leaves. This is why it is important to use organic lettuce.

Lettuces are 90 percent water, which is why they are so low in calories. The remaining ten percent is very nutritious. There is a wealth of vitamins in the leaves – particularly the outer ones: lettuce contains vitamin C, provitamin A, and many B vitamins. The vitamin content decreases inside the lettuce in the leaves near or in the heart. However, the whole lettuce not only contains common minerals like calcium, potassium, and phosphorus, but also rare minerals like iodine, copper, zinc, and selenium, all of which help prevent heart disease and cancer. It is advisable not to eat too much lettuce at lunch time, as it has a calming, soporific effect.

Background: Lettuce seedlings are "started off" in a greenhouse, to ensure that they develop properly. Since 1996 these German "nurseries" have had to conform to organic farming guidelines – after 2002 the seed used will have to be proved to be organically grown.

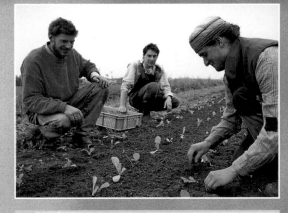

Organic vegetable growers have to do a lot of work by hand. Here they are planting out the lettuce plants.

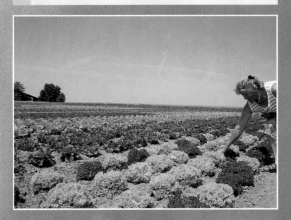

Grooves are made in the soil to mark out the rows where the lettuces will be planted.

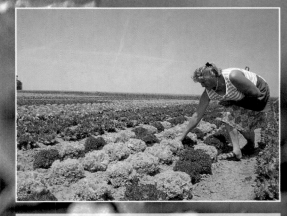

Each head of lettuce shows the care taken to produce it – weeds are removed by hand.

A Glossary of Lettuce

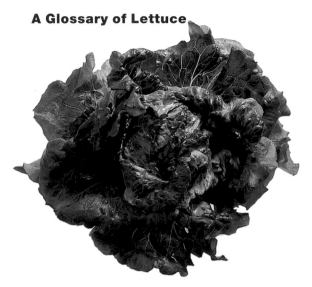

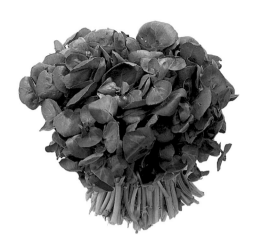

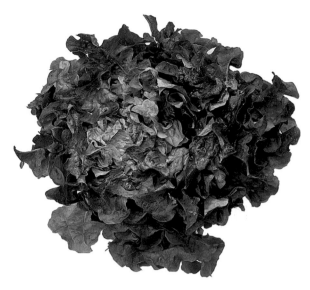

Batavia
An attractive lettuce whose leaves are tinged red at the ends. It is a new, French variety closely related to iceberg. Needs to be grown under warm conditions. A crunchy, crinkly lettuce with a firm structure and peppery flavor.

Watercress
Popular back in the Middle Ages, this water growing plant is used for cooking and medicinal purposes. It purifies the blood, has a peppery flavor, and does not keep well.

Oak Leaf Lettuce
A growing salad that has a delicate structure. The leaves are red at the tips and are the same shape as oak leaves. This lettuce has a delicate, nutty flavor; very good in mixed green salads, wilts quickly.

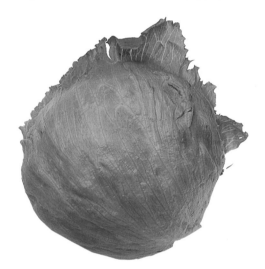

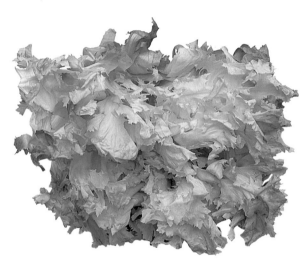

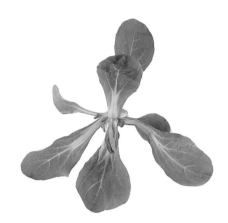

Iceberg Lettuce
Large, firm, roundheads that weigh up to $1^3/4$ pounds (800 g). Pleasantly spicy, very fresh (due to the high water content), fleshy leaves. Keeps well; can be cooked and served as a side vegetable.

Curly Endive
A relative of Belgian endive with green, slightly tough outer leaves and a yellow heart. Slightly bitter in flavor, smooth edged, it is known as escarole and keeps very well; with crinkly edges it is known as frisée.

Lamb's Lettuce
Originally considered to be a weed with small rosette leaves, it is now very popular. Rich in vitamins and iron; has a distinctive nutty flavor.

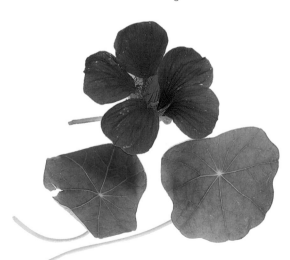

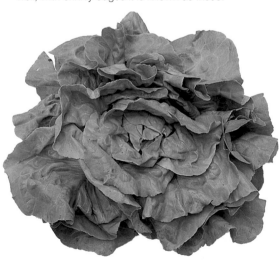

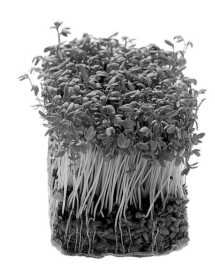

Nasturtium
Very popular garden plant with pretty orange or yellow flowers. Its round leaves have a piquant flavor and can be used for seasoning and salads; the edible flowers make an attractive garnish.

Round Lettuce
One of the most popular types of lettuce; also available in red; bland flavor which makes it ideal for sweet or savory recipes. Also good steamed. Wilts very quickly.

Cress
A quick growing plant that can reach a height of 18 inches (50 cm); cruciferous, with white stalks. Only lives for a few days. Sold in boxes; has a piquant, peppery taste and stimulates the appetite.

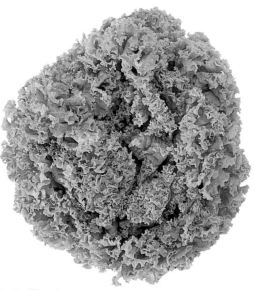

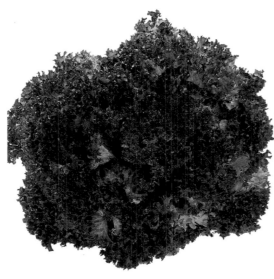

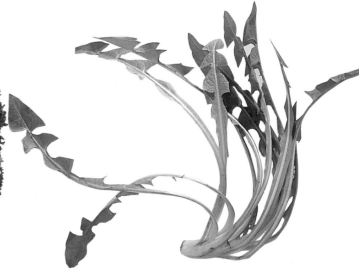

Lollo Biondo
Yellow-green, very crinkly leaves, like the unusually colored Lollo Rosso, which it resembles in its cultivation; comes from Italy. Keeps well and has a delicately mild flavor.

Lollo Rosso
Attractive red, crinkly leaves, very fashionable Italian growing lettuce with an open heart. Goes well in mixed salads; pleasant, mild flavor with a slight nutty taste.

Dandelion
Widely used in folk medicine, widespread weed. Grows in loose soil and forms delicate, white-yellow, long leaves. Has a high vitamin C and essential oil content; very spicy, with a delicate bitterness.

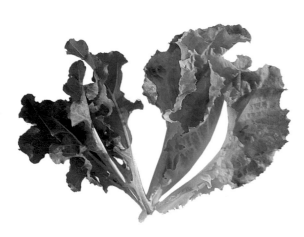

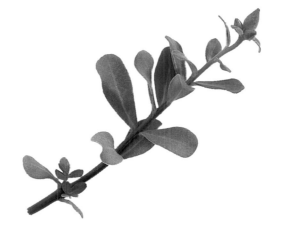

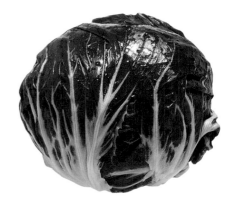

Picking Salad
An early lettuce with long, crinkled leaves, are tender when young. Does not form a heart but grows stalks. Leaves are picked individually; mild flavor. Does not keep.

Common Purslane
An ancient, wild growing vegetable that is having a renaissance. Its round, fleshy, extremely healthy leaves taste nutty, crisp and complement any salad.

Radicchio
Related to chicory and endive; it has a firm, small, red and white head. Contains a bitter substance that is important for the metabolism. Distinctive flavor, very attractive in mixed salads; keeps fairly well.

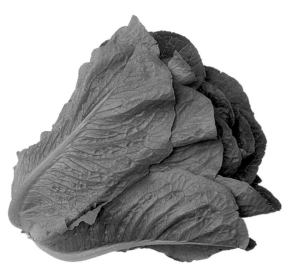

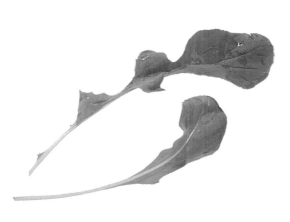

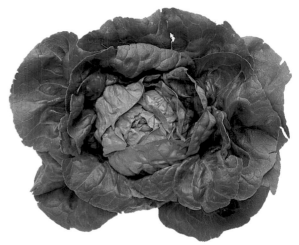

Romaine Lettuce
Has a central stalk from which large, dark green, longish-oval, upright leaves grow. Slightly peppery and crunchy inside; very popular in Mediterranean countries.

Arugula
Widely grown in warm countries, its leaves resemble those of a radish and are dark green if they are grown outside. A characteristically strong, quite hot flavor. It has a stimulating effect on the body.

Sweetheart Lettuce
Not affected by sunlight, this lettuce is grown in southern Europe in the summer as a substitute for round lettuce. A mild, sweetish flavor and a pleasant, firmish leaf structure.

189

Salads

Raw Vegetable Salad

1 small round lettuce
3 Tbs lemon juice
1/2 celeriac
1 sour apple
2 carrots
1 bunch radishes
6 Tbs heavy cream
3 Tbs corn oil
1 tsp raw cane sugar
Coarse salt, black pepper
4 Tbs roasted pumpkin seeds

Wash the lettuce, tear it into large pieces and dry in a salad spinner. Arrange on a large platter. Grate the apple, celeriac, and carrot, sprinkle immediately with lemon juice and put in a bowl. Grate the radishes and add to the vegetable mixture; mix well and add to the lettuce.

Mix the cream with the remaining lemon juice, the oil, sugar, salt, and pepper.

Beat well until it forms a smooth dressing and pour over the salad.

Sprinkle with pumpkin seeds and serve.

Spanish Salad

1 round lettuce
1 red and 1 yellow bell pepper
3 tomatoes
1 red onion
7 oz (200 g) cooked white beans
16 large green olives
8 canned artichoke hearts, quartered
Red wine vinegar
Olive oil
Coarse salt, black pepper

Tear the lettuce leaves, wash and dry in a salad spinner. Cut the bell peppers into strips, slice the tomatoes and the onion.

Arrange the lettuce on large plates and place the bell peppers, tomatoes, onions, and beans on top. Finally, add the artichokes and olives.

Pass the oil, vinegar, salt, and pepper round separately.

Dandelion and Rutabaga Leaf Salad

(Illustration below)

1 large potato
1 tsp caraway seeds
2 eggs
1 onion
2 garlic cloves
1 Tbs sunflower oil
5 oz (150 g) young dandelion leaves
5 oz (150 g) rutabaga leaves
3 Tbs white wine vinegar
3 Tbs sunflower oil
Coarse salt, black pepper

Cook the potato in its skin in boiling water with the caraway until it is tender. Boil the eggs for 4–5 minutes (depending on size) until they are soft-cooked.

Chop the onion and garlic and pan fry in the tablespoon of oil until transparent.

Wash the dandelion and the rutabaga leaves, spin dry and mix together.

Peel the potato and grate over the salad vegetables, then pour over the onion and garlic mixture.

Shell the eggs, place on the salad and break into small pieces using a wooden spoon.

Add the remaining oil and vinegar. Mix all the ingredients together thoroughly, season with salt and pepper, and serve while still warm.

Dandelion and Rutabaga Leaf Salad

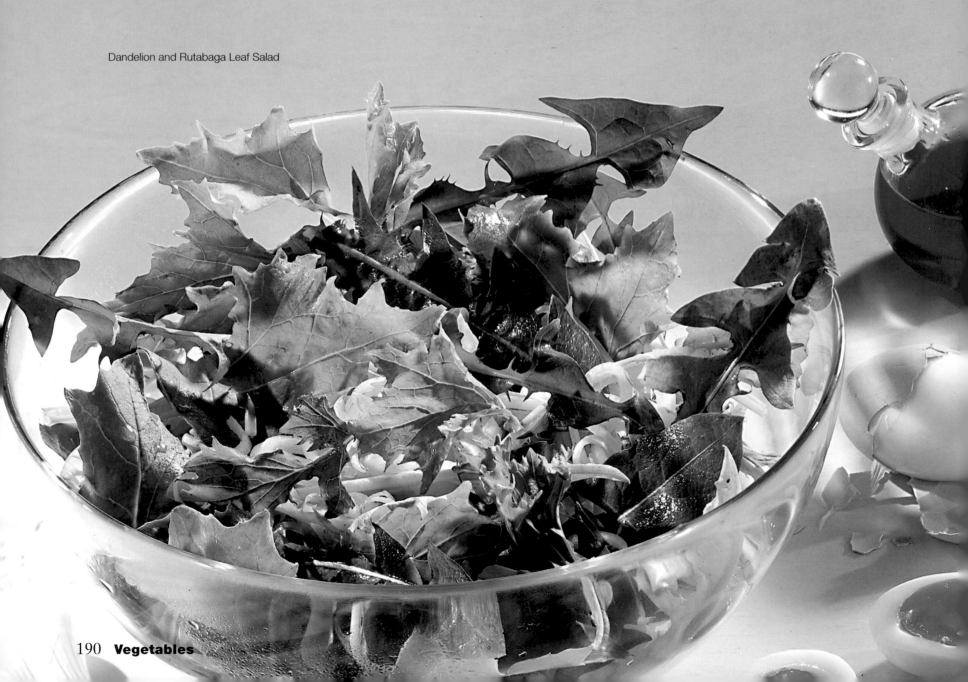

Lamb's Lettuce with Garlic Croutons

3 slices whole wheat toasting bread
2 garlic cloves
2 Tbs butter
1 pinch mustard powder
2 Tbs vegetable stock
4 Tbs wine vinegar
4 Tbs walnut oil
1 finely chopped shallot
1 lb 2 oz (500 g) lamb's lettuce

Cut the bread into small squares.

Halve the garlic cloves and brown in the butter. Remove from the skillet, add the squares of bread to the skillet and fry, stirring frequently. Set aside.

Make a vinaigrette from the mustard powder, vegetable stock, vinegar, and oil, and then stir in the shallot.

Divide up the lamb's lettuce, wash well, and spin dry. Mix with the vinaigrette.

Sprinkle the salad with the garlic croutons and serve.

Romaine Lettuce with Pears and Gorgonzola

1 head romaine lettuce
4 pears
2 Tbs lemon juice
2 oz (50 g) chopped walnuts
3$\frac{1}{2}$ oz (100 g) Gorgonzola
$\frac{1}{2}$ cup (120 ml) light cream
White pepper

Wash the salad, tear into bite-sized pieces, and spin to dry. Arrange on plates.

Slice the pears, sprinkle with lemon juice, and arrange over the lettuce. Sprinkle with the walnuts.

Mash the Gorgonzola and mix with the cream to make a smooth sauce; season with pepper.

Pour the cheese cream over the salad and serve.

Pinzimonio
(Italian Raw Vegetable Salad with a Piquant Dip)

4 carrots
1 red, 1 green, and 1 yellow bell pepper (small)
1 small fennel bulb
2 sticks of celery
1 small salad cucumber
1 bunch radishes

Dip
2 washed anchovy fillets
6 Tbs olive oil
3 Tbs lemon juice
Black pepper

Cut the vegetables lengthways into strips. Leave the radishes whole.

To make the dip: finely chop the anchovies, mix with the remaining ingredients, and place in a small dish.

Place the small dish in the center of a large salad platter. Arrange the vegetables decoratively around the dish.

This dish is an ideal appetizer or side dish.

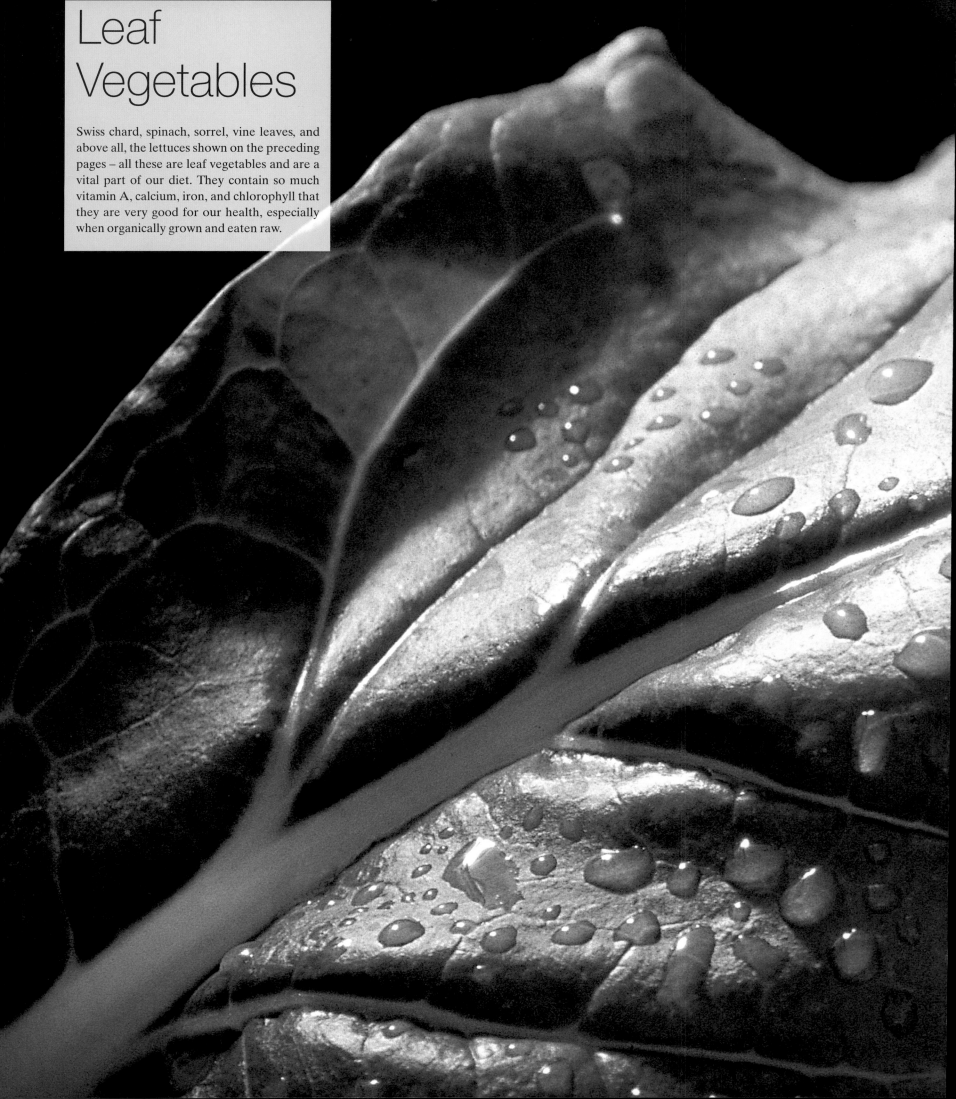

Leaf Vegetables

Swiss chard, spinach, sorrel, vine leaves, and above all, the lettuces shown on the preceding pages – all these are leaf vegetables and are a vital part of our diet. They contain so much vitamin A, calcium, iron, and chlorophyll that they are very good for our health, especially when organically grown and eaten raw.

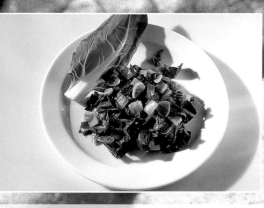 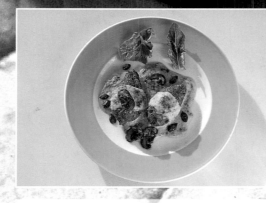 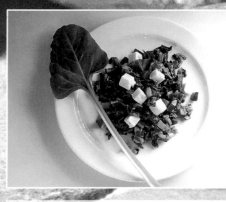

Blanched Swiss Chard with Garlic
(Illustration above)

11 oz (300 g) Swiss chard
1 shallot
3 Tbs olive oil
3 garlic cloves
1 pinch nutmeg
Coarse salt, black pepper

Chop the leaves and stalks of the Swiss chard into small pieces.
Finely dice the shallot and cut the garlic into thin slices. Heat the olive oil in a large pan.
Pan fry the chard stalks in the oil. Add the garlic and onion and fry briefly.
Add a little water together with the Swiss chard leaves; cook until the leaves wilt.
Remove from the heat, add the nutmeg, and season to taste with salt and pepper.
Serve with toast or French bread as an appetizer, or serve as a side vegetable with cereal rissoles.

Warm Potato Salad with Sorrel

2 lbs 3 oz (1 kg) firm potatoes
Coarse salt
1 tsp caraway seeds
7 oz (200 g) young sorrel
1 shallot
$^1/_2$ cup (120 ml) vegetable stock
3 Tbs wine vinegar
4 Tbs olive oil
1 egg yolk
1 pinch mustard powder
White pepper

Cook the potatoes with the caraway seeds in boiling, salted water.
Finely chop the sorrel.
Leave the potatoes to cool slightly, peel, and dice.
Finely chop the shallot and add to the potato.
Make a sauce from the remaining ingredients, season with salt, and mix together with the potatoes. Add the sorrel and serve warm.

Spinach Gnocchi Baked in a Creamy Mushroom Sauce
(Illustration above)

11 oz (300 g) floury potatoes
7 oz (200 g) spinach
1 small onion
1 small garlic clove
1 Tbs olive oil
1 egg
$^1/_4$ cup (30 g) spelt flour
1 pinch nutmeg
Coarse salt, white pepper

Sauce

11 oz (300 g) mushrooms
1 shallot
2 Tbs butter
$^3/_4$ cup (150 g) heavy cream
1 Tbs arrowroot
1 tsp coarse salt
1 pinch white pepper
1 Tbs soysauce
2 Tbs finely chopped flat-leafed parsley

To make the gnocchi: cook the potatoes in their skins, peel and press through a potato sieve or grate, while the potatoes are still warm.
Meanwhile tear the spinach leaves, finely dice the onion, and mince the garlic.
Gently pan fry the onion and garlic in the oil until transparent, then add the spinach and cook gently.
Add the vegetables to the potatoes, add the egg and flour, mix well and season with nutmeg, salt, and pepper.
With damp hands, or 2 spoons form the mixture into small rounds. Cook the gnocchi in boiling, salted water until they float to the surface.
To make the sauce, first slice the mushrooms.
Finely dice the shallot and cook in the butter until transparent.
Add the mushrooms and cook briefly.
Mix the cream with 3 tablespoons of water and add to the mushrooms.
Dissolve the arrowroot in a little water, add to the sauce and stir until it thickens.
Season to taste with salt, pepper, and soy sauce and stir in the parsley.
Serve with the gnocchi.

Spinach Beet with Bell Peppers and Sheep's Milk Cheese
(Illustration above)

1 lb 2 oz (500 g) spinach beet
2 garlic cloves
2 small onions
1 red bell pepper
2 Tbs olive oil
Herb salt
1 tsp sweet paprika
1 pinch cayenne pepper
Black pepper
$3^1/_2$ oz (100 g) sheep's milk cheese

Chop the leaves and stalks of the spinach beet, then chop the bell peppers, onion, and garlic. Pan fry the peppers, garlic, and onion in the oil. Add the spinach beet, cook briefly and add a little water.
Season to taste with the spices.
Dice the sheep's milk cheese and mix in with the vegetables. Serve as an appetizer with French bread.

Broiled Radicchio

3–4 heads radicchio lettuce (about 2 lbs 3 oz/1 kg)
Coarse salt, black pepper
4 Tbs olive oil
Lemon wedges

Preheat the oven to 460 °F (250 °C).
Cut the radicchio heads in half lengthways and place in a heatproof dish with the cut side facing down; season with salt and pepper and drizzle over the olive oil.
Bake in the oven for 5 minutes. Then turn on the broiler and place the radicchio under it for 3 minutes.
Remove the radicchio and leave to cool slightly.
Garnish with lemon wedges.

Background: Swiss chard is a versatile vegetable. The leaves can be used like spinach, added to soups, or used as a filling. The stalks can be cooked and served like asparagus.

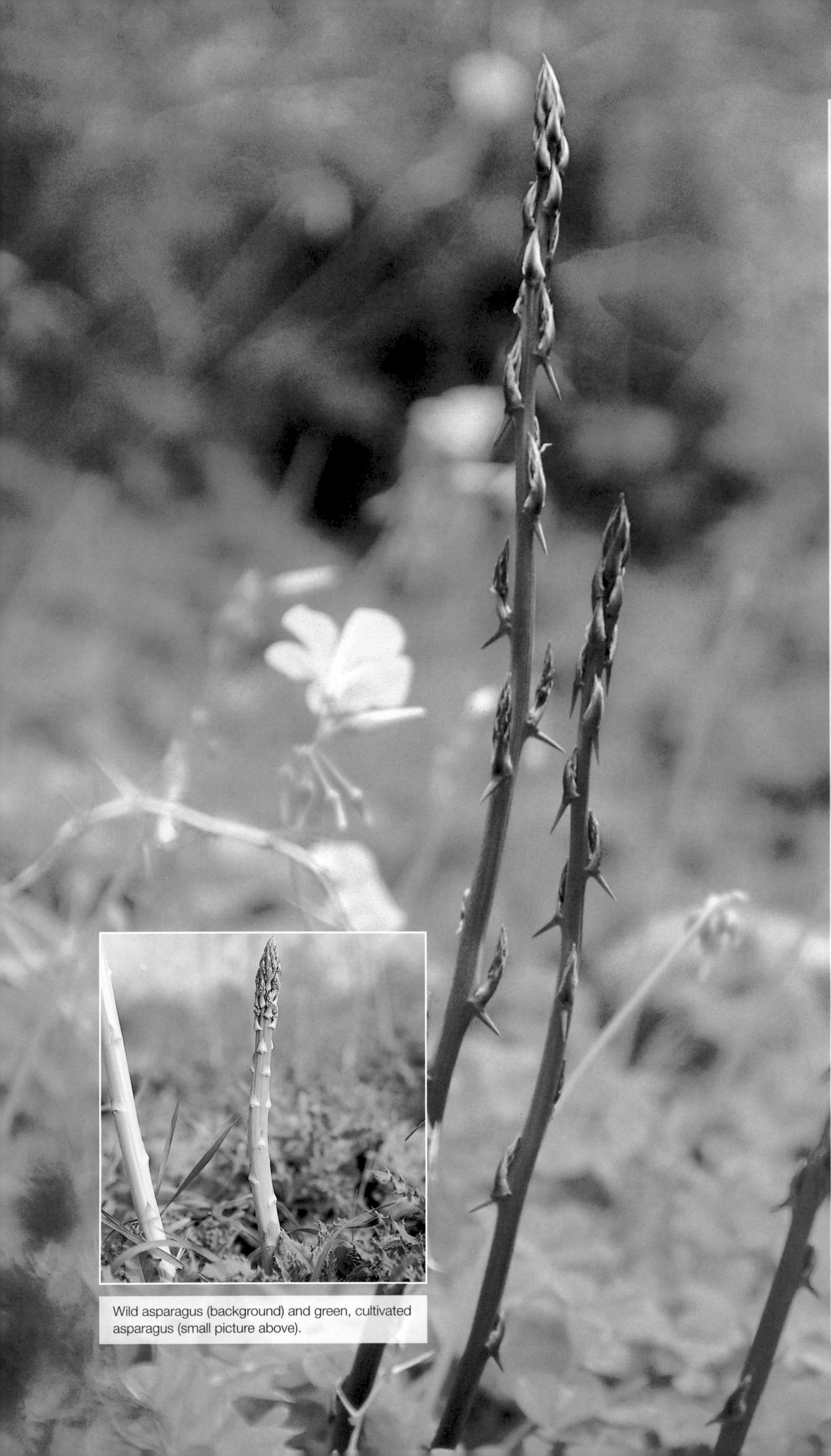

Asparagus

Back in the first half of the 17th century, an English doctor, Nicholas Culpeper, praised the medicinal properties of asparagus. He claimed it removed kidney stones, eased toothache, and aroused desire. Today it is known that asparagus contains vitamin A, many of the B vitamins, vitamin C, as well as minerals and trace elements. The most important substance that asparagus contains is asparagus acid – an amino acid that stimulates the kidneys.

Asparagus, which is related to garlic and is a member of the lily family, has always been prized as a cooking ingredient. Wild asparagus grows throughout the Mediterranean countries, where it is picked and sold in bunches at the side of the road. It is full of flavor, but does not have much texture, so is often used for omelets.

Cultivated asparagus, like wild asparagus, becomes green when it is in contact with the light. Green asparagus is very popular in southern Europe. It has a stronger flavor, does not usually need peeling, and cooks quickly. These are advantages, as every cook knows. Gardeners, too, prefer green asparagus: they do not have to build raised beds for the plants which can be harvested easily, because they are above ground. A few varieties have been found which account for nearly all the green asparagus that is commercially grown.

There are a few special varieties that produce lily white asparagus with tips that are a hand's span in length. The plants are set in rows, which are then heaped up with earth. This method of growing asparagus was invented by Dutch farmers in the 19th century. When the tips of the plants break the surface of the soil, it is time for the asparagus to be cut. If the plants are allowed to grow in the daylight they will discolor and turn mauve. White asparagus must be peeled, and has a milder taste than other varieties. Organic asparagus has a great advantage over traditionally grown asparagus: whether green, white, from the north, or the south, as it has not been treated with pesticides. Chemicals are used in large quantities for conventional asparagus cultivation.

Wild asparagus (background) and green, cultivated asparagus (small picture above).

Tagliatelle with Green Asparagus

1 lb 2 oz (500 g) green asparagus
Coarse salt
11¹/₂ oz (320 g) short tagliatelle
3 egg yolks
5 Tbs heavy cream
2 oz (50 g) freshly grated hard cheese
1¹/₂ oz (40 g) butter

Peel the lower third of the asparagus stalks and remove the woody end. Cut the asparagus into pieces, setting the tips aside.

Bring 15 cups (3 l) of water to the boil with the asparagus pieces. When the water boils, add 3 tsp (15 g) salt and cook the asparagus for 5 minutes. Then add the tagliatelle and the asparagus tips and cook until "al dente."

Meanwhile mix together the egg yolks, cream, and cheese to make a sauce.

Drain the tagliatelle and place in a warmed serving dish. Toss in the butter and cheese sauce and serve at once.

Mixed Leaf Salad with Asparagus and Strawberries

(Illustration below)

Assortment of lettuce leaves (equivalent to one head of lettuce)
3 Tbs white wine vinegar
¹/₂ tsp salt
White pepper
4 Tbs safflower oil
1 Tbs honey
1 sprig tarragon
7 oz (200 g) green asparagus
7 oz (200 g) white asparagus
7 oz (200 g) strawberries

Wash and dry the lettuce leaves.

Make a vinaigrette from the vinegar, salt, pepper, oil, 4 tablespoons (60 ml) of cold water, and honey.

Finely chop the tarragon and add to the vinaigrette.

Peel the white asparagus, and the green, if necessary. Marinate the asparagus in the vinaigrette for 2 hours.

Tear the lettuce leaves into bite-sized pieces and arrange on a large plate.

Cut the asparagus diagonally into pieces about 1 inch (3 cm) long. Arrange these on the lettuce.

Quarter the strawberries and add to the asparagus. Pour the tarragon vinaigrette over the top and serve.

Asparagus – Where, When and How

In southern Europe the first asparagus grows in early spring, while in central and northern Europe the main crop is in May and June. An asparagus field, which may be 10–12 years old, will only be harvested for one month. Any remaining stalks will be left to go to seed. The roots help to return nutrients to the soil ready for the next year's crop, and do not die until the fall.

Asparagus is only delicious when it is young and upright, and can be snapped easily. The stalks should never be dry, and the cut end should not be discolored. It is a bad sign if the tips are open, or loose. To keep asparagus, wrap in a damp cloth and place in the crisper drawer of the refrigerator. The more expensive varieties of asparagus should be eaten as soon after purchase as possible.

Asparagus Gratin

3 lbs 6 oz (1.5 kg) green asparagus
Coarse salt
3 slices whole wheat bread
¹/₂ cup (125 g) soft butter
3¹/₂ oz (100 g) finely grated hard cheese

Peel the lower third of the asparagus stalks and remove the woody part at the end.

Cook the asparagus briefly in boiling, salted water. Remove with a slotted spoon and leave to drain.

Butter a heatproof dish and transfer the asparagus to the dish.

Crumble the bread, and mix with the remaining butter and the cheese. Sprinkle this mixture over the asparagus.

Bake in the oven, or cook under the broiler for 10 minutes.

Asparagus Risotto

14 oz (400 g) green asparagus
14 oz (400 g) white asparagus
Coarse salt
4 Tbs butter
¹/₂ cup (100 ml) light cream
1 small onion
11 oz (300 g) short-grain brown rice
¹/₂ cup (100 ml) dry white wine
3¹/₂ oz (100 g) freshly grated hard cheese

Peel the white asparagus and the lower third of the green asparagus. Cut away the woody ends of the stalks.

Cut the asparagus into pieces, reserving the tips. Cook the white asparagus in 7¹/₂ cups (1.5 l) boiling salted water with 1 tablespoon of the butter. After 5 minutes, add the green asparagus and cook for a further 10 minutes. Remove the asparagus from the cooking water, leave to cool and purée with the cream.

Bring the cooking water back to the boil. Finely chop the onion and pan fry in the remaining butter. Add the rice and cook, stirring frequently. Add the white wine. When the wine has evaporated, add the asparagus water, a little at a time. Leave about 1 cup (200 ml) out of the risotto. Keep adding the water until it has all evaporated. After about 40–50 minutes, add the asparagus purée and the reserved asparagus tips. Simmer for a further 10 minutes.

Stir in the cheese, leave for 1 minute then serve on soup plates.

Asparagus Consommé

1 lb 2 oz (500 g) chicken breast meat
1 shallot
3 Tbs butter
¹/₂ cup (100 ml) dry white wine
2¹/₂ cups (500 ml) chicken stock
14 oz (400 g) white asparagus
14 oz (400 g) green asparagus
7 oz (200 g) sugar snap peas
Coarse salt
1 Tbs finely chopped chives
1 Tbs finely chopped parsley

Remove the skin and fat from the chicken and dice the meat.

Finely chop the shallot and pan fry in the butter until transparent, add the meat and brown.

Deglaze the pan with the white wine.

When the wine has reduced, add the stock and 2 cups (400 ml) water. Simmer gently.

Peel the white asparagus and remove the woody end.

Cut the asparagus stalks into pieces about 1 inch (3 cm) long. Peel the lower third of the green asparagus stalks and remove the woody end. Cut the stalks into pieces the same size as the white asparagus.

Add the sugar snap peas and the white asparagus to the chicken, followed 5 minutes later by the green asparagus. Cook for 15–20 minutes in total, season with salt, sprinkle with the herbs, and serve.

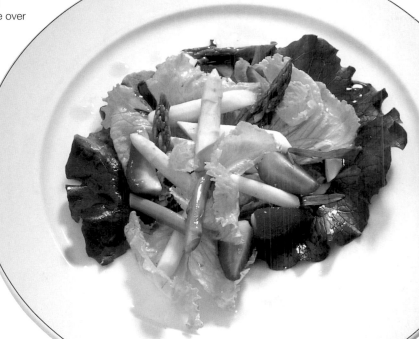

Mixed Leaf Salad with Asparagus and Strawberries

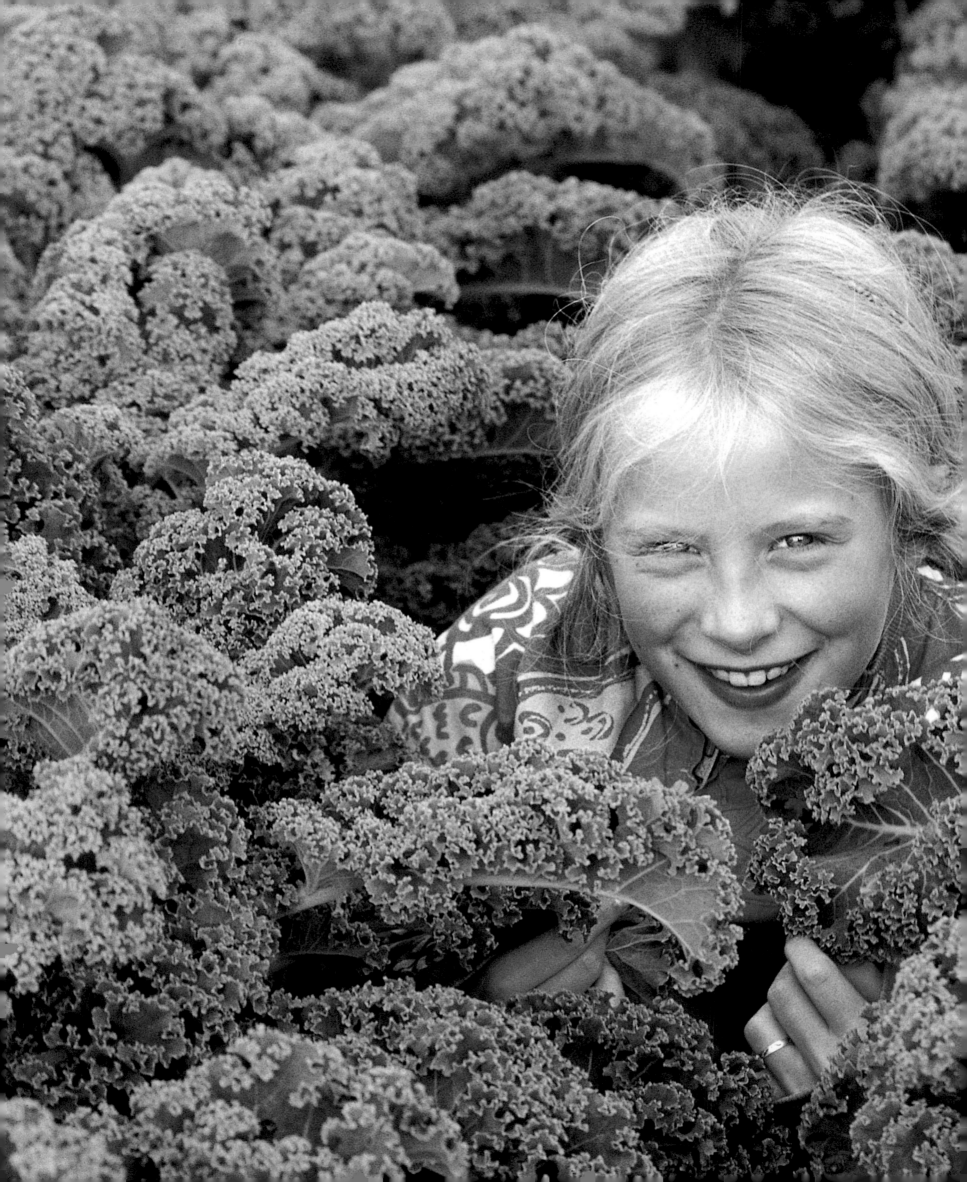

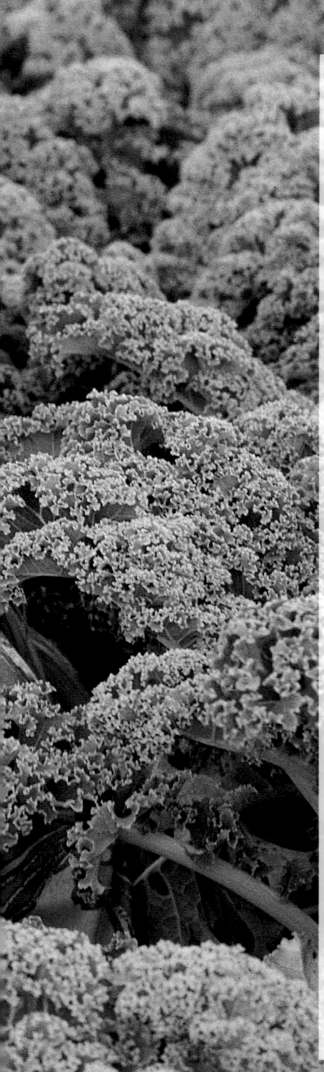

Cabbage

Only carrots have a higher provitamin A content than green cabbage. Provitamin A is important for growth. Green cabbage is one of the richest sources of vitamin C. Despite its nutritional benefits, cabbage is only really popular in northern Europe – particularly with the Germans – despite the fact that it originated in the Mediterranean countries. The dark green color indicates the high content of chlorophyll, a very useful plant substance that appears to have a positive effect on the health and immune system of human beings. Fortunately there are many different varieties of cabbage, all of which grow at different times of year ensuring that cabbage can be eaten all year round. Cabbage is especially popular in the winter, when there is less variety of seasonal vegetables.

Nowadays there seems to be less enthusiasm for cabbage on account of its indigestibility. Cabbage is not naturally indigestible, but it is very sensitive to nitrates, and the amount of nitrates used in modern day fertilizers makes practically all commercially grown cabbages hard to digest. All varieties – whether red, or white, cauliflower or Brussels sprouts – are highly sensitive to nitrates.

Cauliflower and Brussels sprouts belong to the wide-ranging brassica family – which also covers broccoli and other gourmet vegetables. Large cabbages have always been considered food for the people. Practically everywhere in Europe, there was enough food to fill the bellies of the poor. This means that many traditional recipes – whether they come from the north of Ireland or the north of Germany, the Pyrenees or the Balkans – are based around cabbage as the main ingredient. These traditional recipes do tend to be rather heavy, as they were intended to feed people who did hard, physical work. It is not too difficult to adapt them to modern tastes and healthy eating by reducing the quantities of meat for instance, and thus cabbage takes its rightful culinary place.

Cabbage brings many health benefits – it has a remarkably high mineral content and is rich in vitamins. Raw cabbage salads and sauerkraut are the best ways of enjoying the optimum nutritional benefits. They remain in reasonable quantities when the cabbage is lightly cooked, and can be a nutritious treat to be served in many different ways.

Savoy Cabbage Rolls with Gorgonzola

Coarse salt
12 Savoy cabbage leaves
2 oz (50 g) pine nuts
4¼ oz (120 g) mild Gorgonzola
3 Tbs Mascarpone
12 slices air dried ham

In a large saucepan, bring 10 cups (2 l) water to the boil with 2 teaspoons of salt. Blanch the savoy cabbage in the water for 4 minutes and drain. Rinse the cabbage leaves in cold water and leave to drain on paper towels.
Dry roast the pine nuts, leave to cool and chop finely. Mix the Gorgonzola with the Mascarpone to form a smooth paste.
Place a slice of ham on each cabbage leaf, spread the cheese mixture over the top, and sprinkle with pine nuts. Fold the cabbage leaves over the filling and roll them up.
Serve three rolls per person as an appetizer. Serve with lightly chilled rosé wine.

White Cabbage Casserole

2 lbs 4 oz (1 kg) white cabbage
1 onion, 2 garlic cloves
1 sprig rosemary
3 Tbs olive oil
1 cup (200 ml) white wine
Coarse salt, white pepper

Cut the cabbage into quarters, separate the leaves from the stalk and break the leaves into pieces.
Finely chop the onion, garlic, and rosemary and pan fry in the olive oil.
Add the cabbage leaves, pour in the white wine, cover and simmer over a low heat for 60 minutes. Check the cabbage regularly, making sure there is enough liquid in the pan. The dish is cooked when the cabbage leaves turn a light brown color and taste slightly sweet. Season with salt and pepper.

White Cabbage Salad with Dates

1 small white cabbage
1 garlic clove, 1 small onion
1¼ cups (250 ml) sour cream
2 Tbs olive oil
3 Tbs white wine vinegar
1 Tbs honey
1 Tbs turmeric
1 pinch cinnamon
1 tsp ginger powder
1 tsp cardamom
1 pinch cayenne pepper
White pepper
1 tsp coarse salt
5 dates

Cut the cabbage into fine strips. Finely chop the onion and garlic. Make a marinade from the cream, olive oil, vinegar, honey, and spices. Season well, and marinate the cabbage for 60 minutes.
Pit the dates, chop into small pieces, stir into the cabbage, check the seasoning, and serve.

Sauerkraut

Lactic acid fermentation is an ancient method of preserving vegetables. Different types of vegetable are all placed in a stoneware pot or large jar, a little salt water is added, then the pot is sealed and the rest is left to the lactic acid bacteria. This is a complicated process that takes place because of the activity of enzymes. It is a process that retains all the original vitamins and minerals of the vegetables, and adds amino acids and vitamins. The lactic acid bacteria increase in number at a great rate, and help to stop the vegetables spoiling and other bacteria getting into the jar. At the end of the fermentation process – which may take several weeks, depending on the temperature – the ingredients that were put into the container at the beginning will have transformed into an extremely nutritious food.

How to make Sauerkraut

1. The best type of cabbage to use for sauerkraut is white cabbage. It does not make any difference whether the long-lasting round, firm cabbages that can weigh up to 18 pounds (about 8 kilograms) are used or the ruffled Savoy cabbage.
2. Remove the outer leaves, cut the cabbage in half and remove the stalk.
3. There is a special gadget for cutting the cabbage into strips, but it is possible to use a long kitchen knife or a machine for slicing bread.
4. The best container to use is a stone fermenting jar which has a lid and a water rim. The water rim makes it possible to prepare sauerkraut without using salt.
5. Before putting the shredded cabbage into the jar it must be washed thoroughly. Then the salt is added. Traditionally salt made up about 5 percent of the sauerkraut but it is possible to make do with half this amount. Additional spices can be added if desired – juniper berries and caraway seeds help the fermentation process.
6. Fill the jar slightly more than half full with the white cabbage, which will now be so thoroughly shredded that it will produce enough liquid to completely cover the sauerkraut.
7. To ensure that the sauerkraut is successful, make sure that the cabbage is covered by liquid at all stages of the fermentation process. Press the cabbage down with a plate and weigh it down.
8. Fermenting containers are especially designed to keep their contents compact and submerged. Fill the rim with water and place the lid on so that it sinks under the water. This makes the container airtight and ensures that the cabbage will not go moldy. The gases produced can still escape.
9. The cabbage should be stored in a place with an air temperature of about 60–70 °F (18–22 °C) for 14 days. Then it should be moved somewhere cooler with a temperature of about 45–50 °F (6–10 °C). These temperatures help the fermentation process. Sauerkraut takes about 4–6 weeks until it is fully fermented. It tastes delicious raw.
10. If the sauerkraut is stored in its fermentation jar, it should keep from the fall it was made until February of the following year.

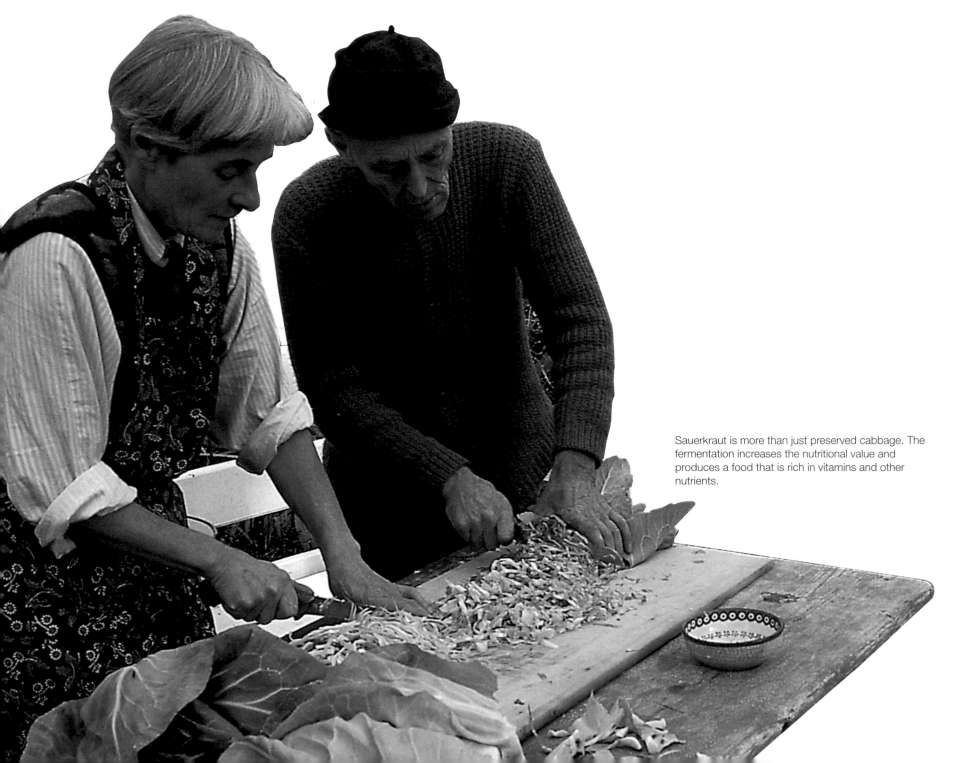

Sauerkraut is more than just preserved cabbage. The fermentation increases the nutritional value and produces a food that is rich in vitamins and other nutrients.

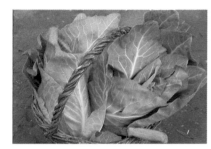

White cabbage is usually used for sauerkraut. There are many different varieties available.

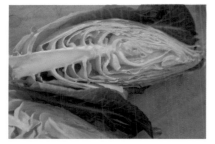

Remove the outer leaves and cut the cabbage in half. This cabbage is a variety with a pointed head.

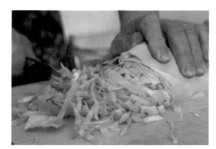

Using a knife or a cleaver, chop the cabbage into thin strips.

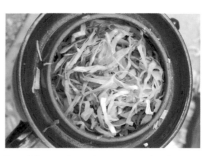

Special sauerkraut jars are made of stone and have a groove for water. The cabbage is packed loosely into the jar.

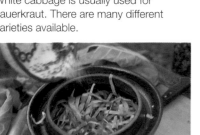

Add coarse salt to taste (salt helps the sauerkraut to keep longer). The salt can be omitted, if preferred.

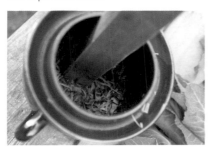

The sauerkraut should be pounded, so that the cabbage releases its juices. There should be enough juice to cover the cabbage.

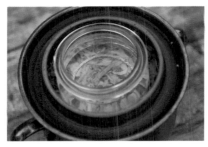

To keep the cabbage submerged during the fermentation process it should be weighted down. A full jam jar is good for this purpose.

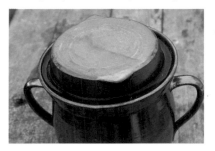

The lid should be placed in the rim, which is filled with water. This ensures that the jar is airtight.

Home made sauerkraut is delicious during the winter months. It can be eaten raw, or cooked.

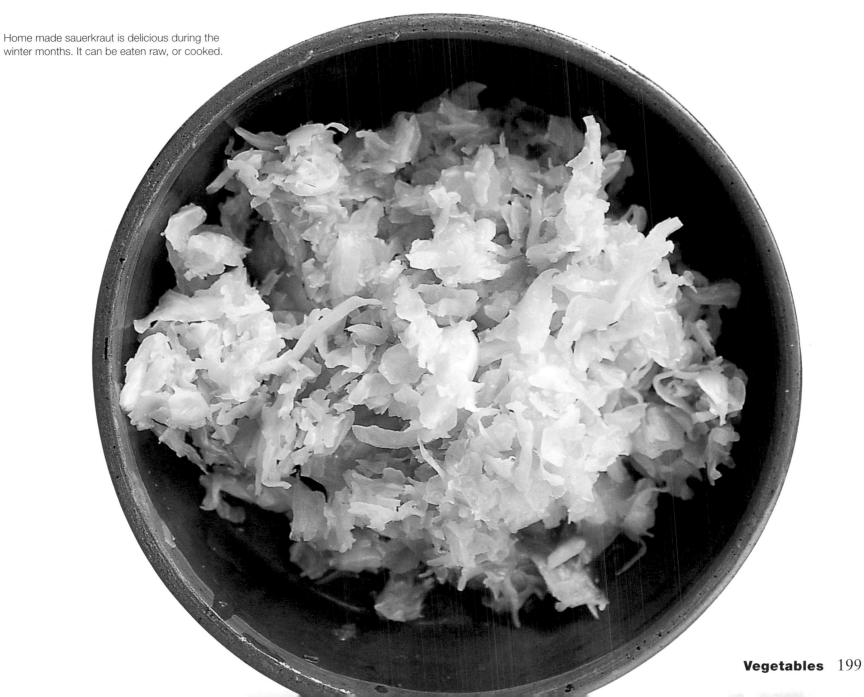

Recipes with Sauerkraut

Cabbage Fritters

Serves 8

2 cups (250 g) spelt flour
1 egg
2 Tbs olive oil
Coarse salt
2 onions
$1^{1}/_{4}$ Tbs (20 g) butter
1 lb 2 oz (500 g) sauerkraut
7 oz (200 g) carrots
1 bay leaf
Black pepper
$^{1}/_{2}$ tsp ground caraway seeds
$^{1}/_{2}$ Tbs honey
1 Tbs lard
5 cups (1 l) vegetable stock

Mix together the flour, egg, olive oil, just over $^{1}/_{4}$ cup (70 ml) water, and a little salt. Knead to make an elastic dough. Cover, and leave to rise at room temperature for 30 minutes.

Meanwhile, finely dice the onions and pan fry in the butter until transparent.

Finely chop the sauerkraut and grate the carrots. Add to the onions with the bay leaf and pan fry. Season with pepper and caraway and stir in the honey. Leave to cool.

Roll out the dough on a floured work surface and spread the sauerkraut mixture over the dough in a thin, even layer. Sprinkle the edges of the dough with water and roll it up to make a strudel.

Cut the roll into pieces 1 inch (3 cm) thick. Fry the pieces in the lard until they are golden brown on both sides. Pour over the vegetable stock, bring to the boil and simmer over a low heat for a few minutes.

Note: Sauerkraut is versatile and can be prepared in many different ways. However, it should not be cooked for longer than 20 minutes, and should only be heated very gently.

Sauerkraut Soup

2 onions
1 scallion
1 red bell pepper
3 Tbs sunflower oil
14 oz (400 g) sauerkraut
5 cups (1 l) vegetable stock
$^{3}/_{4}$ cup (125 ml) dry white wine
1 bay leaf
1 tsp ground caraway seeds
1 Tbs paprika
$^{3}/_{4}$ cup (125 ml) crème fraîche

Finely chop the onions, slice the scallion into fine rings, deseed the bell pepper and chop into short, narrow strips. Pan fry in the oil for about 3 minutes. Add the sauerkraut, pour over wine and stock, then add the bay leaf and caraway. Simmer for 15 minutes.

Stir in the paprika powder just before serving. Garnish with crème fraîche.

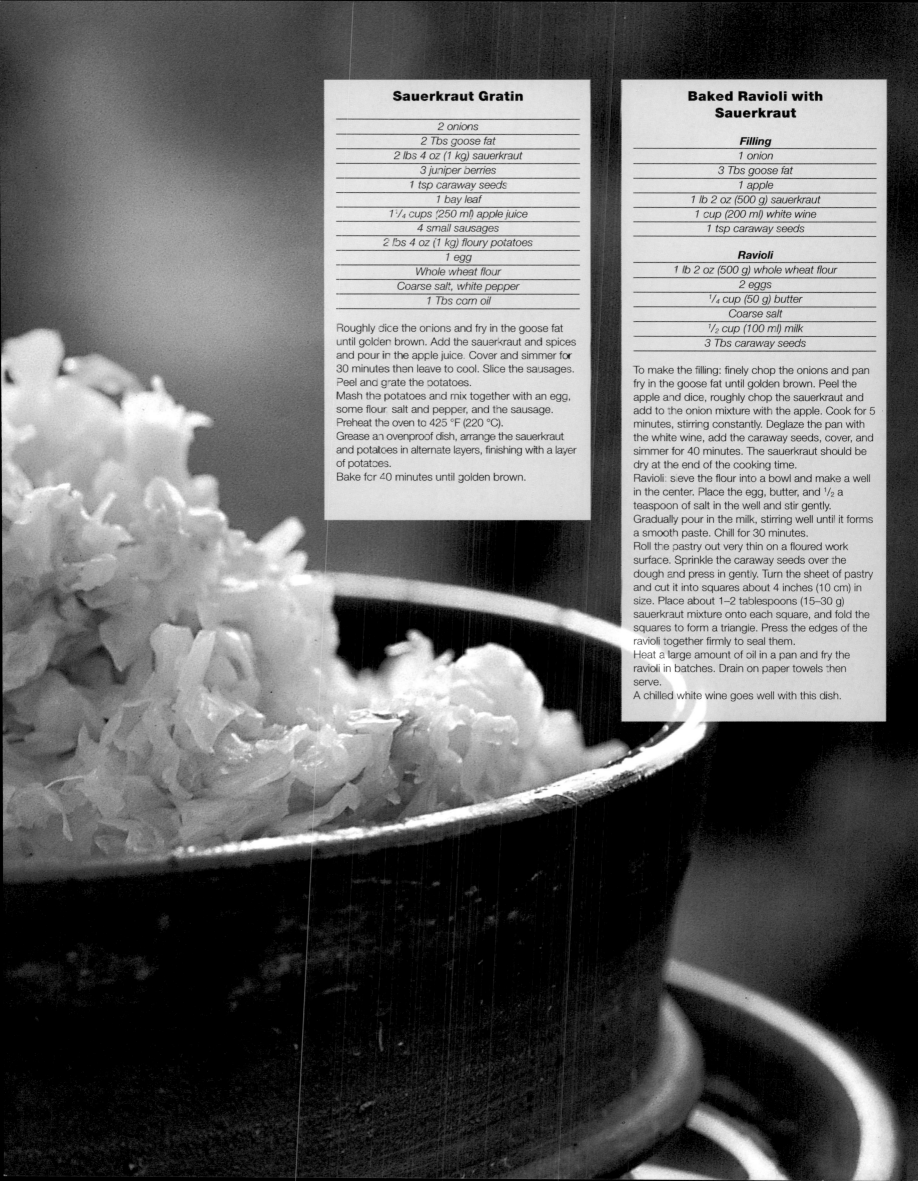

Sauerkraut Gratin

2 onions
2 Tbs goose fat
2 lbs 4 oz (1 kg) sauerkraut
3 juniper berries
1 tsp caraway seeds
1 bay leaf
1¼ cups (250 ml) apple juice
4 small sausages
2 lbs 4 oz (1 kg) floury potatoes
1 egg
Whole wheat flour
Coarse salt, white pepper
1 Tbs corn oil

Roughly dice the onions and fry in the goose fat until golden brown. Add the sauerkraut and spices and pour in the apple juice. Cover and simmer for 30 minutes then leave to cool. Slice the sausages. Peel and grate the potatoes.
Mash the potatoes and mix together with an egg, some flour, salt and pepper, and the sausage. Preheat the oven to 425 °F (220 °C).
Grease an ovenproof dish, arrange the sauerkraut and potatoes in alternate layers, finishing with a layer of potatoes.
Bake for 40 minutes until golden brown.

Baked Ravioli with Sauerkraut

Filling

1 onion
3 Tbs goose fat
1 apple
1 lb 2 oz (500 g) sauerkraut
1 cup (200 ml) white wine
1 tsp caraway seeds

Ravioli

1 lb 2 oz (500 g) whole wheat flour
2 eggs
¼ cup (50 g) butter
Coarse salt
½ cup (100 ml) milk
3 Tbs caraway seeds

To make the filling: finely chop the onions and pan fry in the goose fat until golden brown. Peel the apple and dice, roughly chop the sauerkraut and add to the onion mixture with the apple. Cook for 5 minutes, stirring constantly. Deglaze the pan with the white wine, add the caraway seeds, cover, and simmer for 40 minutes. The sauerkraut should be dry at the end of the cooking time.
Ravioli: sieve the flour into a bowl and make a well in the center. Place the egg, butter, and ½ a teaspoon of salt in the well and stir gently. Gradually pour in the milk, stirring well until it forms a smooth paste. Chill for 30 minutes.
Roll the pastry out very thin on a floured work surface. Sprinkle the caraway seeds over the dough and press in gently. Turn the sheet of pastry and cut it into squares about 4 inches (10 cm) in size. Place about 1–2 tablespoons (15–30 g) sauerkraut mixture onto each square, and fold the squares to form a triangle. Press the edges of the ravioli together firmly to seal them.
Heat a large amount of oil in a pan and fry the ravioli in batches. Drain on paper towels then serve.
A chilled white wine goes well with this dish.

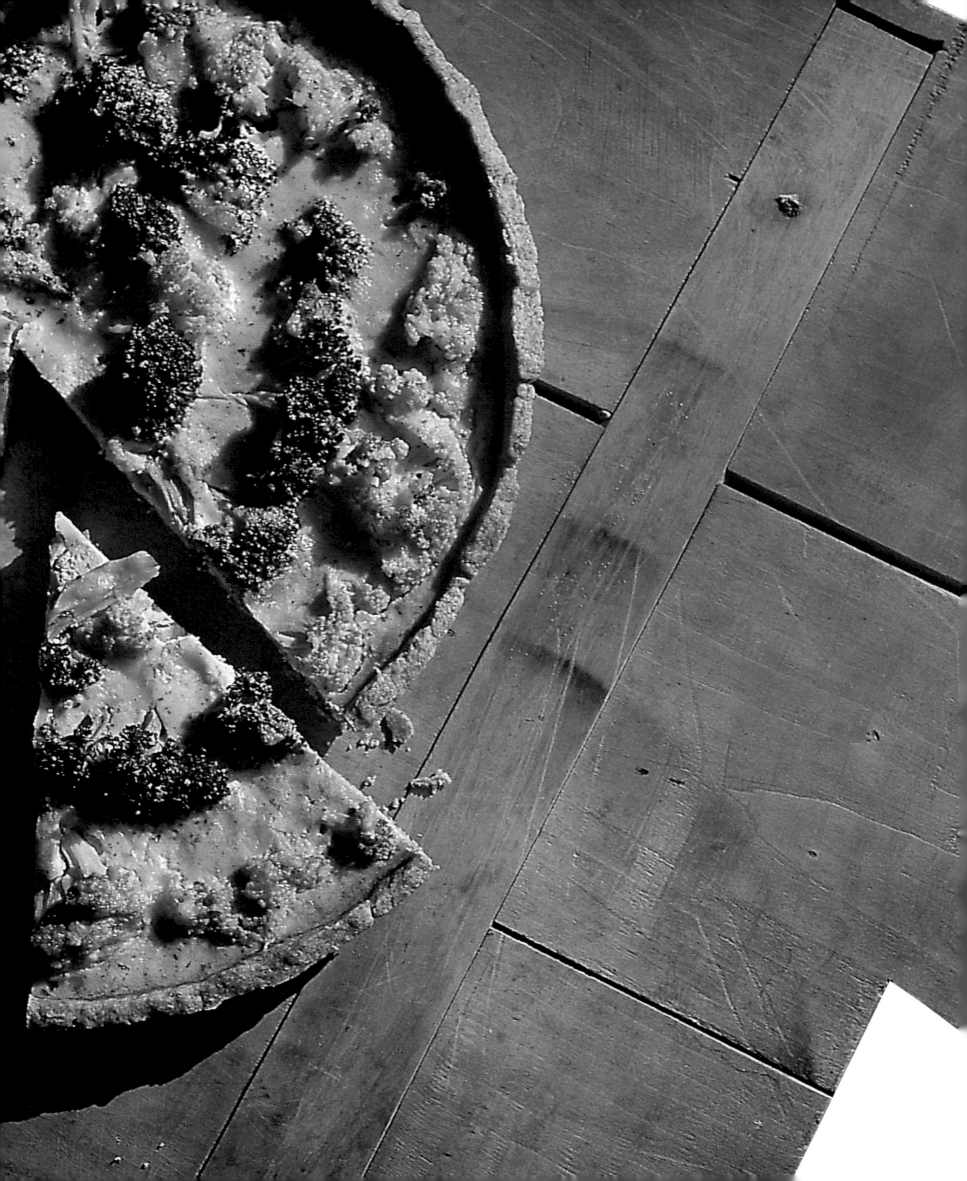

Cauliflower and Broccoli Tart

Cauliflower and Broccoli

Cauliflower and Broccoli Tart
(Illustration left hand page)

Pastry

1³/₄ cups (200 g) spelt flour
¹/₃ cup (80 g) chilled butter
1 pinch coarse salt
1 tsp vinegar

Filling

1 small cauliflower
1 lb 2 oz (500 g) broccoli
2 eggs
1¹/₄ cups (250 ml) sour cream
1 Tbs vegetable stock granules
¹/₂ tsp herb salt
Black pepper
1 tsp soysauce
3¹/₂ oz (100 g) freshly grated hard cheese

To make the pastry: mix together the flour, butter, salt, vinegar, and 4 tablespoons (60 ml) of water and knead until it forms a ball. Chill for 30 minutes.
Roll out the dough on a floured work surface. Butter a round cake pan (about 11 inches – 28 cm – in diameter) and line with the pastry.
Preheat the oven to 375 °F (190 °C).
Break the cauliflower and broccoli into florets and steam until "al dente." Allow to cool slightly.
Arrange the florets decoratively on top of the pastry – you could arrange them in a spiral or like the spokes of a wheel. Beat together the eggs, cream, and herbs and pour evenly over the vegetables. Sprinkle with cheese and bake in the oven for 40 minutes.

Deep Fried Cauliflower

1 large cauliflower
1¹/₃ cups (150 g) spelt or whole wheat flour
³/₄ cup (150 ml) chilled white wine
Coarse salt
2 egg whites
Lemon wedges

Divide the cauliflower into florets and blanch in boiling, salted water for 5 minutes. Drain and leave to cool.
Mix the flour with the wine and ¹/₄ teaspoon of salt so that it makes a thin batter. Chill for 30 minutes.
Beat the egg whites with a pinch of salt until they are very stiff. Fold the beaten egg whites into the batter.
Dip the florets into the batter one by one. Deep fry the cauliflower in plenty of corn oil. Cook the florets in small batches to ensure even cooking.
Garnish with lemon wedges and serve.

Broccoli in Saffron Cream

1 small packet saffron strands
¹/₂ cup (100 ml) cold vegetable stock
1 lb 11 oz (750 g) broccoli
Coarse salt
2 small white onions
2 Tbs butter
¹/₂ cup (100 ml) heavy cream
White pepper

Place the saffron strands in the vegetable stock. Divide the broccoli into florets and remove the stalks. Peel the stalks and slice thinly.
Cook the florets and the stalks in boiling salted water for 5 minutes, drain and plunge into cold water.
Finely chop the onions and fry in the butter until transparent. Pour in the cream and stock and reduce the volume of the liquid by a third. Season with salt and pepper. Add the broccoli. Simmer for five minutes in the saffron sauce.

Broccoli Casserole

4 canned anchovy fillets
2 lbs 4 oz (1 kg) broccoli
3 garlic cloves
Coarse salt
2 dried chili peppers
3 Tbs olive oil
¹/₂ cup (100 ml) white wine

Soak the anchovy fillets in water or milk for 20 minutes. Drain away the liquid, and chop the anchovies finely.
Separate the florets from the broccoli stalks. Peel the stalks and cut into strips 1–1¹/₂ inches (3–4 cm) long. Cut any leaves into strips.
Mince the garlic with the salt, crumble the dried chilis and fry in the oil, together with the chopped anchovies.
Add the broccoli and simmer, stirring frequently, for 5 minutes.
Pour in the white wine, cover the broccoli and cook for a further 10 minutes. Check the seasoning and serve hot.

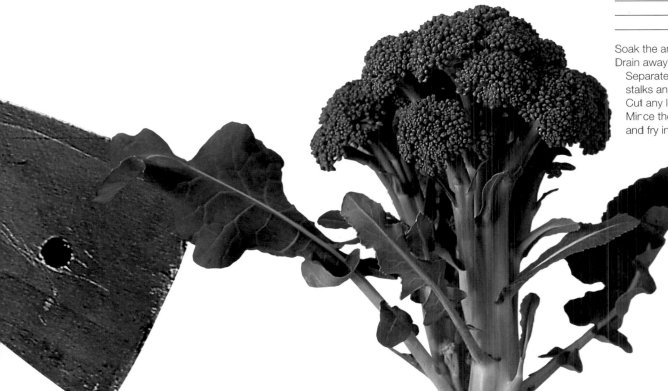

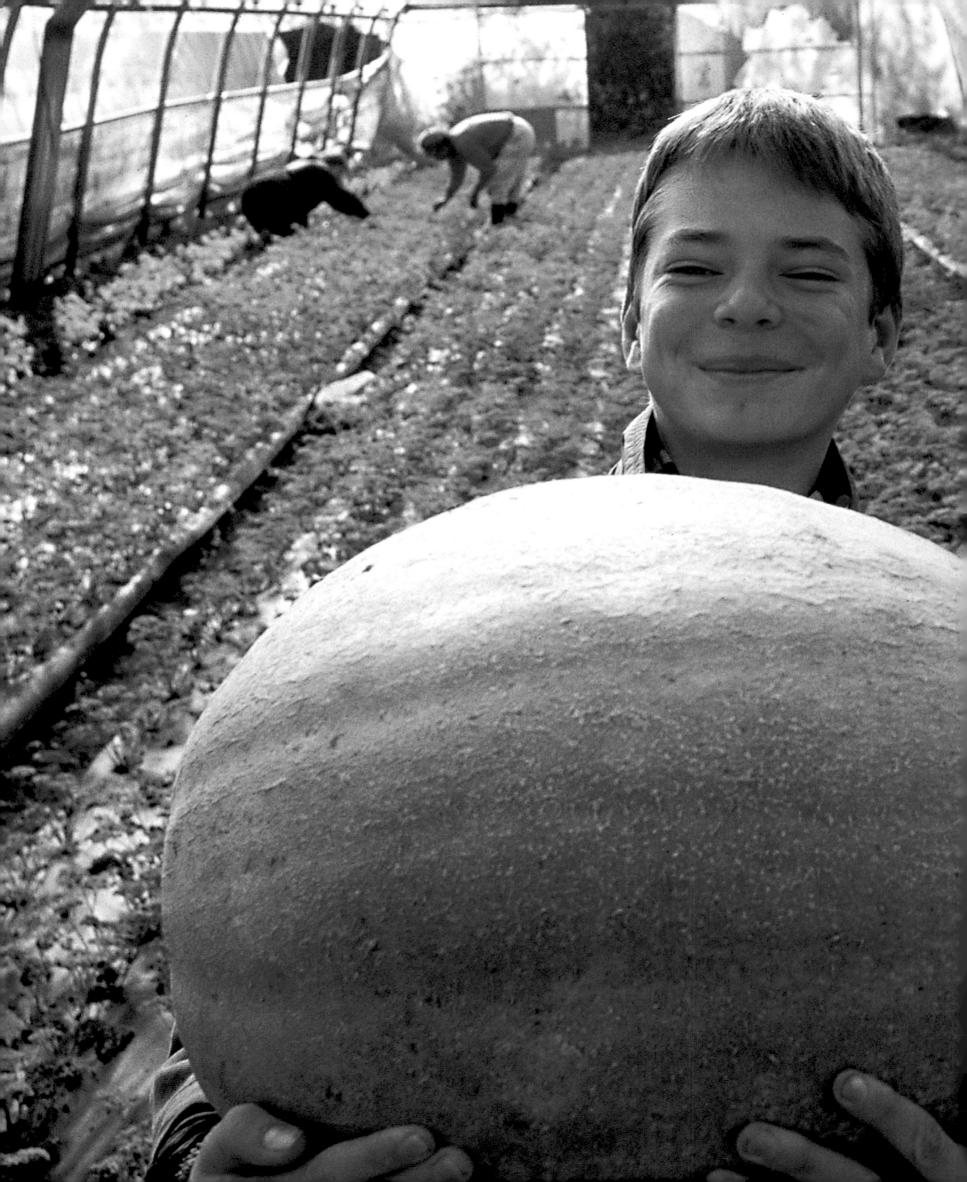

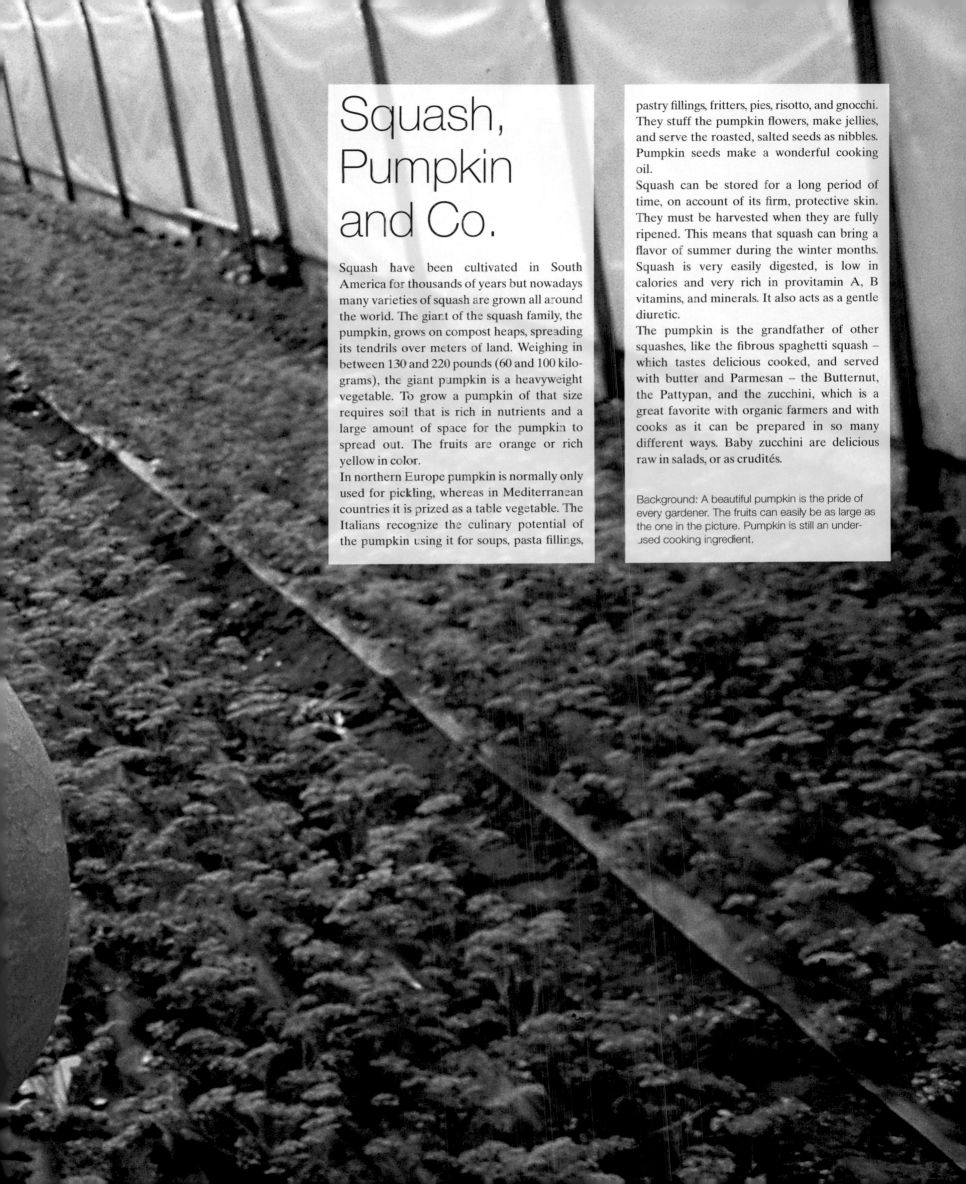

Squash, Pumpkin and Co.

Squash have been cultivated in South America for thousands of years but nowadays many varieties of squash are grown all around the world. The giant of the squash family, the pumpkin, grows on compost heaps, spreading its tendrils over meters of land. Weighing in between 130 and 220 pounds (60 and 100 kilograms), the giant pumpkin is a heavyweight vegetable. To grow a pumpkin of that size requires soil that is rich in nutrients and a large amount of space for the pumpkin to spread out. The fruits are orange or rich yellow in color.

In northern Europe pumpkin is normally only used for pickling, whereas in Mediterranean countries it is prized as a table vegetable. The Italians recognize the culinary potential of the pumpkin using it for soups, pasta fillings, pastry fillings, fritters, pies, risotto, and gnocchi. They stuff the pumpkin flowers, make jellies, and serve the roasted, salted seeds as nibbles. Pumpkin seeds make a wonderful cooking oil.

Squash can be stored for a long period of time, on account of its firm, protective skin. They must be harvested when they are fully ripened. This means that squash can bring a flavor of summer during the winter months. Squash is very easily digested, is low in calories and very rich in provitamin A, B vitamins, and minerals. It also acts as a gentle diuretic.

The pumpkin is the grandfather of other squashes, like the fibrous spaghetti squash – which tastes delicious cooked, and served with butter and Parmesan – the Butternut, the Pattypan, and the zucchini, which is a great favorite with organic farmers and with cooks as it can be prepared in so many different ways. Baby zucchini are delicious raw in salads, or as crudités.

Background: A beautiful pumpkin is the pride of every gardener. The fruits can easily be as large as the one in the picture. Pumpkin is still an under-used cooking ingredient.

Deep Fried Zucchini Flowers
(Illustration below)

2 eggs
$^1/_2$ cup (100 ml) mineral water
$^1/_2$ cup (100 ml) white wine
1 Tbs sunflower oil
Coarse salt, black pepper
1$^3/_4$ cups finest whole wheat flour
16 zucchini flowers with stalks still attached

Separate the eggs. Mix the yolks with the water, wine, oil, salt, and pepper. Beat well, and gradually add the flour to the egg mixture.
Leave the batter to stand for 20 minutes. Beat the egg whites with a pinch of salt until they are stiff. Fold into the batter.
Heat plenty of oil in a large pan. Handle the zucchini flowers very carefully – wipe them clean, do not wash – dip them in the batter and deep fry in batches.
Leave to drain on paper towels.

Deep Fried Zucchini Flowers

Zucchini with Tomatoes

1 onion
3 Tbs olive oil
1 garlic clove
Coarse salt
4 medium zucchini
4 tomatoes
1 pinch raw cane sugar
White pepper
$^1/_2$ bunch basil

Finely chop the onion and pan fry in 2 tablespoons of the oil until golden brown in color. Crush the garlic with a little salt and add to the onion.
Cut the zucchini in half and chop into pieces 1$^1/_4$ inches (3 cm) long. Skin, deseed, and quarter the tomatoes. Add the zucchini to the onion mixture and pan fry for 4 minutes, stirring frequently. Remove from the skillet and set aside.
Put the tomatoes into the skillet, together with the remaining oil and the sugar. Season well with salt and pepper. Add the zucchini and simmer with the tomatoes for 15 minutes. Tear the basil leaves into large pieces and add to the vegetables; check the seasoning and serve.

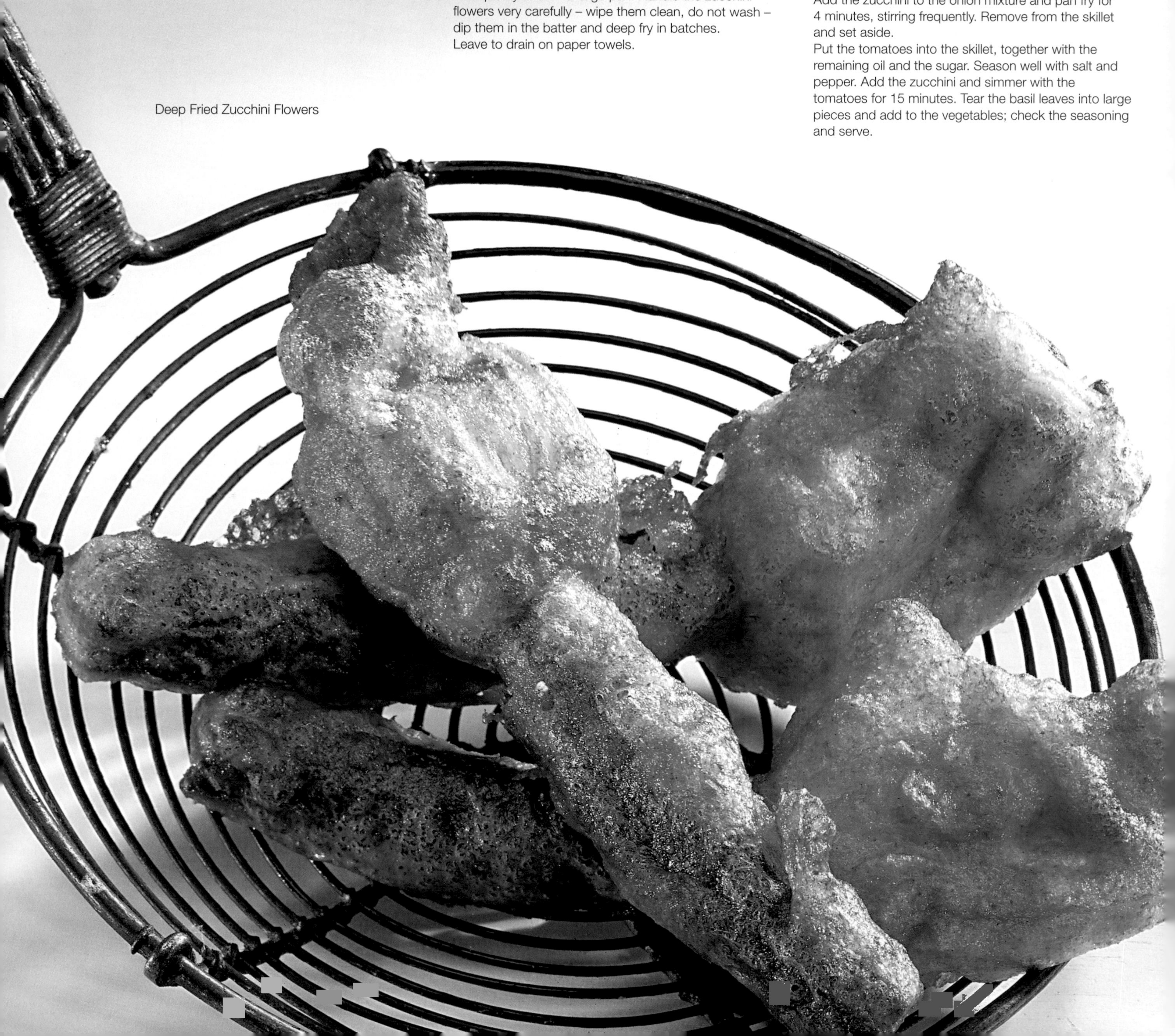

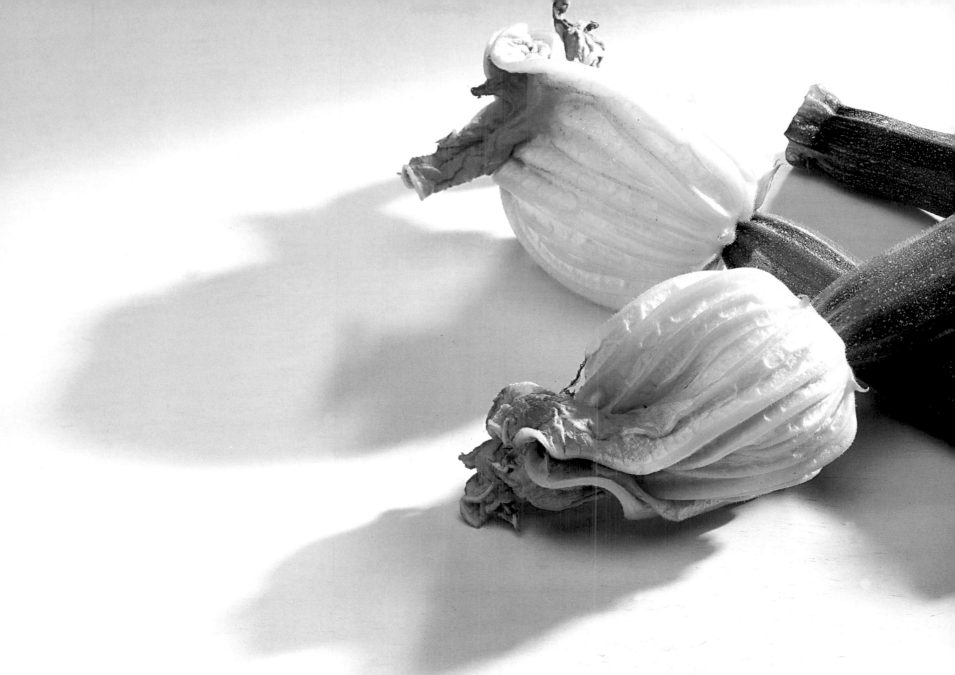

Zucchini Gratin

4 zucchini
3 Tbs butter
1 crushed garlic clove
3¹/₂ oz (100 g) cooked ham
¹/₂ cup (100 g) farmer's cheese with cream
1 egg yolk
2 Tbs chopped parsley
2 oz (50 g) freshly grated hard cheese
Coarse salt, white pepper
¹/₂ cup (100 ml) dry white wine

Cut the zucchini in half, scoop out the flesh and pan fry the flesh in 1 tablespoon of butter together with the garlic. Place in a sieve and leave to cool.
Dice the ham, drain the farmer's cheese and mix with the zucchini, egg yolk, parsley, and cheese. Season with salt and pepper.
Place this mixture in a piping bag with a large nozzle and fill the zucchini skins with this mixture.
Preheat the oven to 350 °F (180 °C).
Butter a heatproof dish and place the zucchini in the dish. Dot the remaining butter on top of the vegetables. Bake in the oven for 15 minutes, pour over the wine, and cook for a further 30 minutes. Serve hot.

Squash Gnocchi

1 lb 11 oz (750 g) butternut squash
Coarse salt, white pepper
1 egg
1²/₃ cups (250 g) whole wheat semolina
5 oz (150 g) freshly grated hard cheese
2 Tbs olive oil
¹/₄ cup (50 g) butter
A few sage leaves

Deseed the squash and scoop the flesh out of the skin. Dice the flesh and cook in salted water. Leave to drain in a sieve.
Purée the squash, then season with salt and pepper. Add the egg, 7 ounces (200 g) of the semolina, and a third of the cheese to the purée, and stir until it forms a solid ball. Add a little more semolina if necessary.
Make a long roll out of the squash mixture. It should be about 1¹/₄ inches (3 cm) in diameter. Cut the roll into pieces ³/₄ inch (2 cm) thick. Press them gently with the back of a fork.
Bring a large pan of salted water to the boil. Add the oil and place the gnocchi in the water. Reduce the heat and cook the gnocchi for 8 minutes.
Brown the butter with a few sage leaves.
Remove the gnocchi from the pan, arrange in a dish and pour the butter over the gnocchi.
Sprinkle with the remaining cheese and serve.

Cream of Pumpkin Soup

1 lb 2 oz (500 g) pumpkin flesh
1 shallot
1 garlic clove
1 oz (30 g) butter
¹/₂ cup (100 ml) dry white wine
5 cups (1 l) vegetable stock
¹/₂ cup (90 ml) crème fraîche
1 Tbs lemon juice
1 Tbs pumpkin oil
2 oz (50 g) roasted pumpkin seeds

Dice the pumpkin flesh.
Finely chop the shallot and the garlic and pan fry in the butter until transparent. Add the pumpkin and pan fry for a further 5 minutes, stirring frequently.
Pour in the stock and simmer for 30 minutes. Then add the crème fraîche and liquidize the soup. Add the lemon juice and oil and season to taste with salt and pepper. Sprinkle with pumpkin seeds and serve.

From Producer to Consumer

Box Schemes

The same question is asked by producers of organic food, whether they grow cereals, vegetables, fruit, or other types of food: what is the most efficient way to deliver the food to the customer? This question is a universal problem that faces every organic gardener or farmer – the marketing and commercial side of their farm or garden. Alternative methods of food production require alternative marketing techniques. In the early years of organic farming, there were no subsidies that would have made a change to these methods of farming easier. People who opted for natural methods of farming were generally making more work for themselves, and found it difficult to find ecologically minded customers for their produce. Even today, there are large numbers of organic farmers who have not managed to find a marketing opportunity for their product, of which milk is a typical example.

The development of organic agriculture went, to some degree, hand in hand with the development of the open market. The more research that the producer carried out on the needs and demands of the consumer, the more he saw the necessity of encouraging customers to visit farms and market gardens. It was important to understand what motivated the customer to buy organic produce. Organic farmers educated the public with information services and open days at farms, farm shops, and market stalls. This helped them to form a firm relationship between producer, and consumer, and to advertise their product.

However much selling produce on the farm strengthens the relationship between the farmer and the customer and makes shopping a pleasure for the customer and their family, it does not encourage city dwellers to buy organic produce as they have to make special trips into the countryside to do their shopping. It does not make ecological sense to transport the produce into the towns, as it involves long road journeys, and this has caused financial problems to many organic farmers.

Initially, shopping cooperatives were formed that would buy large quantities of produce. Some of these cooperatives became whole food shops. This transformation did not essentially alter the relationship between consumer and producer. Nevertheless, a new pattern emerged. Increasingly, customers were asking organic farmers to deliver their fruit and vegetables and this led inevitably to a set procedure where delivery dates were fixed. It was then only a matter of time before this service was extended to include subscription with free delivery. Depending on the structure of the business, and the type of transport and delivery systems available to the farmers, the producers either relied on farm shops with a supplementary income from deliveries, or depended on deliveries alone. This system of delivery is called a Box Scheme. From the beginning, the service consisted of following up customers' requests, and offering a basic assortment of produce. Each order would be different, but would contain a basic amount of produce that would not vary. The basic produce would depend on the varieties of vegetables that the farm had in large quantities. Each farm that participates in Box Schemes offers different sizes of order – which coincide with the needs of particular groups of customers.

One of the Box Scheme pioneers was the Schloss Hemhofen estate in Franconia, Germany. This estate delivers to over 2,000 households in the Erlangen-Furth-Nuremberg area, and its system has been adopted by organic farms all over Germany.

Regular customers, who buy large quantities of vegetables on a regular basis, help the organic farmers to plan their produce and make a living.

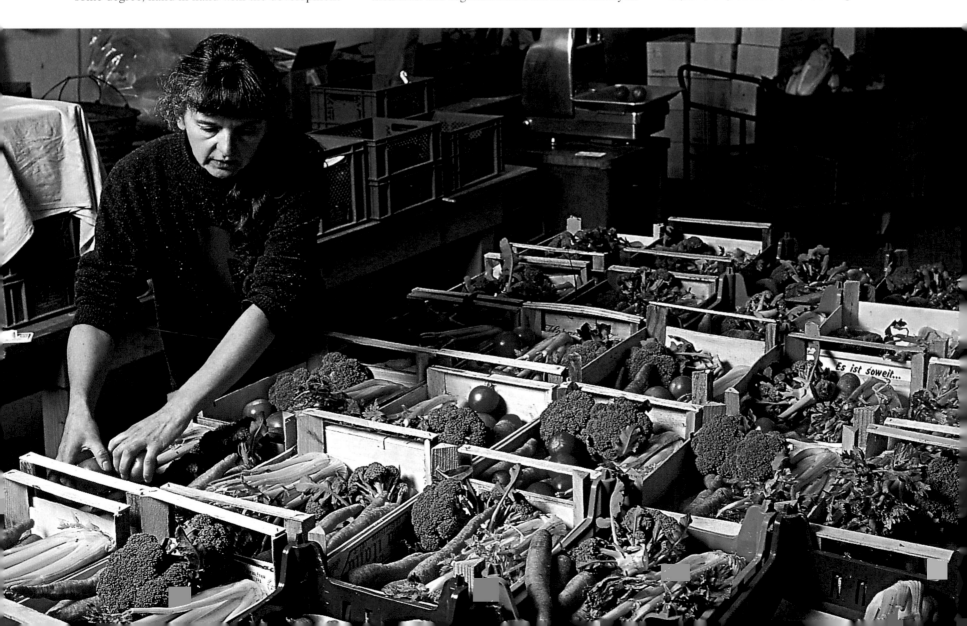

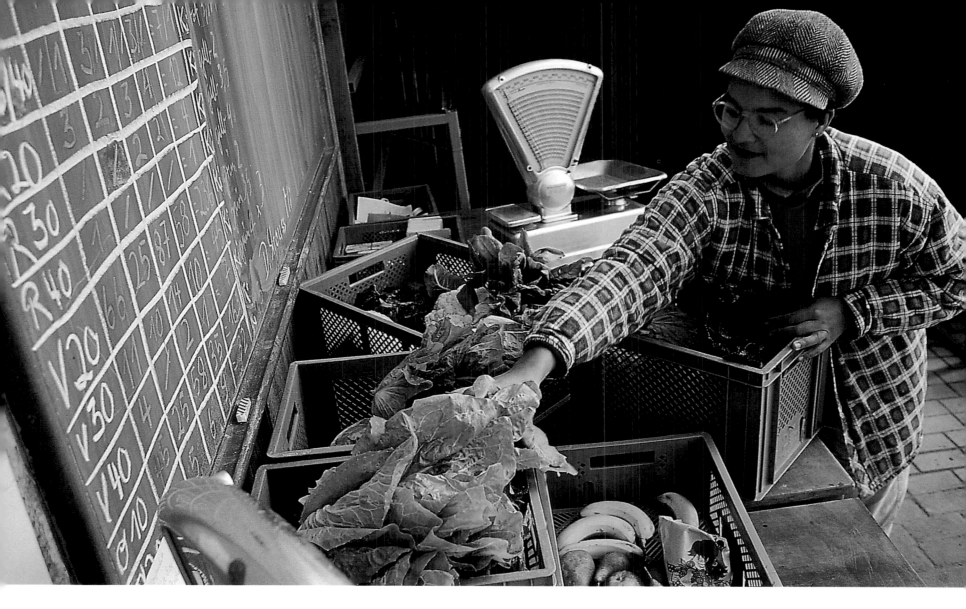

Organic farmers have become accustomed to cater for the wishes of their customers. They offer an attractive range of imported, out-of-season fruit and vegetables.

Schloss Hemhofen offers six different varieties of order in three different sizes. The variety ranges from "the complete range" with vegetables, salad vegetables, and herbs to "simple food" – food that is easy to digest, a special range for mother and baby, that will not upset any sensitive stomachs, a "crudité" selection with lettuces and food that can be eaten raw, a "vegetables only" with no salad ingredients, and a "fruit only" selection. The contents of the boxes vary from season to season depending on what varieties of fruit, vegetables, and lettuces are available.

It is especially good for the producers to sell as much produce as possible from their own farms. The increasing numbers of customers in the Box Schemes has led to greater communication between producer and consumer. Organic farmers are becoming more aware of their customers' needs, and are reorganizing their crops to cater to the tastes of their customers. However, it is not always possible to meet all the demands of the consumers, so the producers often cooperate with other organic farmers in the area to extend the range of produce available to the customers.

Eventually, the farms become "partners" in the scheme. This partnership has many advantages for the producer: it allows for the requirements of the customer to be met, even when one farmer's crop has failed, and it removes the cost that would be incurred by trading with one another. The farm is in a difficult position when it comes to pricing the produce. It wants to offer the customer reasonably priced vegetables, whilst ensuring that the farmers earn enough to continue using organic methods and producing high quality crops.

More business opportunities arise all the time which are as good for the consumer as they are for the organic farmer. The range of "basic" produce is extended, offering the customer different types of organic food, and allowing the farmer to offer products other than fruit and vegetables. The Hemhofen estate now farms beef cattle and pigs. The customers are informed when the animals are to be slaughtered and can order organic meat when they order their vegetables. The farmer then makes contact with a local butcher, who complies with the regulations set down by the German union of organic farmers and the butcher then produces a range of charcuterie from the organic meat. In much the same way, a farm that grows cereal crops can sell its organic flour to a bakery, who will then bake a range of organic bread and bread rolls. Other organic cereal products can also

be made from the flour.

Long lasting organic foods are known as "store cupboard foods" and can often be bought through mail order companies. The definition "store cupboard foods" includes grains, granola, fruit juices, cooking oils, and honey. Seasonal vegetables are always available, and many farms will offer a selection of imported, out of season, organic vegetables to extend their range. Eggs and cheese can often be ordered and sometimes organic farms have types of potatoes and vegetables that are practically impossible to find in a store.

Box Schemes are very popular with people who work full time, particularly families with children where both parents work. Many Box Scheme customers had never bought organic vegetables before.

Mushrooms

Edible wild mushrooms are in short supply because of the heavy soil pollution (see right hand page). There are many types of cultivated mushrooms available, as well as those grown organically. Mushrooms are very nutritious. Cultivation techniques are now so sophisticated that it is possible to grow Japanese shiitake mushrooms as well as oyster and button mushrooms.

Polenta Nests with Chanterelle Ragout
(Illustration below)

1 lb 2 oz (200 g) chanterelles
3¹/₂ oz (100 g) air dried ham
1 shallot
1 garlic clove
2 Tbs olive oil
2 Tbs butter
1 Tbs tomato paste
³/₄ cup (150 ml) dry white wine
1 tsp vegetable stock granules
³/₄ cup (125 ml) crème fraîche
1 Tbs finely chopped parsley
Coarse salt, white pepper

Polenta

1 tsp coarse salt
1¹/₂ cups (250 g) polenta

Clean the chanterelles thoroughly. Dice the ham, finely chop the shallot and the garlic; pan fry in the oil and butter.
Add the mushrooms and brown, stirring frequently.
Mix the wine and tomato paste together and add to the mushrooms, together with the stock granules. Increase the heat and boil until the fluid has reduced. Stir in the crème fraîche and parsley, then season with salt and pepper.
To make the polenta: bring 3³/₄ cups (750 ml) of water to the boil, add salt and a pinch of polenta. Pour in the rest of the polenta slowly and reduce the heat at once. Simmer for 60 minutes, stirring frequently. If the polenta seems too thick, add a little boiling water. Make nests out of the polenta and fill with the chanterelles.
Note: Polenta always sticks to the bottom of the pan. If you soak the pan overnight, the polenta will come away from the pan very easily.

Polenta Nests with
Chanterelle Ragout

Organically Cultivated Mushrooms

Oyster Mushrooms
In the wild these mushrooms love the trunks and branches of deciduous trees, where they grow gray-blue caps. Organically cultivated oyster mushrooms are grown on untreated straw or wood. They often grow like roofing tiles and are usually pale in color. Their white flesh is very good for pan frying. Their gills are pale and the cap can grow up to 6 inches (15 cm) in diameter. They have a delicate but delicious flavor.

Chestnut Mushrooms
Similar in size to button mushrooms, but with a flat, brown cap and violet gills. Because they have a very bland flavor they are not often commercially grown.

Button Mushrooms
Many types grow in the wild, in woods, on fields, and on paths. Cultivated for 350 years, they need to be grown on horse or chicken manure. This manure is not always from organic farms even for organic mushroom cultivation; button mushrooms are usually white; they have firm, round caps with white flesh.

Shiitake
A cultivated mushroom that originated in Japan; cultivated in Japan and China and considered to be the elixir of life. It has always been cultivated on logs from deciduous trees. A polysaccharid – lentinan – that can be extracted from the mushroom, has medicinal benefits. It strengthens the immune system, regenerates the body, and helps prevent cancer and viral infections.
The increasing popularity of shiitake mushrooms in Europe is not least because of its wonderful flavor and delicious consistency. Shiitake mushrooms have caps that vary from light to dark brown in color, and are about 2–3 inches (6–9 cm) in diameter. Because they are members of the mushroom family and grow in dead, organic matter, it is possible to provide them with natural substratum. Shiitake can be grown at home by planting them on the cut surface of a log from a deciduous tree. The mushrooms will grow for many years. They can be eaten fresh and freeze well. If shiitake are dried, their flavor is concentrated and they make an excellent seasoning.

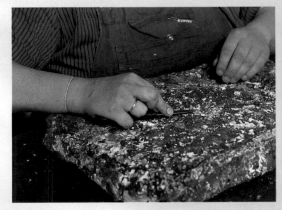

Mushrooms are also grown organically using pads of pressed, treated straw.

Marinated Shiitake Mushrooms
(Illustration below)

11 oz (300 g) shiitake
1 garlic clove
1 shallot
2 Tbs olive oil
2 Tbs soysauce or tamari
1 small bunch flat-leafed parsley
Coarse salt, black pepper
1 small bunch basil

Clean the mushrooms.
Finely chop the shallot and garlic and pan fry in the olive oil. Add the mushrooms, pan fry, and add the soysauce. Chop the parsley and sprinkle over the mushrooms; season with salt and pepper.
Leave for 1–2 hours, then tear the basil leaves into large pieces and sprinkle over the mushrooms. Serve as an appetizer.

Marinated Shiitake
Mushrooms

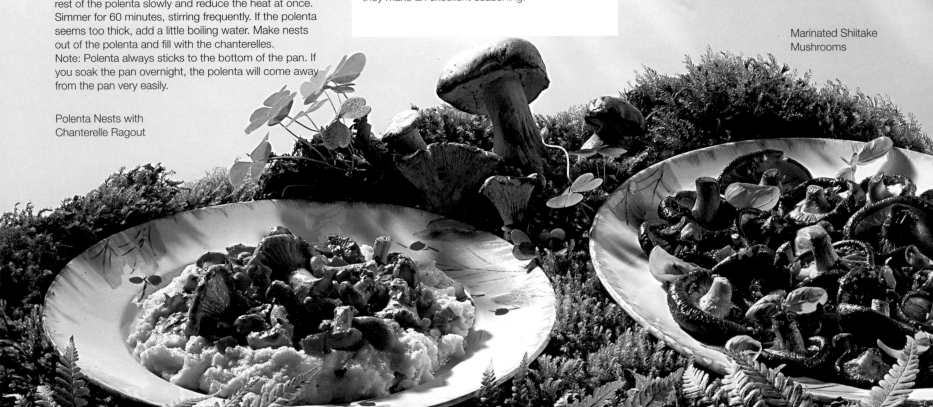

Cep Soup with Small Dumplings
(Illustration below right)

1 lb 2 oz (500 g) fresh ceps
1/4 cup (60 g) butter
2 Tbs olive oil
3 shallots
5 cups (1 l) vegetable stock
1 tsp marjoram
8 slices rustic toasting bread
1 cup (200 ml) milk
1/2 bunch finely chopped flat-leafed parsley
1 egg
1 pinch nutmeg
Coarse salt, white pepper
1 Tbs finely chopped chives

Clean the mushrooms and slice. Heat 2 tablespoons (30 g) of the butter, together with the olive oil. Finely chop 2 shallots and pan fry in the butter/oil mixture until golden brown. Add the mushrooms and braise for 5 minutes, stirring frequently. Pour in the stock, add the marjoram and simmer the mushrooms gently for 15 minutes.

Soak the bread in the milk and squeeze out the excess liquid. Chop the remaining shallot and fry in the remaining butter. Add the parsley. Mix the bread, egg, nutmeg, shallot, and parsley mixture with a little salt and pepper, stirring the mixture well. With damp hands, form the mixture into small balls, place them in boiling, salted water, reduce the heat, and cook for 10 minutes. Check the seasoning in the soup. Remove the dumplings, allow them to drain and place in soup bowls. Pour over the soup and serve sprinkled with the chives.

Stuffed Ceps
(Illustration below left)

8 large ceps
1 small shallot
2 garlic cloves
3 Tbs olive oil
1 tomato
1 egg
3 Tbs freshly grated hard cheese
2 Tbs breadcrumbs
2 Tbs finely chopped parsley
Coarse salt, white pepper

Clean the mushroom caps and remove the stalks. Put the caps to one side and chop the stalks.
Finely chop the shallots, mince the garlic and then pan fry them in 2 tablespoons of olive oil.
Add the mushroom stalks and cook. Skin, deseed, and dice the tomatoes. Add to the mushrooms and cook on a high heat for 3 minutes, until all the liquid has evaporated. Leave to cool.
Add the remaining ingredients to the tomato and mushroom mixture; season with salt and pepper. Stuff the mushroom caps with the filling.
Preheat the oven to 350 °F (180 °C).
Grease a heatproof dish with a little olive oil, and place the mushrooms in the dish. Bake in the oven for about 30 minutes.

How Problematic are Wild Mushrooms?

It is a sad fact that the radioactive leakage from the Chernobyl Nuclear Reactor in the former Soviet Union has taken its toll on nature and that many plants are still suffering. No other type of plant was as badly affected as the mushroom. Mushrooms have a natural affinity for radioactivity, indeed, some mushrooms are naturally slightly radioactive. In 1986 – the year of the Chernobyl disaster – there was a glut of mushrooms in southern Europe, which was not thought to have been affected by the leak. Some sorts had increased their radiation content four fold – the same as their surroundings. This meant that mushrooms contained dangerous levels of heavy metals. In general, mushrooms that have grown in any place that has been contaminated by heavy metals should not be eaten.

As far as radioactive contamination is concerned, in areas that have been particularly affected by the radiation from Chernobyl, mushrooms should not be picked or eaten. The radiation levels have only declined by a minimal amount in the following ten years. In northern and western Europe – areas that were not as severely affected by radiation – there is still some evidence of radiation in mushrooms, but in such small amounts that some mushroom fans are prepared to take the risk and eat the mushrooms. Only the Bay-colored Bolete, which stores radiation in very high quantities, should really be avoided.

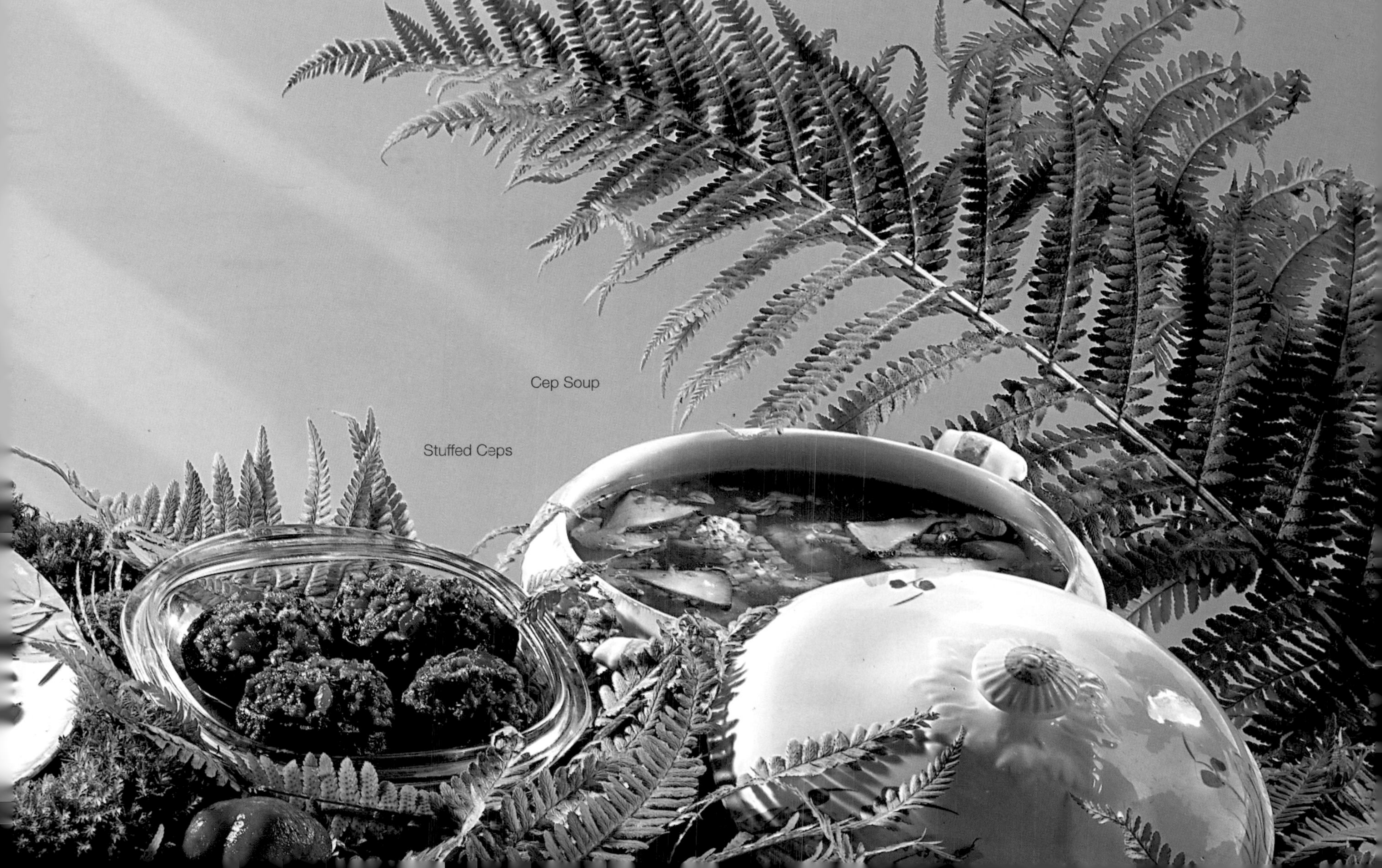

Cep Soup

Stuffed Ceps

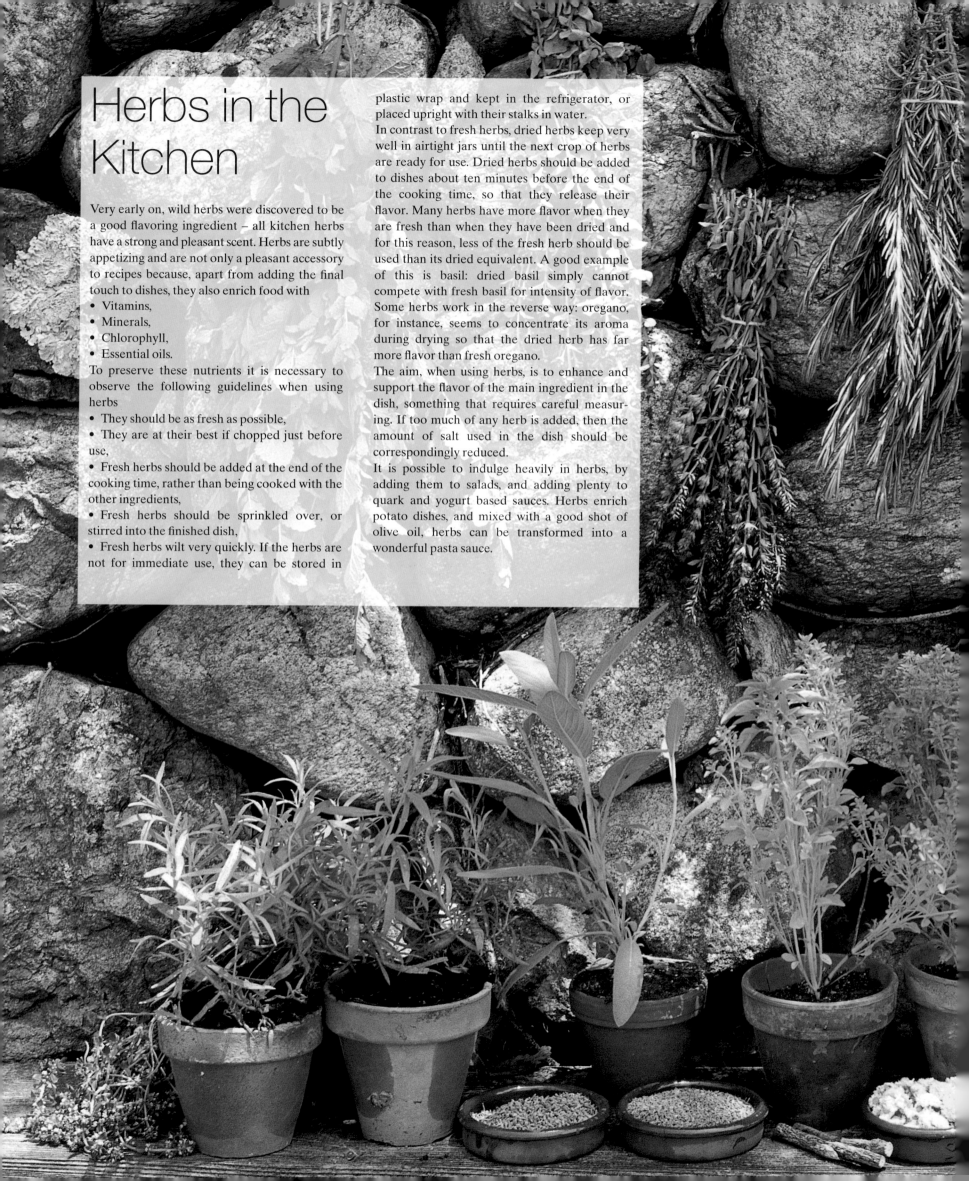

Herbs in the Kitchen

Very early on, wild herbs were discovered to be a good flavoring ingredient – all kitchen herbs have a strong and pleasant scent. Herbs are subtly appetizing and are not only a pleasant accessory to recipes because, apart from adding the final touch to dishes, they also enrich food with

• Vitamins,
• Minerals,
• Chlorophyll,
• Essential oils.

To preserve these nutrients it is necessary to observe the following guidelines when using herbs

• They should be as fresh as possible,
• They are at their best if chopped just before use,
• Fresh herbs should be added at the end of the cooking time, rather than being cooked with the other ingredients,
• Fresh herbs should be sprinkled over, or stirred into the finished dish,
• Fresh herbs wilt very quickly. If the herbs are not for immediate use, they can be stored in plastic wrap and kept in the refrigerator, or placed upright with their stalks in water.

In contrast to fresh herbs, dried herbs keep very well in airtight jars until the next crop of herbs are ready for use. Dried herbs should be added to dishes about ten minutes before the end of the cooking time, so that they release their flavor. Many herbs have more flavor when they are fresh than when they have been dried and for this reason, less of the fresh herb should be used than its dried equivalent. A good example of this is basil: dried basil simply cannot compete with fresh basil for intensity of flavor. Some herbs work in the reverse way: oregano, for instance, seems to concentrate its aroma during drying so that the dried herb has far more flavor than fresh oregano.

The aim, when using herbs, is to enhance and support the flavor of the main ingredient in the dish, something that requires careful measuring. If too much of any herb is added, then the amount of salt used in the dish should be correspondingly reduced.

It is possible to indulge heavily in herbs, by adding them to salads, and adding plenty to quark and yogurt based sauces. Herbs enrich potato dishes, and mixed with a good shot of olive oil, herbs can be transformed into a wonderful pasta sauce.

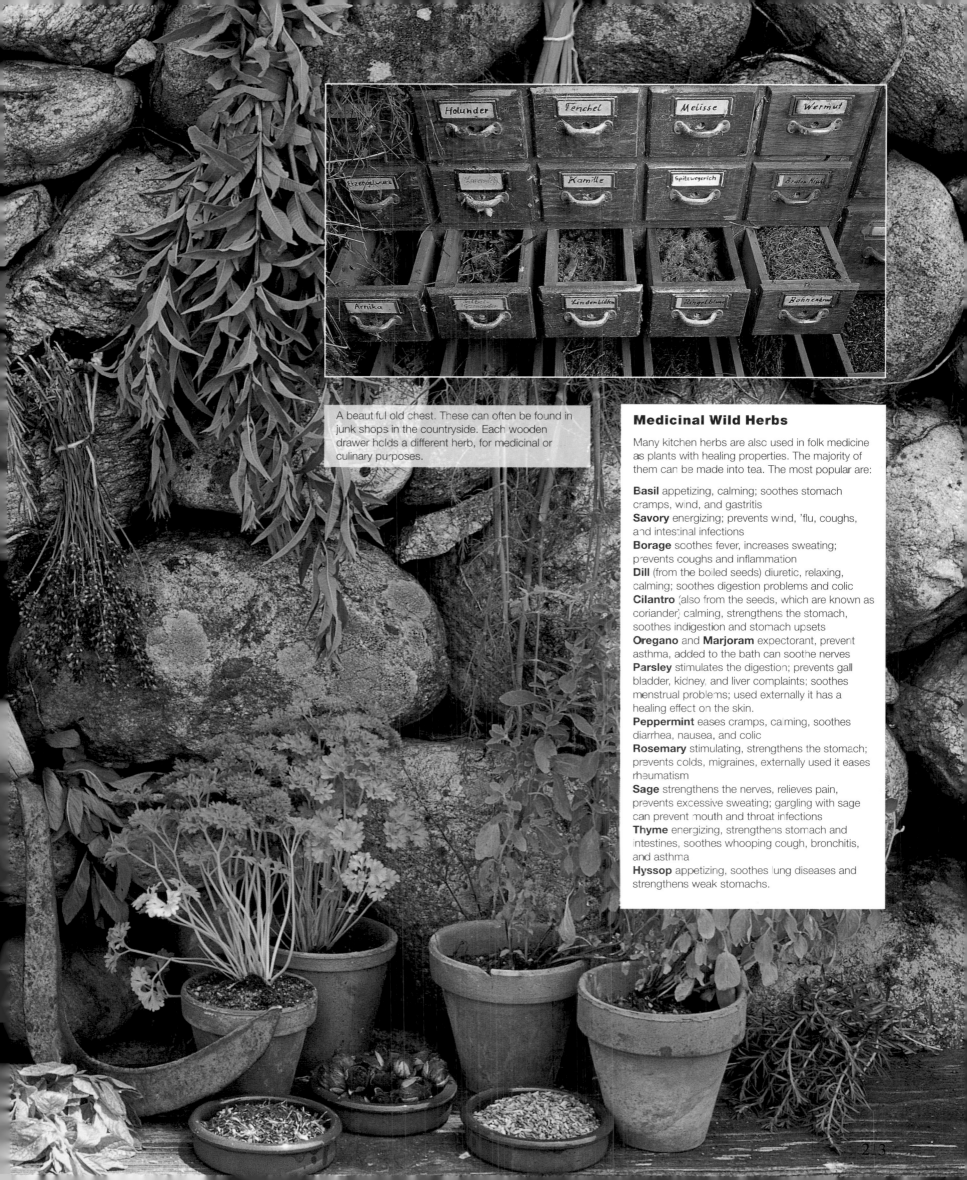

A beautiful old chest. These can often be found in junk shops in the countryside. Each wooden drawer holds a different herb, for medicinal or culinary purposes.

Medicinal Wild Herbs

Many kitchen herbs are also used in folk medicine as plants with healing properties. The majority of them can be made into tea. The most popular are:

Basil appetizing, calming; soothes stomach cramps, wind, and gastritis

Savory energizing; prevents wind, 'flu, coughs, and intestinal infections

Borage soothes fever, increases sweating; prevents coughs and inflammation

Dill (from the boiled seeds) diuretic, relaxing, calming; soothes digestion problems and colic

Cilantro (also from the seeds, which are known as coriander) calming, strengthens the stomach, soothes indigestion and stomach upsets

Oregano and **Marjoram** expectorant, prevent asthma, added to the bath can soothe nerves

Parsley stimulates the digestion; prevents gall bladder, kidney, and liver complaints; soothes menstrual problems; used externally it has a healing effect on the skin.

Peppermint eases cramps, calming, soothes diarrhea, nausea, and colic

Rosemary stimulating, strengthens the stomach; prevents colds, migraines, externally used it eases rheumatism

Sage strengthens the nerves, relieves pain, prevents excessive sweating; gargling with sage can prevent mouth and throat infections

Thyme energizing, strengthens stomach and intestines, soothes whooping cough, bronchitis, and asthma

Hyssop appetizing, soothes lung diseases and strengthens weak stomachs.

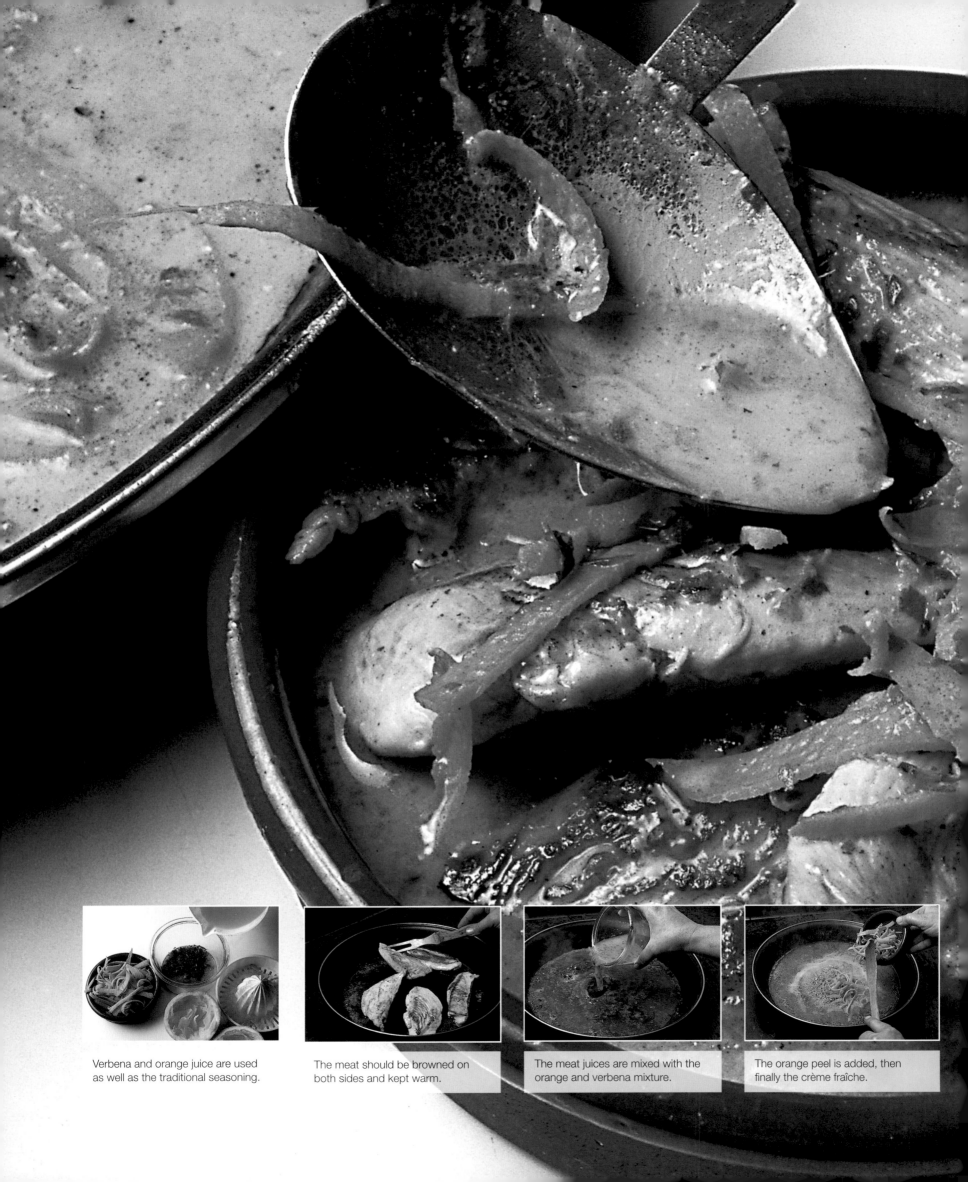

Verbena and orange juice are used as well as the traditional seasoning.

The meat should be browned on both sides and kept warm.

The meat juices are mixed with the orange and verbena mixture.

The orange peel is added, then finally the crème fraîche.

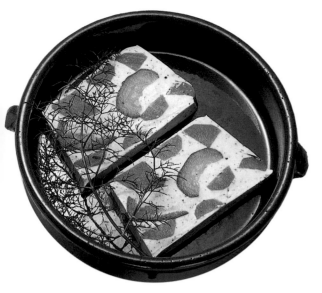

White Vegetable Terrine

Vegetable Purée

1 lb 2 oz (500 g) fennel
$^{1}/_{4}$ cup (50 g) crème fraîche
1 egg white
$^{1}/_{2}$ tsp saffron
1 Tbs milk
Coarse salt

Chop the fennel, setting any fine leaves aside. Steam the fennel in a colander until it is "al dente," then purée. Add the crème fraîche. Beat the egg white until it forms soft peaks then fold into the fennel mixture. Soak the saffron in the milk, mix into the fennel purée and season with a little salt. Garnish with fennel leaves.

Variations
(Illustrations below)

Zucchini purée
1 large pinch nutmeg
A little more salt than the above recipe, no milk

Carrot purée
1 Tbs (15 g) chopped tarragon
3 Tbs (45 ml) milk

Celeriac purée
1 Tbs (15 g) finely grated orange peel
1 pinch nutmeg
2 Tbs (30 ml) milk

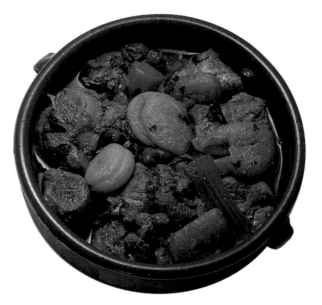

La Gallimafrée

La Gallimafrée
(Eaten for pleasure)
A 17th century recipe
(Illustration above)

$^{1}/_{2}$ cup (100 ml) red wine
$^{1}/_{2}$ Tbs honey
3 oz (80 g) raisins
16 dried apricot halves
2 carrots, 3 celery stalks
1 onion
2 lbs (800 g) shoulder of pork
2 Tbs vinegar
1 tsp finely chopped peppermint
Coarse salt, black pepper
$^{1}/_{2}$ tsp caraway seeds

Mix the red wine with the honey and soak the raisins in the mixture. Soak the apricots in water.
Chop the carrots and celery into pieces $1^{1}/_{4}$ inches (3 cm) long. Slice the onion into rings.
Brown the pork in a cast iron casserole without adding any extra fat; wait until the pork fat melts. Remove the meat and set aside. Deglaze the pan with the vinegar, add the vegetables, and pan fry. Add the meat, sprinkle with mint, season with salt and pepper, and pour in enough water to cover. Cover the pan and simmer for 60–90 minutes.
Drain the raisins and apricots. Add the raisins to the meat and cook for another 10 minutes. Then add the apricots and caraway and cook for a further 10 minutes. Serve with puréed vegetables.

Recipes with Herbs

White Vegetable Terrine
(Illustration above)

9 oz (250 g) young carrots
9 oz (250 g) small zucchini
1 cup (250 g) farmer's cheese
1 cup (250 g) crème fraîche
1 Tbs finely chopped peppermint
$^{1}/_{2}$ Tbs finely chopped dill
Coarse salt
Organic gelling agent (pectin based)
$^{1}/_{2}$ cup (100 ml) vegetable stock
1 sprig dill

Halve the carrots lengthways, or cut into quarters. Steam in a colander, together with the zucchini. Mix together the farmer's cheese, crème fraîche, and the herbs. Mix the gelling agent with the stock and add to the cheese mixture. Season with salt.
Layer the vegetables and cheese mixture alternately into a terrine dish. Finish with a layer of the mixture. Garnish with dill and serve with bell pepper sauce (see recipe on right).

Turkey Breasts with Orange and Verbena
(Illustration left hand page)

1 tsp chopped verbena
2 oranges
4 turkey breast fillets
1 Tbs lard
Coarse salt, black pepper
8 whole verbena leaves
1 Tbs crème fraîche

Put the chopped verbena in a jar, squeeze the oranges and pour the juice into the jar.
Peel two orange halves, making sure that there is no pith on the peel, and slice the peel. Blanch in boiling water for 5 minutes.
Cook the turkey in the lard on both sides until golden brown and then season with salt and pepper. Remove the turkey from the skillet and keep warm.
Deglaze the skillet with the orange juice, add the orange peel and the verbena leaves. Reduce the liquid slightly, then add the crème fraîche. Arrange the meat on plates and pour over the sauce, making sure that the orange peel and verbena leaves are evenly distributed.

Carrot Purée

Zucchini Purée

Red Bell Pepper Sauce

1 large red bell pepper
$^{3}/_{4}$ cup (150 ml) olive oil
Coarse salt

Halve, deseed, and steam the peppers. Keep the cooking water. Remove the skin from the peppers, chop the flesh into small pieces and purée. Using a whisk, beat the pepper mixture, and gradually add $^{3}/_{8}$ cup (75 ml) of the cooking water and all the olive oil, so that the pepper mixture has the consistency of a thick runny cream. Season with salt. Good served cold with White Vegetable Terrine.

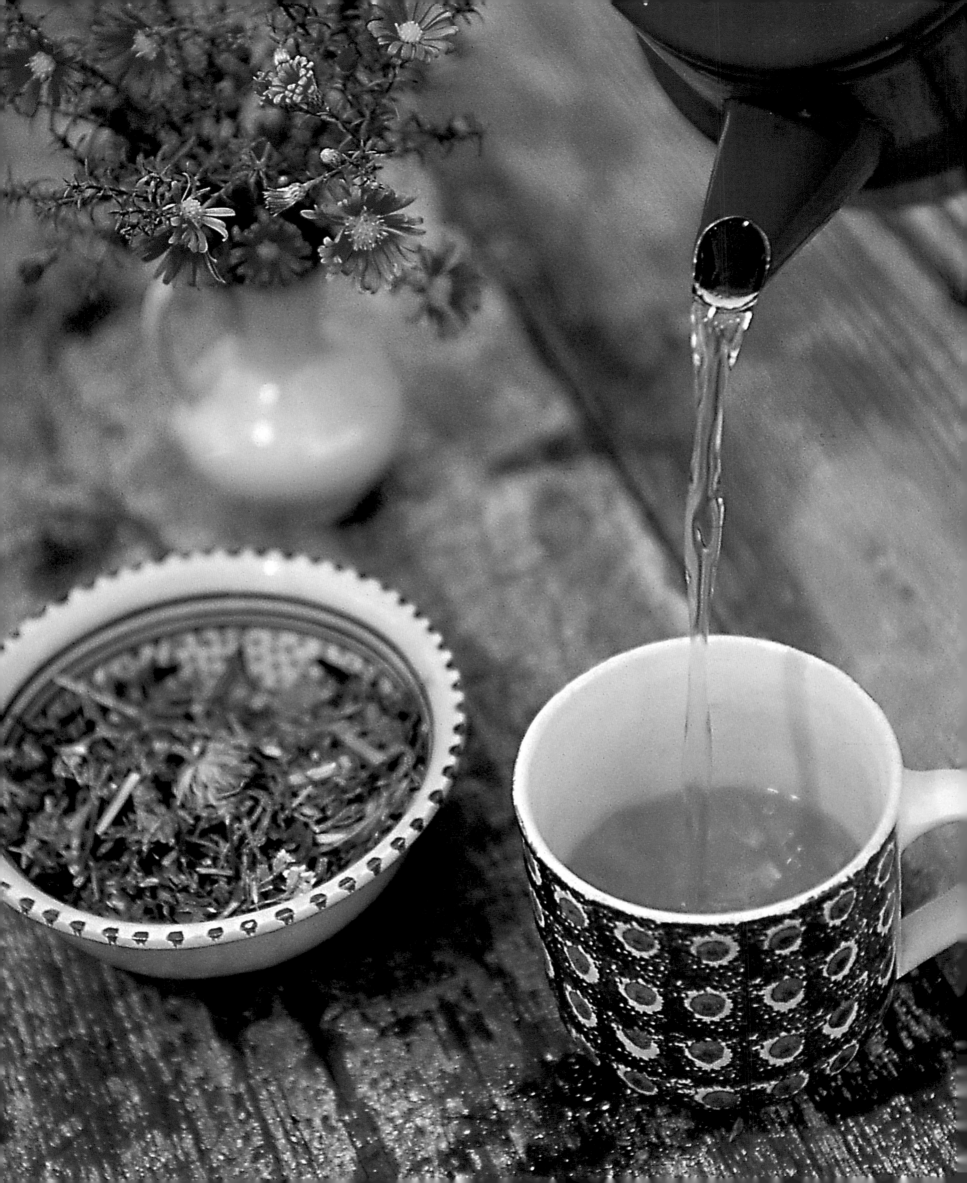

Herbal Teas

Long before black and green teas from China, India, and Ceylon came to Europe, people made infusions from herbs, flowers, and leaves. These drinks had an important role in folk medicine, where they were used to treat colds. Some plants were only used to treat specific illnesses, but a wide range of herbs, particularly cooking herbs, and berries were kept to make pleasant, usually hot drinks.

In many countries, children are given weak herbal tea as a thirst quenching drink which is thought to strengthen their resistance to disease. In some countries, herbal teas are an important part of everyday life – in France, *tisanes* are very popular, and are drunk after the evening meal or served in elegant glasses in restaurants.

The range of flavors and medicinal benefits of herbal teas is astounding. There are teas for all occasions and requirements: stimulating teas made from rosemary, peppermint, or raspberry leaves; teas that calm the nerves, made from balm or hyssop; teas that soothe nasty coughs, made from aniseed or thyme; teas that ease cold symptoms, made from fennel and elderberries; teas that soothe the stomach, made from camomile and yarrow; sleep-inducing teas, made from hops or black currant. Many of these teas have other beneficial effects.

If herbal tea is to be drunk purely for pleasure, it should be made fairly weak, and not have too much of any one herb as an ingredient. To keep a supply of herbs for tea all the year round it is necessary to have a large supply of dried herbs in stock. When drying herbs, they should be picked after a long period of sunshine, in the morning when the dew has gone. It is important, when making tea, to use the uppermost leaves of the plants, or in the case of borage, camomile, marigold, and linden, pick the flowers themselves. To dry the herbs successfully, tie the stalks together so that the herbs form a loose bunch and hang up to dry in an airy, shaded place. The buds and flowers should be spread out on cloths or frames. It is very useful to invest in drying machines or drying cupboards. A basic rule to follow is that the temperature should not exceed 90 °F (35 °C) as this destroys the essential oils in the plant, and the herb will lose its flavor and healing properties.

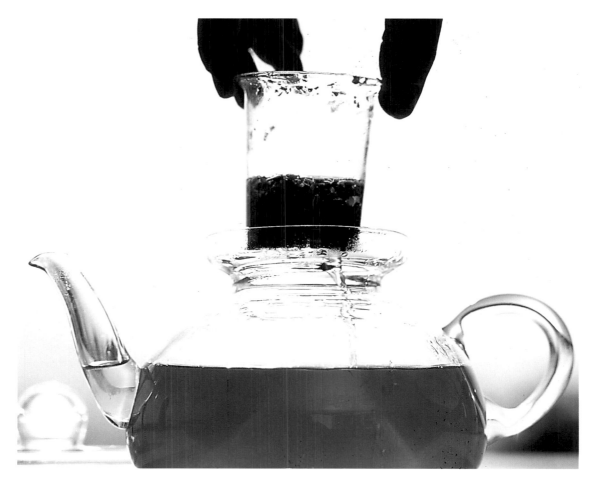

Herbal tea is best made in a pot with a removable strainer and left to steep for between 5–10 minutes.

Herbal Teas

Teas Made From Dried Herbs
4 tsps (20 g) to 5 cups (1 l) water – put the tea in the tea pot pour over boiling water, and leave to brew for 5–10 minutes.

Teas Made From Fresh Herbs
1 cup leaves to 5 cups (1 l) water – put the tea in the pot, pour over boiling water, and leave to brew for 3–5 minutes.

Tea Made From Your Own Garden Herbs
Use basil, borage, fennel, marjoram, balm, mint, rosemary, sage, yarrow, thyme, verbena, hyssop, and lemon thyme.

Tea From Assorted Herbs
For instance: basil and sage; balm and rosemary; balm, verbena, and lemon thyme. The following combinations of plants make a good basis for any herb mixture: raspberry, black currant, and blackberry leaves; also linden, marigold, and white thorn flowers. Apple, orange, and lemon peel gives a refreshing taste to any tea.

Herbal Tea From the Meadows

Veit Lucewig, one of the pioneers of organic farming in the former German Democratic Republic, uses 30 different dried plants to make his delicious tea:

1. Arnica
2. Blackcurrant
3. Camomile
4. Yarrow
5. Thyme
6. Elderflower
7. Raspberry leaf
8. Beech leaf
9. Sage
10. Lemon balm
11. Lavender
12. Common Rue
13. Basil
14. Heather
15. Coltsfoot
16. Stinging nettle
17. Horsetail
18. Dandelion
19. Yarrow
20. Peppermint
21. Fennel
22. Angelica
23. Mugwort
24. Hyssop
25. Oregano
26. Savory
27. Marigold
28. Wood Sage (or the closely related Water Germander)
29. Tarragon
30. Rose leaf

Dips

Dips have always been a part of healthy eating and vegetarian cookery. The traditional Italian dish Pinzimonio consists of fresh, raw vegetables that are sliced, or cut into strips. It was not practical to pour the salad dressing over the vegetables and often they were too hard to pick up with a fork. So the vegetables were picked up in the fingers and dipped into the sauce. Gradually more sauces were offered with the dish so that a different sauce could accompany each type of vegetable. This was how the dip was born. People soon discovered that bread, chips, plain and cheese crackers were good for dipping. Now the dip has advanced from its early state as a traditional vinaigrette to a wide range of exotic flavors with a creamy consistency. Whole food stores have a large range of healthy dips. Home made dips are particularly delicious, so here are a selection of recipes as a source of inspiration.

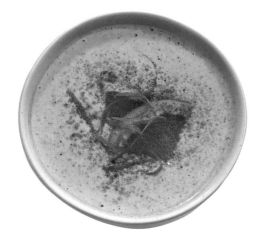

Curried Honey and Orange Dip

2 garlic cloves
Just over ¹/₂ cup (120 g) mayonnaise
¹/₂ cup (100 g) crème fraîche
2 heaping tsp curry powder
1 pinch ground coriander seeds
2 Tbs orange juice
1 tsp firm honey
1 pinch cayenne pepper
Coarse salt

Mince the garlic and liquidize the remaining ingredients. If the dip seems too thick, add a little more orange juice.
Serve with blanched cauliflower and poultry.

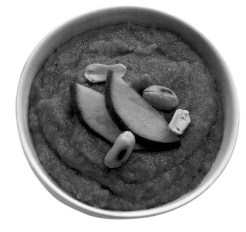

Curried Peanut and Mango Dip

3¹/₂ oz (100 g) peanuts without skins
Coarse salt
1 small onion, 1 garlic clove
1 mango
¹/₂ tsp coriander seeds, 2 tsp curry powder
¹/₄ cup (50 g) mayonnaise
1 tsp honey

Dry roast the peanuts and add salt. Coarsely chop the onion and garlic. Juice the mango and crush the coriander seeds. Liquidize ¹/₄ cup (50 ml) mango juice together with the coriander, curry powder, onion, garlic, peanuts, and mayonnaise. Gradually add the remaining mango juice and sweeten with honey.
Serve with Belgian endive, poultry, and cooked fish.

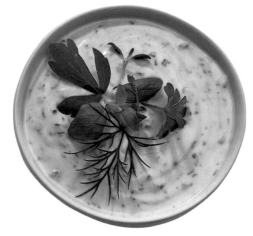

Herb Dip

1 bunch curly parsley
¹/₂ bunch dill
5 sprigs thyme
5 sprigs marjoram
1 sprig lovage
1 sprig hyssop
1 garlic clove
1 pot yogurt
1 pot crème fraîche
2 Tbs mayonnaise
Coarse salt, white pepper

Finely chop the herbs and garlic. Purée with the remaining ingredients and season generously with white pepper.
Serve with any dish: particularly tasty with bread sticks.

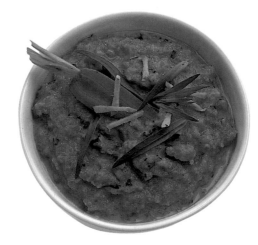

Carrot and Ginger Dip

3 tomatoes
3 carrots
1 garlic clove, 2 small onions
2 tsp freshly grated ginger
3 sprigs thyme
3 sprigs tarragon
¹/₄ cup (50 ml) heavy cream
1 tsp vegetable stock granules
A little lemon juice
Nutmeg
Coarse salt, white pepper

Dice the carrots and tomatoes. Finely chop the onion and garlic and pan fry in the oil. Add the carrots, tomatoes, ginger, and herbs. Liquidize with the cream and add the remaining ingredients; leave to cool.
Serve with vegetables, tofu, and meat dishes.

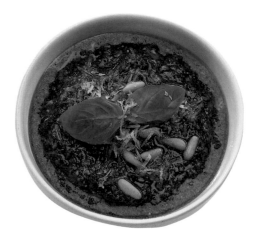

Pesto

About 1 Tbs (10 g) pine nuts
4 garlic cloves
2 bunches basil
1 pinch grated lemon peel
Black pepper
Nutmeg
³/₄ cup (150 ml) olive oil
4 oz (120 g) freshly grated Parmesan
Coarse salt

Dry fry the pine nuts and crush them well. Finely chop the garlic and cut the basil into thin strips. Mix together with the lemon peel, pepper, nutmeg, and olive oil. Season to taste with salt.
Serve with pasta and vegetable soups.

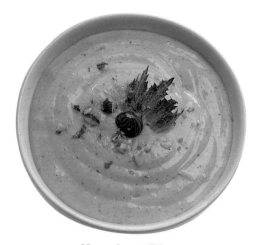

Hazelnut Dip

About 1 Tbs (10 g) hazelnuts
$^1/_4$ cup (50 ml) balsamic vinegar
1 small garlic clove
2 tsp pear juice concentrate
$^3/_4$ cup (150 g) mayonnaise
Nutmeg
Coarse salt, black pepper

Dry roast the hazelnuts, rub them between two pieces of paper towel to remove the skins and roughly chop the nuts. Liquidize with the other ingredients and season to taste with nutmeg, salt, and pepper.
Serve with blanched cauliflower, broccoli, and Brussels sprouts.

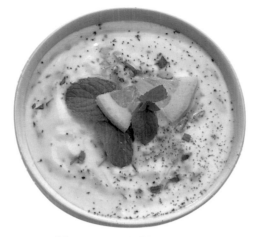

Yogurt and Mint Dip

1 bunch fresh mint
1 pot yogurt
1 pot crème fraîche
A little lemon juice
Coarse salt
Nutmeg

Finely chop the mint leaves. Mix together with the yogurt, crème fraîche, and lemon juice. Season to taste with salt and nutmeg.
Serve with millet balls or other cereal burgers. When thinned with a little water the dip becomes a refreshing soup.

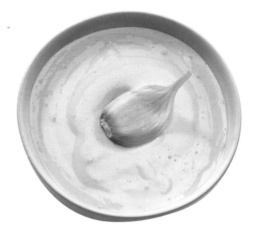

Garlic Mayonnaise

5 garlic cloves
$^3/_4$ cup (150 g) mayonnaise
A little lemon juice
Coarse salt

Roughly dice the garlic and liquidize with the mayonnaise. Season to taste with lemon juice and salt. If a thinner consistency is desired, stir in a little yogurt.
Serve with tomatoes and broiled fish.

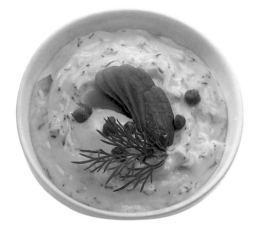

Remoulade

1 small shallot
2 small dill pickles
10 capers
1 bunch dill
$^1/_2$ cup (100 g) mayonnaise
1 tsp Dijon mustard
1 Tbs yogurt
$^1/_2$ tsp apple juice concentrate
Coarse salt, white pepper

Finely chop the shallot, dill pickles, and capers, and slice the dill. Mix all the ingredients together and season to taste with salt and pepper.
Serve with leeks, raw cucumber, and potatoes.

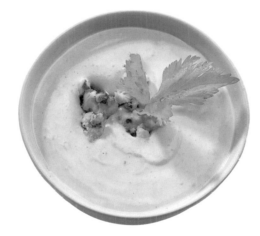

Roquefort Dip

1 oz (30 g) Roquefort
1 pot crème fraîche
2 pots yogurt
White pepper

Crumble the Roquefort. Liquidize with the crème fraîche and yogurt. Season to taste with white pepper.
Serve with baked potatoes or use as a salad dressing.

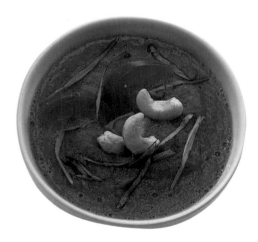

Red Bell Pepper Dip

1 garlic clove
2 medium onions
2 Tbs soya oil
2 bay leaves
2 red bell peppers
2 tomatoes
About 1 Tbs (10 g) cashew nuts
1 tsp each of salt and yeast extract
1 Tbs chopped basil

Dice the onion and the garlic and pan fry in the oil over a high heat with the bay leaves. Deseed the peppers and chop into small pieces. Add to the onions and pan fry. Dice the tomatoes, and add to the peppers with the cashew nuts. Cover and simmer for 60 minutes. Remove the bay leaves, stir in the salt and yeast extract. Liquidize the vegetables, leave to cool, and stir in the basil.

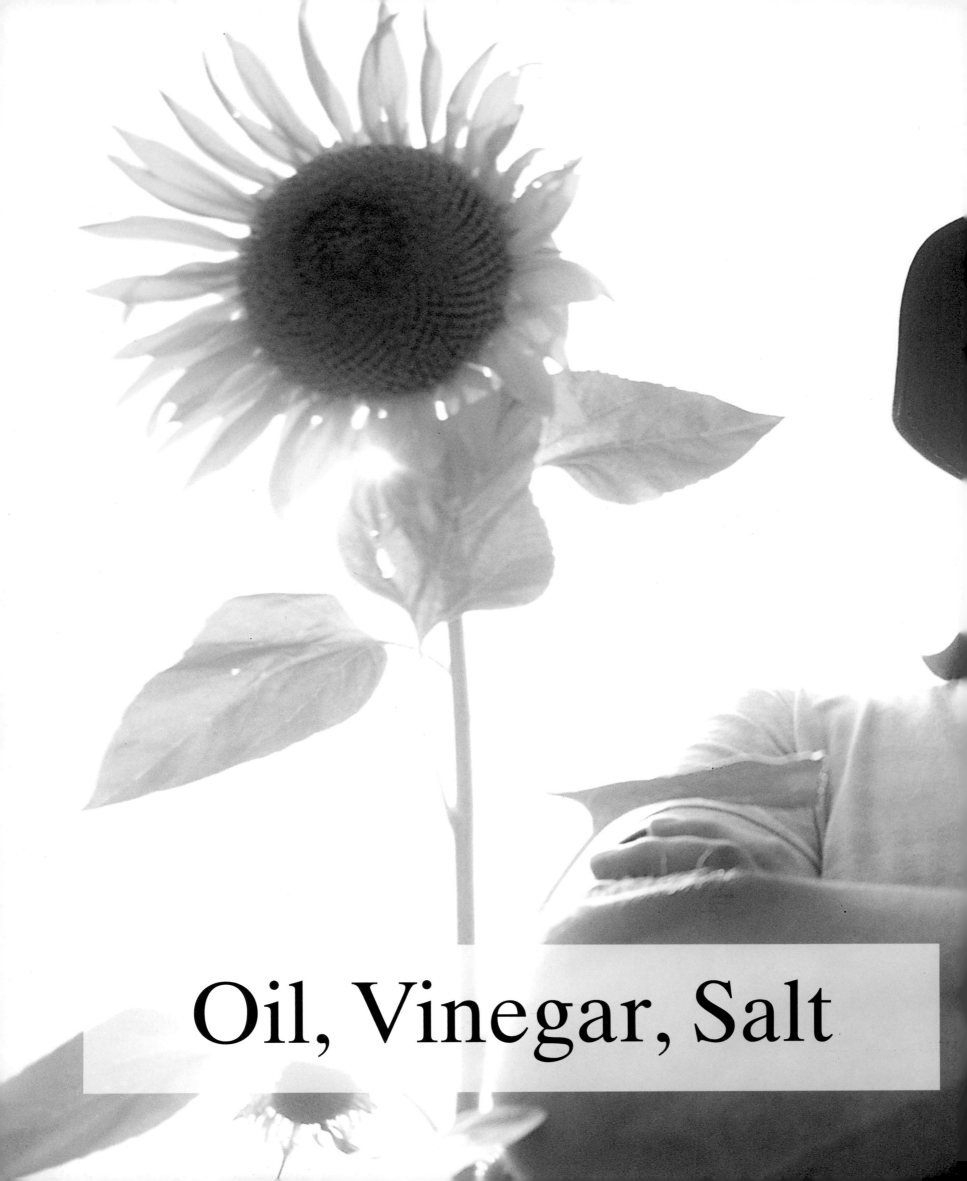

Oil, Vinegar, Salt

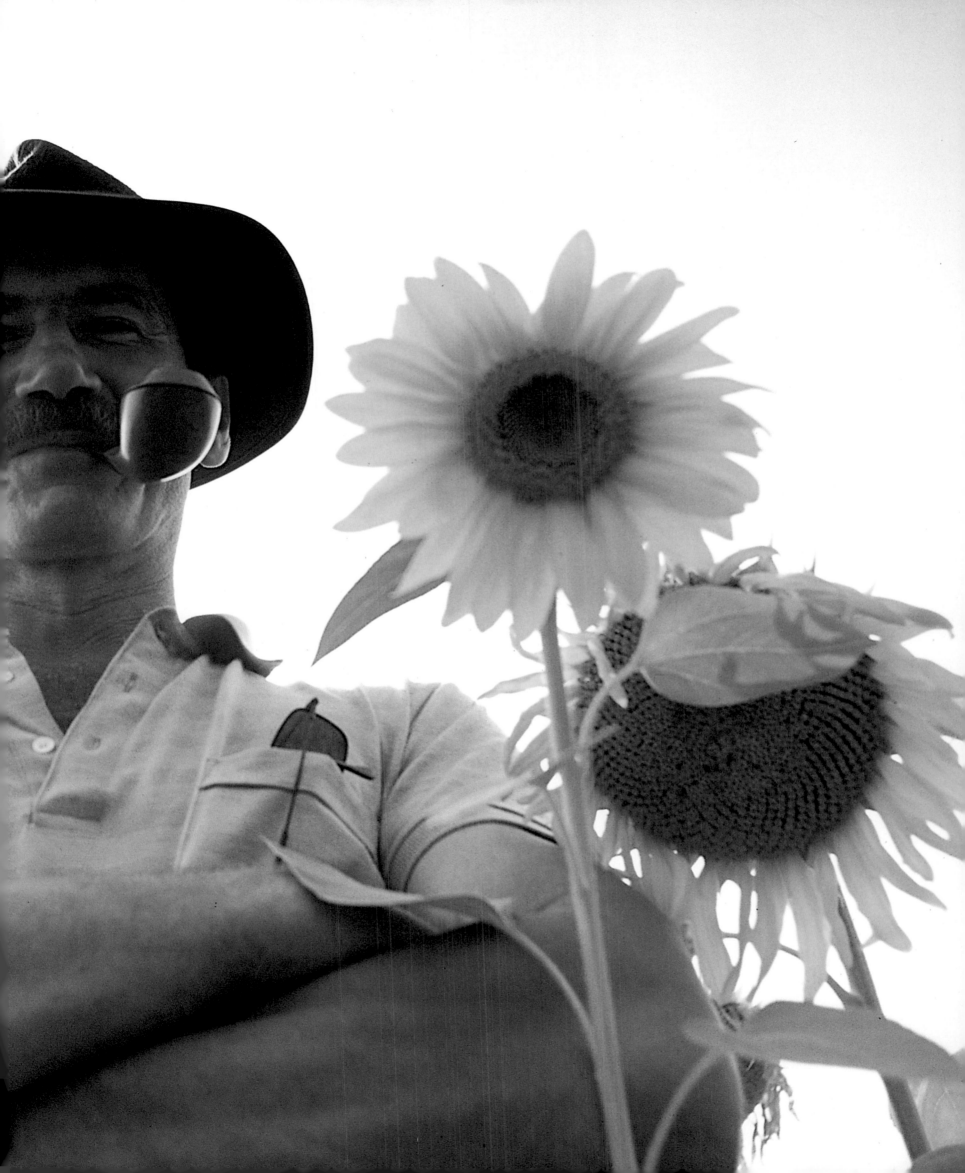

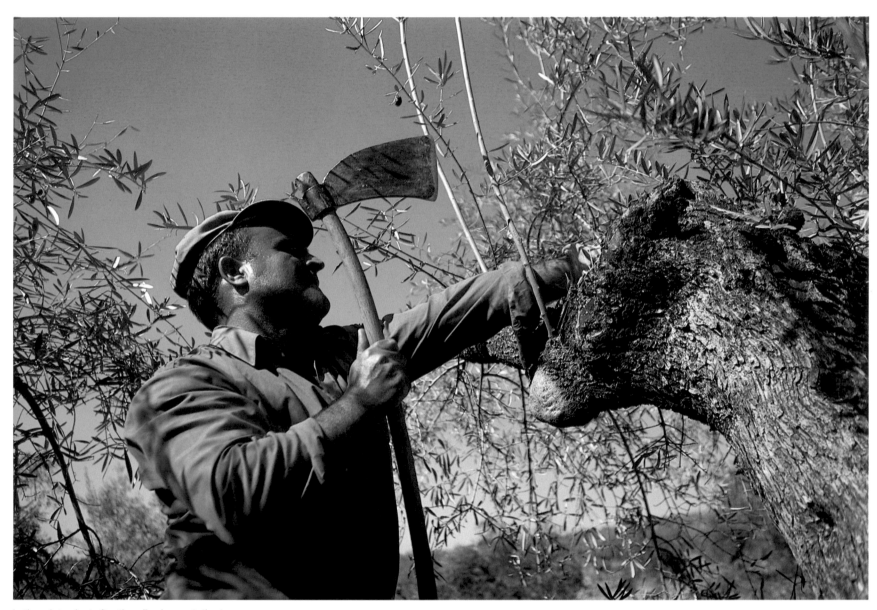

In the winter, just after the olive harvest, the trees are
thinned out and any rotten branches are removed: this
is done every three or four years.

Previous double page: When sunflowers are this tall,
promising excellent oil, the farmer will be satisfied.

Plant oils are one of the great mysteries of life. Thousands of years ago, people in Asia and the Mediterranean countries – the cradle of civilization – discovered that some seeds, nuts, and fruits contained a thick, golden juice that had amazing properties. It provided energy and immunity to disease, improved the health of the sick, made the complexion smoother and more beautiful, enhanced the flavor of food, and gave light when it was lit. Oil was precious, and was often offered up to the gods to obtain their favor. Babies, brides and bridegrooms, and the dying were annointed with oil as were priests and kings. Oil became a symbol of the essence of life. This is not surprising, as the fatty acids that oil contains are vital components of our bodies, and without these fats the human organism would not survive. Only cold-pressed oils contain all the beneficial substances that contribute so greatly to our diets. They also contain many fat-soluble vitamins. These nutrients are the reason vegetable oils are such an important part of nutrition. They are designed for pan frying as they have distinctive flavor, but are far more useful in wholefood cookery before they have been heated. They are important for salad recipes, make good spreads for bread and delicious dips. Oils are a good flavoring ingredient for boiled vegetables. Naturally produced oils, in contrast to refined oils, often have a distinctive flavor that increases their culinary value. Up until now, oil has not been given the recognition it deserves. The same applies to vinegar. Just like cold-pressed oil, high-quality vinegars, made from good wines or fruit juices that have been untreated by chemicals and left to ferment for a long time are hard to find and very expensive. Used sparingly, they are very good flavor enhancers and excellent seasoning ingredients. Vinegar stimulates the metabolism and has a natural antibiotic effect. This has made vinegar a popular natural medicine. Like many seasoning ingredients, vinegar is only good when used in the right quantities. Vinegar should be used sparingly, but it always adds flavor. So many wholefood recipes would be insipid without a little pinch of coarse salt, or a drop of vinegar.

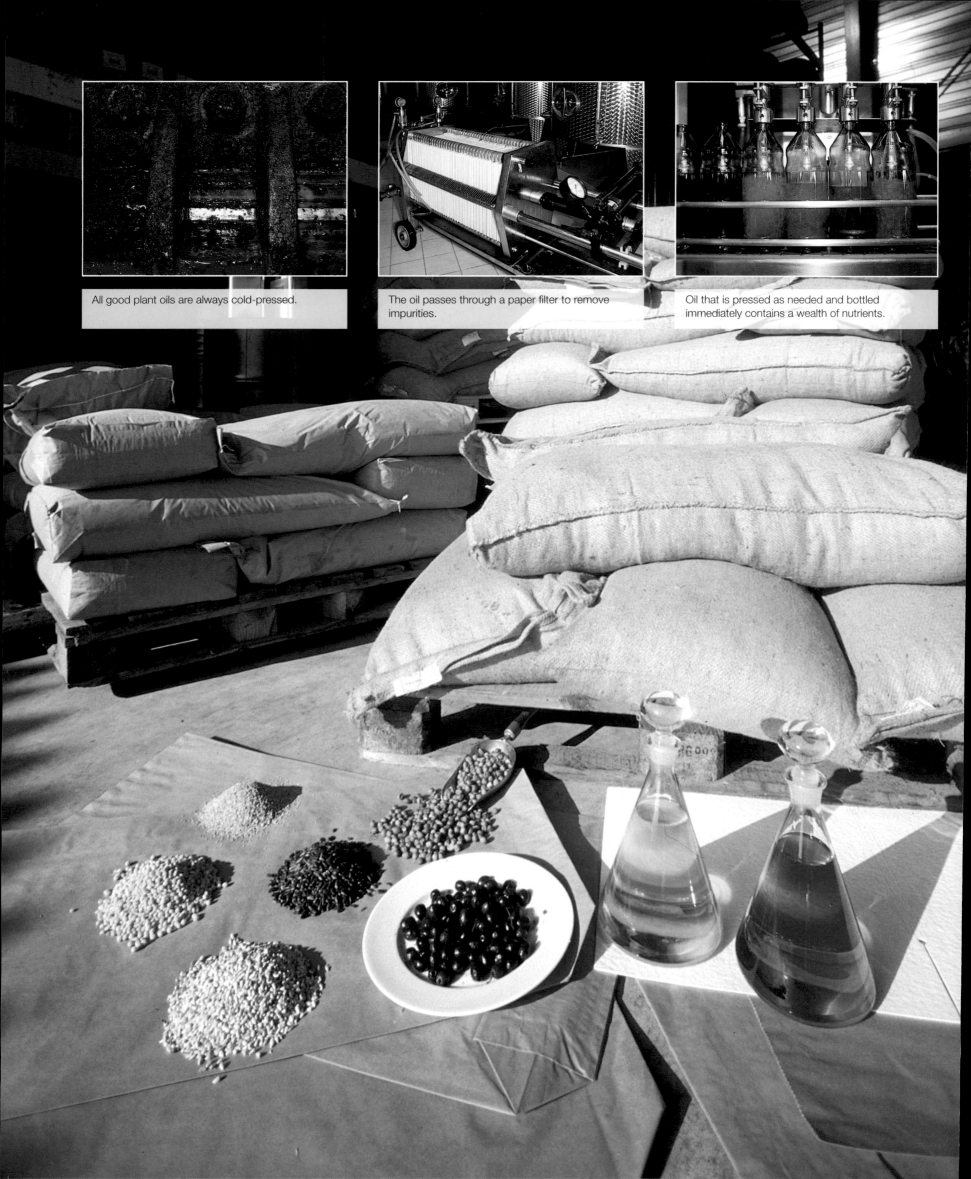

All good plant oils are always cold-pressed.

The oil passes through a paper filter to remove impurities.

Oil that is pressed as needed and bottled immediately contains a wealth of nutrients.

Liquid Gold

Cold-Pressed Edible Oils

Cold-pressed oils – especially olive oil – are a Mediterranean legend. In earlier times they were obtained in a lavish but gentle manner. To begin with, the oil-giving seeds and fruits were pounded into a mulch that was then pressed to release the juice. Later the fruits were simply ground, and this then became the pressing process.

As long as oil is not overheated, it retains all its nutrients and special characteristics. Recent technology enables the optimum amount of oil to be extracted from the fruits without spoiling its quality. Refined oils have been through a process that involves the use of chemicals to make physical changes to the oil. Refining produces a clear, stable, neutral cooking fat which should have no place in wholefood cookery. Unrefined, cold-pressed oils that have only been pressed once have a very high content of unsaturated fatty acids, enzymes, hormones, and nutrients and are liquid gold for cooking and health.

To obtain good quality oil, it is important to have high quality ingredients. There is no point in using special pressing techniques if the oil-giving plants are poor quality, have been raised on artificial fertilizers, grown in soil polluted by chemicals, and had their leaves, fruits, or seeds sprayed with chemicals. Even if the oil seeds are well protected by nature, as in the case of grape seeds, pumpkin seeds or nuts, the effects of chemical sprays can penetrate through the protective layers around the seed. For the best oil, only organically grown seeds or fruits should be put into the press. This has led to partnerships between oil producers and farmers, although some farmers have obtained the equipment to produce their own oil. Oil-giving fruits or seeds must be stored in cool, dark surroundings. Before pressing takes place, the seeds and kernels are carefully sorted to remove any impurities. In the case of nuts or sunflower seeds, it is necessary to remove the shells. During the sorting process there are a few other factors which are important – how likely the seeds are to germinate, the amount of moisture they contain, and the smell of the seeds.

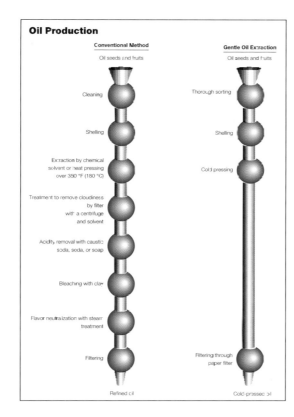

Oil Production

Conventional Method — Oil seeds and fruits
- Cleaning
- Shelling
- Extraction by chemical solvent or heat pressing over 350 °F (180 °C)
- Treatment to remove cloudiness by filter with a centrifuge and solvent
- Acidity removal with caustic soda, soda, or soap
- Bleaching with clay
- Flavor neutralization with steam treatment
- Filtering

Refined oil

Gentle Oil Extraction — Oil seeds and fruits
- Thorough sorting
- Shelling
- Cold pressing
- Filtering through paper filter

Cold-pressed oil

Continuous pressing means that the oil cannot be stored for very long, but should be bottled as soon after pressing as possible. Pressing is usually carried out a few days before distribution. Oil can be obtained most easily when the seeds are at a temperature of 68 °F (20 °C); if they are below this temperature then they should be warmed up before pressing takes place. Pressing is done mechanically, usually in a spiral press, which grinds the seeds or fruits with a continual action from a screw, which gradually increases the pressure. Smaller presses ensure that the temperature of the seeds does not increase significantly because the pressure increases at a slower rate. With smaller presses the oil extraction process takes longer, but the quality, flavor, and nutritional content of the oil is significantly higher than that of oil produced from a larger press.

Not every cold-pressed oil remains cold during pressing. Usually four-fifths of the volume of oil becomes no hotter than 100 °F (40 °C), but towards the end of the pressing, the temperature can rise to more than 130 °F (50 °C). This has a negative effect on the flavor and the vitamin content of the oil, but with good equipment and careful supervision this rise in temperature can be avoided. The oil is left to stand for a few days and becomes cloudy. It is then passed through a paper filter and collected for immediate bottling, thus ensuring that the oil retains its natural characteristics and all its nutrients. Oil obtained by these gentle methods has an intense, distinctive flavor. Cold-pressed oils – in contrast to industrially produced oils, are a valuable culinary ingredient.

Are Fatty Acids Important?

Fats, also known as lipids, consist of three different fatty acids:
- Saturated fats – these include palmitin, stearin, and butyric acid. They are found in all animal fats (also palm oil and coconut oil) and are produced by the human body. They are often solid at room temperature, do not react and are very difficult to digest.
- Monounsaturated fats are generally found in oil. They occur in practically all foods that contain fats, both animal and vegetable. They are generally liquid at room temperature, react and can be metabolized by the body.
- Polyunsaturated fats – like linoleic acid (bisaturated), linolenic acid (tri-saturated), and arachidon acid (vitamin F) are almost always vegetable fats. They are liquid, react easily, and are essential for the human organism. They help the body regulate all its functions and, as the body cannot produce these fats itself, they are an important part of the diet.
The levels of these three fats in different cooking oils determines their quality.

Fatty Acid Content in Oils
Amount as a percentage of the oil

Oil Type	Saturated Fat	Mono-unsaturated Fat	Poly-unsaturated Fat
Rape seed	11	55	34
Safflower	9	14	77
Peanut	16	46	38
Hazelnut	6	79	15
Pumpkin seed	17	30	53
Linseed	9	18	73
Corn	12	31	57
Almond	7	72	21
Poppy seed	11	19	70
Olive	15	75	10
Sesame	14	42	44
Soya	13	25	62
Sunflower	12	25	63
Grape seed	11	21	68
Walnut	9	20	71
Wheat	12	27	63
In comparison:			
Butter fat	64	28	3
Coconut oil	90	8	2

Edible Oils in the Kitchen

Pan Frying, Braising

High temperatures have a negative effect on good quality oil. It is therefore recommended to use small quantities, or to dry fry ingredients.

Flavoring

To season salads, sauces or other recipes it is good to use oils that have been flavored with fresh herbs. Whole sprigs of herbs look very appealing in bottles of oil, but more flavor is gained from torn and salted herb leaves.

Deep Frying

This method of cooking is not recommended, as the high level of heat can produce tarring that may be carcinogenic. This cancels out the beneficial effect of the vitamins and polyunsaturated fats in the oil. Deep fried foods are enclosed in a layer of fat that is very difficult to digest. If you must deep fry, do be careful not to let the oil temperature rise above 375 °F (190 °C) and do not allow the oil to smoke.

Baking and Pastry Making

Whether it is used to grease a tin or added to pastry, butter and oil lose their vitamins and polyunsaturated fats at high temperatures, even though baking temperatures are not high enough to produce carcinogens.

Marinating

Whether it is just for an hour, overnight, or for several days, marinating seals the ingredients in a protective film and protects them from oxidation. The addition of herbs and spices enhances the flavor of the food, and adds extra flavor of its own. As the marinade absorbs extra flavors, it can be used as a sauce or the basis of a sauce.

Mayonnaise

Since mayonnaise is prized for its flavor, stronger tasting oils are the best to use to make mayonnaise. Only olive oil should be used when making Aïoli or garlic mayonnaise (see p. 180).

Raw Vegetables

The addition of oil to raw vegetables not only enhances their flavor but also enables the fat-soluble vitamins to be used by the body. Raw vegetables are at their best when served with oil, lemon juice, vinegar, and herbs, and left for 30 minutes before serving so that the flavors have a chance to develop.

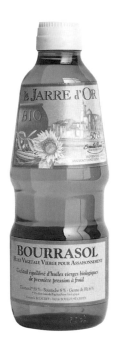 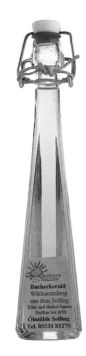 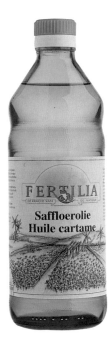 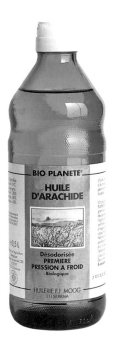 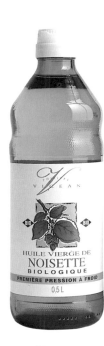 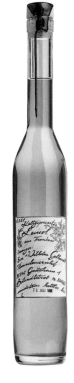

Bourass Oil

A mixture of sunflower and 6 percent each of wheat and borage oil. Known for its healing properties since the Middle Ages, it has a beneficial effect on female hormones. Use for salad dressings, mayonnaise, and cold sauces.

Beech Nut Oil

In Europe after the Second World War, beech nuts were collected from the woods and turned into oil. Now this oil is very rare, because of the decrease in the beech nut harvest. It is golden yellow in color, it is slow to oxidize and has an exquisite flavor.

Safflower Oil

When dyers were processing these plants 300 years ago, to obtain the natural red color, they noticed that the flowers produced a mild-tasting oil with a high percentage of polyunsaturates. This is one of the most valuable oils, and is especially recommended for heart and circulation problems.

Peanut Oil

Peanuts were grown for their oil in South America many years ago; now they are grown in all hot countries of the world. When it is cold-pressed it retains its typical peanut flavor. It can be used when cold, and is also good when heated as it does not add too much of its own flavor to the ingredients.

Hazelnut Oil

Hazelnuts originated in Mediterranean countries and were used to produce oil in the Middle Ages. The oil is easy to obtain, has a delicate flavor and is perfect for salad dressings and baking. It stimulates the body and is easy to digest. Hazelnut oil is also a good massage oil.

Linseed Oil

This oil, which has the highest linoleic acid content of any cooking oil (30–64%), is very healthy. Its intense, smooth flavor combines well with hearty salads and is good mixed with milder oils for a blander taste.

Salads

One of the best ways to enjoy the individual flavor of oil is to serve it with green salads. The salad leaves should be salted just before serving, drizzled with vinegar or lemon juice and finally dressed with salad oil. When the leaves are dressed in this order, they will not wilt.

Vinaigrette

Oil and vinegar form the basis of this well-known sauce. Vinaigrette is a good accompaniment to warm or cold cooked vegetables, as well as to salads. It is generally made in the ratio of 3:1 oil to vinegar. If a strongly flavored oil is used, it should be combined with a traditional wine vinegar. If a neutrally flavored oil is used it can be mixed with a stronger flavored vinegar. To give the dressing more complexity and refinement, and to maximize the polyunsaturated fat content, more than one type of oil can be mixed with the vinegar.

Seasoning Oil

Aromatic oil with a distinctive flavor enriches all types of dishes. This oil should be drizzled sparingly over the dish just before serving. Olive oil is especially good for flavoring fish and vegetable dishes, as are nut and sesame oil. Seasoning oil retains all its nutrients as it is not exposed to heat.

Storing Cooking Oils

Because cooking oils are naturally high in polyunsaturated fats, naturally obtained oils react quickly to their surroundings. This also means that they deteriorate comparatively quickly although their vitamin E content protects them to some degree. The vitamins in oil are sensitive to light. Cold-pressed oils should be:
• properly sealed,
• kept in dark glass containers or containers made of high-grade steel,
• kept cool, but not below 50 °F (10 °C).
In these conditions oil will keep for 8–12 months. It is best to buy oil in small quantities, and to use it quickly.

Olive Oil Quality

• The best olive oil is "extra virgin" obtained from the first pressing. This oil has no more than 1% free fatty acids (fatty acids that are not combined to glycerin and affect the flavor) and often contains only 0.5 % or less.
French: Huile d'olive vierge extra
Greek: ΕΞΤΡΑ ΠΑΡΘΕΝΟ ΕΛΑΙΟΛΑΔΟ
Italian: Olio d'oliva extra vergine
Portugese: Azeite de oliveira extra virgem
Spanish: Aceite de oliva virgen extra
• Good quality oil is known as "virgin cold-pressed." It is obtained from the first pressing and may contain up to 2% free fatty acids.
French: Huile d'olive vierge
Greek: ΠΑΡΘΕΝΟ ΕΛΑΙΟΛΑΔΟ
Italian: Olio d'oliva vergine
Portugese: Azeite de oliveira virgem
Spanish: Aceite de oliva virgen

Other types that are described as pure olive oil are not organically produced, as they may contain oil that has been refined and extracted with the use of chemicals. Only mechanically extracted oil can be described as organic oil

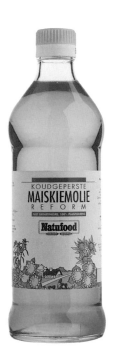

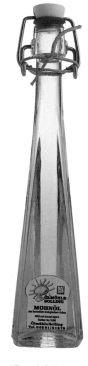

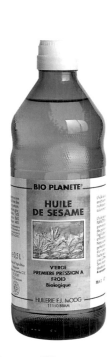

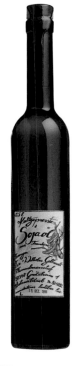

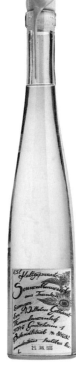

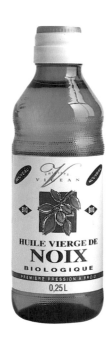

Corn Oil

Maize is the cereal crop of South America and its kernel contains more than 40% oil. Over half of the fat content is made up of polyunsaturated fats. When fresh, it has a sweet, corn flavor and is also good for pan frying.

Poppy Seed Oil

It is possible that poppies were grown in Oriental countries for their oil back in the Stone Age. Later they were cultivated in Europe and Asia. This oil lowers the cholesterol level in the blood. It has a very delicate flavor and should only be eaten cold, preferably on salads.

Sesame Oil

Sesame has been grown for thousands of years in warm countries. It was considered to be a sacred plant and was used to make oil. Its gentle nutty flavor has a high linoleic acid content and contains lecithin which helps open the arteries. Use for salads and for pan frying.

Soy Oil

Soybeans are not only a rich source of protein, but they also contain polyunsaturated fats. In contrast to mass produced soy oil, which has a neutral flavor, organic soy oil has an intense bean flavor. It is best used cold to preserve its flavor.

Sunflower Oil

The sunflower originated in America and was grown in Europe from the 18th century. It was a very popular crop in Russia and was grown for its oil. Organic sunflower oil can help prevent arteriosclerosis. Sunflower oil is very aromatic and tastes best in salads.

Walnut Oil

The walnut tree is grown all over the world, but is especially common in France. Walnuts give an excellent oil that is very good for the health and has a delicious flavor. It is very good in warm salads and also in cakes. It becomes rancid relatively quickly.

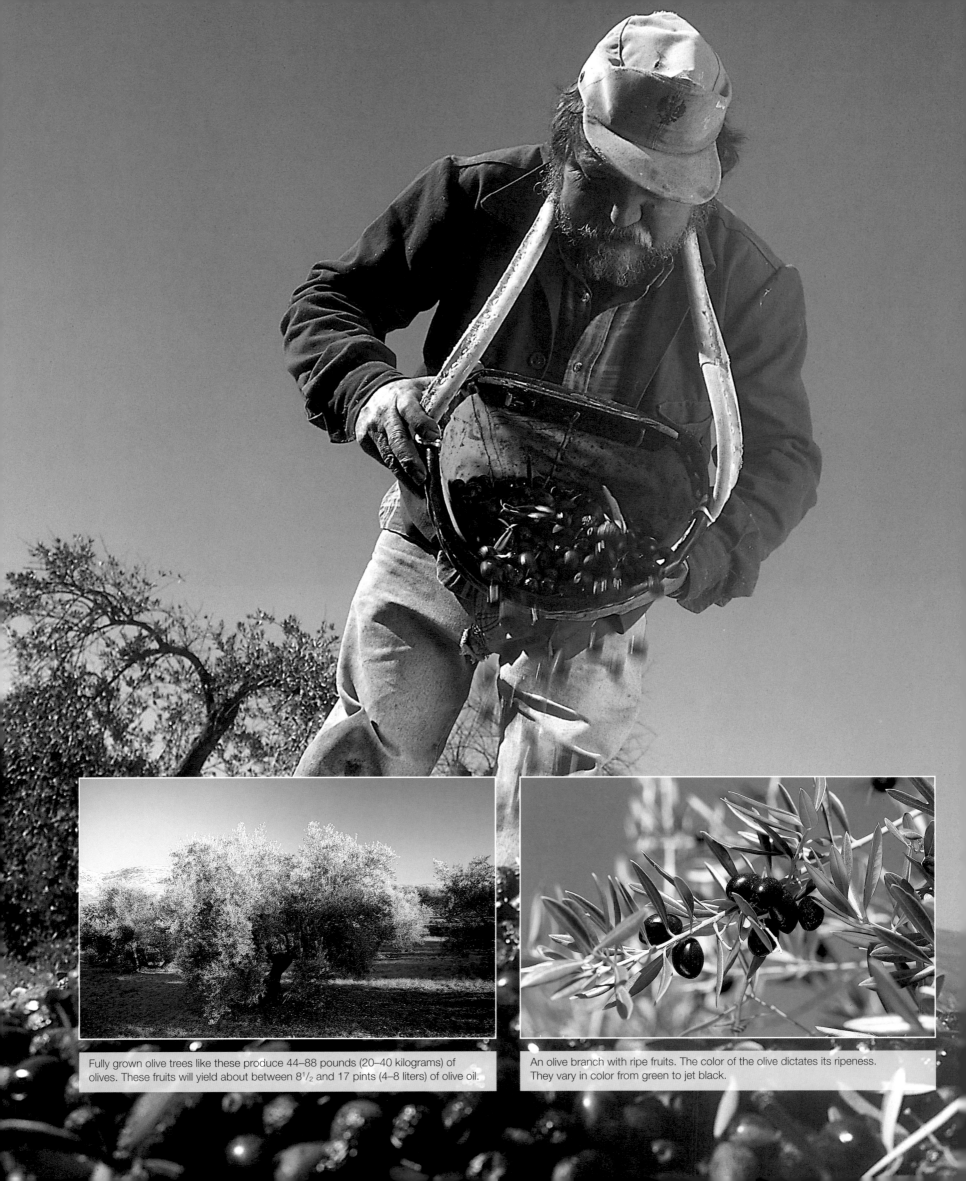

Fully grown olive trees like these produce 44–88 pounds (20–40 kilograms) of olives. These fruits will yield about between 8 1/2 and 17 pints (4–8 liters) of olive oil.

An olive branch with ripe fruits. The color of the olive dictates its ripeness. They vary in color from green to jet black.

In the Olive Grove

The olive tree *Olea europaea* is an evergreen tree that loves the Mediterranean climate with dry summers and mild winters. Olive trees can live for a thousand years and do not grow very fast. They can be between 10 and 30 feet high (3–10 meters) and their branches thicken, and become gnarled over the decades. Olive trees have many twigs and grow long, leathery leaves with a dark green upper side and a silvery lower side. In earlier times, as other crops were sometimes grown between the trees, they were planted 30 feet (10 meters) apart and sometimes they grew more than one trunk. Today, even olive trees have to bow to modern practices. Saplings with one stem are planted, and about 60 trees are planted to the acre (150 per hectare), often even more. It takes 4–10 years before the trees bear fruit, after 30–35 years they reach their peak productivity, but by the age of 75 productivity dwindles noticeably.

Olive trees are similar to vines both in their requirements and cultivation. Olive trees have to be pruned carefully because the fruit grows best from the young branches. If the trees do not bear too much fruit, they live for longer, and produce better flavored fruit. The difference between organic and non organic olive cultivation lies in the type of fertilizer used. Sheep manure and natural compost make good fertilizers, and good pruning protects the trees from fungal and insect infections. The greatest threat to the olive crop is the olive fly although it is possible to control this pest by using an organic insecticide.

In the early part of the year the olive trees form panicles which bear small white flowers, which are pollenated by the wind. It is very rare for pollenation not to take place. From September the first green olives are picked. These are for eating. From November the oil olives are harvested and this can continue through March, depending on the climate of the region. The earliest olives are a violet color, while towards the end of the harvest they are black and a little wrinkled. As the olives ripen, they darken in color. Semi ripe olives produce an oil that is delicately flavored, fruity, and spicy with a peppery flavor. However, semi ripe olives produce less oil, so the oil is more expensive. Fully ripe olives give a blander, nuttier, smoother, and milder oil and produce larger quantities.

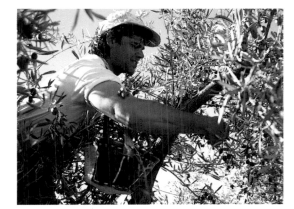

Despite practice and speed, experienced olive pickers do not harvest more than 88 pounds (40 kilograms) of olives each day.

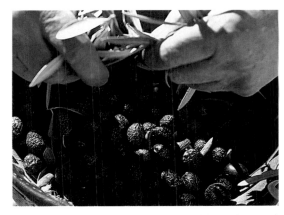

For the best quality oil, the olives should be undamaged and clean.

For top quality oil, the tiny olives are picked by hand. Even an experienced olive picker cannot collect more than 88 pounds (40 kilograms) of olives in a day. In a good year, this quantity of olives will yield 8 to 16 pints (4 to 8 liters). For lower quality oil, the olives are obtained by beating the trees with sticks, and are caught in nets to prevent damage to the fruit. Olive skin is sensitive; once it is broken the juice begins to ferment which increases the fat content of the oil and causes the nutrients to spoil. It is becoming more common, in intensive olive cultivation, to collect the olives using specially made tractors. This has not been the case in organic cultivation as it has adverse effects on the health and longevity of the trees.

Olive Oil

Olive oil has always been associated with Mediterranean cuisine. Up until a few decades ago it was only available in northern Europe from drugstores as a massage oil, or known only to gourmets, and available in specialist stores. Since then it has gained in popularity. This began with the interest in Italian, Provençale, Spanish, and Greek cookery, all of which use olive oil. Now it is well known that olive oil has a beneficial effect on the health:

• It is easily digested, has a positive effect on the stomach and intestines, and prevents ulcers and gallstones.

• Its high content of monounsaturated fatty acid which, at 75 percent, is not only better than animal fats but also most other vegetable oils, keeps the arteries elastic and so reduces the risk of heart and circulatory diseases.

• Olive oil has a high level of antioxidants, and can withstand greater temperatures than other oils. Olive oil does not release dangerous substances when it is heated, unlike other animal and vegetable fats. It is possible that olive oil helps prevent cancer in the human body.

The great culinary advantage that olive oil has is its broad range of flavors. The flavor depends on the type of olive (of which there are at least a dozen), the time of the harvest, the climate, and the type of soil. This is another way in which olive oil is similar to wine. The differing tastes of olive oil are well known in Italy, but in the other lands where oil is produced, the variety of flavors is less understood. This is changing, and hopefully in the future there will be an even greater range of organically produced olive oils on the market. To fully appreciate the nuances in the oil's flavor, it should simply be poured over finished dishes.

• The most common flavors to be found in olive oil are: almond, nut, artichoke, fresh grass, hay, wild herbs, asparagus, sometimes tomato or apple, pear, lemon and orange peel. The best oils have a taste that is compared to pepper, cayenne, or even tannin.

• Olive oil is sensitive to heat, air, and humidity. It should always be kept firmly sealed, in a bottle that does not let in the light, and stored in a cool dark place. It should not be kept in the refrigerator. It keeps very well for 9–12 months, after which time the flavor begins to weaken. Olive oil should not be kept for more than 18 months.

Left hand page: Once picked, the olives are collected in nets and taken to the olive press as quickly as possible, so that they do not lose their delicate flavor.

In the Oil Mill

When the harvest has been gathered in, the farmer has to move quickly, as olives are very sensitive fruits. Like grapes, they tend to oxidize very quickly, and their delicate flavor does not withstand contact with oxygen. Before pressing can take place, the olives have to be washed. In hot, dry, places where olives are grown, it is common to find that the olives are covered in a layer of dust. This dust has an adverse effect on the flavor of the olives. Any leaves or bits of twig are also removed at this stage of the oil making process.

When the olives have been cleaned, the grinding process can begin. Large, round granite stones roll over the olives, which have been spread out in a thin layer. The stones press the olive flesh and pits into an even, fatty, and damp paste. Nowadays these stones are powered by machines, but the grinding process has hardly changed over the last thousand years. It is simply the best way to extract oil from the fruit. Some modern methods use steel rollers instead of granite which makes the extraction quicker and easier, but allows the olives to become too hot. When the oil reaches a temperature above 80 °F (30 °C) it loses its essential oils.

To obtain high quality oil, the paste is placed into cylinders which are carefully rocked backwards and forwards. The oil drips through a fine-meshed sieve and does not need any extra pressure. Modern methods not only press the olives for a second time but also pierce the fruit. Oil that is produced using gentle methods does not taste bitter. About 26 pounds (12 kilograms) of olives are required to produce 1³/₄ pints (1 liter) oil. Conventional pressing methods require the olives to be spread out on round mats known as *capachos*. These were traditionally made of velvet, and are now made of nylon. The mats are stacked up under a hydraulic press and held in place by a steel or iron rod. The liquid that is collected is a mixture of fruit juice and oil. This liquid is placed in a centrifuge to separate the oil.

The old "decanting" method is rarely used today. This worked on the principle that oil is lighter than water. The juice and oil mixture was left to stand until the oil floated to the surface. The oil was then removed from the surface and tipped from one container to another. This was a natural way to separate

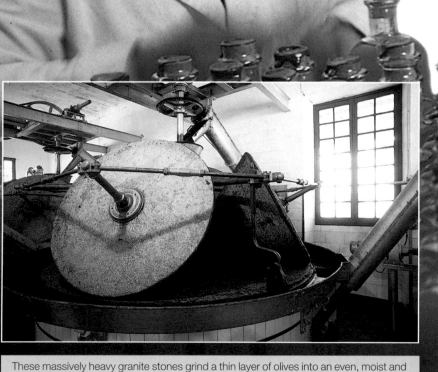

In Andalusia, the high-grade oil is bottled by hand, then sealed and identified with a numbered label

These massively heavy granite stones grind a thin layer of olives into an even, moist and oily paste.

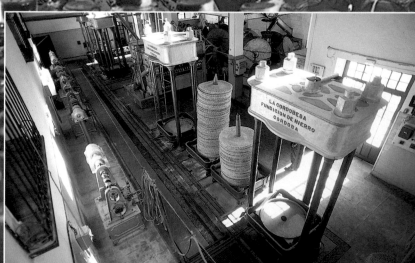

Stacked up under the hydraulic press (foreground) lie a pile of *capachos* – round mats spread with crushed olives.

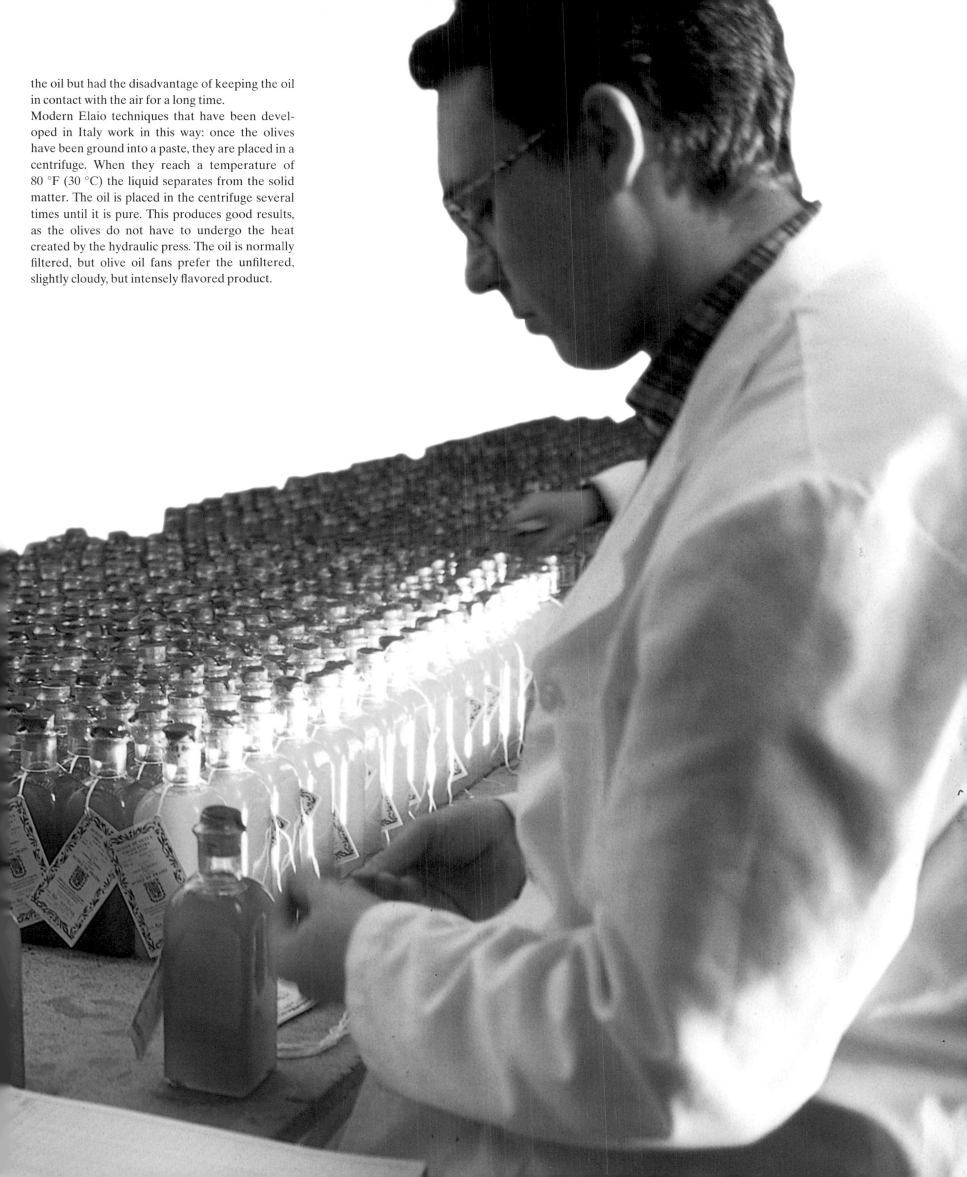

the oil but had the disadvantage of keeping the oil in contact with the air for a long time.

Modern Elaio techniques that have been developed in Italy work in this way: once the olives have been ground into a paste, they are placed in a centrifuge. When they reach a temperature of 80 °F (30 °C) the liquid separates from the solid matter. The oil is placed in the centrifuge several times until it is pure. This produces good results, as the olives do not have to undergo the heat created by the hydraulic press. The oil is normally filtered, but olive oil fans prefer the unfiltered, slightly cloudy, but intensely flavored product.

Naturally Fermented Vinegar

Vinegar has been known since ancient times, especially in regions with a mild climate, where vinegar occurred naturally. Wherever fluid that contained sugar began to ferment there were acetates "lurking" in the air. When yeast finally transformed the sugar in the liquid into alcohol, and the liquid was left to stand, the acetates started to work. The bacteria consumed the alcohol, leaving acetic acid behind. Our ancestors rarely drank pure wine, as it had generally transformed itself into vinegar. Vinegar was very popular in ancient times. It was diluted and drunk to quench the thirst, and used to season food. Soon people discovered that vinegar could be used to preserve meat, vegetables, and fruit.

But vinegar had even more uses. In olden days it was used to treat wounds and inflammation, and was recommended for chest and stomach complaints. Vinegar was put into dirty water to make it drinkable and was used for washing. The Greeks and Romans refined its culinary uses, mixing vinegar with herbs and spices, and used vinegar for medicinal purposes. In the Middle Ages it was a basic household ingredient and an important trading commodity. It was only in the 19th century that it was discovered how wine could be made into vinegar. The French chemist and biologist Louis Pasteur (1822–1895) discovered acetate and this led him to investigate microorganisms during fermentation which explained how wine and vinegar could be made.

It was quite difficult to make vinegar. Often unpleasant smells were produced or the liquid went moldy. There was a great demand for vinegar so Pasteur's discovery was seized upon by vinegar producers. It was then discovered that vinegar could be made in large barrels, provided that they were kept at the right temperature for the acetic acid to take effect and that there was enough air for fermentation to take place. Sometimes bacteria are grown and mixed in with the wine so that fermentation can take place within 24–36 hours. Sometimes, industrial acetic acid is simply diluted.

Good quality and organic vinegars are always fermented in the traditional way. When the first alcoholic fermentation has taken place, the fruit or grape wine is poured into open, or well-aired barrels, often containing a starter of acetic acid. The bacteria in the air ensure that the vinegar fermentation takes place by attacking the surface of the wine. The quality of the vinegar depends

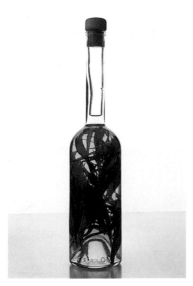

Tarragon – white wine vinegar

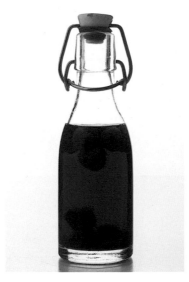

Raspberry – red wine vinegar

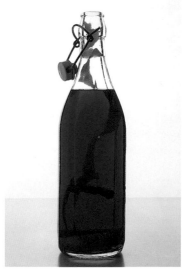

Orange – red wine vinegar with cinnamon and cloves

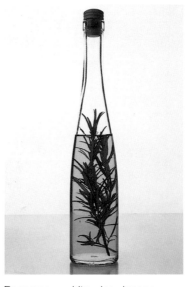

Plum – white wine vinegar

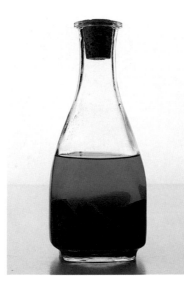

Rosemary – white wine vinegar

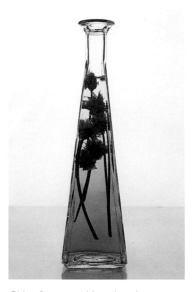

Chive flower – white wine vinegar

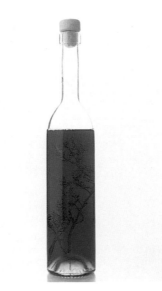

Thyme – red wine vinegar

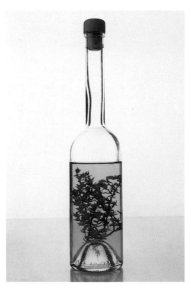

Thyme – white wine vinegar

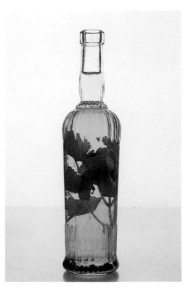

Lemon balm – white wine vinegar

very much on the quality of the wine to start with. This also applies to the nutritional content of the vinegar. Old wooden barrels that contain a natural oxidant but no tannin improve the bouquet and the flavor of the finished product. Old, traditionally fermented vinegars are a rarity today. For whole food nutrition, only high quality, naturally produced vinegars made from organically grown fruits should be consumed. These are the different types of vinegar:

• Fruit vinegar: made from fruit juice, the most popular being apple vinegar. Mild in flavor, when sweetened with honey, it makes a good medicine. Real fruit vinegars are sometimes confused with fruit flavored vinegar.

• Real wine vinegar: made from red or white wine, the flavor of the vinegar depends on the age and quality of the wine. Extremely versatile and the basis for seasoned vinegars. In many European countries the term vinegar is reserved for wine vinegars. This is not the case in England or Germany.

• Seasoned vinegars: these should be made from wine vinegar, which has had spices, herbs, fruits or fruit juices added. Depending on the additional ingredients these are known as herb or fruit flavored vinegar. The flavoring limits their culinary uses.

• Balsamic vinegar: from Modena, in Italy, comes *aceto balsamico tradizionale* or *naturale,* a vinegar made from juice that has been fermented over several years and further aged in wooden barrels before it is used. It is a precious, very expensive seasoning that is also used medicinally. It is usually about 12 years old and is normally sold in small $3^1/_2$ fluid ounce (100 ml) bottles. Many Balsamic vinegars on sale are not *naturale* or *traditionale* but just imitations.

• Vinegar seasoning: home made vinegar often does not have the 5% acid content that it is required to have by law and is known as vinegar seasoning. This also applies to rice vinegar, Genmai Su and the red Ume Su which is a by-product of the fermentation of Umeboshi, a paste made from the Japanese salted apricot.

How to Use Vinegar

Vinegar belongs in the hand of a wise man – so says an Italian proverb. A sensible amount of vinegar can add sophistication and flavor to a dish, but too much can ruin it. When using flavored vinegars it is important to consider if the flavor of the vinegar will overpower that of the dish. When using pure, naturally fermented vinegars it is important to familiarize oneself with the flavor, acidity, and strength of the vinegar before using it in a recipe. Vinegar is an essential flavor enhancer and a subtle seasoning.

Vinegar can be used in hundreds of dishes:
• in salads and raw vegetable dishes with cold-pressed oil,
• in small quantities in soups and sauces,
• in legume dishes,
• to prevent vegetables oxidizing,
• in cold marinades with oil and herbs or spices for vegetables, meat, and fish,
• to preserve and pickle vegetables, when thinned with water and seasoned with herbs,
• mixed with oil, to preserve goat's cheese and other fresh cheeses,
• as a piquant addition to chutneys and tasty spreads,
• a few drops added to fresh fruit salads,
• in juice or water as a refreshing drink.

Aromatic Vinegars

Fruit Vinegar

11–14 oz (300–400 g) fruit
3³/₄ cups (750 ml) white wine vinegar

Take the fruit, which can be raspberries, cherries, black currants, strawberries, blueberries etc, wash and dry it well. Remove any pits and cut in half. Place in a screw top jar, fill with vinegar and put the lid on the jar. Leave to macerate for at least 4 weeks. Filter the vinegar and decant into a bottle.
Fruit vinegar is very good sprinkled over fruit salad.

Herb Vinegar

Several sprigs of fresh herbs
3³/₄ cups (750 ml) white wine vinegar

Put about three sprigs of herbs (for instance tarragon) into a bottle of white wine vinegar, close it and leave to macerate for at least 4 weeks; then filter it.
Many herbs are suitable for herb vinegar. It is a good idea to make small quantities of individual types of herb vinegars. Use them in salad dressings and sauces.

Garlic Vinegar

12 garlic cloves
3³/₄ cups (750 ml) white wine vinegar

Peel and halve the garlic cloves. Place in the vinegar and leave to macerate for at least 4 weeks. Filter. Very good for deglazing and making sauces and mayonnaise.

Vinegar – Homemade

Even those who like wine rarely empty every bottle. There is a very good use for the left overs – turn them into home made vinegar.
You will need:
• about 10–15 cups (2–3 liters) wine,
• a large glass container with a wide neck,
• a large piece of gauze or muslin to cover the container,
• a long piece of string or a rubber band to secure the gauze,
• 2–3 bottles naturally fermented vinegar.
To make vinegar, pour the wine into the container and leave it uncovered by a sunny window. If you live in a wine producing area, the wine will ferment by itself, as there are acetates in the air. When there is a lot of sunlight, warmth, and oxygen, the wine will ferment quickly. It is important to ensure that the wine is not exposed to too much heat. The acetate likes warmth, but should not be exposed to temperatures over 99 °F (37 °C). After a few days, cover the container with the gauze and secure it well. The time of year will determine how quickly fermentation occurs. After about 14 days, the surface of the wine will become covered with a layer of vinegar. The top layer needs to be left for a while until it has destroyed all the alcohol. The vinegar is ready for use after about three months. To ensure that fermentation takes place in areas where wine is not made, it is advisable to add naturally produced vinegar to the wine. It is best to use unfiltered vinegar for this purpose, which has residue in the bottom of the bottle. It is also advisable to use organic wine that has a low sulfur content and has not been pasteurized.
The quality of the vinegar depends on the quality of the wine or wines that are used. Wine that has been fermented in barriques – the name given to the 59 gallon (225 liter) casks – or wines that are high in tannins are not as suitable for making vinegar as a fruity young wine. Vinegar that has a high tannin content is very acidic when first made and should be used sparingly. Vinegar is much better for ageing, so it is as well to have a small oak barrel for this purpose.
When the vinegar is no longer required, tip away the bottom of the vinegar and retain the film on the top. It is good to use a barrel with a tap on it for this purpose. The film can be used as a starter for later batches of vinegar, and will keep for about a year.

A Pinch of Sun, Wind, and Sea

Atlantic Salt

There is so much salt in the ocean that if it were dried it could cover the earth in a layer of salt 120 feet (37 meters) thick. Salt used to be such a rare commodity, and so difficult to obtain, that it became extremely precious. Salt was often the motive for the conquest of other lands and there were salt routes to the most inaccessible places. Salt trading led to contact with other cultures and thus to the exchange of knowledge. Salt is not only a valuable seasoning and preserving ingredient but is used to make enamel and soap, and is invaluable for the tanning industry and for alchemists.

Salt is mined from large rock salt supplies, from salt springs or from sea water. Rock salt is almost pure sodium chloride, whereas sea salt is made up of about 80 different salts, minerals, and trace elements. Mined rock salt is not a living substance, which is why sea salt (also known as coarse salt) is used in wholefood cookery.

Sea salt in Europe is taken from the Atlantic coasts of Portugal, France, and Spain. 83 percent of French Atlantic sea salt is obtained on the Guérande peninsula in southern Brittany. The salt works stretch over 5,000 acres (2,000 hectares). The Romans discovered the salt supplies there and evidence from three wells shows that they used it to make Garum, a spicy sauce made from pickled fish.

Since the 9th century or earlier, salt has been obtained from there in the same way, just as the special architecture of the salt gardens, five of which were made under the rule of Charlemagne, have hardly changed, and are still in use. There is a system of canals and lakes that were dug in the flat clay soil. A complicated system enables the salt farmer, the *paludier*, to let fresh sea water into the lakes every two weeks when there is a high tide. The water is collected in a deep pool, a *vasière*, in which the salt farmer opens a *trappe* – a large gate. Many salt reserves are formed from the 4–16 inch (10–40 centimeter) pool which contains many impurities. In the summer, evaporation begins. $1^3/_4$ pints (1 liter) sea water contains about $1^1/_5$ ounces (34 grams) salt. Over the summer it becomes more concentrated – to about $1^1/_2$ ounces (40 grams). In the salt pond, the *corbier*, the salt content is about 2 ounces (50 grams) as the water clarifies. The water travels through a watercourse, the *tour d'eau*, into the precise system of lakes, the *fards,* that are only $1^3/_4$–2 inches (4–5 centimeters) deep. Through the heat of the sun, the water temperature rises to 81 °F (32 °C). The water is contained in the rivers, held in by a series of dams. This speeds up evaporation. With the salt content now at 7 ounces (200 grams) per $1^3/_4$ pints (1 liter) or 20° Beaumé, the water flows out of the final *fard* into the *adernes*. These lakes hold the daily supply of salt solution for the *oeillets.* They are just over $1/_4$ inch ($1/_2$ centimeter) deep in the middle and about 83 square yards (70 square meters) in size and it is here that the salt crystallizes. Every day during the salt harvest – which begins in June and ends in September – the *paludier* pushes the contents of the lake to one side with a long rake. The harvest consists of large, gray, irregular crystals. On the surface of the lake fine white crystals settle, from the water which now contains 11–14 ounces salt (250– 300 grams) per $1^3/_4$ pint (1 liter). These crystals are known as salt flower, the top quality salt, the *fleur du sel,* and are the best salt available.

Paludiers have the same status as farmers. In a large salt works there are about 60 *oeillets* from which about 1.3 tonnes (1.43 tons) of salt are produced. The salt farmer is busy all year round, keeping the lakes clean and maintained, regulating the water or harvesting the salt. The salt harvest depends on the summer weather; it can double in a good year or reduce by a half or more in bad weather. Sea, sun, and wind are the three ingredients for a good harvest. Good airy surroundings keep away pollution in a natural way. Apart from grinding, the salt requires no more attention and is ready to be packaged and sold.

Background: In the salt gardens of Guérande, a *paludier* is pushing the crystallized salt on the surface carefully to the edge of the pool.

Salt and Health

Salt, sodium chloride, is essential for human life. It is a component of body tissues and regulates the bodily fluids. We excrete $1/_{10}$–$1/_8$ ounce (3–5 grams) of salt every day, so we should aim to replace the same quantity every day. Salt is contained naturally in many foods, so we consume the right quantity without having to add salt to our food. Too much salt is not good for the health, as it can lead to high blood pressure. The Japanese, known for their large salt intake, have a considerably higher rate of hypertension than other nations. Hypertension can lead to heart disease and strokes. It is not so much the salt that we use to season foods that is the danger, as hidden salts. Milk products, cheeses, biscuits, breads, preserved vegetables, and olives, smoked and pickled fish, sausage, and hams contain huge amounts of hidden salt. The "record holder" for hidden salt is that seasoning loved by wholefood recipes – soysauce.

To season food, the best salt to use is the magnesium rich complex natural product – sea salt, with its special flavor. Apart from seasoning foods it can be used for gargling, inhalations, dental care, baths, and foot baths as well as to disinfect wounds.

Composition of the Coarse Salt from Guérande*

Moisture	6.75 %	Magnesium	0.71 %
Insoluble		Sodium	35.20 %
matter	0.34 %	Copper	2.5 mg/kg
Sulfates	1.90 %	Zinc	5.0 mg/kg
Chloride	54.50 %	Manganese	6.8 mg/kg
Potassium	0.20 %	Iron	85.0 mg/kg
Calcium	0.12 %	Iodine	trace

* As analyzed by the Loire Atlantique Field Studies Station

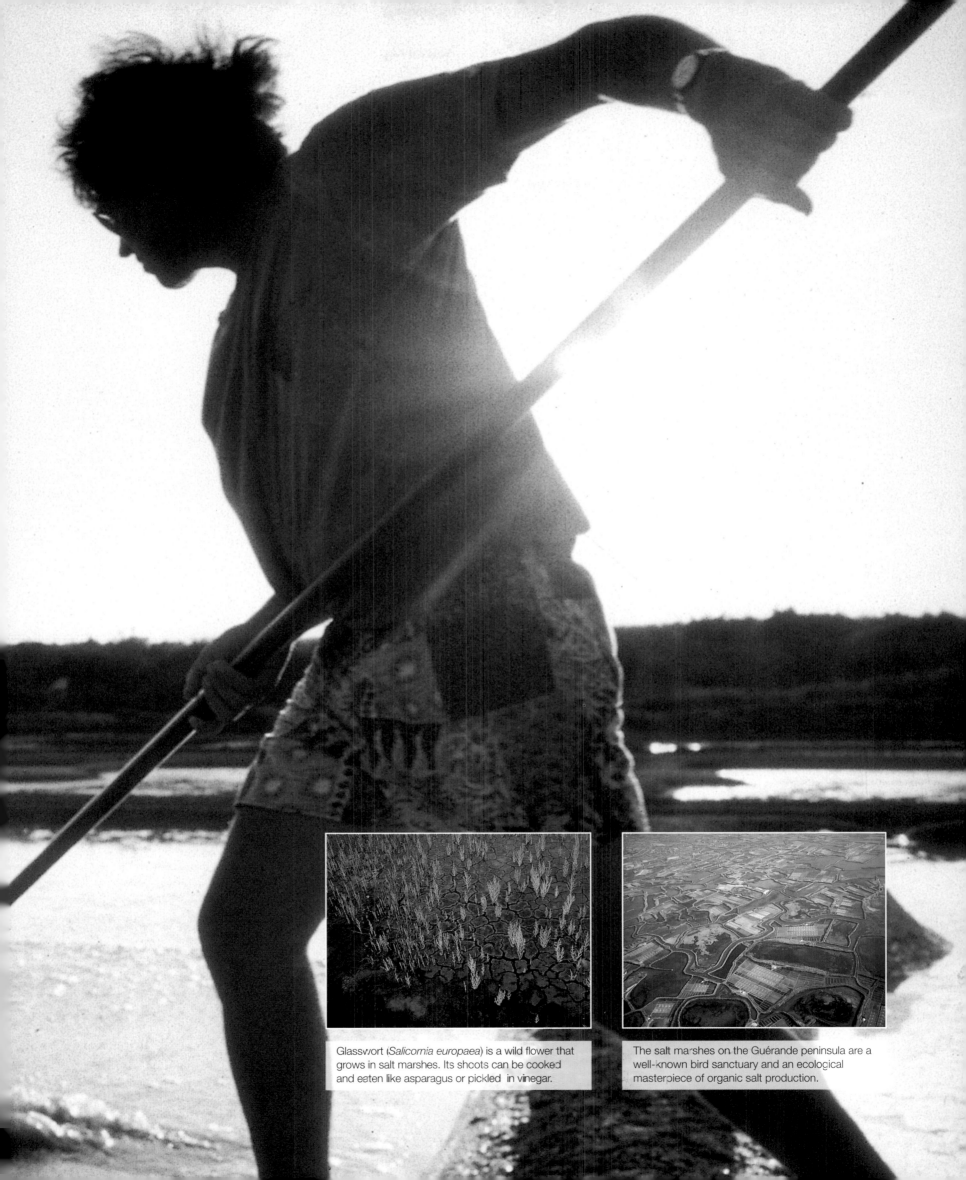

Glasswort (*Salicornia europaea*) is a wild flower that grows in salt marshes. Its shoots can be cooked and eaten like asparagus or pickled in vinegar.

The salt marshes on the Guérande peninsula are a well-known bird sanctuary and an ecological masterpiece of organic salt production.

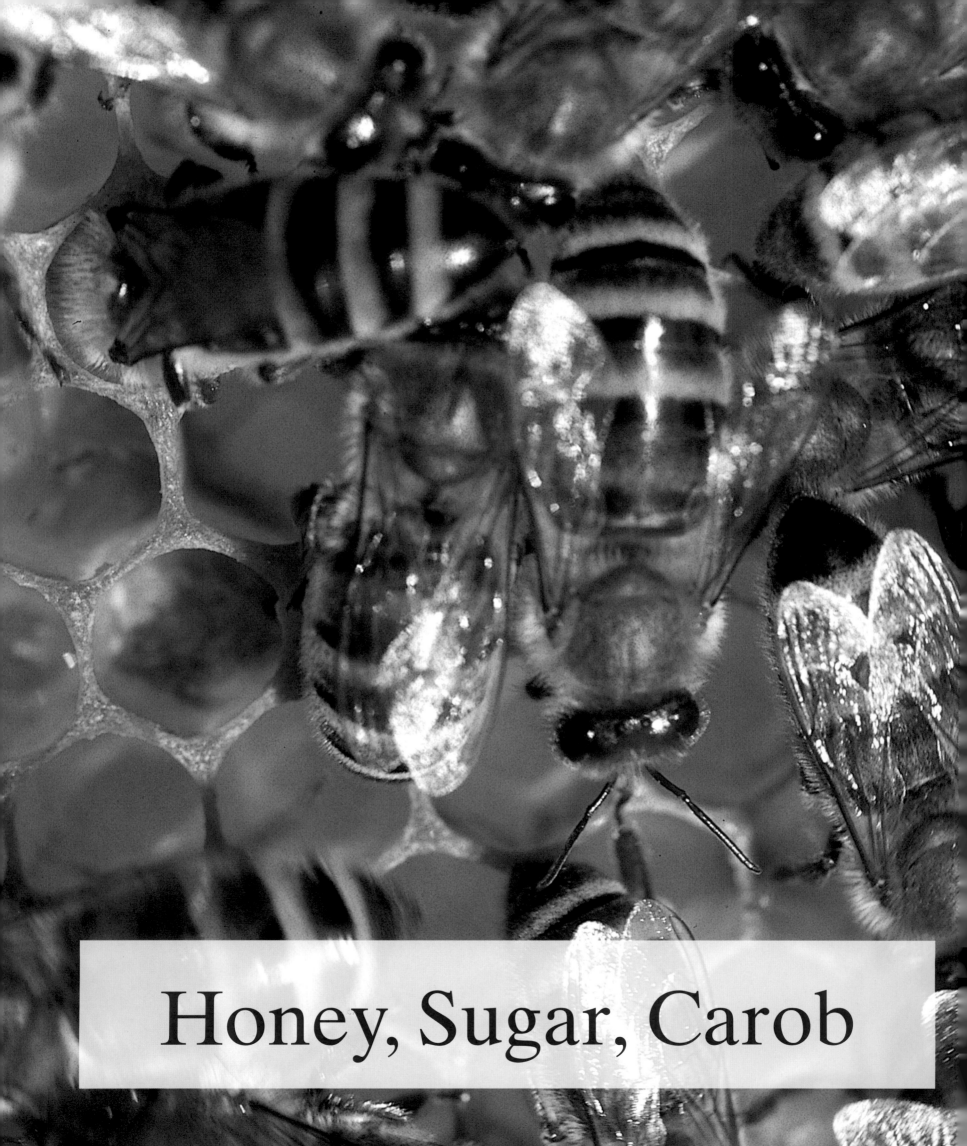

Honey, Sugar, Carob

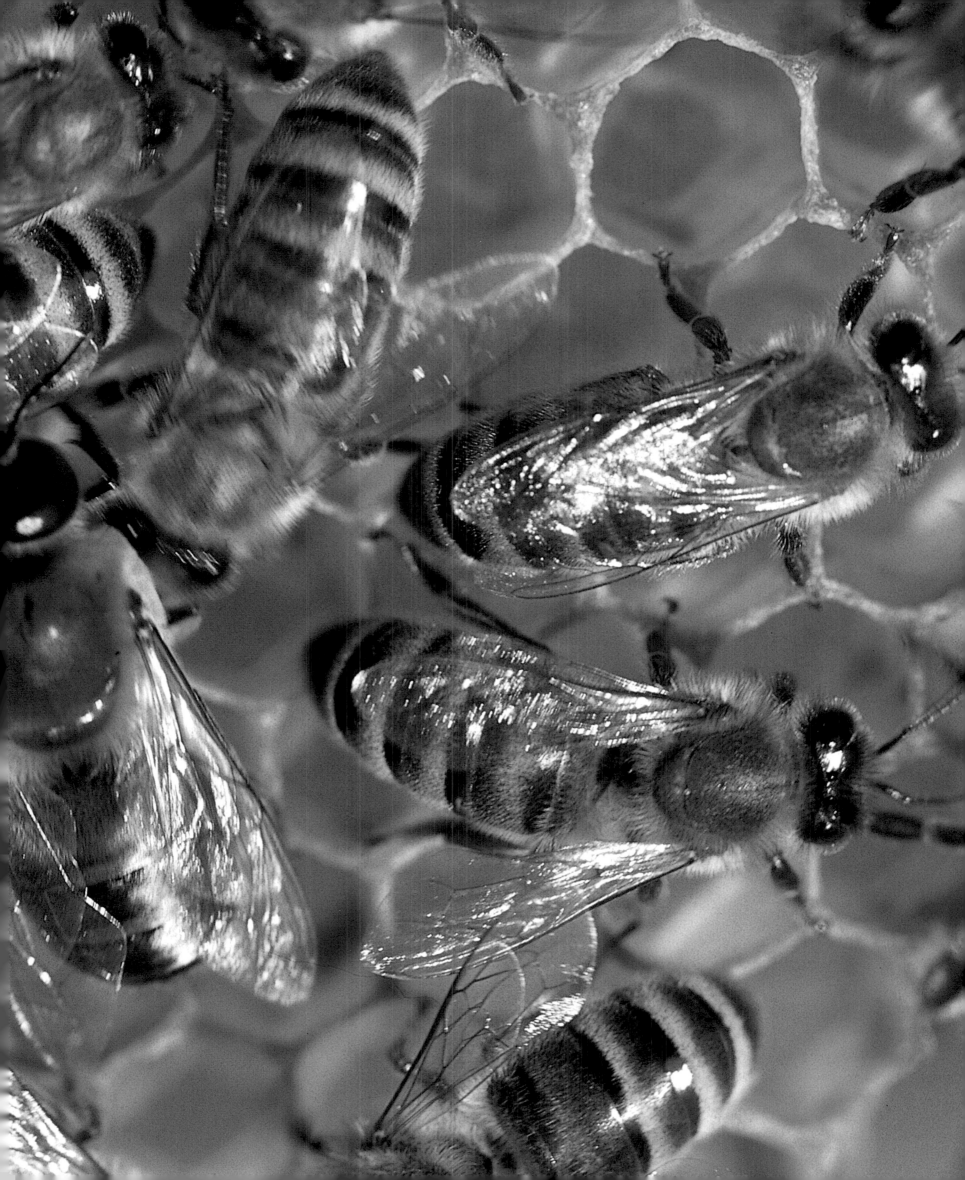

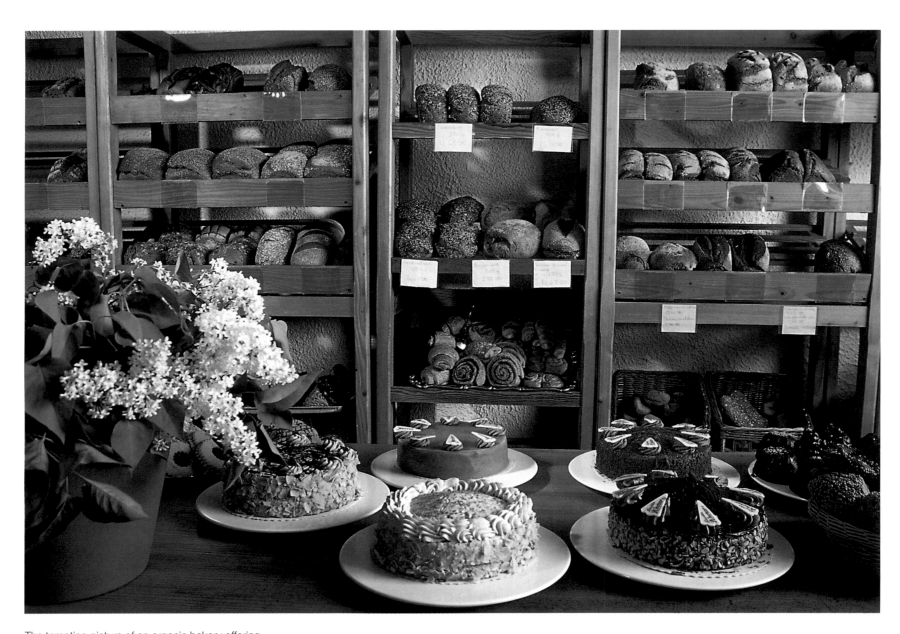

The tempting picture of an organic bakery offering
gateaux, flans, cakes, and cookies, all sweetened with
honey and fruit juice concentrates. Carob is used
instead of chocolate and cocoa.

Previous double page: The industrious worker bees are
filling the cells with honey, which they have converted in
their bodies from flower nectar or honeydew.

Bees have a hard time of it. In large areas of Europe the great wealth of plants that used to grow there have been driven out by monotonous industrial agriculture, as well as by chemical pollution. The decline in natural flora has had an adverse effect on the bee population. Because of the lack of flora, and the pollution of the environment, these insects have decreased in numbers – insects which play an important part in the food chain, as they are responsible for the pollination of many types of flower. Without bees, many varieties of fruit and flowers would simply not exist. For this reason it is commendable that so many bee keepers have made a great effort over the last decade to give bees the respect they are due. The fact that honey has improved in quality is reward enough for showing more restraint towards nature. Nutritionists advise people to only eat honey in small amounts, and to avoid sugar completely. No other food causes such heated debate, although there is plenty of evidence to suggest that sugar is a cause of many diseases. Sugar is concealed in many different foods: baby drinks, breakfast cereals, coffee whitener, jellies, ice cream, fruit yogurts, fruit drinks, ketchup, and sauces, even in sausages and bread and many other types of food. Eternally popular cookies and candy, that people nibble on in their free time, ensure that we consume far more sugar (and calories) than are good for us. It is unfair to expect people to give up sweet treats completely and it is possible to make delicious candies using ingredients from wholefood stores. These can be eaten (almost) without guilt. Organic bakeries create delicacies that allow us to enjoy sweet foods without worrying that they are doing us harm. Wholefood cookery relies on people changing their eating habits and experimenting with new flavors. A little sweetness goes a long way.

A Gift of the Gods

Honey

Just as animal farming techniques have become industrialized over the last fifty years, bee keeping methods have altered to keep up with the times. To increase honey production, forward-thinking bee keepers have made new discoveries about the natural cycle of the bee population. It is possible to put ready made honeycomb into the hive, contain swarms, breed artificial queen bees, and to use artificial fertilization. Bee breeding has been endangered by the Varroa mite, which causes a disease that infects the whole population. Instead of researching the causes of the mite, conventional bee keepers simply eradicate the mite using chemicals, which naturally increases the amount of residue in the honey.

To produce honey that has no residue requires special bee keeping techniques. Bees are raised in accordance with guidelines set down by organic agriculture. In the case of bees – which are communal insects – each bee should be treated as an individual. Bees have very particular behavior patterns and have a strict division of labor within their community.

The queen is responsible for producing and raising the new bees, laying some 1,200 eggs every day.

• Five to eight drones (who have no stingers) are allowed to fertilize the queen when she is ready to conceive. They are then killed in the "drone abattoir."

• The worker bees build the hive in which the summer bees carry out a range of different duties during their six-week lives. They feed the queen, the drones, and the brood, and build hexagonal chambers using wax that they produce from a special gland. These chambers hold the eggs, pollen, and honey. As well as these duties, the worker bees bring pollen and plant resin – known as propolis – into the hive.

When the first spring flowers appear, the bees' new life begins. The bees bring food, the queen lays eggs, drones appear, the hive grows until there are up to 50,000 inhabitants. A new queen is raised, fed on special food, the old queen swarms, taking some of the bees with her, and sets up a new hive.

Organic bee keeping is based on the philosophy that the bee keeper allows the bees their freedom to reproduce naturally, and to build their own honeycomb. For this purpose he provides a custom-made frame on which the bees can build their honeycomb. This means that all the honeycombs are the bees' own work and the honeycomb is the right size to meet the bees' demands. This ensures that the bee keeper will have beeswax of the highest quality.

The bee keeper intervenes when the bees begin to swarm. Just before the old queen leaves the hive, the bee keeper removes her and divides up the bee population. This is entirely different to the process of artificial fertilization and artificial breeding mentioned earlier. Natural methods produce new queens without resorting to complicated techniques. To combat the Varroa mite organically, natural acids are used, like lactic or formic acid. These acids occur naturally in honey. When the bee keeper extracts the honey from the honeycomb, he leaves some honey behind in the breeding chamber. During the late summer and fall the bee population decreases its numbers to between 15,000 and 20,000. Finally breeding takes place and the bees cluster themselves together for the winter. The winter bees live from September through April or May of the following year. After the final honey collection, the bee keeper increases the winter food supply by adding a mixture of honey, sugar, herbal tea, and salt.

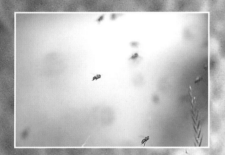

Bee hives can be placed in a field, so that the bees have direct access to nectar from flowers.

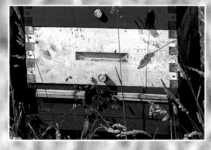

With impressive speed the bees swarm out of the hive to collect food for the colony.

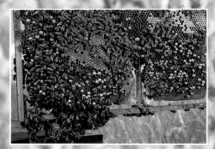

In organic bee keeping, the frames are large enough to allow the bees plenty of room to build their nests.

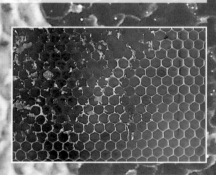

Summer bees spend half of their six-week lives filling the combs with honey.

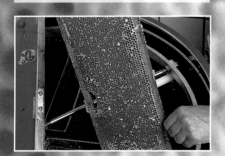

The frames with honeycombs are placed in the extractor; they are rarely sold as honeycomb.

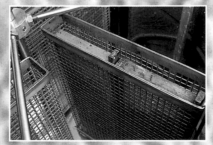

Honey comes out of the wax chambers when it is rotated in the drum.

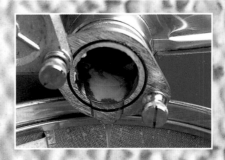

The honey passes through a filter, which removes any impurities.

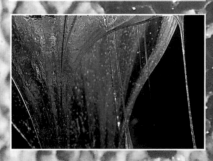

Honey contains 20 different types of sugars and 180 other substances, including enzymes and hormones.

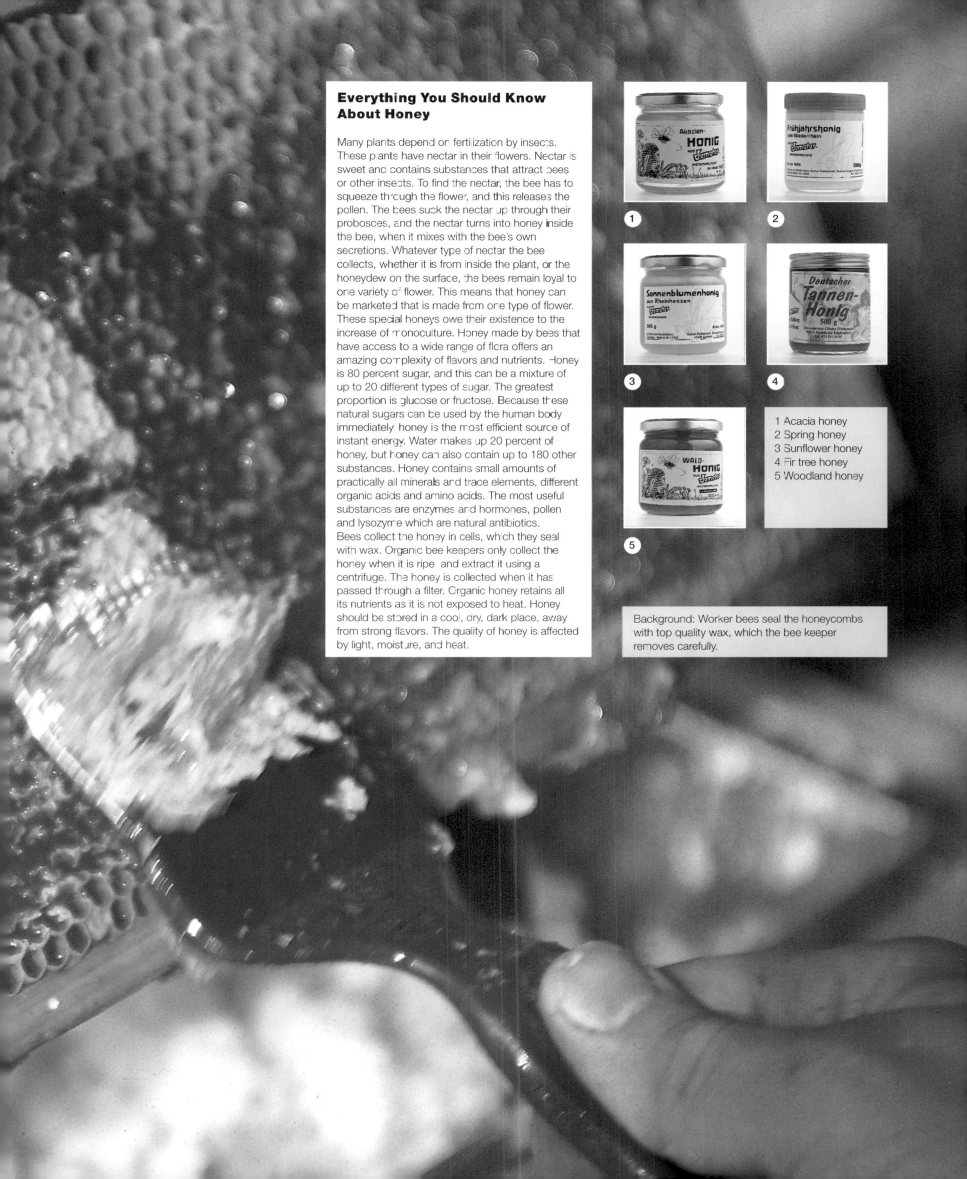

Everything You Should Know About Honey

Many plants depend on fertilization by insects. These plants have nectar in their flowers. Nectar is sweet and contains substances that attract bees or other insects. To find the nectar, the bee has to squeeze through the flower, and this releases the pollen. The bees suck the nectar up through their proboscis, and the nectar turns into honey inside the bee, when it mixes with the bee's own secretions. Whatever type of nectar the bee collects, whether it is from inside the plant, or the honeydew on the surface, the bees remain loyal to one variety of flower. This means that honey can be marketed that is made from one type of flower. These special honeys owe their existence to the increase of monoculture. Honey made by bees that have access to a wide range of flora offers an amazing complexity of flavors and nutrients. Honey is 80 percent sugar, and this can be a mixture of up to 20 different types of sugar. The greatest proportion is glucose or fructose. Because these natural sugars can be used by the human body immediately, honey is the most efficient source of instant energy. Water makes up 20 percent of honey, but honey can also contain up to 180 other substances. Honey contains small amounts of practically all minerals and trace elements, different organic acids and amino acids. The most useful substances are enzymes and hormones, pollen and lysozyme which are natural antibiotics.

Bees collect the honey in cells, which they seal with wax. Organic bee keepers only collect the honey when it is ripe and extract it using a centrifuge. The honey is collected when it has passed through a filter. Organic honey retains all its nutrients as it is not exposed to heat. Honey should be stored in a cool, dry, dark place, away from strong flavors. The quality of honey is affected by light, moisture, and heat.

1 Acacia honey
2 Spring honey
3 Sunflower honey
4 Fir tree honey
5 Woodland honey

Background: Worker bees seal the honeycombs with top quality wax, which the bee keeper removes carefully.

Sugar

Life without sugar would be unthinkable. Sugar is the product of photosynthesis: plants create sugar by means of a reaction between sunlight, the chlorophyll in their leaves, the carbon dioxide in the air, and the water in the ground. Sugar is also known as carbohydrate. There are simple sugars, that are made up of a single molecule, like glucose and fructose and disaccharides (two-molecule sugars). Sugars that are made up of two molecules are sucrose, maltose, and lactose. Sucrose consists of one glucose molecule and one fructose molecule. Sucrose is the same as refined white sugar. Starch is made of a combination of different sugar molecules, as is cellulose, which cannot be digested by the human body. These are polysaccharides, or complex sugars.

Carbohydrates have to be transformed into simple sugars for the body to metabolize, for it is only in this simple form that they can be absorbed into the bloodstream. Other substances are needed for this process: vitamins, minerals, enzymes, and hormones. Cereals, vegetables, and fruits naturally contain these nutrients, so the natural sugars in these foods are quickly absorbed by the body. When refined sugar is obtained from natural sources, the nutrients are removed. The body, however, needs vitamin B1 to process sugar.

Refined sugar, that is derived from sugar cane or sugar beet, consists almost entirely of sucrose. It is not only used in home cookery, but is concealed in a large number of mass-produced foods: Lemonade, fruit drinks, chocolate, candy, bread, cakes, desserts, ice creams, compotes, breakfast cereals, snacks, and jellies all contain large quantities of sugar. On average, western Europeans consume about 100 pounds (45 kilograms) of sugar per person every year. This means that many children eat more than their body weight in sugar. Because so many vitamins – especially vitamin B1 – are required to process such large quantities of sugar, excessive sugar consumption can lead to an imbalance of nutrients in the body. This imbalance in turn leads to diet-related diseases like obesity, diabetes, and stomach and digestive disorders. Scientists have long been warning people that sugar consumption may lead to life-threatening diseases like cancer, heart attacks, and arteriosclerosis.

High sugar consumption has other serious effects on the body: when the blood sugar level rises very quickly, the pancreas reacts by producing large quantities of insulin. This turns the sugar into insulin, and leads to a low blood sugar level – known as hypoglycemia. The symptoms of hypoglycemia are low concentration span, tiredness, and inability to work. Extensive research into the effect of sugar on the teeth has shown that eating

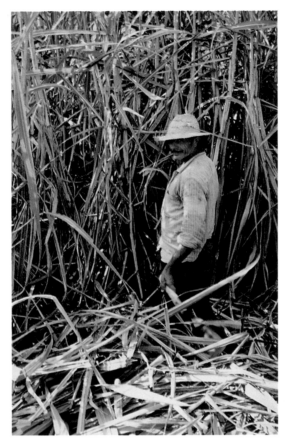

Harvesting sugar cane with a machete is a technique that has to be learnt. The leaves and stalks are cut away, while the rhizome must be left intact.

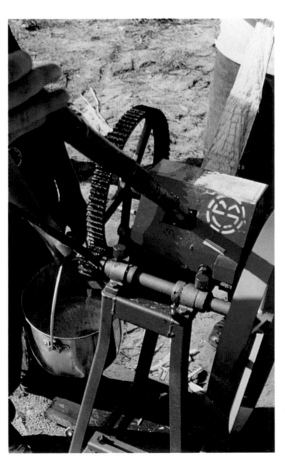

This small press demonstrates how the juice is extracted from the cane. Large presses work on the same principle.

sugar produces bacteria in the mouth which form an acid that attacks the tooth enamel. This leaves a fissure in the tooth, which makes the inside of the tooth decay. Tribes who eat no sugar, have no caries.

Wholefood cookery advises against the use of refined sugar. Refined sugar is an umbrella term for household sugar, which is known as granulated, superfine, lump, cane, beet, and white sugar. Other types of sugar claim to be different, but have the same chemical structure: these are preserving sugar, confectioners' sugar, sugar crystals, and rock candy. "Raw sugar" is no different, having simply been given a dash of molasses to change its color.

A Short History of Sugar

Man has always had a sweet tooth. Concentrated sugar was, however, a rarity, existing only as honey. From all the sweet tasting fruits and vegetables, one was discovered that was far sweeter than the rest – the sugar cane. It grew in Polynesia. The Indians discovered a way to concentrate the sweetness of the plant by boiling it. In the Persian empire, this technique was developed further and the Moors took this method with them to Spain. In the Middle Ages, the merchants in Venice made their fortune trading in spices, and sugar was considered to be a spice. When America was discovered, the West Indies became the main producers, and millions of slaves worked in the sugar plantations. Sugar remained, both there and in Europe, one of the most valuable commodities and created huge profits. This all changed at the beginning of the 19th century when sugar beet was first grown on a large scale in Germany. Sugar beet processing – developed by the German chemist Franz Carl Achard (1753–1821) – was seized upon by the rest of Europe and became a large industry. A small revolution occurred: sugar, which had once been a luxury and an expensive delicacy, now had the status of a basic foodstuff. Nowadays, the yearly sugar production world wide is more than 110 million tons (100 million tonnes).

Using Sweeteners in the Wholefood Kitchen

Whatever form it comes in, large or small quantities, concentrated or not, sugar is always an unhealthy food. The fact that people are conditioned to like highly sweetened flavors is a disadvantage to the enjoyment of natural products. Refined sugar, or sugar substitutes, have no place in wholefood nutrition. Sugar should never be eaten in conjunction with whole cereals or raw food as it causes problems with digestion. If it is necessary to sweeten foods, do so with discretion, even when using the "healthy" sweeteners below.

• Fruit: in fruit salads, granola, or with milk products. Ripe fruits contain so much natural sugar that no additional sweetener is required. Fruit is a healthy sweet.

• Dried fruits: add a gentle sweetness to many recipes. Dried fruits should not be eaten in excessive quantities as overconsumption can lead to caries.

• Honey: when organically produced it is the one natural sweetener that has a large quantity of nutrients and simple sugars. These nutrients are sensitive to heat, so honey should not be heated or poured over hot foods. Honey should be used sparingly.

• Apple and pear concentrate: made from the evaporation of fruit juice, they contain simple sugars and more nutrients than are present in sugar. It is advisable to buy organic apple and pear concentrate. Use very sparingly.

• Sugar beet syrup: made by steaming or boiling the beet. This should be bought from an organic supplier. Contains many vitamins and minerals but is over 60% sugar. Use very sparingly.

• Whole cane sugar: made from thickened cane syrup and contains high quantities of potassium, magnesium, phosphorus, and iron as well as vitamins B1, B2, and B6, niacin, and panthenoic acid. It does have a high sucrose content and should be used very sparingly.

• Maple syrup: comes from wild growing maple trees in Canada. An alternative that is rich in minerals, but does not make ecological sense because of the waste of energy the syrup making incurs. Once opened maple syrup will keep for a few weeks in the refrigerator. Use very sparingly.

• Eco sugar: refined sugar made from organic sugar beet. Differs from regular household sugar only in that the beets are organically grown. Not recommended.

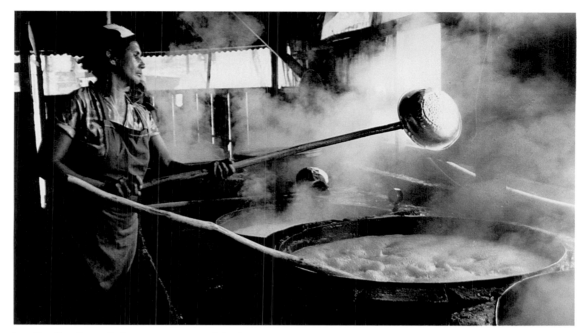

In a Brazilian Fazenda the raw sugar cane juice is put into large vats where it is thickened. The vats are heated by compressed residues.

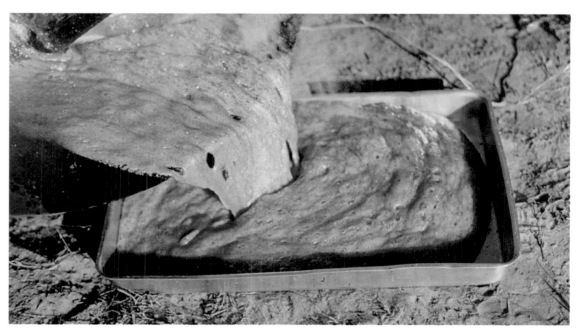

Earlier, the sugar was poured into molds and sold by the block. Today it is sold once it has been finely ground.

Sugar Cane

Despite the large numbers of sugar beet plantations in Europe, they account for only a third of all sugar production. The other two-thirds is provided by sugar cane. Brazil is one of the top sugar cane growers. In the mid 1980s, the first organic sugar cane plantations were set up. Since then, the trend has been to plant beans with the cane. Sugar cane consumes a lot of nutrients from the soil, and cattle manure helps to fertilize the soil and increase the harvests.

In a good year the reed-like plants will grow to heights of 13–23 feet (4–7 meters). The stalks have a diameter of 2 inches (5 centimeters). The canes are harvested from May through September, by which time they will have formed thick fluids in their sap.

The sugar canes are carefully trimmed, taking care not to damage the rhizome as the canes should last for 4 or 5 years in the same fields. All leaves and tips should be removed. Once it has been cleaned, the sugar cane is pressed in three stages. The juice is filtered and cleaned with a small amount of chalk, then it is boiled until it forms a syrup. The leftover foliage or "Bagasse" is used to fuel the large vats in which the syrup is cooked. The sugar syrup is cooked until it crystalizes. Originally it was made into blocks called "Rapadura" and sold in the shops in its block form. Today the terms "rapadura", "supersweet", or "succanat" refer to whole raw sugar. Whole raw sugar is made from unrefined thickened sugar cane syrup.

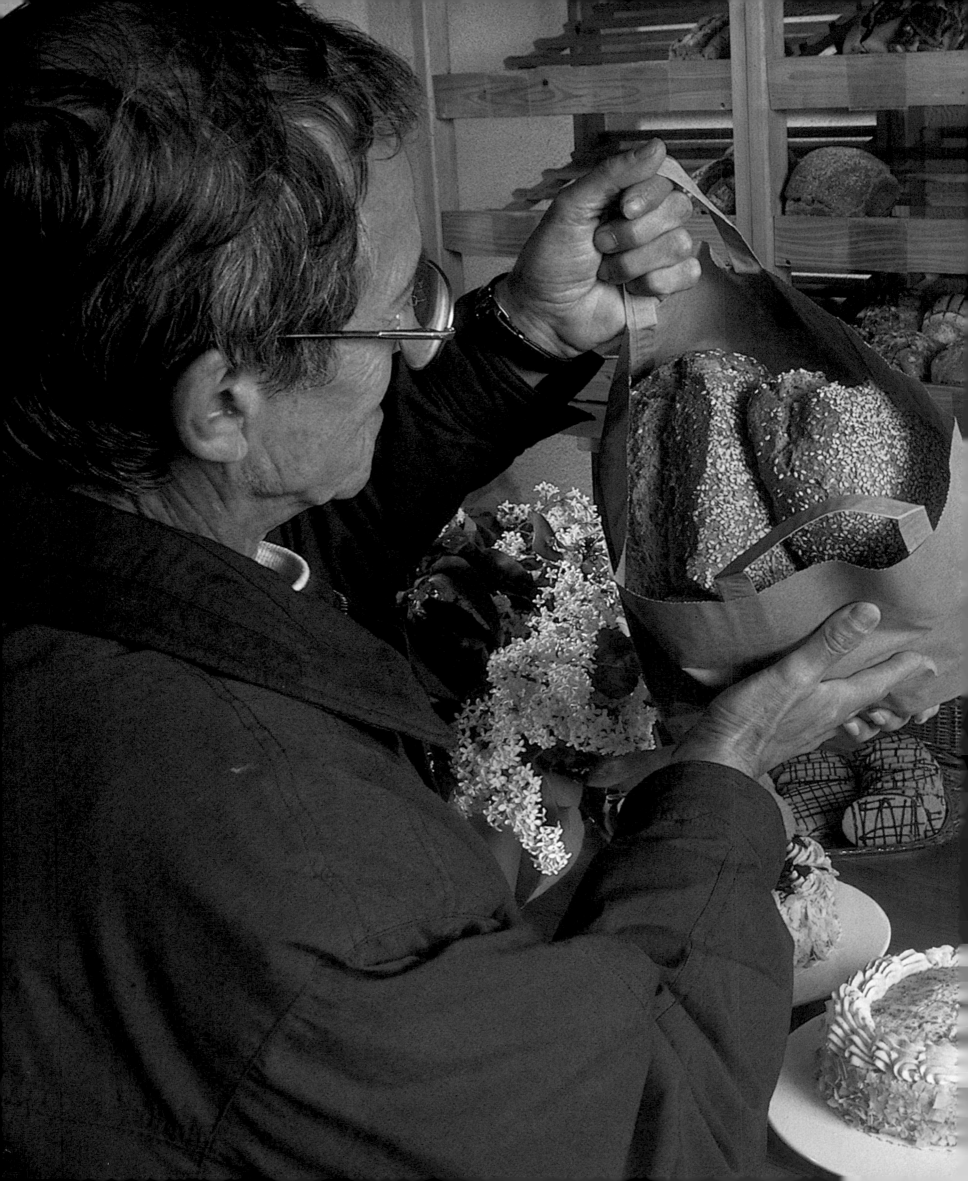

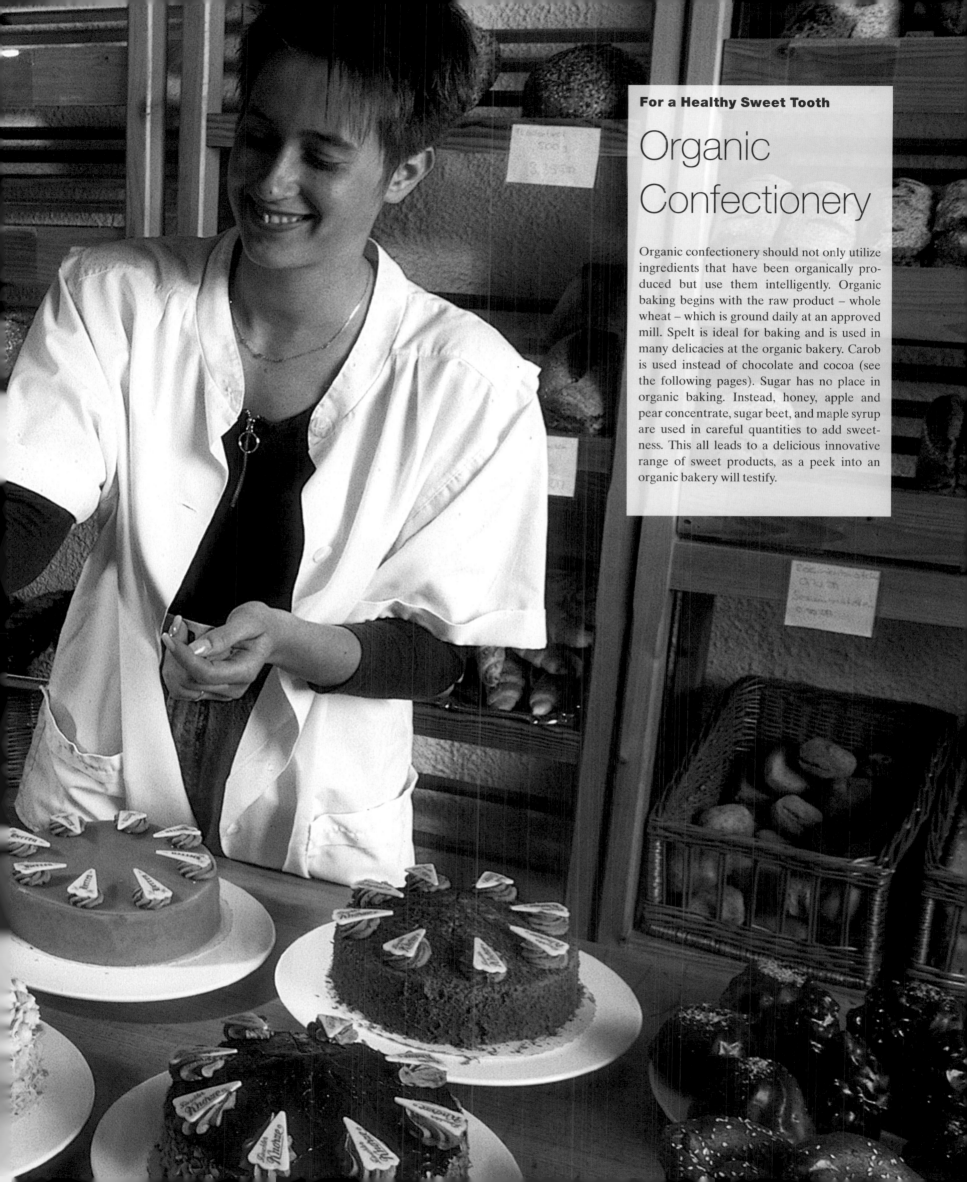

Organic Confectionery

Organic confectionery should not only utilize ingredients that have been organically produced but use them intelligently. Organic baking begins with the raw product – whole wheat – which is ground daily at an approved mill. Spelt is ideal for baking and is used in many delicacies at the organic bakery. Carob is used instead of chocolate and cocoa (see the following pages). Sugar has no place in organic baking. Instead, honey, apple and pear concentrate, sugar beet, and maple syrup are used in careful quantities to add sweetness. This all leads to a delicious innovative range of sweet products, as a peek into an organic bakery will testify.

For Spoiling and Enjoying
Cookies and Crackers

What would the most popular festival of the year be like without cookies and crackers to share with friends and relatives? What would childhood be like if one could not delve into the cookie jar? It would be a sad kitchen that never wafted the scent of freshly baked cookies around the house. Unfortunately our society has made these special treats, once reserved for the biggest event of the year, into everyday occurrences. It is not only the enjoyment of these treats that disappears with overindulgence, overconsumption of sweet foods is very bad for the health. With this in mind, it is not necessary to forego cookies and sweet things entirely, and it is permissible to enjoy the occasional sweet treat made from good quality ingredients. Spelt flour is often used for good reason (see p. 52), being especially suitable for baking.

Shortcrust Pastry Cookies

2 cups (250 g) fine spelt flour
5/8 cup (150 g) butter
2 Tbs honey
1/2 tsp vanilla extract
Zest of 1 lemon
1 egg (optional)

Mix all the ingredients together to make a dough.
Cover the dough and chill for at least 30 minutes.
Roll out the pastry until it is about 1/4 inch (5 mm) thick.
Cut out shapes using a variety of cookie cutters.
Preheat the oven to 350 °F (180 °C).
Put the cookies on a greased baking sheet and cook in the oven for about 20 minutes.
Place the cookies on a cooling tray and leave to cool.

Viennese Whirls

2/3 cup (175 g) butter
1 egg
2 Tbs honey
2 1/2 oz (75 g) ground almonds
1/2 tsp vanilla extract
2 cups (250 g) fine spelt flour

Beat together the butter, egg, and honey until they are creamy.
Add the vanilla, almonds, and flour and stir well to form a smooth mixture.
Preheat the oven to 340 °F (175 °C).
Put the mixture in a piping bag with a large nozzle and pipe the mixture into different shapes such as rings, stars, S-shapes, or pretzels onto a well-buttered baking tray.
Bake in the oven for 15 minutes.

Cinnamon Stars

3 egg whites
1/4 tsp vanilla extract
1 tsp ground cinnamon
2 cups (250 g) whole raw sugar
11 oz (300 g) ground almonds

Beat the egg whites until they are very stiff. Stir in the sugar and spice. Place a large cup of egg white mixture to one side, to decorate the cookies.
Preheat the oven to 340 °F (175 °C).
Stir the almonds into the egg white mixture. Roll out the pastry, cut out star shapes and spread with the reserved egg white. Bake for 30–40 minutes.

Aniseed Cookies

2 eggs
4 Tbs honey
1/2 tsp vanilla extract
1 2/3 cups (200 g) fine spelt flour
3 tsp aniseeds

Beat the eggs with the honey and vanilla until they have a creamy consistency. Stir in the aniseed and the flour and mix together well.
Using a teaspoon, make small heaps of cookie mixture on a well-buttered baking sheet. Flatten them slightly, cover and leave to dry out for about 6 hours.
Preheat the oven to 335 °F (170 °C).
Bake in the oven for 15 minutes.

Coconut Macaroons

2 egg whites
2 1/2 Tbs honey
Juice and zest of 1/2 lemon
6 oz (175 g) desiccated coconut
30 cookie papers of diameter 1 1/2 inches (4 cm)

Beat the egg whites until they are very stiff, stir in the honey, lemon zest and juice and mix in the coconut.
Chill the mixture for 2 hours.
Preheat the oven to 350 °F (180 °C).
Using a teaspoon, make small heaps of the mixture in the cookie papers. Bake for 10–15 minutes.

Heidesand

1 cup (250 g) butter
2 Tbs honey
1 tsp vanilla extract
Zest of 1 lemon
Pinch coarse salt
3 Tbs (45 ml) heavy cream
2 1/3 cups (300 g) spelt flour
Just over 1/2 cup (75 g) buckwheat flour
1 tsp baking powder

Brown the butter and leave to cool. Beat the honey, vanilla, lemon zest, salt, and cream with the melted butter until it becomes foamy. Mix the spelt and buckwheat flours with the baking powder and mix into the butter; knead well.
Make a roll about 1 1/4 inches (3 cm) thick. Wrap in foil and chill through.
Preheat the oven to 350 °F (180 °C).
Using a sharp knife, slice the pastry roll into pieces about 1/4 inch (5 mm) thick. Place on a greased baking sheet and bake in the oven for 20 minutes.

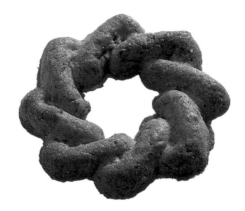

Apple and Cinnamon Crowns
Ingredients: whole wheat flour, baking powder, honey, whole raw sugar, butter, vegetable fat, apples, and cinnamon

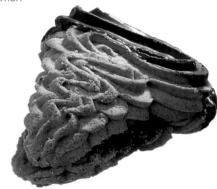

Flaming Hearts
Ingredients: whole wheat flour, honey, butter, raspberry jam, carob cake covering

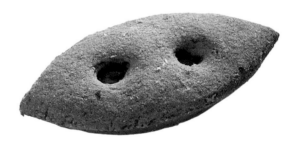

Nut Boats
Ingredients: whole wheat flour, baking powder, honey, butter, hazelnuts

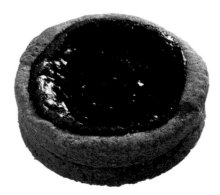

Plum Tarts
Ingredients: whole wheat flour, baking powder, honey, butter, hazelnuts, plum purée

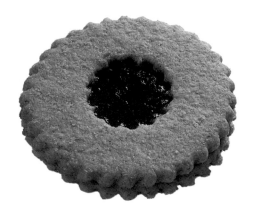

Spelt Cookies with Raspberry Jam
Ingredients: whole spelt flour, baking powder, honey, butter, raspberry jam

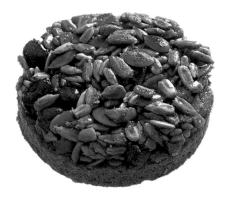

Florentines
Ingredients: whole wheat flour, baking powder, honey, butter, pumpkin seeds, sunflower seeds, sesame seeds, hazelnuts

High Quality Cocoa Substitute

Carob

Carob is made from the dried fruit of the carob tree which is deseeded and ground. Carob pods are green, grow to a length of 8 inches (20 centimeters) and can be wider than a thumb's width. When they are ripe, the carob pods dry out, harden to a certain degree and become a black-brown shiny color. These pods are sold as carob, and are available in markets in southern Europe as well as in wholefood stores in northern Europe and the United States. The pods have an over-poweringly sweet flavor and an individual scent.
In the lands where carob grows, it is a cheap foodstuff used as a syrup, basis for alcoholic drinks or as animal fodder. The seeds of the plant, known by the Latin name *Ceratonia*, weigh about 0.18 gram and in earlier times were sold by the carat – the weight used for diamonds. These imposing, decorative legumes were not only known in Egypt, Israel, and Arabic countries but also on the European side of the Mediterranean, where carob grew wild and was cultivated. Due to increase in demand, many organic farms have converted to carob cultivation as the bacteria in the carob bulbs fertilize the soil. It is important to buy organic carob, as conventionally produced carob is chemically treated to prevent damage by insects.

The advantages of carob over cocoa that make it such a popular ingredient in wholefood cookery are based on four facts:

1. Carob is very low in fat, containing only 1% whereas cocoa is 30% fat.
2. Carob contains less caffeine than cocoa.
3. Carob does not have to be roasted. This means that carob does not absorb any of the unhealthy irritants which cocoa does during the roasting process.
4. Carob has a high fructose content (30–50%) which means that it does not require additional sweetening.

Carob powder behaves like cocoa powder and can be used to make cookies, cakes, and desserts as well as drinks and sauces. Wholefood stores offer a wide range of carob products.

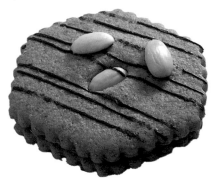

Almond Cookies
Ingredients: whole wheat flour, honey, butter, almond paste, almonds, carob cake covering

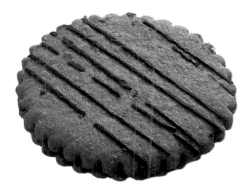

Carob Cookies
Ingredients: whole wheat flour, baking powder, honey, butter, carob and hazelnut spread, carob cake covering

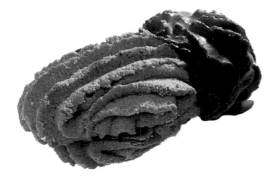

Carob Whirls
Ingredients: whole wheat flour, honey, butter, carob and hazelnut spread, carob powder, carob cake covering

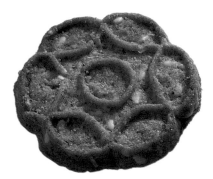

Sesame and Hazelnut Cookies
Ingredients: whole wheat flour, baking powder, honey, whole raw sugar, vegetable fat, sesame seeds, hazelnuts

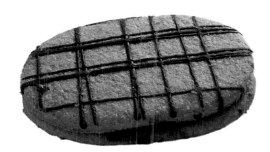

Spelt and Carob Cookies
Ingredients: whole spelt flour, baking powder, honey, butter, carob and hazelnut spread, carob cake covering

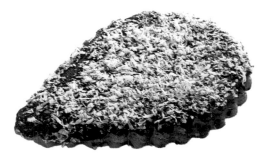

Coconut and Carob Cookies
Ingredients: whole wheat flour, butter, desiccated coconut, carob and hazelnut spread, honey

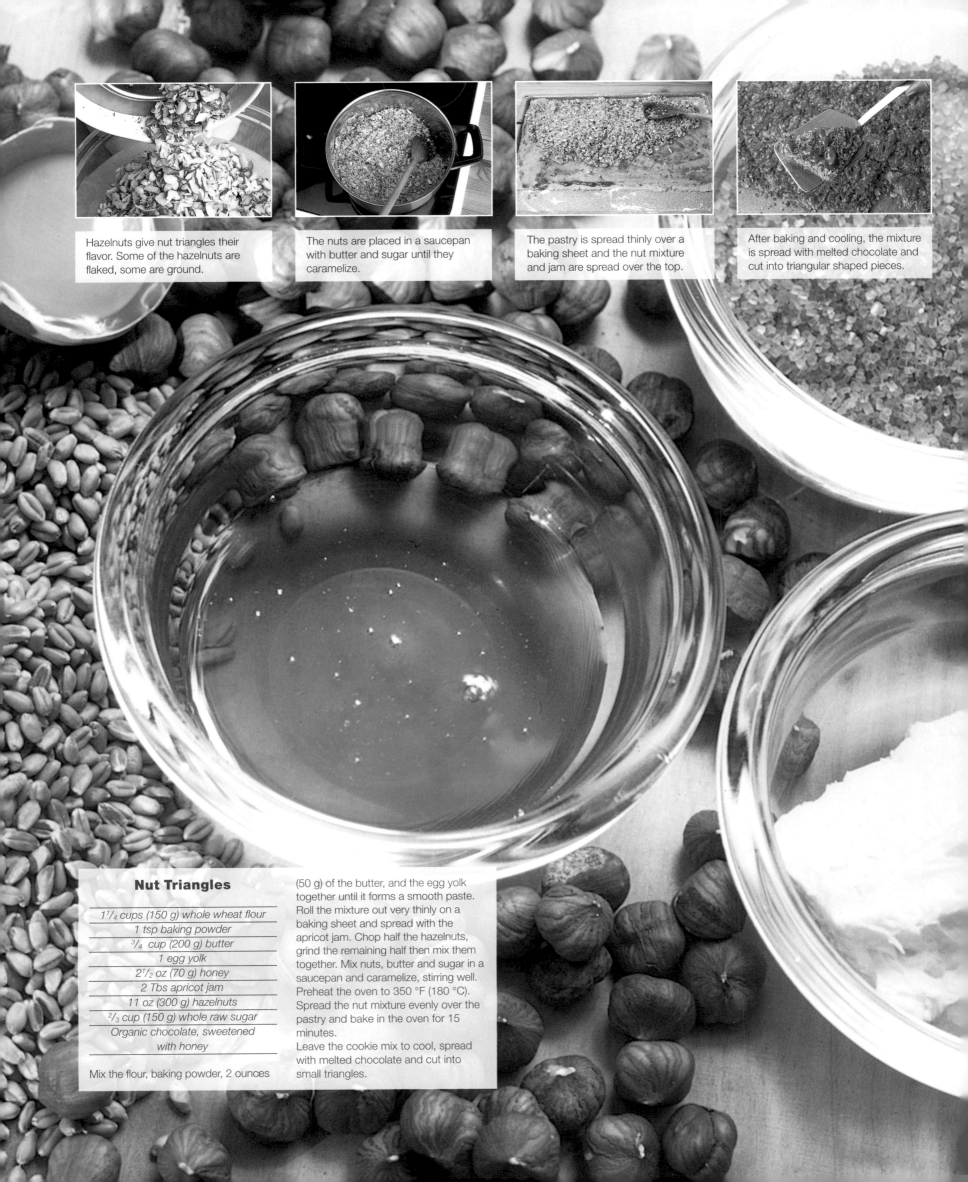

Hazelnuts give nut triangles their flavor. Some of the hazelnuts are flaked, some are ground.

The nuts are placed in a saucepan with butter and sugar until they caramelize.

The pastry is spread thinly over a baking sheet and the nut mixture and jam are spread over the top.

After baking and cooling, the mixture is spread with melted chocolate and cut into triangular shaped pieces.

Nut Triangles

1¹/₄ cups (150 g) whole wheat flour
1 tsp baking powder
³/₄ cup (200 g) butter
1 egg yolk
2¹/₂ oz (70 g) honey
2 Tbs apricot jam
11 oz (300 g) hazelnuts
²/₃ cup (150 g) whole raw sugar
Organic chocolate, sweetened
with honey

Mix the flour, baking powder, 2 ounces (50 g) of the butter, and the egg yolk together until it forms a smooth paste. Roll the mixture out very thinly on a baking sheet and spread with the apricot jam. Chop half the hazelnuts, grind the remaining half then mix them together. Mix nuts, butter and sugar in a saucepan and caramelize, stirring well. Preheat the oven to 350 °F (180 °C). Spread the nut mixture evenly over the pastry and bake in the oven for 15 minutes.
Leave the cookie mix to cool, spread with melted chocolate and cut into small triangles.

With Herbs, Seeds, and Cheese

Savory Baking

Finely seasoned crackers and cookies, puffs and biscuits are ideal accompaniments to a long, refreshing drink be it water, juice, cider, or wine. Shortcrust pastry is extremely versatile, not only for making sweet cakes and pastries, but it can also be flavored with herbs and spices, salt and cheese. Choux pastry can be used to create wonderful savory recipes.

Fill savory pastry with cheese creams, healthy spreads, luxurious dips (pp. 218–219) or garlic mayonnaise (p. 180).

Cheesy Crackers
(Illustration right)

5¼ oz (150 g) mature Gouda
5¼ oz (150 g) Parmesan
¾ cup (200 g) butter
2⅓ cups (300 g) whole wheat flour
Pinch coarse salt
3 Tbs crème fraîche
1 egg yolk
Caraway, sunflower seeds, sesame seeds, and poppy seeds

Finely grate the cheeses and mix together. Add the butter, flour, salt, and crème fraîche and stir until it forms a smooth pastry. Cover and chill for 1–2 hours. Roll out the cheese shortcrust pastry until it is thin. Cut out shapes with cookie cutters. Beat the egg yolk and brush the cookies with the beaten egg.
Preheat the oven to 340 °F (175 °C).
Divide the crackers into four groups and sprinkle each group with different seeds.
Bake the cheesy crackers for about 20 minutes.

Herb Crackers

2⅓ cups (300 g) spelt flour
½ tsp baking powder
5 oz (150 g) cold butter
1 tsp coarse salt
1 Tbs finely chopped parsley
1 Tbs finely chopped basil
1 Tbs finely chopped oregano
2 finely chopped garlic cloves
1 egg
3 Tbs crème fraîche
1 egg yolk
2 oz (50 g) freshly grated Parmesan
1 Tbs dried thyme

Sift the flour with the baking powder into a large bowl. Add the butter in pieces, then the salt, fresh herbs, garlic, egg, and 1 tablespoon (15 ml) of the crème fraîche. Mix the ingredients together to form a smooth dough. Chill for 60 minutes. Roll the pastry out thinly

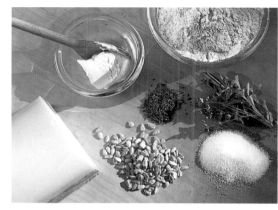

Cheesy crackers require nearly a dozen ingredients, but they are worth all the hard work.

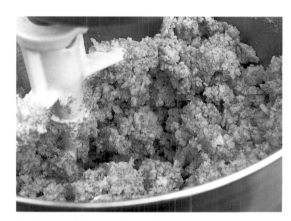

Finely grated cheese, butter, flour, salt, and crème fraîche are kneaded together to make the pastry.

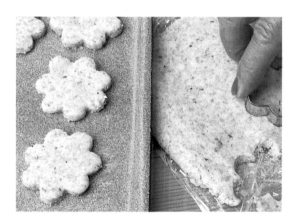

After rolling the dough out thinly, cut out shapes using cookie cutters.

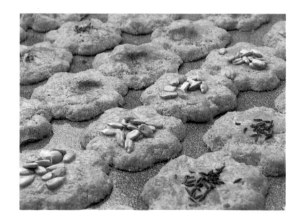

Vary the crackers by sprinkling them with different seeds and herbs.

and cut out shapes using cookie cutters. Place the crackers onto a buttered baking sheet.
Preheat the oven to 350 °F (180 °C).
Beat the remaining cream with the egg yolk and brush the cookies with the egg and cream mixture. Mix together the thyme and Parmesan and sprinkle over the crackers.
Bake the herb crackers in the oven for 15–20 minutes.

Spelt Puffs with Creamy Goat's Cheese Filling

Choux Pastry
½ cup (100 g) butter
½ tsp coarse salt
1 cup (125 g) fine spelt flour
4 eggs
1 egg yolk

Goat's Cheese Cream
11 oz (300 g) fresh goat's cheese
2 oz (50 g) crème fraîche
1 Tbs olive oil
Black pepper
1 tsp herb salt

To make the pastry: cut the butter into small pieces and melt in 1¼ cups (250 ml) of water, with some salt. Remove the pan from the heat.
Sift the flour and stir into the butter and water mixture, until it forms a ball of dough. Place the pan back on the hob and beat with a wooden spoon until the dough comes away from the sides. Remove the pan from the heat and stir in one egg then the remaining three eggs.
Preheat the oven to 400 °F (200 °C).
Place the choux pastry mixture in a piping bag with a large nozzle. Make walnut sized mounds of the mixture onto a buttered baking sheet and brush with beaten egg yolk.
Bake in the oven for 15 minutes.
In the meantime, mix the goat's cheese with the crème fraîche, olive oil, pepper, and herb salt. Stir well until all the ingredients are combined.
Allow the spelt puffs to cool slightly. Fill a piping bag with the creamy cheese mixture and, using a medium sized nozzle, carefully fill the puffs.

Crackers with Nuts and Seeds
(Illustration overleaf)

7 oz (200 g) farmer's cheese
⅓ cup (75 g) soft butter
¾ cup (125 ml) olive oil
1 tsp coarse salt
2⅓ cups (300 g) whole wheat flour
1 tsp baking powder
1 egg yolk
Pumpkin, sunflower, sesame, and poppy seeds
1 Tbs coarse salt

Drain the farmer's cheese well and mix with the butter, oil, and salt.
Mix the flour and the baking powder, add to the cheese mixture and mix to form a smooth dough.
Preheat the oven to 400 °F (200 °C).
Roll the pastry out thinly and cut out different shapes using cookie cutters. Brush the crackers with egg yolk and sprinkle with different seeds. Grind the salt and sprinkle over the crackers.
Bake in the oven for 15 minutes.

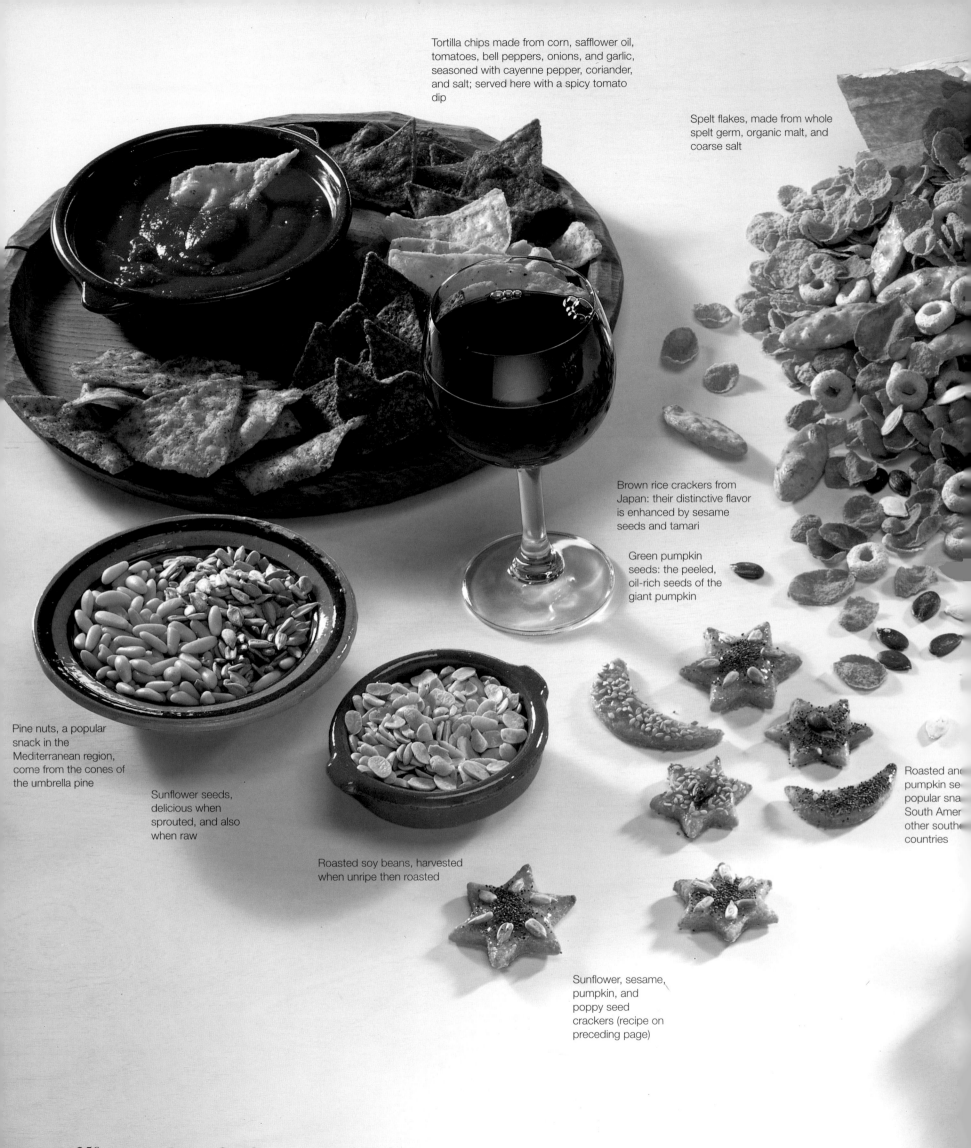

Tortilla chips made from corn, safflower oil, tomatoes, bell peppers, onions, and garlic, seasoned with cayenne pepper, coriander, and salt; served here with a spicy tomato dip

Spelt flakes, made from whole spelt germ, organic malt, and coarse salt

Brown rice crackers from Japan: their distinctive flavor is enhanced by sesame seeds and tamari

Green pumpkin seeds: the peeled, oil-rich seeds of the giant pumpkin

Roasted and pumpkin se popular sna South Amer other southe countries

Pine nuts, a popular snack in the Mediterranean region, come from the cones of the umbrella pine

Sunflower seeds, delicious when sprouted, and also when raw

Roasted soy beans, harvested when unripe then roasted

Sunflower, sesame, pumpkin, and poppy seed crackers (recipe on preceding page)

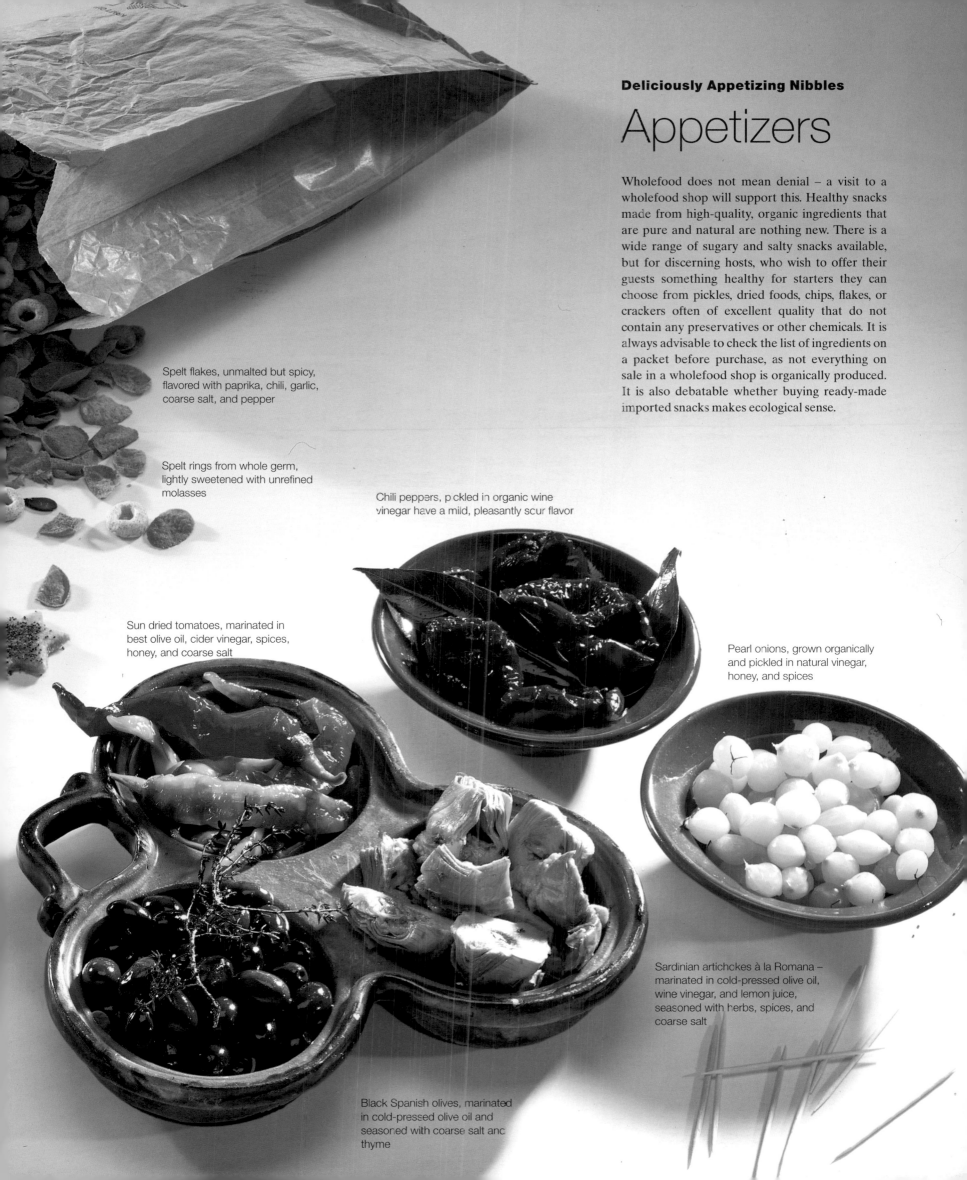

Deliciously Appetizing Nibbles

Appetizers

Wholefood does not mean denial – a visit to a wholefood shop will support this. Healthy snacks made from high-quality, organic ingredients that are pure and natural are nothing new. There is a wide range of sugary and salty snacks available, but for discerning hosts, who wish to offer their guests something healthy for starters they can choose from pickles, dried foods, chips, flakes, or crackers often of excellent quality that do not contain any preservatives or other chemicals. It is always advisable to check the list of ingredients on a packet before purchase, as not everything on sale in a wholefood shop is organically produced. It is also debatable whether buying ready-made imported snacks makes ecological sense.

Spelt flakes, unmalted but spicy, flavored with paprika, chili, garlic, coarse salt, and pepper

Spelt rings from whole germ, lightly sweetened with unrefined molasses

Chili peppers, pickled in organic wine vinegar have a mild, pleasantly sour flavor

Sun dried tomatoes, marinated in best olive oil, cider vinegar, spices, honey, and coarse salt

Pearl onions, grown organically and pickled in natural vinegar, honey, and spices

Sardinian artichokes à la Romana – marinated in cold-pressed olive oil, wine vinegar, and lemon juice, seasoned with herbs, spices, and coarse salt

Black Spanish olives, marinated in cold-pressed olive oil and seasoned with coarse salt and thyme

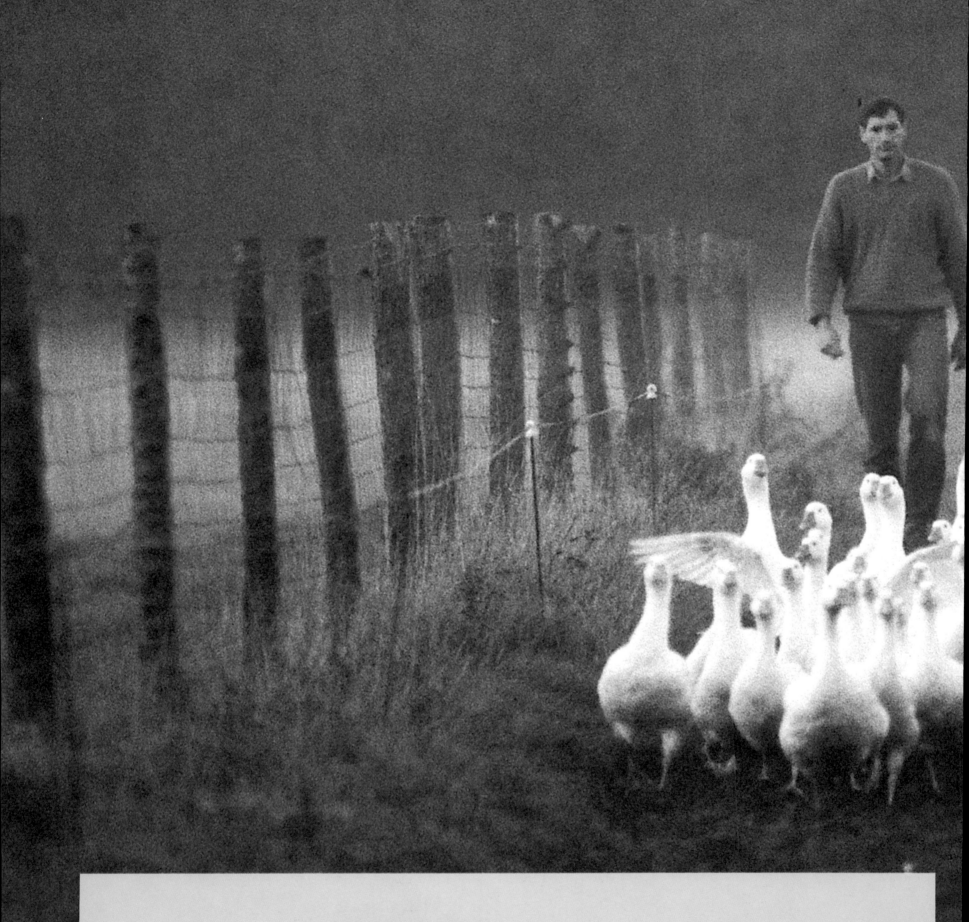

Meat, Poultry, and Eggs

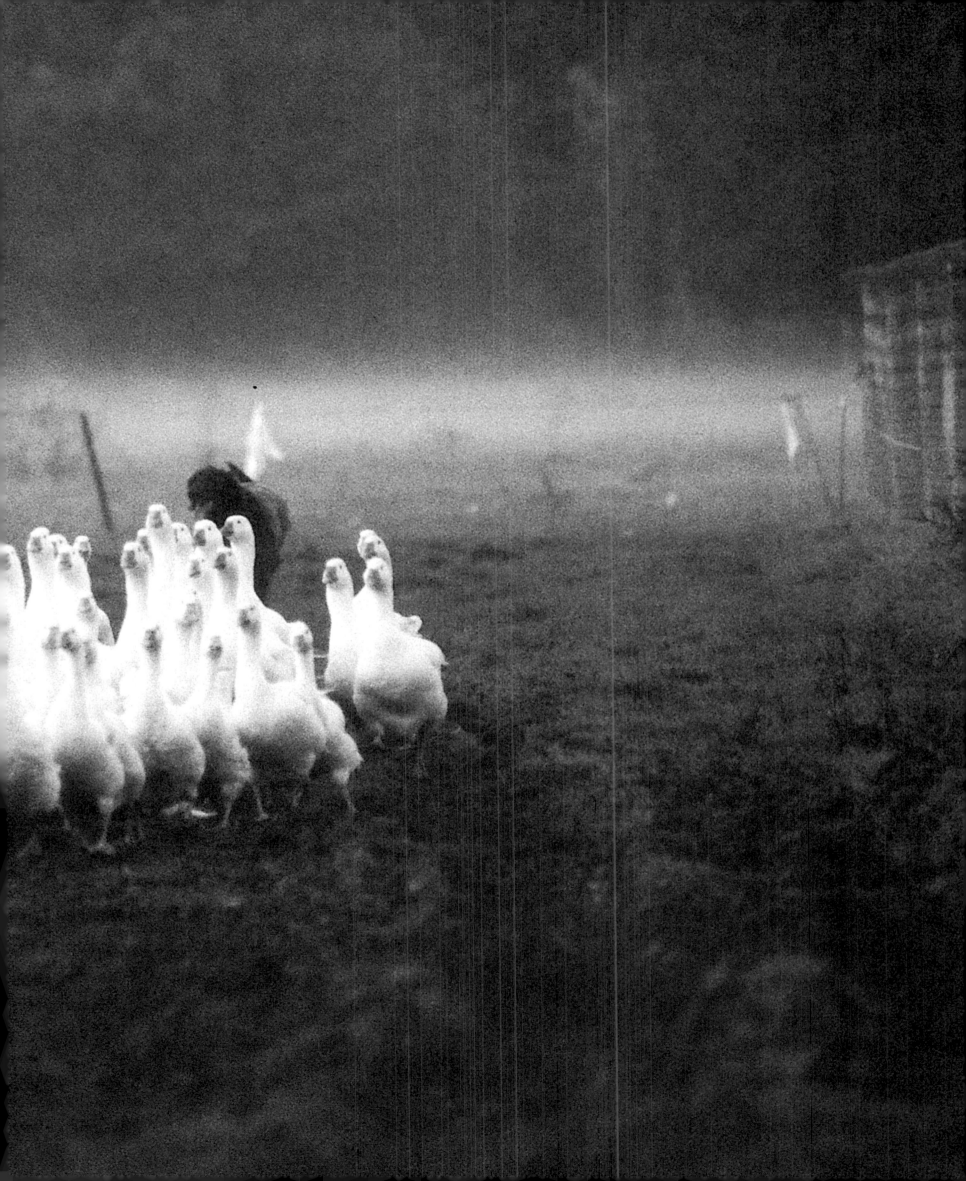

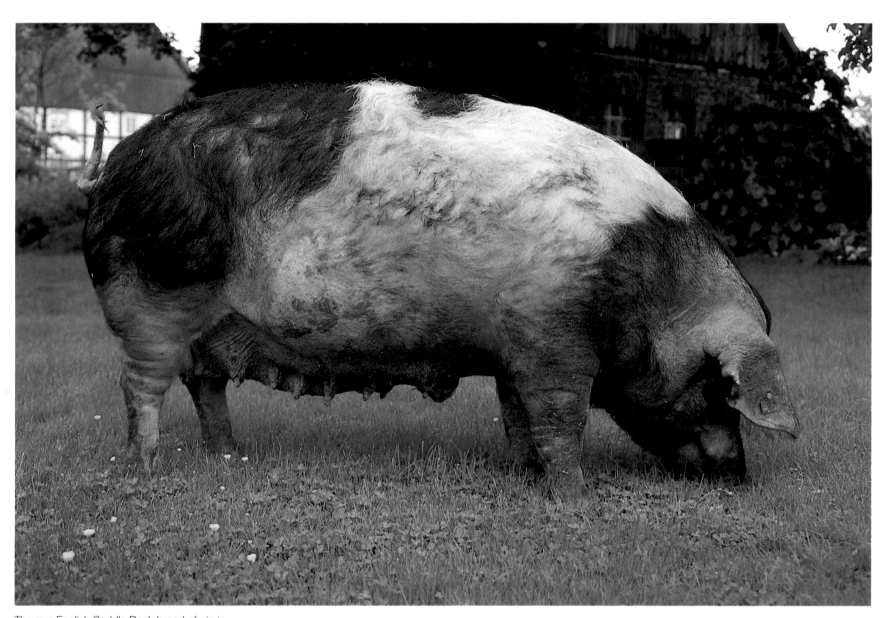

The rare English Saddle Back breed of pig is
experiencing a renaissance on organic farms.

Previous double page: Geese in Westphalia. These
animals live a humane existence before they are killed.

Animals play an important role in the organic farm. Many farmyards work on the principle that the cows, pigs, sheep, or goats are as important as the farmer and his assistants. Animals on organic farms are treated with respect and even deference. The animals are important for the soil as well as providing meat themselves. Animal manure guarantees that the plant life of the farm will be well fed. This includes the many field vegetables, fruits, and other vegetables that come from organic producers. Animals live a humane existence where they feel comfortable and are healthy. A farm that works on this principle and uses techniques that are thousands of years old – which have been developed to adjust to the changing times – gives meat an entirely different value to industrial meat farming. Only recently there was uproar at the cruel methods of keeping, transporting, and slaughtering animals, not to mention the salmonella scare, and the threat of B.S.E. Fortunately, there are more and more farmyards where the animals are being well treated. The consumer's attitude has also changed. Healthy eating is possible without eating any meat at all, certainly it is a good idea to cut down on meat consumption. Eating too much meat, which includes cold meats, is known to be a contributing factor to many diseases, ranging from rheumatism, to obesity, to increased risk of heart attacks. "We only eat meat once or twice a week" says a beef farmer, whose animals spend up to two months of every year outdoors. He recommends that his customers cut down on meat as well. Meat that has been humanely produced has a quality that cannot be found in conventionally produced meat. Meat in a diet based on wholefoods can make every meal in which it features, a meal fit for a celebration.

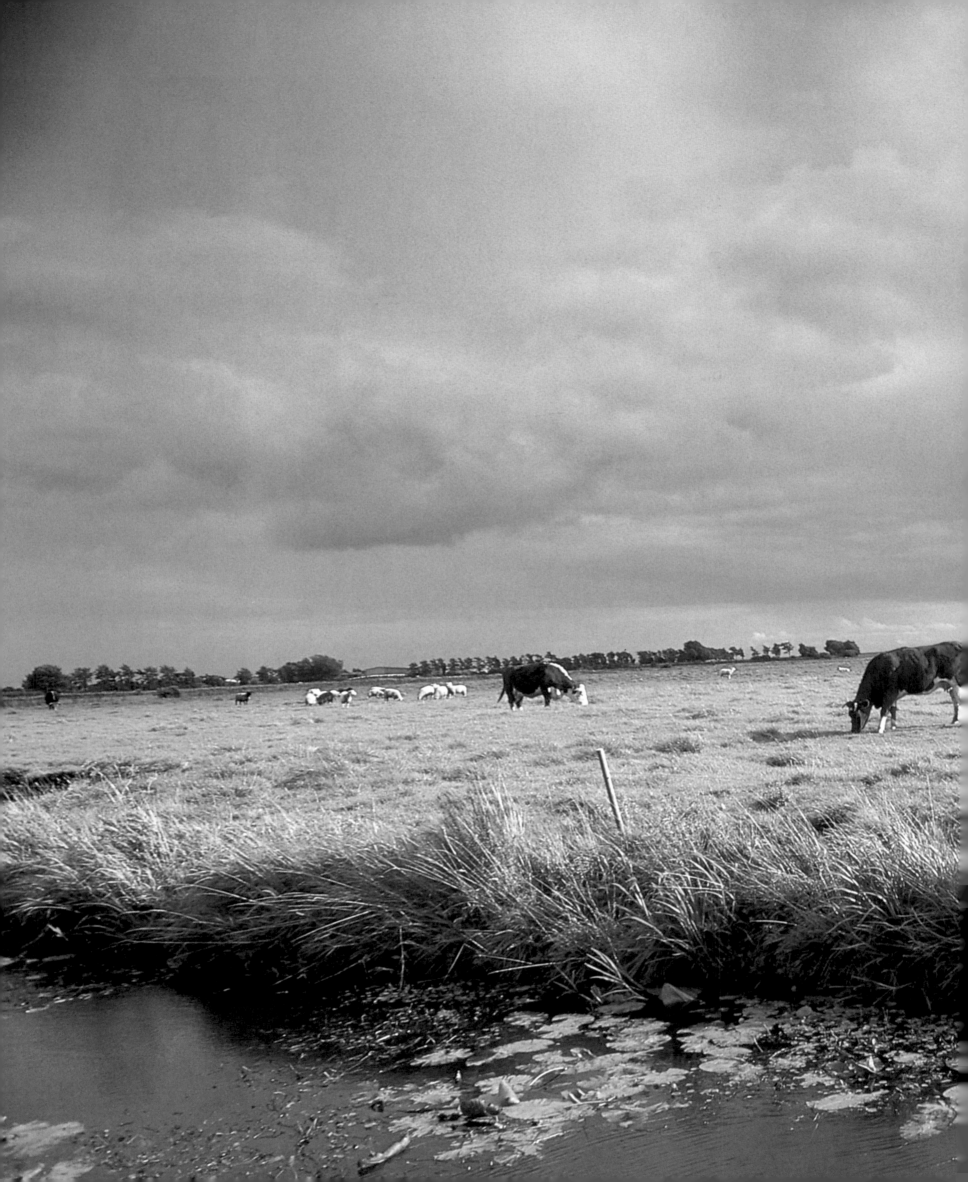

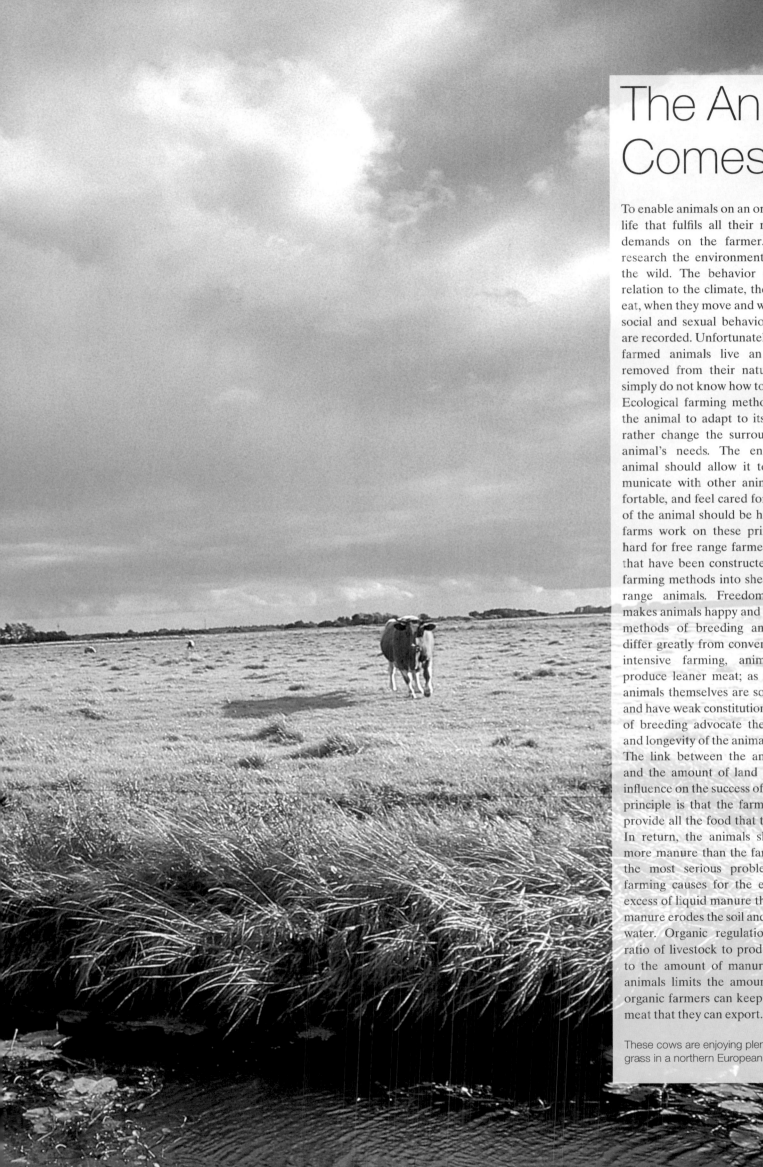

The Animal Comes First

To enable animals on an organic farm to live a life that fulfils all their needs makes great demands on the farmer. Organic farmers research the environment of the animals in the wild. The behavior of the animals in relation to the climate, the type of feed they eat, when they move and when they rest, their social and sexual behavior, all these factors are recorded. Unfortunately, many intensively farmed animals live an existence so far removed from their natural one that they simply do not know how to behave.

Ecological farming methods do not require the animal to adapt to its surroundings, but rather change the surroundings to suit the animal's needs. The environment of the animal should allow it to move, eat, communicate with other animals, rest, be comfortable, and feel cared for. The environment of the animal should be hygienic. Free range farms work on these principles. It is often hard for free range farmers to convert sheds that have been constructed for conventional farming methods into sheds suitable for free range animals. Freedom to move about makes animals happy and contented. Organic methods of breeding and rearing animals differ greatly from conventional methods. In intensive farming, animals are bred to produce leaner meat; as a consequence the animals themselves are sometimes deformed and have weak constitutions. Organic methods of breeding advocate the health, hardiness, and longevity of the animal as a priority.

The link between the amount of livestock, and the amount of land available has great influence on the success of the farm. The basic principle is that the farm should be able to provide all the food that the animals require. In return, the animals should not produce more manure than the farm requires. One of the most serious problems that intensive farming causes for the environment, is the excess of liquid manure that it produces. This manure erodes the soil and poisons the ground water. Organic regulations concerning the ratio of livestock to production of food, and to the amount of manure produced by the animals limits the amount of livestock that organic farmers can keep and the amount of meat that they can export.

These cows are enjoying plenty of room and lush grass in a northern European meadow.

Irreplaceable Helpers

Cattle

Cattle belong in the fields. Only they and other ruminants are capable of converting cellulose – from grass and plants – into valuable foodstuffs like meat and milk. Their steady grazing keeps large areas of grassland neat and tidy. This is why cattle are, and always have been, an important feature of central and northern European agriculture. Hopefully, cattle will always fulfil this role, as agriculture would never have been possible without the assistance of the cow. The most important contribution that cattle make to agriculture is not their production of milk and meat, but rather their rich manure. Without this natural fertilizer, farmers throughout time would not have been able to keep the same land productive. This would have meant that farmers could not have produced enough cereal and vegetables to feed the population.

It always used to be the most important consideration that cattle led a healthy life, had a varied diet and had enough to eat. Cow manure ensured that the ground received in nutrients what the cows took from it in the form of vegetation. Artificial fertilizers and the use of chemicals on the soil have upset the natural balance, which has led to the soil becoming poor, or even barren, just as intensive breeding methods have caused cattle and other farm animals to become weaker and more susceptible to illness.

When these factors are taken into consideration, it is easy to understand why organic animal farmers consider their cattle to be of such great value.

In a farming system that is as self-sufficient as possible (see p. 428 f.) to ensure that the soil is fertile, cattle are a vital link in the chain. Very few organic farms exist, that do not rely heavily on the

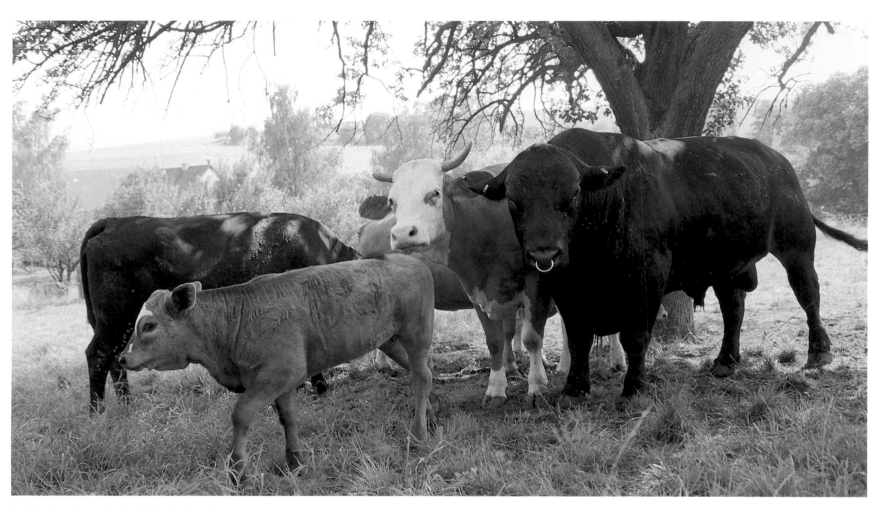

An Aberdeen Angus bull with his family: a happy example of organic animal farming.

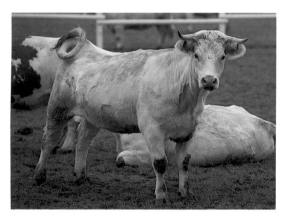

Charolais cows, from Burgundy in France, are undemanding animals that produce excellent meat.

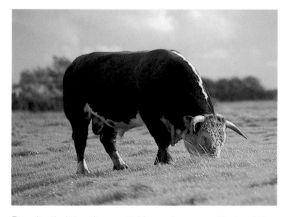

Despite their tender meat, Limousins can withstand the coldest of climates.

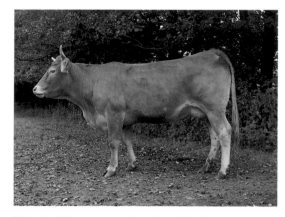

When building up an outdoor herd, it is important to choose resilient, rustic breeds of cattle.

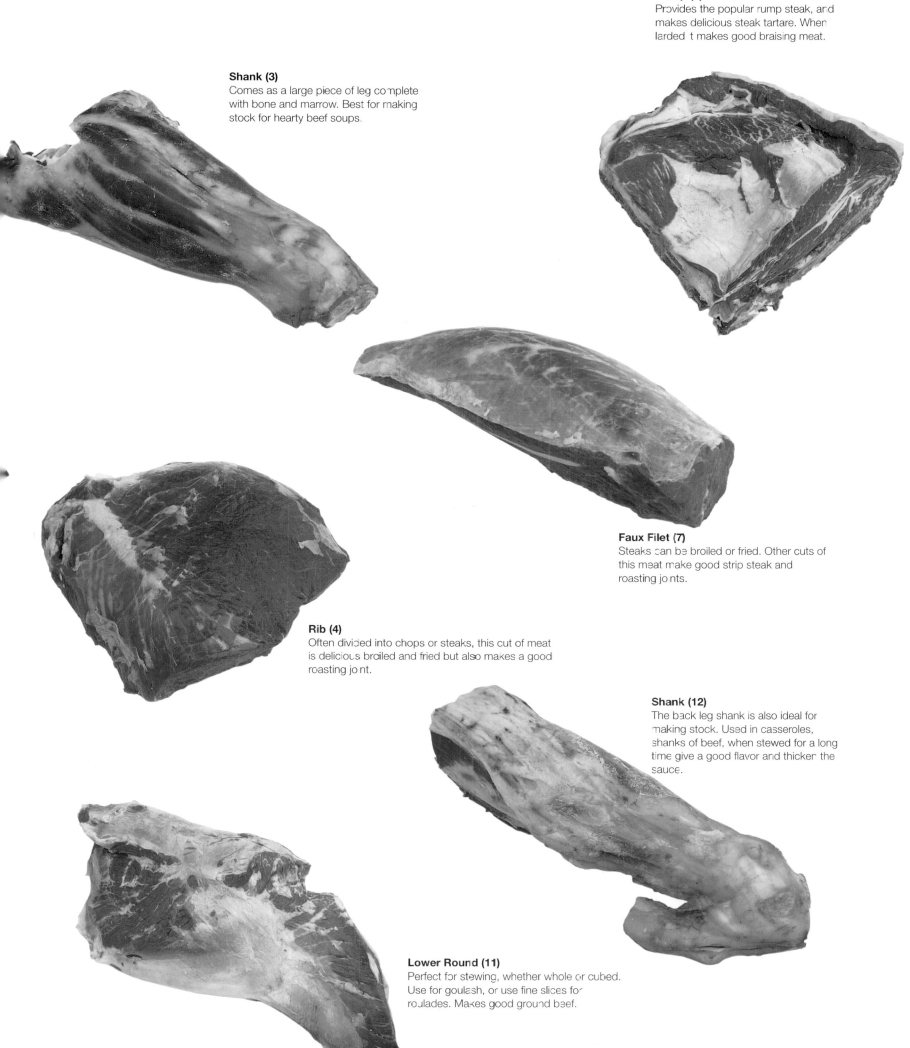

Rump (8)
Provides the popular rump steak, and makes delicious steak tartare. When larded it makes good braising meat.

Shank (3)
Comes as a large piece of leg complete with bone and marrow. Best for making stock for hearty beef soups.

Faux Filet (7)
Steaks can be broiled or fried. Other cuts of this meat make good strip steak and roasting joints.

Rib (4)
Often divided into chops or steaks, this cut of meat is delicious broiled and fried but also makes a good roasting joint.

Shank (12)
The back leg shank is also ideal for making stock. Used in casseroles, shanks of beef, when stewed for a long time give a good flavor and thicker the sauce.

Lower Round (11)
Perfect for stewing, whether whole or cubed. Use for goulash, or use fine slices for roulades. Makes good ground beef.

261

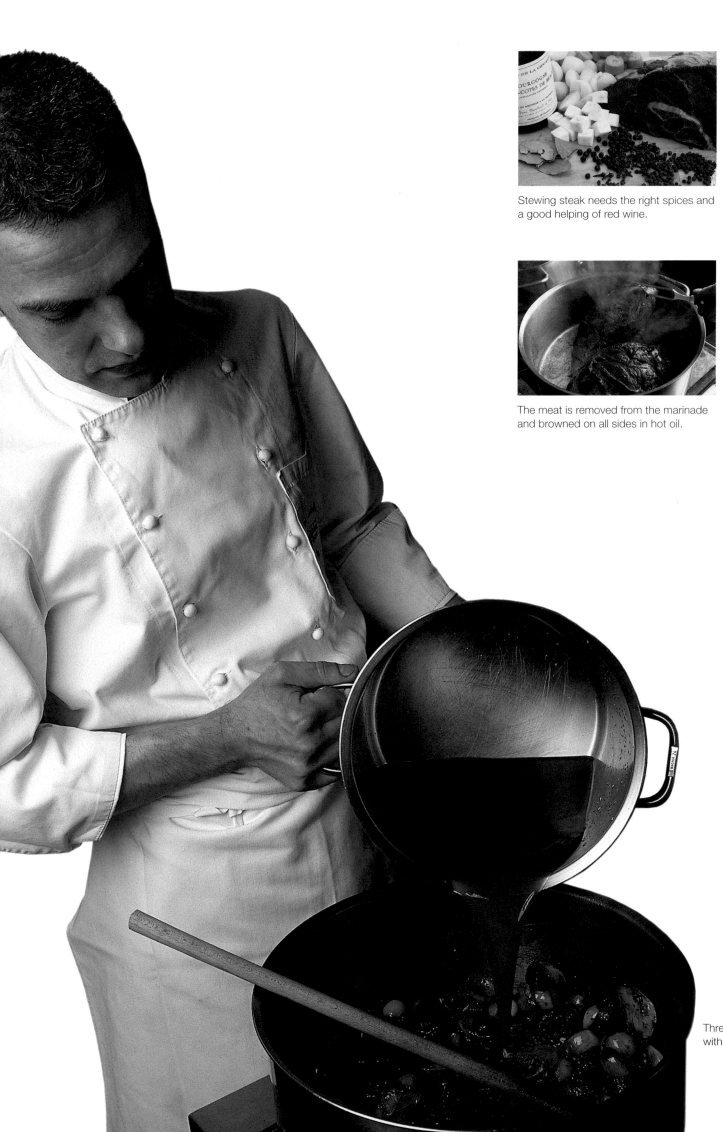

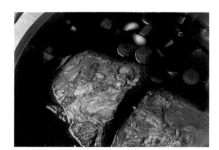

Stewing steak needs the right spices and a good helping of red wine.

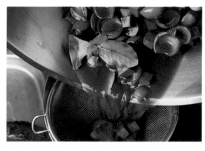

The meat is placed in a dish with all the ingredients and is left to marinate for three days.

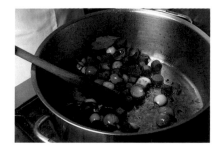

The meat is removed from the marinade and browned on all sides in hot oil.

The marinade is strained into another bowl and the vegetables are saved.

The vegetables are pan fried in a skillet and mixed with tomato paste.

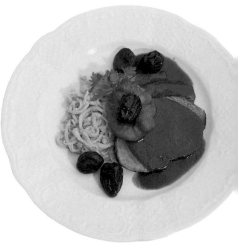

The meat is added to the vegetables, followed by the marinade, the casserole is covered and placed in the oven.

Three days of waiting is rewarded: Braised Beef with Pickled Fruits.

Braised Beef with Pickled Fruits

2 lbs 4 oz (1 kg) shoulder of beef

Marinade

5 oz (150 g) carrots
3 medium onions
1/4 celeriac
1 small parsley root
1 garlic clove
3 cloves
1 bay leaf
10 peppercorns
Coarse salt
1 Tbs raw cane sugar
1 3/4 pints (1 l) full-bodied red wine

Pickled fruits

2 oranges
6 cloves
1 cinnamon stick
7 oz (200 g) mixed, dried fruit
2 1/2 cups (500 ml) black tea

Preparation

Coarse salt
Black pepper
1 Tbs groundnut oil
1 Tbs tomato paste
Pinch raw cane sugar

Place the meat in a bowl. Add all the marinade ingredients and pour over the red wine. Leave in the refrigerator for at least three days.
The day before cooking the dish, pickle the fruit. Cut the oranges into pieces and place in a bowl with the spices and the dried fruit. Pour over the tea and chill. Remove the meat from the marinade and season with salt and pepper. Heat some oil in a heatproof casserole dish, add the meat and brown on all sides. Remove and set aside.
Remove the vegetables from the marinade and drain. Place in the casserole with the tomato paste and pan fry. Pour in the marinade and add the meat. Cover and place in the medium oven 400 °F (200 °C) and cook until tender, turning the meat frequently. Remove the meat and keep warm. Purée the vegetables and liquid, season to taste with salt, pepper, and sugar. Chop the meat and pour the sauce over the meat. Heat the pickled fruit, together with its marinade, remove the fruit with a slotted spoon and arrange around the meat. Best served with home made noodles.

Boiled Fillets of Beef with Vegetables, Beet, and Creamed Horseradish

2 beets
1 Tbs red wine vinegar
Coarse salt, pepper
2 carrots
2 parsley roots
1/4 celeriac
1 leek
7 oz (200 g) string beans
5 cups (1 l) beef stock
4 slices beef fillet, each weighing about 6 1/2 oz (180 g)
8 slices beef marrow
1 tsp natural gelling agent (pectin based)
1 Tbs chopped parsley

Creamed Horseradish

1 1/4 cups (250 ml) whipping cream
3 1/2 oz (100 g) prepared horseradish
1 tsp white wine vinegar
Coarse salt

Clean the beet and boil in water with the vinegar, salt, and pepper until the beets are "al dente." Chop into diamonds. Clean the remaining vegetables, cut into diamonds and keep the remaining vegetable pieces that are not diamond-shaped. Cook the vegetable diamonds in the beef stock and set aside. Place the vegetable offcuts and the beef fillets (preferably Charolais) into the stock, reduce the heat, and leave for 8 minutes. The stock should not be boiling as this will prevent the meat from remaining juicy. Remove the fillets and keep warm. Reduce the stock by a third, strain and reheat, place the pieces of beef marrow in the stock and leave for 3 minutes. Remove the marrow and keep warm. Dissolve the gelling agent in a little cold water and add to the sauce to thicken. Add the vegetables with the beet and reheat them. Place the beef on warmed soup plates, season with salt and pepper. Add two pieces of beef marrow to each plate, pour over the stock, arrange the vegetables around the beef, and sprinkle with a little parsley.
Beat the cream, mix in the horseradish, season to taste with salt and pepper. Serve the sauce separately from the beef.

Best Veal with Bouillon Potatoes and Salsa Verde

2 lbs 4 oz (1 kg) best veal
Coarse salt
2 carrots
1/4 celeriac
1 leek
1 bunch parsley
1 unpeeled large onion
Peppercorns
2 bay leaves
Black pepper

Sauce

2 bunches flat-leafed parsley
3/4 cup (150 ml) olive oil
Coarse salt, black pepper

Potatoes

7 oz (200 g) firm potatoes
1 Tbs finely diced celeriac
1 Tbs finely diced leek
1 Tbs finely diced carrot
1 Tbs finely chopped parsley
Coarse salt

Soak the veal for 30 minutes in cold water. Remove, place in a pan, and fill with cold water until the meat is covered. Bring to the boil and skim the water. Add salt, vegetables, parsley, and spices and simmer just below boiling point until tender.
Meanwhile, prepare the salsa verde. Put parsley, salt, and 1/2 cup (100 ml) of cooled meat stock into a liquidizer and purée, gradually adding the olive oil. Place the sauce in the refrigerator and leave to cool.
Peel the potatoes and cut into 1/2 inch (1.5 cm) dice Remove 2 1/2 cups (500 ml) of stock from the cooking pot and cook the potatoes in the stock for about 15 minutes. Then add the diced vegetables and cook for a further 5 minutes. Sprinkle with parsley just before serving.
Arrange the potatoes, slice the meat, season lightly with salt and pepper, and garnish with a little salsa verde.

Handling Delicate Meat

• Keep meat cool at a temperature of 41 °F (5 °C). Do not wrap in plastic wrap or aluminum foil, rather store it in a porcelain or steel dish.
• Remove meat from the refrigerator an hour before cooking, otherwise it will be tough.
• Meat keeps better and is more tender when it has been marinated in an acidic marinade. It should always be kept in the refrigerator.
• Tenderize steaks before pan frying. This makes the muscle fibers shorter and tears the connective tissue; if the meat is not tenderized, the fibers bind together during cooking and the juices flow out. Do not tenderize fillet.
• The shorter the cooking time, the more nutrients and flavor will remain in the meat.
• With meat that is enclosed in fat and connective tissue, make cuts in the outside. The cuts will close up during cooking as the meat swells.
• Only broil meat on the stove. Grilling over wood and coal embers can produce carcinogens.
• Steaming is a good and gentle way of cooking meat.
• When boiling meat, always place it straight into boiling stock – this is the ideal way to boil meat – then reduce the temperature. This method of cooking is also suitable for very good cuts of meat.
• When serving meat that has been cooked in liquid, try to use the liquid in the recipe, as the liquid contains many nutrients.
• Never pierce roasting meat with a fork. This causes juices to flow out, and the meat to lose nutrients.
• Add salt to steaks, cutlets, and fillets either during or after cooking; roasting joints and stewing meat should be salted just before cooking.
• Roasted joints should be allowed to rest before carving, so that the juices can distribute themselves evenly throughout the meat.

Roast Beef Rolls Stuffed with Gorgonzola

1 lb 11 oz (800 g) beef sirloin
11 1/2 oz (320 g) Gorgonzola
16 large basil leaves
Coarse salt
Black pepper
Oil for browning
1 1/2 cups (300 ml) veal gravy
1 Tbs butter

Cut the sirloin into 8 equal slices. Divide the cheese into eight equal sized slices, wrap each piece of cheese in two basil leaves and place on top of a slice of beef. Roll up the meat and season with salt and pepper on the outside. Either secure with a cocktail stick or use cooking thread to tie them up. Heat up some oil in a skillet until it is very hot. Pan fry the beef rolls in the oil so that they are evenly browned. Place the skillet, with the rolls in it into a preheated oven – 400 °F (200 °C) and cook for a further 5 minutes. Remove the rolls and leave to stand. Pour the gravy into the skillet and deglaze. Mix with the butter. Serve 2 rolls per person on warmed plates; cut one of the rolls open so that the cheese runs appetizingly out of the meat.

Special Occasion Beef Recipes

Veal Roulades with Sun-dried Tomatoes

3¹/₂ oz (100 g) sun-dried tomatoes
16 pitted black olives
2 Tbs small capers
2 garlic cloves
2 egg yolks
2 Tbs chopped parsley
Coarse salt
White pepper
4 thin veal fillets
8 slices bacon
Butter for greasing the pan
¹/₂ cup (100 ml) white wine
7 oz (200 g) mixed salad leaves
4 Tbs olive oil
1 Tbs white wine vinegar

Cook the sun-dried tomatoes in a little water for about 5 minutes, then drain. Finely chop the tomatoes, olives, capers, and garlic and mix well with the parsley and egg yolks. Season to taste with salt and pepper. Cover the veal fillets with the stuffing, roll them up and wrap each roulade in two slices of bacon. Preheat the oven to 460 °F (250 °C). Butter a heatproof dish, place the roulades in the dish with the open side facing down. Cook for 15 minutes. Then pour over the white wine and cook for a further 30 minutes. Remove the meat from the dish, allow to cool and cut diagonally into pieces ¹/₃ inch (1 cm) thick. Wash the salad. Make a vinaigrette from the olive oil, vinegar, salt, and pepper. Dress and toss the salad, arrange on plates, and surround with pieces of roulade.

Beef Roulades with Spinach and Roquefort Sauce

(Illustration below)

1 lb 9 oz (750 g) leaf spinach
2 garlic cloves
4 Tbs (60 g) butter
4 slices of beef
Coarse salt
White pepper
12 small slices mild, cured ham
¹/₂ cup (100 ml) white wine
4¹/₂ oz (125 g) Roquefort
1 cup (200 ml) light cream
1 tsp vegetable stock granules

Pick over the spinach, wash it and wilt in a large saucepan. Drain in a sieve allowing all the water to drain away. Peel and halve the garlic cloves and pan fry in half the butter in a wide cooking pan. Remove, place the drained spinach in the pan and cook for 2 minutes, then remove, set aside, and allow to cool.
Tenderize the slices of beef until they are quite flat and cut them into three pieces. Season with salt and pepper and cover each roulade with a piece of ham, and 2 tablespoons (30 g) of spinach. Roll up the roulades and secure with a cocktail stick lengthways.
Heat the remaining butter in a pan, brown the roulades on all sides and remove from the pan. Deglaze the pan with white wine and bring to the boil. Crumble the Roquefort, mix with the cream and the vegetable stock granules and pour into the pan. Place the roulades in the sauce and simmer for 20 minutes until the sauce has thickened. This dish is especially good with broiled polenta.

Stewed Beef with Shallots and Peas

1 lb 9 oz (750 g) beef shoulder
1 onion
2 sticks celery
1 garlic clove
1 tsp finely chopped rosemary
6 Tbs olive oil
4 Tbs tomato paste
1 cup (200 ml) red wine
1 tsp vegetable stock granules
1 lb 2 oz (500 g) shallots
1 oz (30 g) butter
11 oz (300 g) fresh peas from the pod
Coarse salt
White pepper

Roughly dice the beef. Finely chop the onion, celeriac, and garlic and sweat in the oil, together with the rosemary. Pour in the red wine and ¹/₂ a cup (100 ml) of water. Add the tomato paste and stock granules, stir, cover the pan, and leave to stew. After an hour, peel the shallots and sweat in the butter, then add to the meat and stew for a further 10 minutes. Season to taste with salt and pepper and serve at once. Serve with rustic bread and a mixed salad.

Beef Roulades with Spinach and Roquefort Sauce

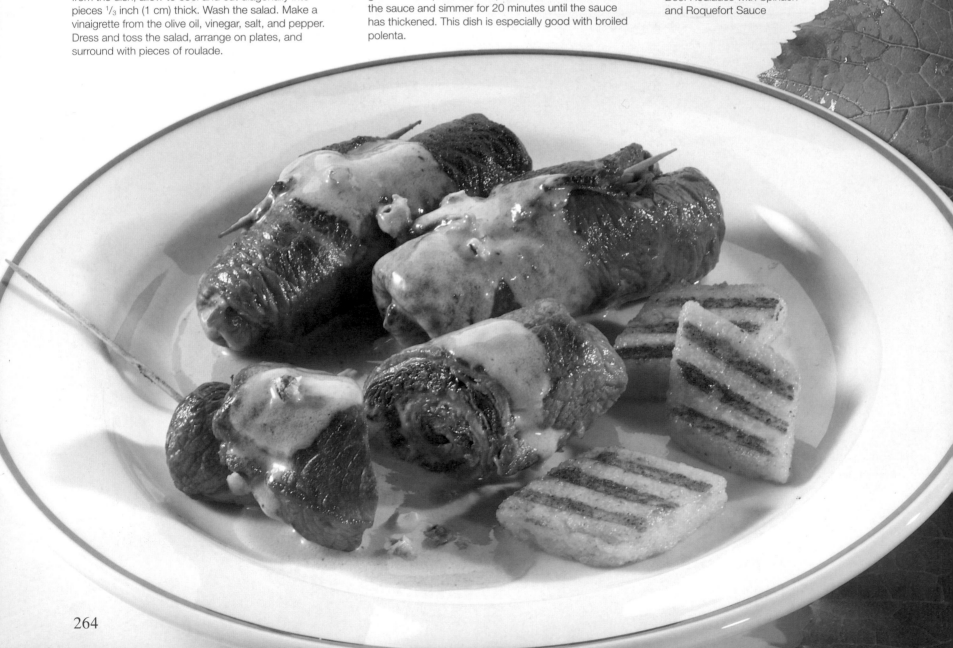

Nutritional Content of Meat in Comparison with Lentils

Nutrients	Beef	Pork	Lamb	Chicken	Duck	Lentils
Protein (in g)	17	14	16	18	16	23
Fat (in g)	15	26	12	9	12	1
Cholesterol (in mg)	57	59	60	60	70	0
Vitamin B1 (in mg)	0.1	0.8	0.1	0.1	0.2	0.5
Vitamin B2 (in mg)	0.2	0.15	0.2	0.15	0.15	0.3
Vitamin B3 (in mg)	5.3	3.2	3.8	5.8	2.6	1.9
Vitamin B6 (in mg)	0.4	0.4	0.3	0.2	–	0.6
Calcium (in mg)	9	7	7	12	8	70
Potassium (in mg)	290	280	250	210	240	820
Magnesium (in mg)	20	23	18	16	16	72
Phosphorus (in mg)	150	160	155	140	145	395
Iron (in mg)	2.3	1.8	1.8	1.4	1.6	6.7
Kilojoules	850	1200	800	550	750	1450
Kilocalories	200	285	190	130	180	345

Gourmet Veal Ragout
Bocconcini di vitelle buongustaio
(Illustration below)

· 1 lb 9 oz (750 g) leg of veal
---
1 lb 2 oz (500 g) ripe tomatoes
---
1 lb 2 oz (500 g) zucchini
---
1 garlic clove, 2 white onions

Coarse salt
---
1 dried chili pepper

A little flour
---
2 oz (60 g) butter
---
3 Tbs olive oil
---
1 cup (200 ml) white wine

White pepper

$^1/_2$ bunch finely chopped flat-leafed parsley

Dice the meat roughly. Skin, deseed, and dice the tomatoes. Wash the zucchini and cut into $^1/_3$ inch (1 cm) slices. Finely dice the onion. Pound the garlic, together with a little salt and the chili, in a mortar until it forms a paste. Lightly coat the meat cubes in the flour. Heat 2 tablespoons (30 ml) of olive oil and 2 ounces (50 g) of butter in a casserole, brown the meat in batches, remove from the casserole and set aside. Pan fry the onions until they are transparent, add the garlic paste and pour in the wine. After 2 minutes, add the meat and diced tomato, cover and simmer for 45 minutes. Pan fry the zucchini in the remaining fat and add to the meat. Season to taste with salt and pepper, stir in the parsley and serve at once. This dish is good served with firmly cooked brown rice.

Gourmet Veal Ragout

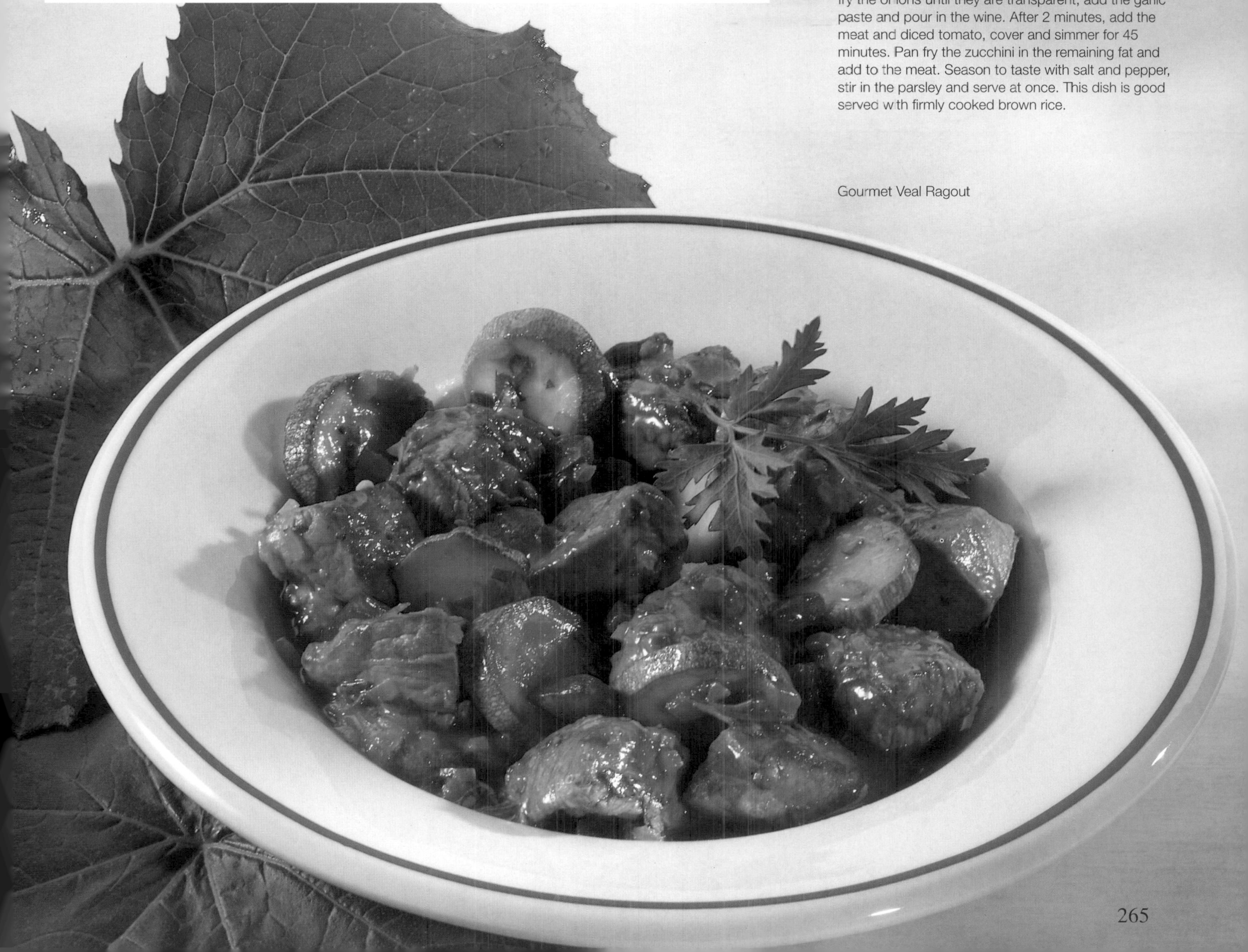

265

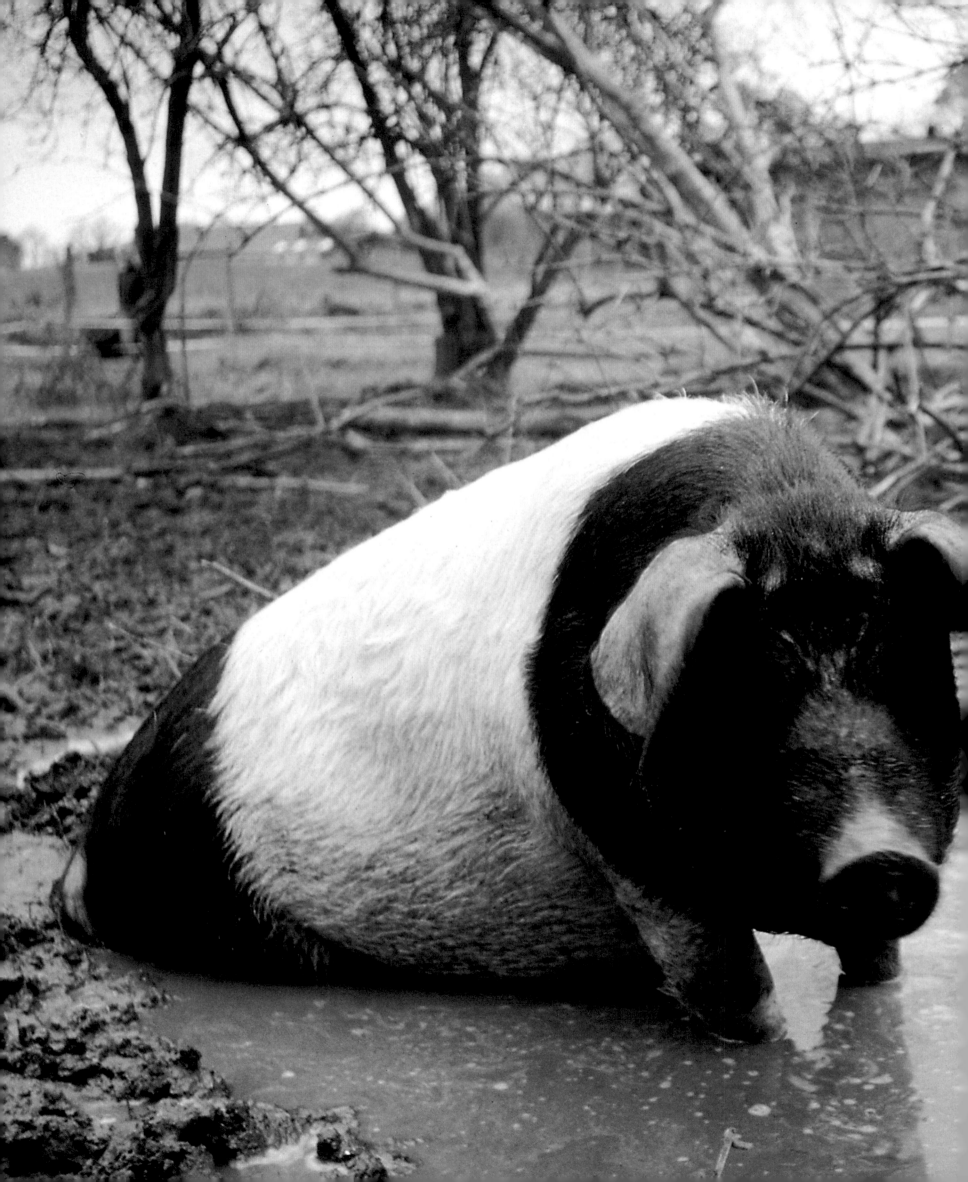

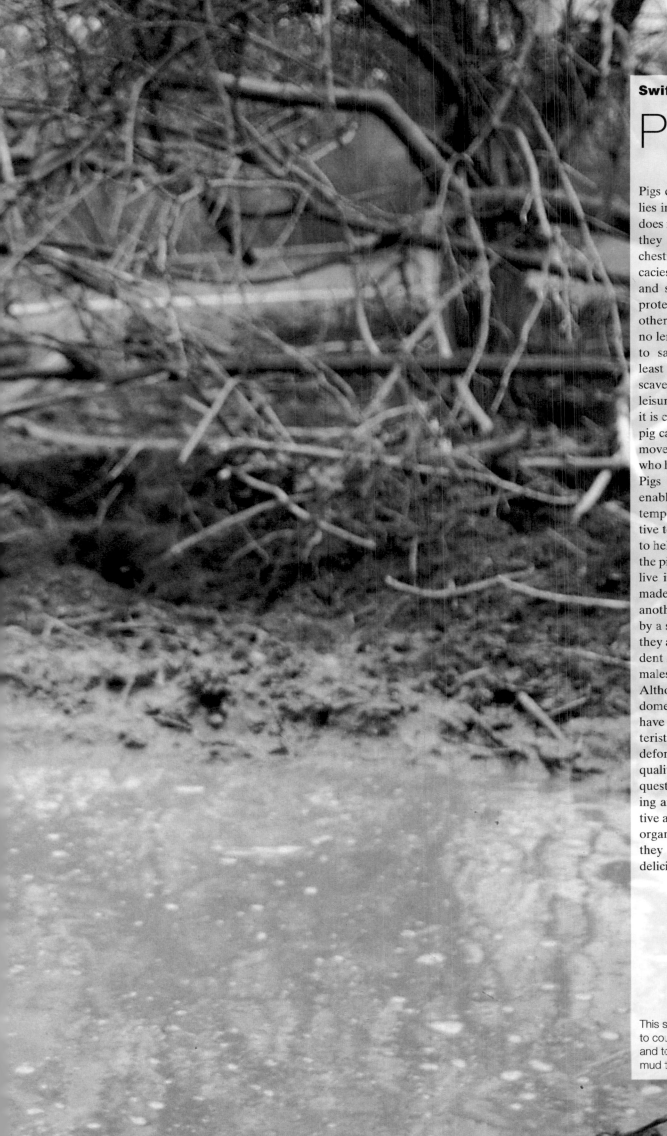

Pigs

Pigs come from the forest. Their ideal home lies in the shade of the trees. Their thin skin does not like too much sun. In the leafy shade they graze on greenery, as well as acorns, chestnuts, beech nuts, and other forest delicacies. They dig up roots from the ground, and snuffle through the earth in search of proteinous foods like worms, larvae, and other smaller or larger living things. There are no lengths to which a pig will not go in order to satisfy his appetite, and he spends at least half his days looking for food. When scavenging for food the pig moves in a leisurely fashion, but if confronted by danger, it is capable of amazing speed and stamina; a pig can easily outrun a cow. This swiftness of movement is particularly noticeable in piglets who have just been weaned.

Pigs have a very well insulated skin which enables them to withstand very cold temperatures. This means that they are sensitive to extreme heat, and they wallow in mud to help themselves to cool off. Moisture helps the pig to rid its body of excess heat. Wild pigs live in herds of 30 to 40 animals. These are made up of sows that are related to one another and their offspring. The herds are led by a sow. Male animals leave the herds when they are ready to reproduce and live independent lives. However, when the sows fight, the males get involved.

Although pigs have probably been kept as domestic animals for over 10,000 years, they have not retained many of their wild characteristics, as can be seen from deviant and deformed breeds that exist. The fact that the quality of pork as a meat has been called into question is due to the cruel methods of farming and the unfair way in which these sensitive animals are so frequently handled. On an organic farm, the pigs are treated well, and they reward the farmer with good quality, delicious meat.

This strong Saddle Back pig is wallowing happily, to counteract the strong heat of the summer sun, and to lower its body temperature. The layer of mud that coats the pig helps to insulate its skin.

Delighted

To be a pig

It is fun to watch pigs wallowing in mud. Part of the fun is knowing that the pigs are making themselves cool and comfortable. Because pigs have very set criteria for their comfort, free range farming methods have very high standards. Freedom to move about is the most important consideration. A cow does not enjoy being kept in a small area, but a pig finds it a living hell. Pigs also like to decide for themselves whether they are going to live inside or outside. All free range farmers take these considerations into account. Visitors are always astounded that the pigs do not smell; that well known piggy smell is a result of cramped living conditions imposed by intensive farming methods. Pigs are generally super clean.

The most appropriate type of environment for pigs to live in would be a proper meadow, that would allow the pigs to live a life similar to their former woodland existence. This is not very common in northern and central Europe. In contrast, free range pigs of the unspoilt or occasionally cross bred *Cerdo ibérico* breed in Spain and Portugal frequently enjoy an outdoor life. Further

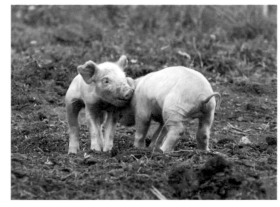

Pigs need a lot of space to move about in, as these playful piglets demonstrate.

north, the pigs prefer to have some sort of shelter, and many organic farms provide outdoor living, with huts for the pigs to take shelter from the cold. Most farms offer huts for the pigs to live in at the coldest times of the year. This way, the pigs can roam freely in the field, and shelter in the huts if they so wish.

Pigs like to live in herds, which is important for their health, provided that they have enough space to establish their own hierarchy. Their curly tails are a good indicator of their happiness. Pigs that are intensively farmed have their tails docked, as there is a danger that the pigs will bite each

others' tails off in their cramped surroundings. Organic farming methods would never condone tail docking, just as they do not permit farmers to make pigs wear rings in their noses or file down the piglets' teeth.

Sows are only kept apart from the herd when they are farrowing. At this important time, the sow is given somewhere comfortable to rest. Piglets, weaned piglets, and fattening pigs all like plenty of straw to dig about in. The pigs trample and soil the straw, which rots and becomes hard. Over the course of the year, the straw rots and forms excellent fertilizer. Organic farming uses a composting agent to make the rotting of the manure coincide with the time the animals are kept inside. Once a year the stall is thoroughly mucked out and the straw and manure is piled up. Another composting agent is used to help the piles of straw to rot more. After a year, the compost is ready and can be scattered over vegetable fields and grassland and worked into the soil where it improves its quality and fertility.

In these stalls, the pigs can choose whether to live inside or outside.

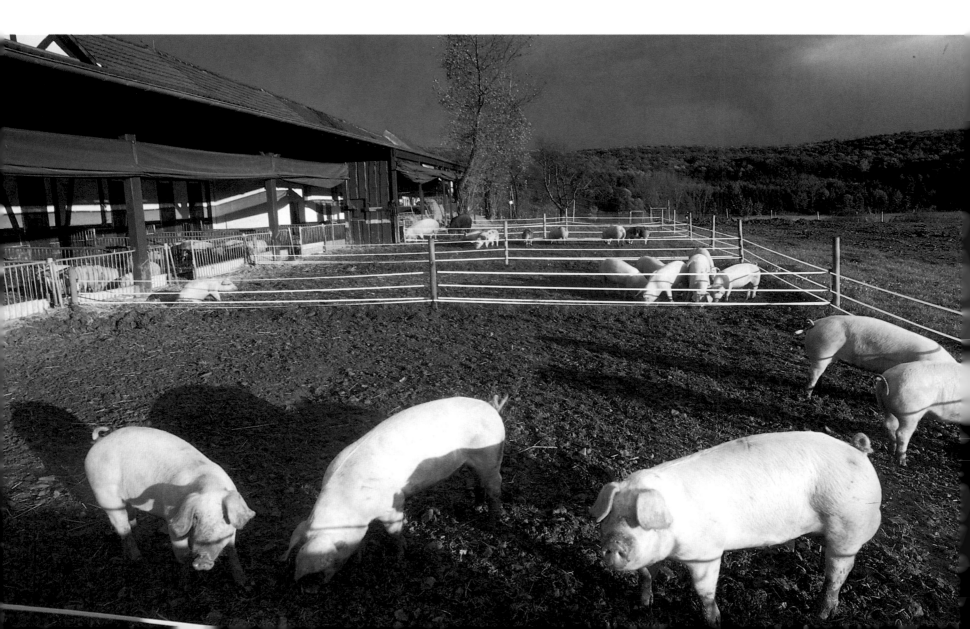

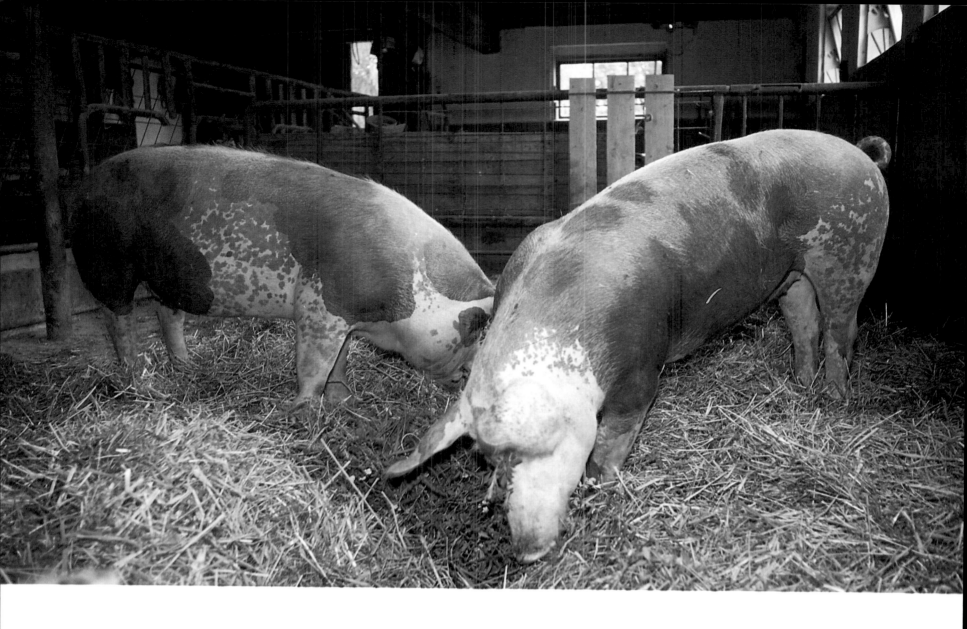

If pigs feel comfortable in their pens, they are less likely to bite at each others' tails.

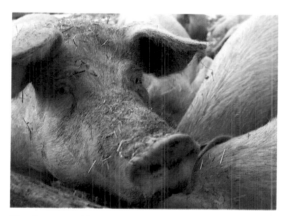

Pigs have specific criteria for their existence. They are only healthy when these criteria are fulfilled.

Pigs are omnivorous and require a varied diet. To supply protein, the best types of fodder are sweet lupins, peas, and fava beans. Piglets enjoy plant compost, which they can eat very early on in their lives. Plant compost provides the piglet with trace elements, particularly iron. Organically raised pigs often benefit from the varied produce that organic farmers grow, and may enjoy carrots, potatoes, lettuces, or other vegetables that are not good enough to sell at market. Any farmer with the patience to allow his pigs to forage on newly plowed fields can rid himself of beetles that eat the potato crop. Growth hormones, antibiotics, medicines, animal, and fish derivative foods have no place in organic pig farming. The pigs are not slaughtered until they are a year old – in contrast to six months in intensive farming – and their meat is delicious. When they are taken to be slaughtered, they are not cramped together with 20 or 30 other pigs, but have a straw lined space shared with, at the most, six or seven others. Everything is done to avoid causing the animals unnecessary distress, as this has a bad effect on the meat.

Breeds of Pig

In the old days, pet pigs were free to roam or were kept in large fields. At the beginning of the 19th century pig pens became popular, and pig breeders put more emphasis on breeds that would be most productive. Intensive farming has led to pig breeds with up to 16 ribs, buckled front legs and low life expectancy. This applies to the Large White pig – which was a breed found in Yorkshire, England and is now bred throughout Europe – or any other German or Belgian breed. Of the greatest importance to intensive farmers was to obtain the greatest quantity and the leanest type of meat from one animal. Pietrain, a new breed that was developed in Belgium after 1960, had all these attributes. The results of these economically successful breeds: short life expectancy, infertility, fewer piglets in a litter, birthing problems, lameness, high stress levels etc., not forgetting poorer quality meat.

Organic pig farming favors the following breeds of pig.
- The Schwäbisch-Hallisch pig,
- English Saddle Backed pigs,
- Hampshire pigs.

Ecologically minded pig farmers strive to breed more robust pigs through cross breeding. Their customers respond by increasing their demand for good quality meat.

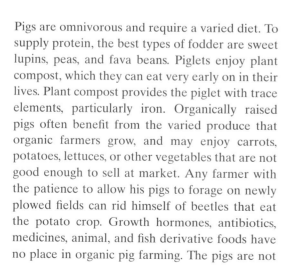

Organic Home Slaughtering

It is no longer rare to find an organic farm that carries out its own slaughtering. The goal of organically butchered, organic meat, is drawing nearer.

Usually the butcher comes to the farm to kill and butcher the animals. All the necessary pots and pans have to be prepared, not just to hold the meat for immediate consumption or meat for the freezer, but because many parts of the animal will be used to make sausage straight away. Many kinds of salami are made from raw meat, which is dried and/or smoked. Frankfurter sausages use finely chopped meat that is boiled in the sausage skin. Cooked sausages like liver sausage and black pudding (blood sausage) use meat that has been parboiled before the skins are filled, then the stuffed skins and the precooked meat are boiled again.

Cuts of Meat from Organic Home Slaughtering

(Illustration below)

1 Cutlet or Spare Rib Fillet
Broil, stew, or pan fry, sliced or whole

2 Fat Rib
Part of a spare rib, for pan frying or broiling

3 Neck
Can be pan fried whole or divided into chops

4 Bacon Belly
A very fatty cut that is often boiled

5 Lard
Belly fat that can be melted and used to brown meat

6, 8 Hock, Front and Back
Broiled, pan fried, roasted, boiled, or stewed whole

7, 9 Trotters, Front and Back
For stews and brawn

10, 11, 13, 14 Ham
Whole hams can be salted, dried or smoked, boiled or baked

12 Shoulder
Prepared for pan frying, or for stews

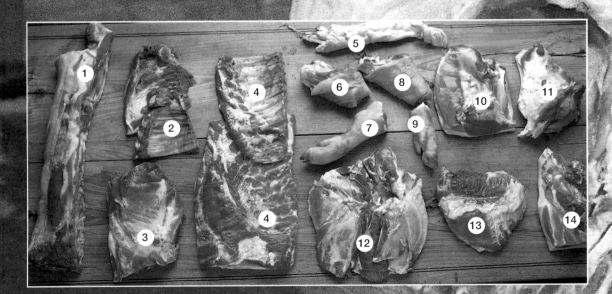

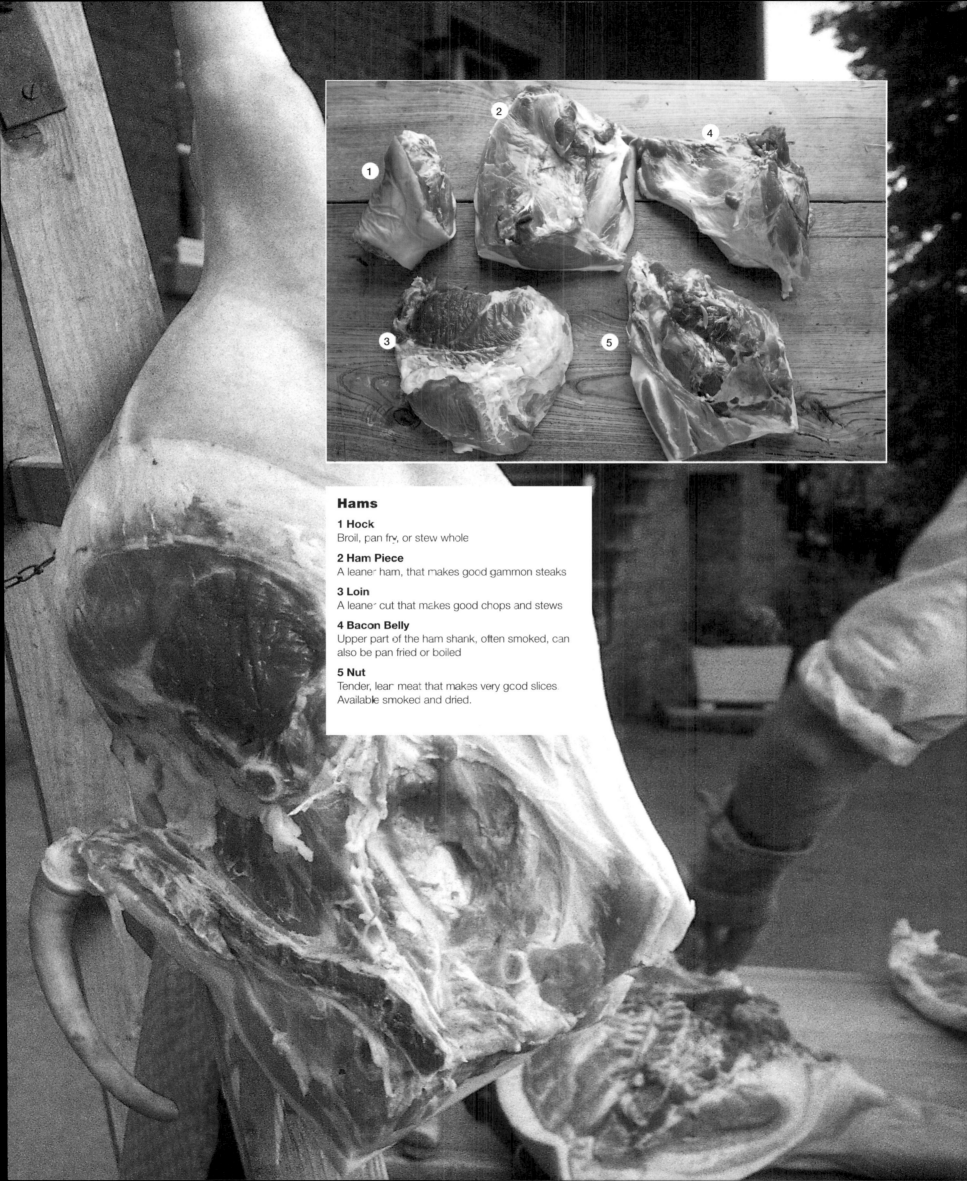

Hams

1 Hock
Broil, pan fry, or stew whole

2 Ham Piece
A leaner ham, that makes good gammon steaks

3 Loin
A leaner cut that makes good chops and stews

4 Bacon Belly
Upper part of the ham shank, often smoked, can also be pan fried or boiled

5 Nut
Tender, lean meat that makes very good slices. Available smoked and dried.

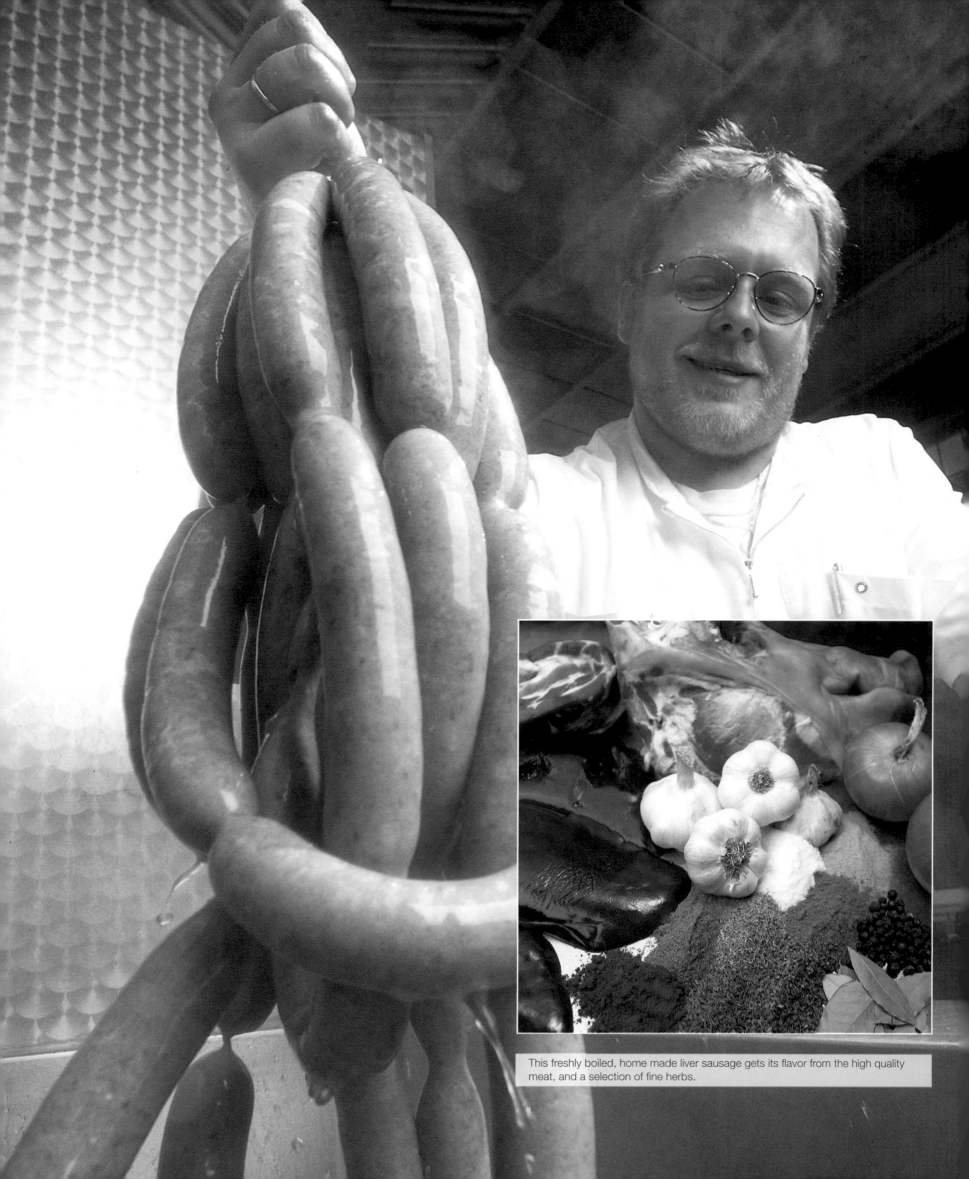

This freshly boiled, home made liver sausage gets its flavor from the high quality meat, and a selection of fine herbs.

Healthy Sausages

There is growing scepticism towards mass produced sausages. This is because of animal epidemics, intensive farming, and the objectional methods of abattoirs. At the end of the day, the consumer never knows exactly what is in the sausages they buy. Anything that the consumer would prefer not to see disappears in the grinding process. This includes all the parts of the animal that cannot be sold as a complete piece or in slices, then all the additives, low quality eggs, gelatine, blood plasma, then finally, quite apart from salt, sugar, and spices, a whole mass of other additives, reddening agent like pickling salt or salt peter, preservative and softening agent, flavor enhancer, and phosphate. Hardly any butchers make their own sausages.

Organic sausages have to be made from meat that comes from humanely reared healthy animals that are fed on organically produced fodder and have not been treated with antibiotics, hormones, or other medicines. A further advantage is that organic sausage does not contain pickling salt or any chemical colorings, preservatives or other additives. This applies to all types of sausage:

• Raw sausage like Mettwurst, and salami made from raw meat, that are preserved by drying or smoking the meat. Salami includes spreadable sausages like Mettwurst and Teewurst.

• Stewing sausages: Once made, these sausages are cooked in boiling water. They do not keep for long. Types of stewing sausage are Fleischwurst, Fleischkäse, Lyoner and also includes Bockwurst, Frankfurters, Wieners, Strasbourger, frying sausages, meat pâtés, and Mortadella.

• Boiling sausages: liver sausage, black pudding. These are made from precooked meat and are cooked again when the sausage has been put together. This includes aspic and corned beef. Meat products from organic farms are handmade. Many farms make their own sausage under close supervision of a highly trained butcher. Sometimes whole animals are given to a good butcher, and the parts that are not sold as pieces of meat are transformed into sausage. The recipes are very simple. Meat, fat, coarse salt, herbs, spices, and natural gut are the ingredients required. Depending on the region where the sausage is made, the meat is either air dried or smoked over untreated wood. Even sausages can be a healthy treat.

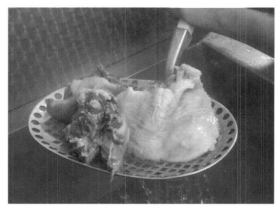

To make liver sausage requires fatty belly pork and leaner pork. This must be cut into pieces.

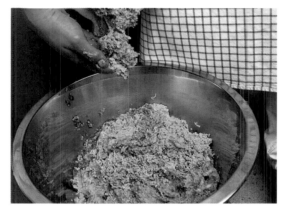

Meat, garlic, and onion are ground together and mixed well.

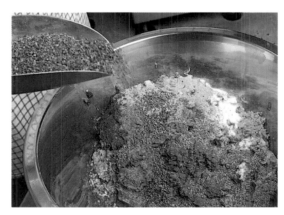

At this point ground spices and finely chopped herbs are added and thoroughly mixed into the meat mixture.

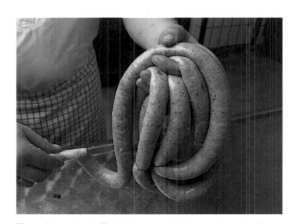

The mixture is stuffed into natural skins and cooked in boiling water to help it keep longer.

Why Pickling Salt is Bad for Your Health

The organic soil growers' association has guidelines that prevent the use of pickling salt in products that are sold as organic. There is a good reason for this. Salt peter, or sodium nitrate can combine with amino acids and form carcinogens. Pickling salt overconsumption can lead to dilation of the arteries that causes a massive drop in blood pressure and the collapse of the patient. This has been known for a long time. Brockhaus discovered in about 1960 that pickling salt caused the substance in red blood cells (hemoglobin) to transform into hemiglobin, and so starve the internal organs of oxygen. The nitrate content of salt is not allowed to exceed 0.5%. Pickling salt was used to preserve meat products as it protected the meat from bacterial and fungal infection. It also reddens the meat, as it causes the meat to produce a red oxygen product: oxydymoglobin. This gives the meat its attractive red color. Organic sausages often look rather gray in color because no pickling salt is used. Some organic farmers do not like the color that their sausages appear and reach for the nitrate laden salt. The test for the customer is: if the sausage is red and looks like it has come from a supermarket shelf, then it is likely that the producer is not adhering to organic guidelines, to the detriment of our health.

Home Made Mettwurst

Per sausage

1 lb 2 oz (500 g) more lean than fatty pork
$1/2$ oz (12 g) coarse salt
$1/20$ oz (1.5 g) black pepper
$1/20$ oz (1.5 g) glucose (optional)
Pinch (0.25 g) dried garlic
$1/4$ tsp mustard seeds

Mix all the ingredients together well and grind finely. Knead the mixture for 5 minutes. Stuff the mixture into natural skins, naturine skins, or silk skins.

Thin sausages need 7 days at lukewarm room temperature to dry properly, while thicker sausages may need up to 14 days. The room should be lukewarm as too much heat in the first three days of drying can lead to fermentation. After this the sausage can be smoked twice, or simply eaten as it is: air dried sausage.

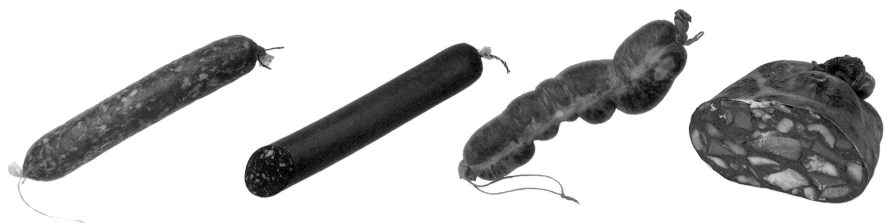

German Country Sausage
A classic smoked sausage made from raw, not too fatty meat

Stewed Black Pudding
Raw ingredients are placed in natural skins, then the whole sausage is cooked

Smoked Blood Sausage
Made from diced belly pork, onions, fresh pig's blood, and spices

Coarse Blood Sausage
With large pieces of meat and pork belly, blood, and spices

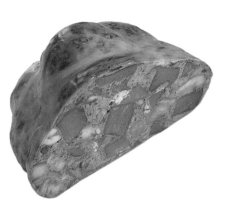

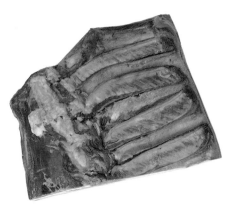

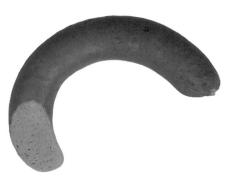

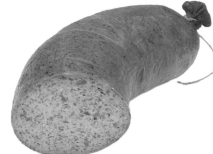

White Blood Sausage
Bound together with egg

Dried Pork
Dry cured, and air dried

Mixed Meat Sausage
A stewing sausage made from pork and beef

Fine Herzwurst
A delicate version of the south German variety, made with heart

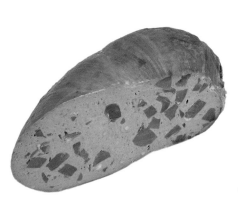

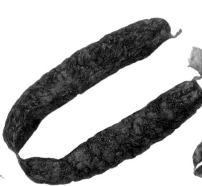

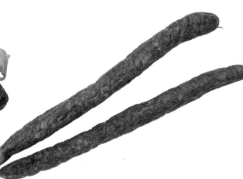

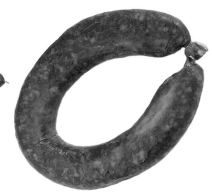

Coarse Herzwurst
Coarsely chopped variety meats and other meat

Knacker (Smoked)
Strongly smoked raw sausage made from medium coarse pork

Knacker
Made from pork and pork belly, dried and smoked

Garlic Sausage
A stewing sausage made from finely ground, garlic flavored meat

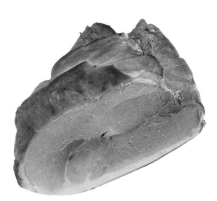

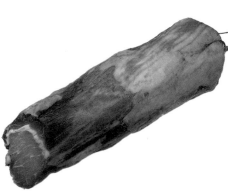

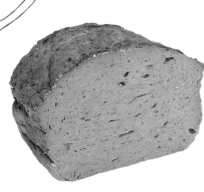

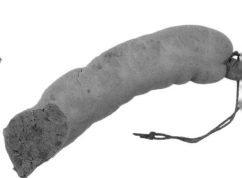

Cooked Ham
From the saddle, salted, pressed, and poached

Smoked Ham
Quick smoked, dry cured pork sausage

Liver Terrine
Baked mixture of liver, meat, pork belly, eggs, and spices

Liver Sausage
Liver and cooked meat are ground and boiled

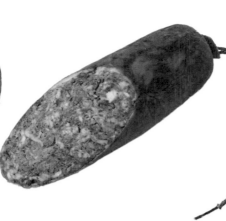

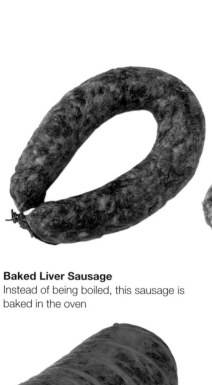

Baked Liver Sausage
Instead of being boiled, this sausage is baked in the oven

Coarse Liver Sausage
Made from coarsely cut ingredients, strongly spiced, lightly smoked

German Sausage
To make it easy to spread, the meat is finely ground

Smoked German Sausage
Made from raw meat and belly pork, dried and smoked

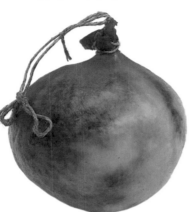

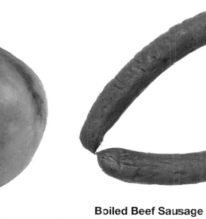

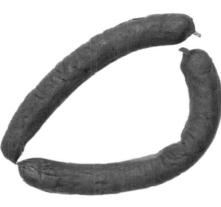

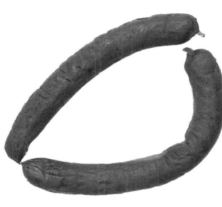

Presskopf
A large jellied sausage made from pork and blood

Presswurst
A Bavarian specialty made from cooked meat

Boiled Beef Sausage
Finely ground beef cooked in the skin then smoked

Raw Beef Sausage
From coarser cut meat and fat

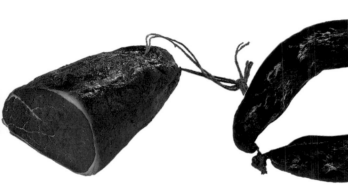

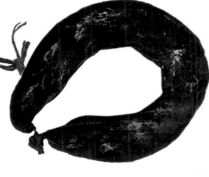

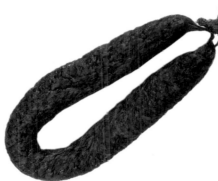

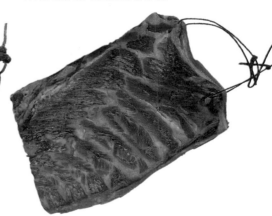

Smoked Beef
A succulent piece from the leg, mildly cured and smoked

Beef Salami
Dried and matured in the skin. Made from raw, medium fine beef and fat

Lamb Salami
Air dried, made from lean and fatty ground lamb

Bacon
A special, leaner and cold smoked piece of pork belly

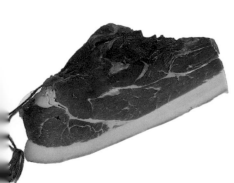

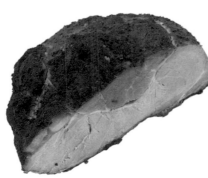

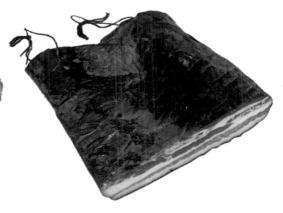

Raw Ham
Cured and cold smoked boned ham

Roast Pork
Thinly cut, eaten cold with mustard and pickled cucumbers

Streaky Bacon
Dry cured, smoked, fairly lean pork belly

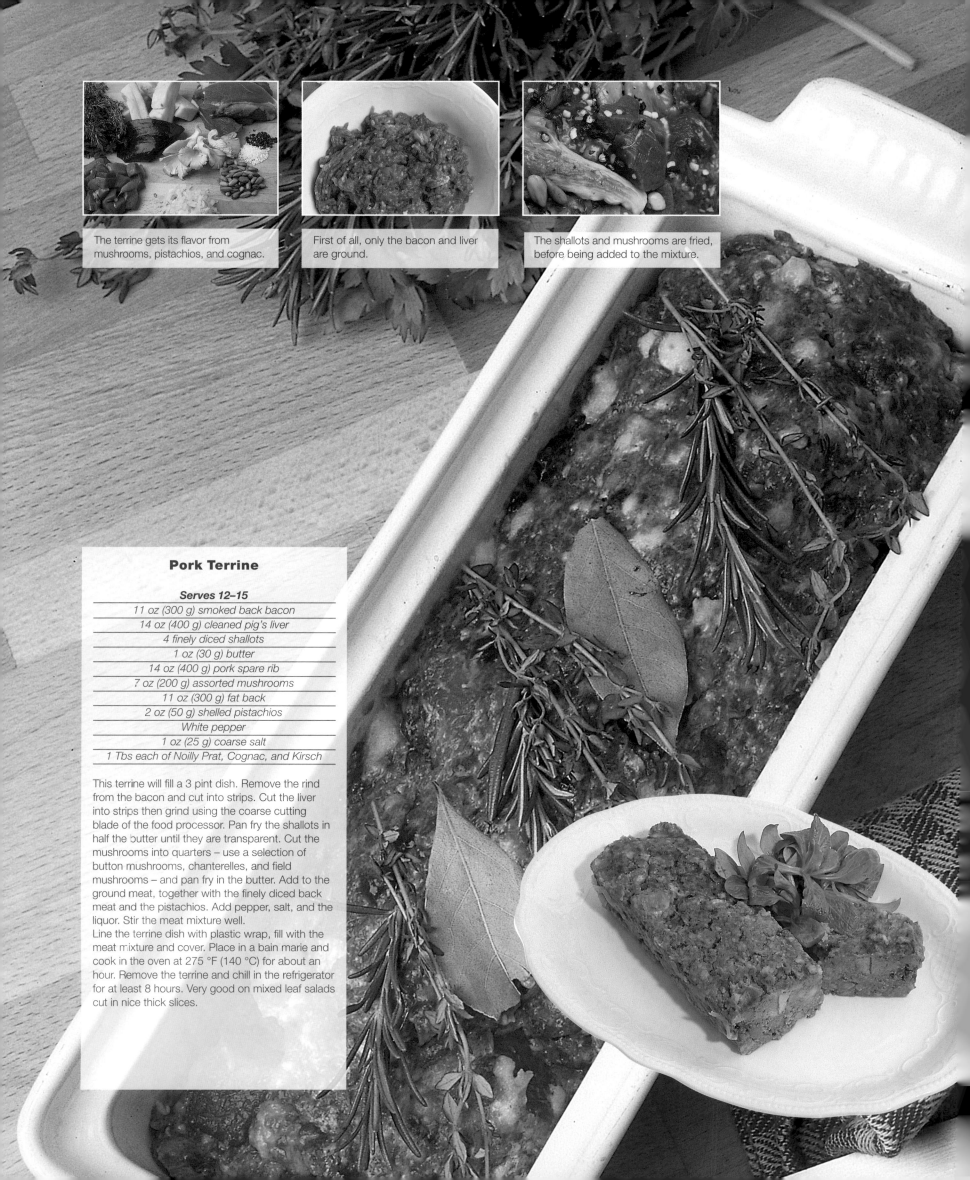

The terrine gets its flavor from mushrooms, pistachios, and cognac.

First of all, only the bacon and liver are ground.

The shallots and mushrooms are fried, before being added to the mixture.

Pork Terrine

Serves 12–15

11 oz (300 g) smoked back bacon
14 oz (400 g) cleaned pig's liver
4 finely diced shallots
1 oz (30 g) butter
14 oz (400 g) pork spare rib
7 oz (200 g) assorted mushrooms
11 oz (300 g) fat back
2 oz (50 g) shelled pistachios
White pepper
1 oz (25 g) coarse salt
1 Tbs each of Noilly Prat, Cognac, and Kirsch

This terrine will fill a 3 pint dish. Remove the rind from the bacon and cut into strips. Cut the liver into strips then grind using the coarse cutting blade of the food processor. Pan fry the shallots in half the butter until they are transparent. Cut the mushrooms into quarters – use a selection of button mushrooms, chanterelles, and field mushrooms – and pan fry in the butter. Add to the ground meat, together with the finely diced back meat and the pistachios. Add pepper, salt, and the liquor. Stir the meat mixture well.

Line the terrine dish with plastic wrap, fill with the meat mixture and cover. Place in a bain marie and cook in the oven at 275 °F (140 °C) for about an hour. Remove the terrine and chill in the refrigerator for at least 8 hours. Very good on mixed leaf salads cut in nice thick slices.

Recipes with Pork

(illustration left)

Roast Pork

2 lbs 3 oz (1 kg) leg of pork
1 Tbs coarse salt
1 tsp caraway
Black pepper
1 Tbs pork dripping
4 onions
2 carrots
Corn starch

Using a sharp knife, make cuts in the rind of the pork. Rub the joint with salt, caraway, and black pepper. Heat the dripping in a large roasting pan and brown the meat in it on all sides. Peel the onions and cut into eighths, clean the carrots and cut them into large pieces. Put the vegetables in the pan and pan fry them briefly. Turn the joint so that the skin is facing downwards. Pour over 1¼ cups (250 ml) boiling water. Cover the roasting pan and place in a preheated oven at 350 °F (180 °C). After 30 minutes, turn the meat. Uncover the pan and baste the meat frequently. After 90 to 100 minutes take the meat out of the oven, and place on a baking sheet with the skin facing upwards. Sprinkle the skin with a little cold water and place the meat back in the oven. Pour off the fat, strain the meat juices, season, and thicken with a little corn starch if required. Serve with potato dumplings.

Potato Dumplings

2 lbs 3 oz (1 kg) potatoes
3½ oz (100 g) whole wheat flour
1 egg
Pinch nutmeg
White pepper, coarse salt
2 stale bread rolls
1 Tbs dripping
A little extra flour

The day before serving, boil the potatoes in their skins, plunge into cold water, and peel. Sieve the potatoes and place in the refrigerator. The next day, sieve the flour into the potatoes, add the egg, a pinch of pepper, nutmeg, and a little salt and mix thoroughly. Flour your hands and roll out the potato mixture on a well floured work surface so that the potato forms a long sausage shape. Cut the potato roll into slices about 1¼ inch (3 cm) thick. Heat the fat and pan fry small cubes of the stale rolls. Season with a little salt. Place a few cubes of bread in the center of each potato slice and roll the potato between your hands to form dumplings. Bring a large pan of salted water to the boil, place the dumplings in the water and simmer gently for about 20 minutes.

Assorted Meat Platter with Sauerkraut

Serves 6–8

2 onions
1 Tbs pork dripping
2 lbs 3 oz (1 kg) sauerkraut
10 juniper berries
3 bay leaves
Pinch caraway
1 glass Franken wine
1 lb 2 oz (500 g) belly pork
1 lb 2 oz (500 g) boiled pork
1 large liver sausage
12–18 Nuremberg frying sausages

Peel the onions, dice finely, and pan fry in the hot dripping. Add the sauerkraut, juniper berries, bay leaves, and caraway. Pour in the wine and season to taste with salt and pepper. Add the belly and boiled pork, cover and simmer over a low heat for about an hour. Then add the liver sausage, cover again and simmer for another good 30 minutes. Just before serving, broil the Nuremberg sausages. Arrange the meat on the sauerkraut and surround with the sausages.

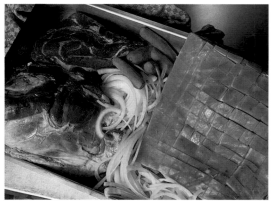

There is no stinting with the onions when roast pork is being made.

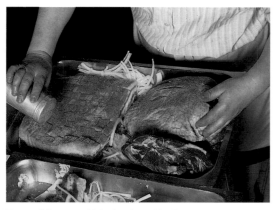

The well-browned joint is placed in the oven and turned frequently during cooking.

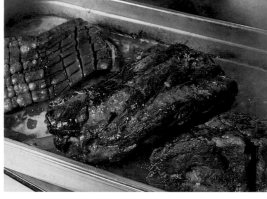

A 2¼ lb (1 kg) joint needs about 1 hour 40 minutes cooking time until the outside is crispy and the inside is juicy.

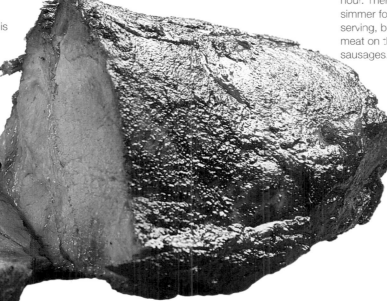

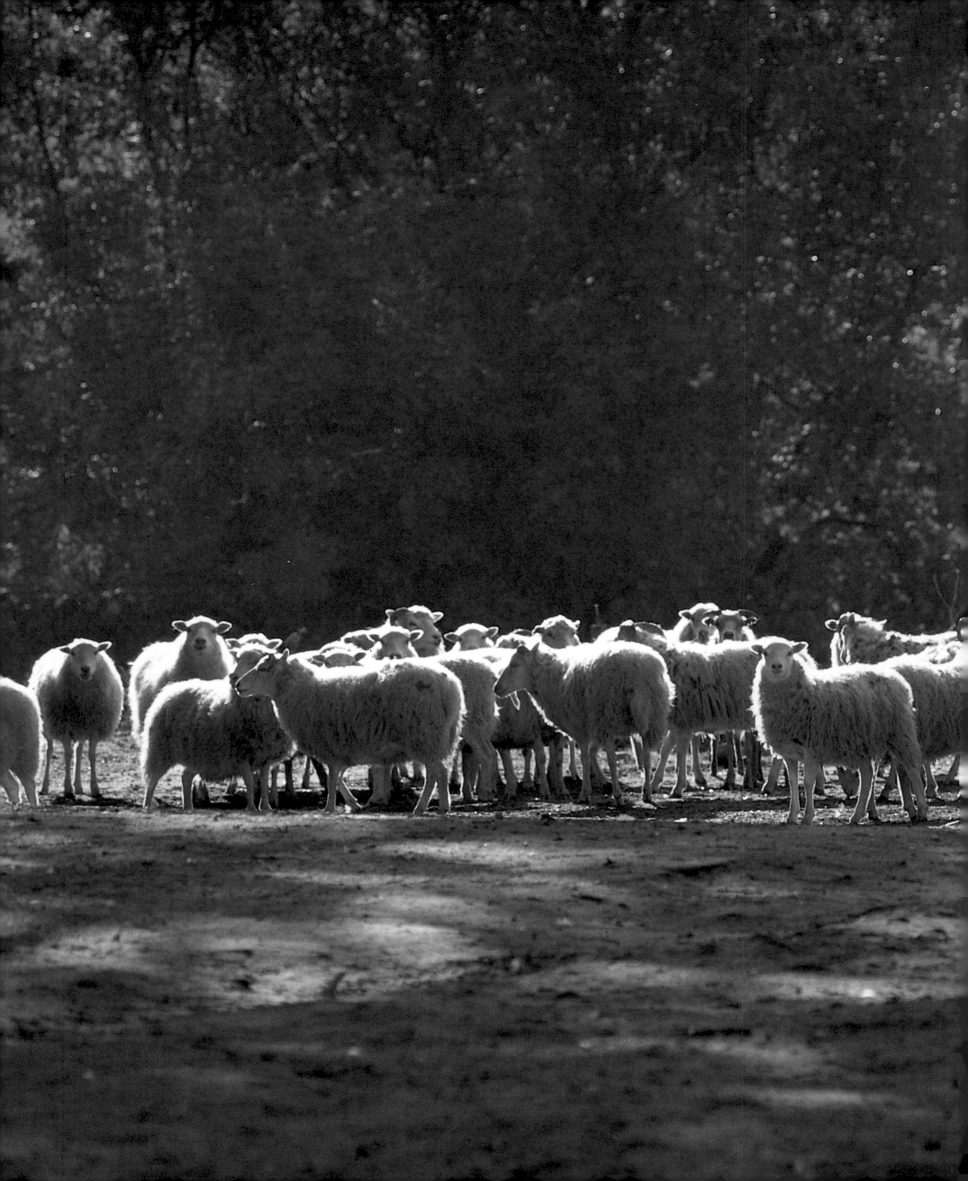

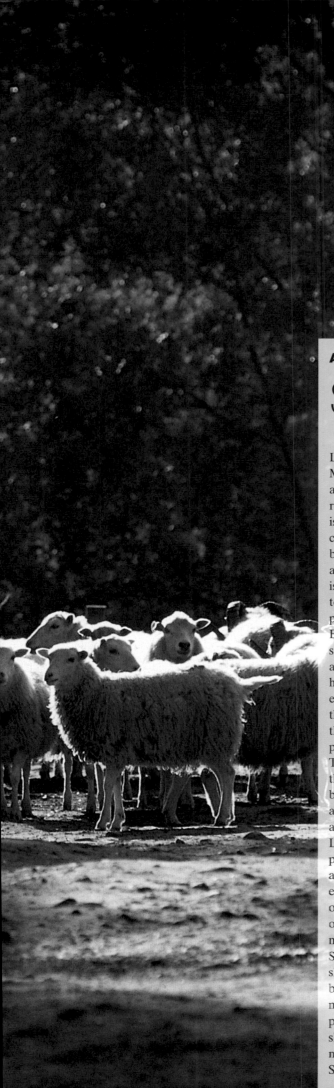

An Endangered Breed of Sheep

Skudden

Large areas of Europe are grazed by sheep. In Mediterranean countries, freely grazing sheep are a common sight. In northern Europe, the role of the shepherd seems rather anachronistic. There are an increasing number of countryside and town open spaces which are being maintained by sheep as they are almost as easy to look after as goats. The advantage is that they prefer eating grass and greenery, to stripping trees and bushes. Sheep also prefer flat ground to graze. In every region in Europe over the last centuries the breeds of sheep have adapted themselves to the flora and climate. There have been changes that have threatened some breeds of sheep with extinction. The main factor is the decline of the wool market, and a contributing factor is the increase in demand for meat from particular breeds of sheep.

The rare Skudden sheep have been victims of these changes. They are a very old country breed of sheep that was farmed in East Prussia and Baltic countries. Their habitat was the area around the Baltic sea from western Lithuania to the Vistula river. This area had poor soil and sparse vegetation but the animals were used to this and were hardy enough to be kept outdoors all year long. The only shelter they required was a roof to keep off the wind and rain during the coldest months of the year.

Skudden are one of the smallest breeds of sheep. Their withers – the highest part of the back – are only 19 to 23 inches (50–60 centimeters) tall. They weigh, on average, about 77 pounds (35 kilos). Skudden have wedge shaped heads with wide foreheads, delicate noses, and incredibly small ears. Usually Skudden have a grayish white fleece but occasionally they are darker in color, and can even be black, brown, or gray. The positive attributes of Skudden sheep are their robustness, vitality, independence, fertility, loyalty to their habitat, and the quality of their wool. Their wool is a mixture of fibers: underhair, fine wool fibers, and long hair. It is very good for spinning and in earlier times it was used to make excellent woollen cloth, which was sought after by merchants from England and France, German traders from the Rhine and cloth marketeers in eastern Germany. The world exhibition held in Paris in 1867 showed the high esteem that the Skudden wool cloth had achieved. Once wool was needed that was easier to use in mass production of cloth, an attempt at cross breeding with Merino sheep was made. This was unsuccessful, as were any attempts to cross breed Skudden with heavier breeds in order to obtain more meat. There was no longer any demand for this breed of sheep. Thanks to the efforts of a few idealists, there are now about 1,000 Skudden in west and central Germany and about 200 in Austria and Switzerland.

Apart from regions where sheep can graze unpolluted soil and satisfy organic meat standards, Skudden are very popular with organic farmers because of their modest needs. There is also a growing interest in the Skudden's delicious meat, which is becoming more popular every year.

Now there are herds of Skudden in eastern Germany. Skudden are a lowland breed that was once farmed in Baltic countries.

Recipes with Lamb

Lamb Chops
(Côtelettes d'agneau)
(Illustration below)

Serves 2

6–8 cutlets of very young lamb
3 minced garlic cloves
Coarse salt
Black pepper
2 Tbs olive oil
1 tsp finely ground savory

Preheat the broiler. Rinse the chops and pat dry. Rub with the garlic and drizzle with olive oil. Season with salt and pepper on both sides.
Broil for 1–1¹/₂ minutes then turn. Sprinkle the broiled side with savory and cook the other side for 1–1¹/₂ minutes. Serve on warmed plates with ratatouille (see p. 143).

Huntsman's Lamb
Agnello alla cacciatore

1 lb 11 oz (800 g) boned shoulder of lamb
1 lb 2 oz (500 g) ripe tomatoes
1 lb 2 oz (500 g) potatoes
2 onions
9 oz (250 g) fresh mushrooms
4 garlic cloves
1 dried chili pepper
1 tsp dried oregano
Coarse salt
4 Tbs olive oil
1 cup (200 ml) red wine

Cut away all the fat from the lamb and dice the meat. Skin and quarter the tomatoes. Peel and quarter the potatoes. Clean and slice the mushrooms. Peel the garlic cloves and mince with the chili. Preheat the oven to 240 °F (170 °C). Put the meat and the vegetables in an ovenproof dish, add the herbs and spices, and mix together well. Drizzle with olive oil and pour over the red wine. Cover and stew in the oven for 2 hours until cooked.

Lamb Goulash with Fried Noodles

1 lb 2 oz (500 g) boned shoulder of lamb
3 Tbs (45 ml) olive oil
Coarse salt
Black pepper
3 finely chopped onions
1 garlic clove
¹/₂ tsp cumin
¹/₂ tsp sweet paprika
1 tsp tomato paste
¹/₄ cup (40 ml) red wine
1¹/₄ cups (250 ml) lamb stock
1¹/₄ cups (250 ml) chicken stock
11 oz (300 g) spelt tagliatelle

Dice the lamb, heat 2 tablespoons of olive oil and pan fry the lamb. Season with salt and pepper. Add the garlic and onion and brown lightly. Sprinkle with paprika and cumin and stir in the tomato paste. Pour in the red wine and allow to come to the boil. Pour in the lamb and chicken stock. Cover the pan and stew in the oven at 350 °F (180 °C) for 40 minutes.
Cook the tagliatelle until it is "al dente," drain, and leave to dry. Heat the remaining olive oil, pan fry the tagliatelle in the oil and arrange on individual plates. Check the seasoning of the goulash, arrange on top of the tagliatelle and serve.

Lamb Chops

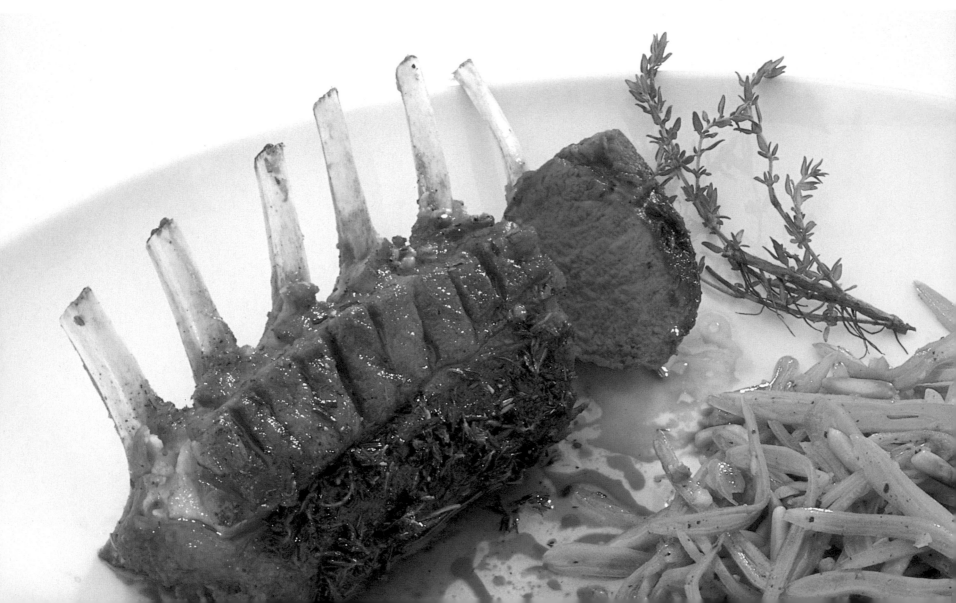

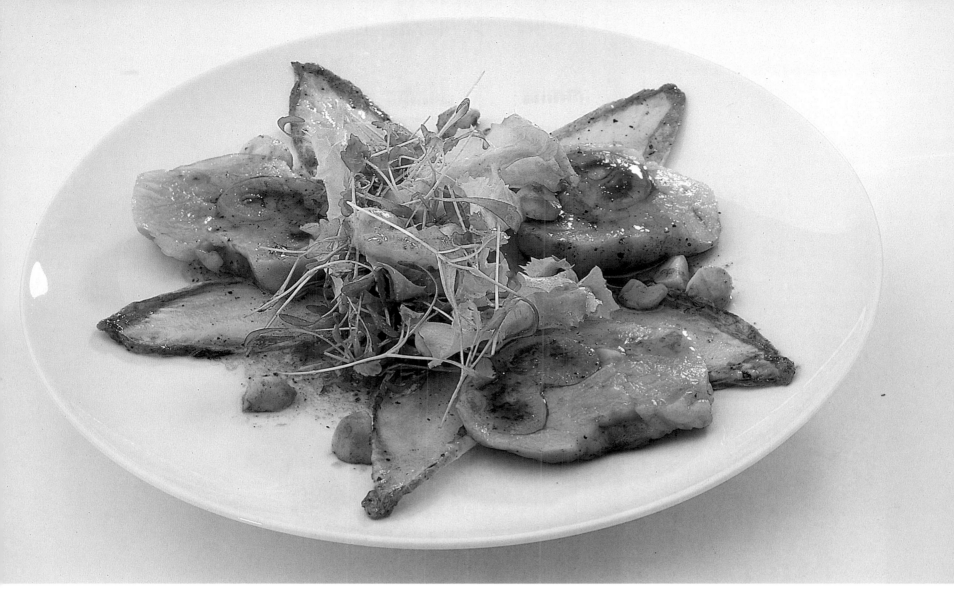

Warm Salad of Lambs' Kidneys and Braised Belgian Endive

Fricassee of Lamb with Artichoke Hearts

Agnello in fricassea con carciofi

1 lb 11 oz (800 g) boned lamb
4 Tbs olive oil
2 finely chopped garlic cloves
1¹/₂ cups (300 ml) dry white wine
1 jar artichoke hearts
3 Tbs finely chopped parsley
3 egg yolks
Juice of 1 lemon
Pepper, coarse salt

Cut the lamb into medium sized cubes. Heat the oil in a casserole, pan fry the garlic in the oil for about a minute, then add the meat and brown thoroughly. Pour in a third of the white wine, cover and simmer over a low heat for 60 minutes. Check to make sure there is sufficient cooking liquid, adding a little water if required. Rinse the artichokes, drain, and cut into quarters. Add the artichokes to the meat and simmer for 5 minutes. Mix the egg yolk with the lemon juice, add to the casserole and stir until it thickens. Serve the fricassee straight from the casserole with whole wheat bread and a fresh green salad.

Warm Salad of Lambs' Kidneys and Braised Belgian Endive

(Illustration above)

6 lambs' kidneys in their own fat
Coarse salt
Black pepper
1 Tbs olive oil
1 Tbs butter
30 Belgian endive leaves
1 Tbs sunflower oil
¹/₂ tsp honey
¹/₂ head frisée
2 oz (60 g) garden cress
1 tsp walnut oil

Balsamic Vinaigrette

3 Tbs halved macadamia nuts
1 tsp butter
¹/₄ cup chicken stock
¹/₄ cup (40 ml) lamb gravy
¹/₈ cup (20 ml) sunflower oil
¹/₈ cup (20 ml) walnut oil
Pinch coarse salt
Plenty of black pepper
¹/₈ cup (20 ml) balsamic vinegar
2 tsp (10 ml) hazelnut oil
1 bay leaf
1 small cinnamon stick

Season the kidneys with salt and pepper and sear in the olive oil on all sides until the fat becomes a rust brown color. Remove from the heat and leave to rest for 5 minutes. Place the kidneys into a preheated oven at 350 °F (180 °C) and cook for 6 minutes until they are pink in color. Leave to rest for another 5 minutes. Meanwhile pan fry the Belgian endive leaves in sunflower oil and butter, and season with salt and pepper. Sweeten with the honey, caramelize lightly, and place on plates immediately.

To make the vinaigrette, roast the macadamia nuts in butter. Mix the other ingredients together well, add the nuts and put the vinaigrette in a warm place.

Wash the frisée and tear into bite sized pieces. Wash the cress, spin it dry and mix with the lettuce. Season with plenty of walnut oil, salt, and pepper. Arrange the lettuce in the middle of the plates. Halve the kidneys, place on the lettuce, and drizzle the warm dressing over.

Kid

Kid is a specialty that is associated with the celebration of Easter. Its tender, flavorsome meat is highly prized by the Greeks, Italians, Spanish, and French. Goat meat is not as easily available as other types of meat beacause goats are kept principally for their milk. Organic goat farming leads to the production of goats' cheese but occasionally kids are sold to private customers. It is very rare to find organic goat meat in a store.

This recipe requires a lot of preparation and makes a wonderful festive meal.

A Party Roast: Roast Kid

Serves 6–8

Preparation of the Meat

Back Meat
Remove any ligaments and bones, cut away any untidy scraps of meat. Trim tendons and fat leaving the meat clean and fatless.

Leg and Shoulder
Cook whole.

Belly Cuts and Ribs
Using a sharp knife, loosen the thin layers of meat from between the ribs without completely removing them. Turn down the meat so that there is a broader surface of meat to work with.
• Spread the belly meat with stuffing, leaving the bones free.
• Roll up the spine and ribs.
• Fold the belly meat with stuffing over the other meat.
• Tie the joint up with butcher's thread.

$^1/_2$ kid weighing between $6^1/_2$ and $7^1/_2$ pounds (3–3.5 kg)
4 Tbs olive oil
Coarse salt
Black pepper
1 small cauliflower
6 carrots
1 small celeriac
12 shallots
2 lbs 3 oz (1 kg) firm potatoes
2 Tbs butter, cut into pieces

Stuffing

$^1/_2$ stale bread roll
7 oz (200 g) kid meat from neck and shank
2 oz (50 g) fresh belly pork
2 oz diced onion
1 Tbs olive oil
Black pepper
Coarse salt
A few drops chili oil

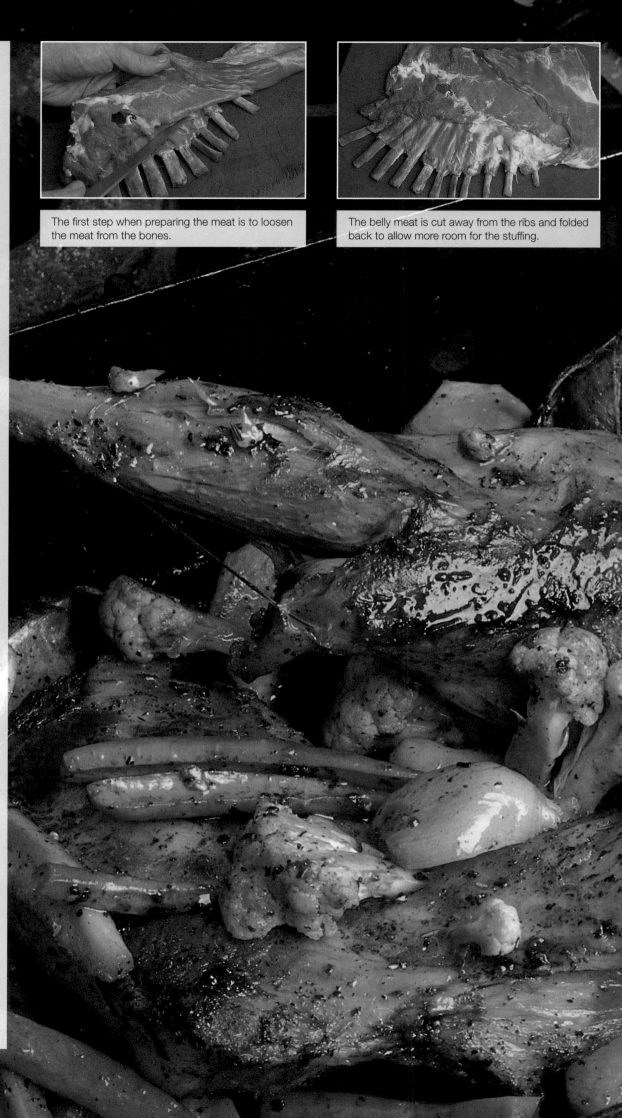

The first step when preparing the meat is to loosen the meat from the bones.

The belly meat is cut away from the ribs and folded back to allow more room for the stuffing.

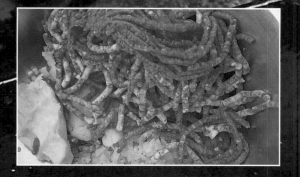

To make the stuffing, take neck and shank meat, belly pork, stale bread, and diced onions. Grind well.

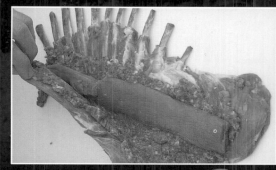

The belly meat is spread with the stuffing, leaving the bones free.

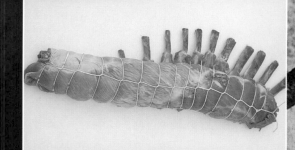

The back meat is rolled up towards the ribs, the belly meat is wrapped around and the whole joint is tied up securely.

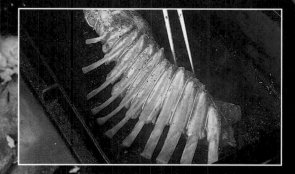

The stuffed kid joint is browned in very hot olive oil.

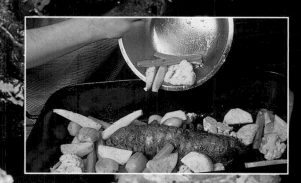

The vegetables are chopped and added to the meat. Both are roasted until cooked through.

Stuffing

Soak the bread roll in water and squeeze out any excess liquid. Fillet the kid neck meat, dice the meat, dice the belly pork, and grind using the fine blade of the food processor. Pan fry the diced onion in the oil, add to the meat and mix together well. Season to taste with salt, pepper, and chili oil.

Gravy

Backbone and neckbone of the kid
1 Tbs olive oil
2 carrots
1/4 celeriac
2 onions
2 garlic cloves
1 Tbs tomato paste
1 bay leaf
10 peppercorns
1/2 cup (100 ml) red wine
1 tsp dried Provençal herbs
Coarse salt

Gravy

Finely chop the bones and deep fry until browned. Peel the carrots and celeriac, retaining the skins, and dice the flesh.
Finely chop the onions and 1 clove of garlic. Add the vegetables to the bones and fry. Then put the bones and vegetables in a sieve and shake off the excess fat. Drain the fat from the pan, put the bones and vegetables back in the pan and caramelize with the tomato paste. Add the bay leaf and the crushed peppercorns, pour in the red wine and bring to the boil. Fill the pan with water so that the ingredients are covered and simmer for 45 minutes. Keep checking the pan. When the 45 minutes have passed, turn down the heat and cook, just below boiling point for another 30 minutes. Strain through a cloth and place back into the pan. Add the dried Provençal herbs, the second garlic clove and the vegetable peelings. Cook slowly, skimming the surface of the stock frequently until the volume of the liquid has reduced to a fifth. Remove the peelings and season with salt. Lamb gravy can be made in the same way.

Method

In a large roasting pan, brown the rolled belly joint, the leg and the shoulder in 2 tablespoons (30 ml) hot olive oil. Cover with aluminum foil and roast in the oven for 25 minutes at 350 °F (180 °C). Clean the vegetables, cut the cauliflower into large florets and cut the carrot and celeriac into large sticks. Dip the vegetables in the remaining olive oil, season well with salt and pepper. Add the vegetables to the meat, cover the roasting pan with aluminum foil and roast for a further 55 minutes.
Remove from the oven and leave to rest at a temperature of 110 °F (45 °C). Dot with pieces of butter, place the pan under the broiler and cook until browned.
Carve the meat, serve with the vegetables, and pour over the gravy.

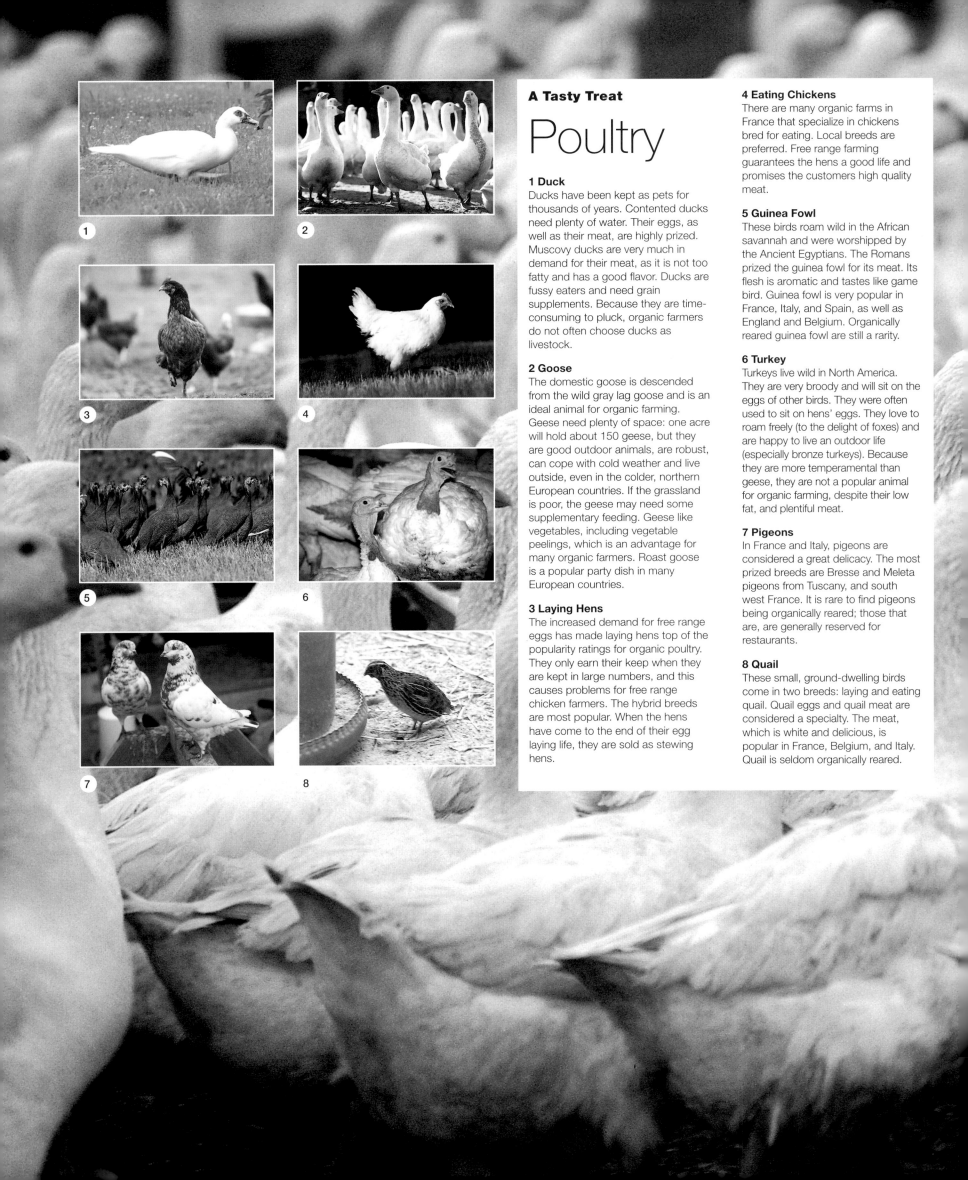

A Tasty Treat

Poultry

1 Duck

Ducks have been kept as pets for thousands of years. Contented ducks need plenty of water. Their eggs, as well as their meat, are highly prized. Muscovy ducks are very much in demand for their meat, as it is not too fatty and has a good flavor. Ducks are fussy eaters and need grain supplements. Because they are time-consuming to pluck, organic farmers do not often choose ducks as livestock.

2 Goose

The domestic goose is descended from the wild gray lag goose and is an ideal animal for organic farming. Geese need plenty of space: one acre will hold about 150 geese, but they are good outdoor animals, are robust, can cope with cold weather and live outside, even in the colder, northern European countries. If the grassland is poor, the geese may need some supplementary feeding. Geese like vegetables, including vegetable peelings, which is an advantage for many organic farmers. Roast goose is a popular party dish in many European countries.

3 Laying Hens

The increased demand for free range eggs has made laying hens top of the popularity ratings for organic poultry. They only earn their keep when they are kept in large numbers, and this causes problems for free range chicken farmers. The hybrid breeds are most popular. When the hens have come to the end of their egg laying life, they are sold as stewing hens.

4 Eating Chickens

There are many organic farms in France that specialize in chickens bred for eating. Local breeds are preferred. Free range farming guarantees the hens a good life and promises the customers high quality meat.

5 Guinea Fowl

These birds roam wild in the African savannah and were worshipped by the Ancient Egyptians. The Romans prized the guinea fowl for its meat. Its flesh is aromatic and tastes like game bird. Guinea fowl is very popular in France, Italy, and Spain, as well as England and Belgium. Organically reared guinea fowl are still a rarity.

6 Turkey

Turkeys live wild in North America. They are very broody and will sit on the eggs of other birds. They were often used to sit on hens' eggs. They love to roam freely (to the delight of foxes) and are happy to live an outdoor life (especially bronze turkeys). Because they are more temperamental than geese, they are not a popular animal for organic farming, despite their low fat, and plentiful meat.

7 Pigeons

In France and Italy, pigeons are considered a great delicacy. The most prized breeds are Bresse and Meleta pigeons from Tuscany, and south west France. It is rare to find pigeons being organically reared; those that are, are generally reserved for restaurants.

8 Quail

These small, ground-dwelling birds come in two breeds: laying and eating quail. Quail eggs and quail meat are considered a specialty. The meat, which is white and delicious, is popular in France, Belgium, and Italy. Quail is seldom organically reared.

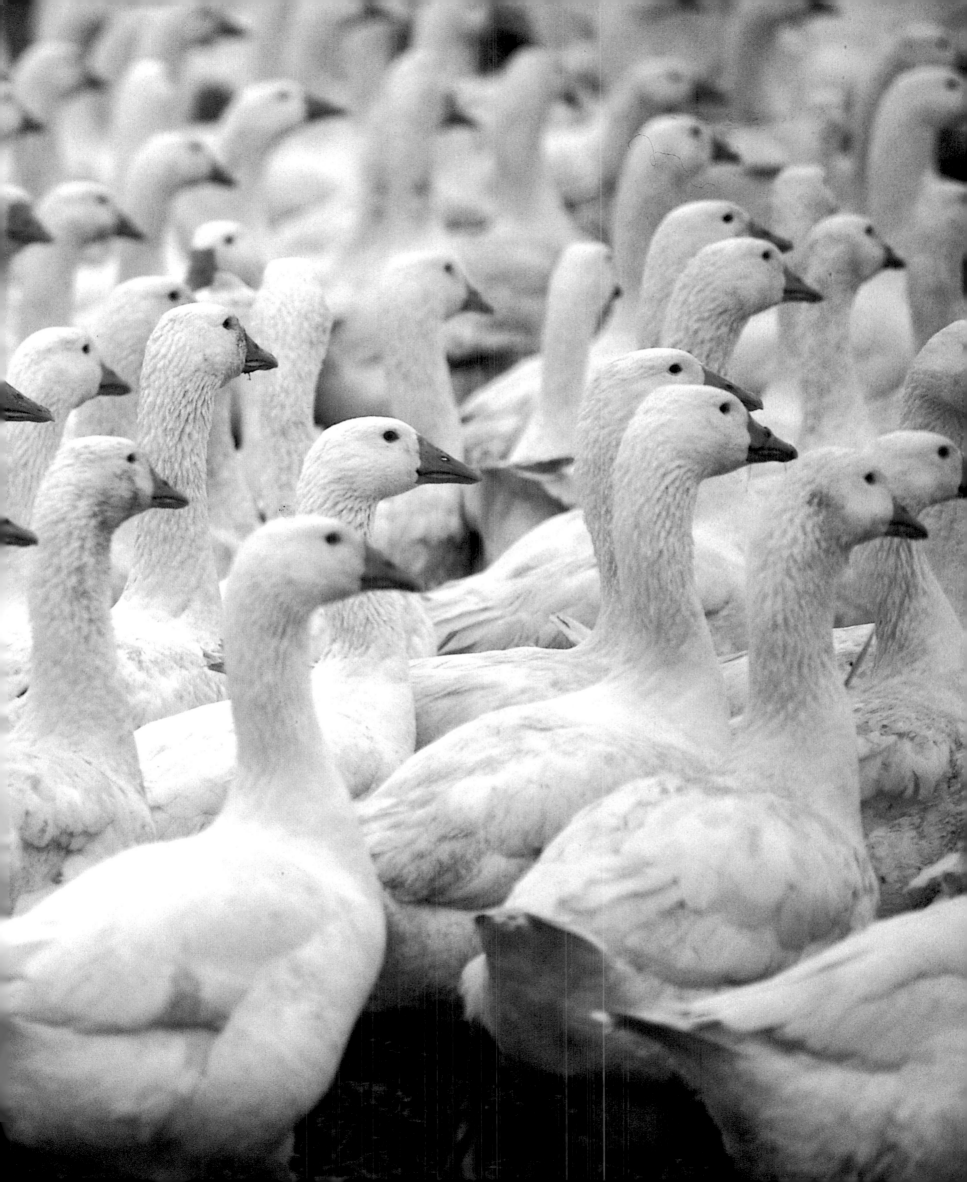

Bresse Poultry

If the German emperors had only known! Where once the land was tilled to supply them and their entourage in the nearby Ingelheim Imperial Palace, now the fattening poultry display the French national colors. Young hens and cockerels strut around on blue feet, have gleaming white feathers, and sport blood-red combs: the unmistakable features of France's tastiest chicken breed from the Bresse region. The Mechtildshausen farm, one of the largest organic farms in Europe, succeeded in obtaining breeding pairs from the poultry haven just outside Lyons.

The prestige chickens from the fertile farming region between Burgundy and Jura are an old, particularly resistant breed. As the lush meadows were used mainly for dairy farming, poultry was really only a secondary concern to the farmers' wives. What they had in mind above all were the big family gatherings at the end of the year. Nothing was regarded as too good or too costly for fattening up the cocks and hens. The Bresse poultry thrived so well that in 1957, the French parliament conferred on the breed the only "Appellation d'Origine Contrôlée" ever awarded to poultry. This distinction is otherwise reserved for wines, cheeses, and remarkably few other delicacies.

As part of this, each individual chicken was officially allocated an area of 12 square yards (10 square meters), the number of birds was limited to 500 per enclosure, and they were guaranteed a life of at least four months. In keeping with the established customs, they now have to be fed with corn softened in milk and are allowed out to pasture from the age of 35 days at the latest. Before being served up as the special occasion roast, they are confined to cages and given extra rations to ensure they have the optimum layer of fat when they go into the oven.

The fact that these exquisite chickens can be reared outside of their traditional region, and, what is more, on an organic farm, is something of a revolution. The positive features of a breed are here being consciously combined with the special requirements of rearing animals according to the needs of the species, without acting solely in the interest of the gourmet. Now the superbly robust and healthy birds peck and scratch around contentedly under the Hessian fruit trees or enjoy a snooze in the shade of the fruit bushes. They live like royalty. A 25 acre (10 hectare) fenced-in orchard is available where the 3,000 birds a year can run around. Here they can move about freely. They live in ten cheerful caravans parked by the fruit trees or at the edge of the field. They are so accustomed to their mobile living quarters that they never stray more than 100 yards from them. This accommodation creates a lot of work for the team, both in moving the vans occasionally and with regard to cleaning and daily feeding. The food that the chickens find for themselves is supplemented with organic corn and wheat as well as a little milk and milk powder.

After about 15 weeks, when the young cockerels weigh at least 3¼ pounds (1.5 kilograms), they are taken to meet their fate at the on-site slaughterhouse. From there it is only a few yards to the farm shop, where there is keen demand from ecologically conscious families and gourmets alike. These are, after all, the most exquisite poultry raised on German soil. Not even an emperor could expect better!

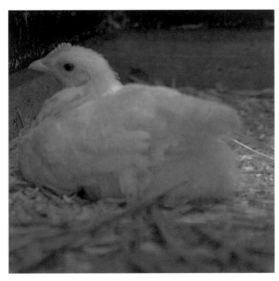

Chickens as robust and healthy as those from the Bresse region are a rarity.

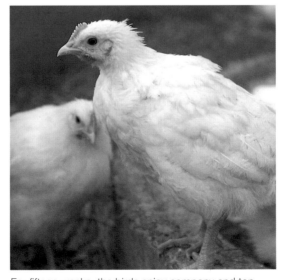

For fifteen weeks, the birds enjoy company and top quality food and can run around freely.

Recipes with Poultry

Bresse Chicken Braised in Red Wine

Serves 4–6

1 Bresse chicken weighing about 4 lbs (1.8 kg)
Coarse salt, Black pepper
7 oz (200 g) smoked bacon
11 oz (300 g) mushrooms
2 oz (50 g) butter
7 oz (200 g) small shallots
1 bottle red Burgundy
2½ cups (500 ml) chicken stock
1 small carrot
¼ celeriac
1 small leek
1 Tbs flour
1 Tbs butter

Divide up the chicken, separate the legs and cut through the joints. Separate the breasts with the wings and divide into two pieces. Season the meat with salt and pepper. Cut the bacon into strips. Clean and quarter the mushrooms. Heat the butter in a skillet and brown the chicken pieces on both sides. Add the onions, mushrooms and bacon and cook until browned. Add the red wine and chicken stock and simmer for about 15 minutes until the breast meat is cooked. Remove the breast pieces from the pan. Dice the vegetables finely. After a further 10 minutes, add the diced vegetables and about 10 minutes later, remove the cooked leg pieces. Now pass the sauce through a sieve and continue cooking until reduced by about half. Knead together the flour and softened butter and gradually add enough of this paste to bind the sauce while it is simmering. Heat the meat through briefly in the sauce, then put the meat on the plates and pour over the sauce. This can be served with homemade noodles or brown rice.

Traditional Roast Goose

Serves 6–8

2 russet apples
4 onions
1 goose weighing about 8¾ lbs (4 kg)
Coarse salt
Black pepper
3 sage leaves
Juice of 2 oranges

Peel and core the apples and cut them into eighths. Peel and quarter the onions. Season the inside of the goose generously with salt and pepper, then fill it with the apples, onions and sage. Truss the bird with kitchen string. Pour about an inch (3 cm) of water into a large roasting pan then place the goose in the pan. Roast in the oven at 400 °F (200 °C) for 2–2½ hours. While the goose is cooking, skim off some of the fat produced from time to time. This can be used for preparing red cabbage. To ensure the goose gets a nice crispy skin, baste it every 15 minutes with the roasting juices. When it is cooked, take the goose out of the roasting pan and pour off the fat. Deglaze with the orange juice and reduce slightly.

The goose should be carved at table, and served with traditional accompaniments such as red cabbage, chestnuts, dumplings and baked apples.

Right-hand page: This proud Bresse cock wears the French national colors; red, white, and blue.

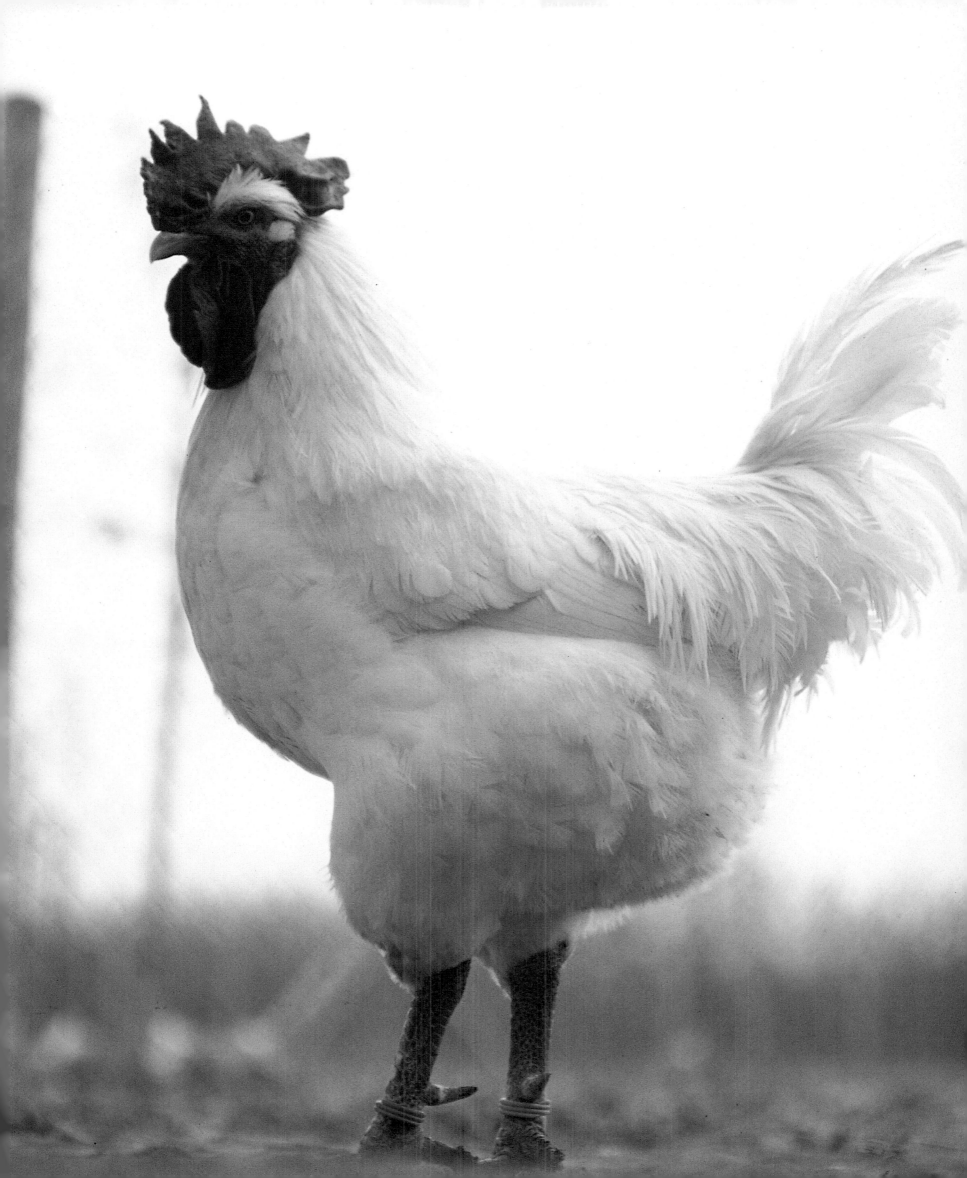

Lean Ducks

The Mallard, which occurs in the wild in Europe, Asia and North America, is the ancestor of most common breeds of domestic duck. It was domesticated long ago in China and ancient Egypt. Amongst its brownish colored plumage, it has a characteristic blue mark on the wings and in the breeding season, the shining green coloring on the drake's head is an impressive sight.

Forms of Mallard are widespread in Europe today, whilst in Britain, the Aylesbury duck is very popular in the world of gastronomy. Muscovy ducks, which originated in South America, and were brought to Europe by the conquering Spanish, are also beginning to gain popularity as

eating ducks. These ducks are very susceptible to cold. They may be identified by the reddish warts at the base of the beak and by the eyes. Apart from plenty of space, the main requirement for keeping domestic and Muscovy ducks under correct conditions is free access to water, ponds or rivers, as these water birds will suffer if they are unable to bathe regularly and preen themselves thoroughly.

Compared with Mallards, Muscovy ducks have more meat on them, and this meat is lower in fat and very juicy and aromatic. The famous Barbary duck came about by crossing the domestic duck with a leaner wild drake and combines the advantages of both. But above all, ducks have another culinary trump which has allowed them to surpass their relations, the geese, in terms of numbers: they are smaller.

They make a good meal for four to six people; in other words, a quantity to suit any household. More organic farmers ought to come round to this idea in future.

Duck Breast in a Salt Crust

| 2 large duck breasts (at least 11 oz/300 g each) |
| 4 lbs 2 oz (2 kg) coarse salt |

Cut the skin of the duck breasts in a criss-cross pattern and fry for 2 minutes until golden brown, then remove them and let them drain. Cover the bottom of a small heatproof dish with a layer of salt about 1/2 inch (1 centimeter) deep. Lay the duck breasts in the dish next to one another, and sprinkle generously with salt and just a little water. Preheat the oven to 460 °F (250 °C). Cook for about 20 to 25 minutes (they should still be pink inside), remove from the oven and leave to stand for a further 5 minutes. Then remove the salt crust, cut the meat into slices and serve.

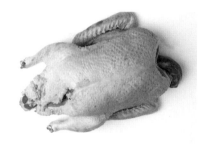
When you buy a duck, ...

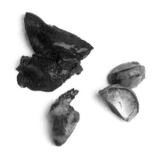
... the liver, heart and stomach are already separated. If the duck is not going to be roasted whole, ...

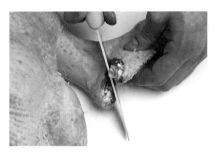
... first cut through the lower wing joint, ...

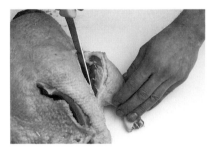
... then the upper joint ...

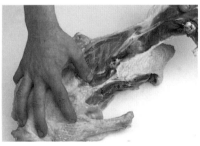
... and pull it off.

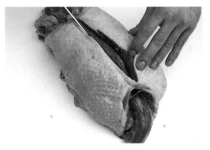
Then cut lengthwise along the body, ...

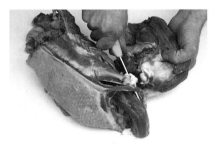
... and cut deep into the breast, ...

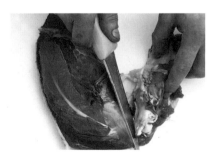
... in order to cut through the leg joint, ...

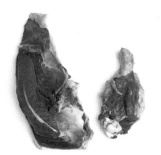
... so that the breast and leg can be separated.

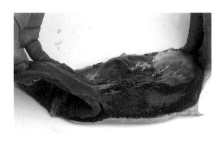
Once you have removed the fillet from the breast, ...

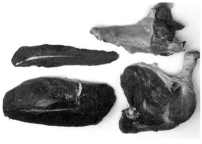
... the fillet, breast, upper wing joint and leg are ready to be used in the following recipes.

Exquisite Duck
(Illustration below left)

5 medium-sized fresh figs
5 oz (150 g) black currants
1/2 cup (100 ml) good red wine
1/2 cup (100 g) unrefined cane sugar
1/2 cup (100 ml) Crème de Cassis
4 small duck breasts each weighing 6 1/2 oz (180 g)
2 Tbs oil
Coarse salt, black pepper
3/4 cup (150 ml) chicken stock

Remove the skins from the figs and place the figs in a small bowl. Boil the black currants, red wine and sugar together and purée them in a blender, pour the mixture over the figs, add the Crème de Cassis, and let the figs marinate in the refrigerator for two days. Slit the skin of the duck breasts in a criss-cross pattern to prevent it bulging out during cooking. Heat the oil in a pan, then place the duck breasts in the pan, skin side down, brown them and then turn them onto the other side. Cook them just once more with the fat side downwards until they are a lovely golden brown color. Keep them warm in the oven. Pour the stock into the pan, add 2 tablespoons of the fig marinade and season to taste.

Heat the figs in the remaining marinade. Arrange the duck breasts on the plates, pour over the juice, and garnish each breast with a fig.

Duck Legs on a Bed of Salad with Mushrooms
(Illustration below right)

4 medium-sized duck legs
Coarse salt, black pepper
2 lbs 3 oz (1 kg) goose or duck dripping
1 small carrot
1/4 celeriac
1 onion
1 bouquet garni of rosemary, thyme and parsley
1 tsp black peppercorns
1/2 tsp juniper berries
2–3 bay leaves
2 unpeeled crushed garlic cloves
11 oz (300 g) oyster mushrooms and plain mushrooms
2 Tbs butter
2 finely chopped shallots
Various types of salad, to garnish

Season the duck legs, which should weigh about 5 ounces (150 g) each, with salt and pepper. Heat some of the dripping in a skillet and brown the duck legs on both sides. Dice the carrot, celeriac, and onion finely. Add the diced vegetables, bouquet garni, seasoning ingredients, garlic cloves, and the remaining dripping to the pan and cook, covered, for about 1 hour on a low heat. Then remove the lid and simmer until the juice produced has evaporated and only the dripping is left. Place the legs in an earthenware dish or similar and pour over the strained dripping.
The meat can be kept covered in a cool place or in the refrigerator for several weeks to enhance the flavor.
To serve, first clean and slice the mushrooms, heat the butter, cook the shallots in it until they become transparent, brown the mushrooms, and season with salt and pepper. Heat the duck legs in a little dripping. Arrange a selection of fresh lettuce leaves such as escarole, oakleaf and lollo rosso on the four plates, place one leg in the middle of each plate, arrange the mushrooms around it and trickle the butter from the pan over the salad.

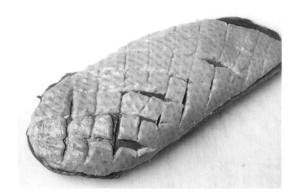

First cut the skin of the duck breast in a criss-cross pattern.

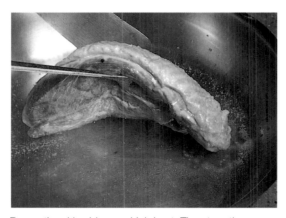

Brown the skin side on a high heat. Then turn the breast over and brown it on the other side too.

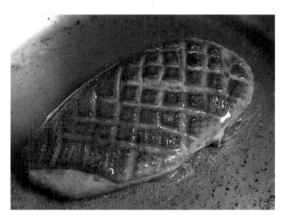

Once the duck breast has been fried for about 3 minutes on each side, it is brown and crispy on the outside and still pink on the inside.

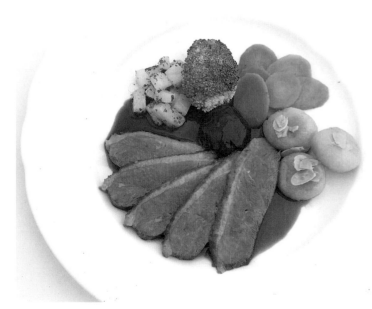

Exquisite Duck

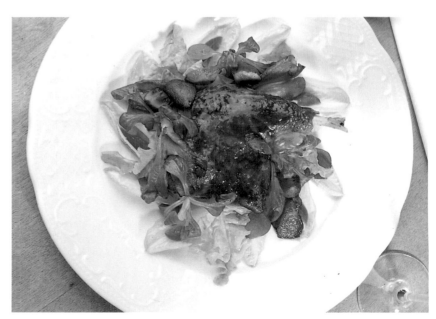

Duck Legs on a Bed of Salad with Mushrooms

Egg Farming

Eggs have always appealed to us humans, both for nutrition and as a symbol of life itself or of fertility and wholeness. According to the Hindu story of creation, the universe was created from an egg. And in the Christian religion, the egg is seen as a symbol of Christ's resurrection. The Bankiva breed chickens living in the Asian Steppes, from which domestic chickens descended, were probably first kept as domestic animals in China, the Malayan islands and India. From there they spread via Babylonia to Egypt and on to Europe. Nowadays most western European countries keep about half as many egg-laying chickens as there are inhabitants, and more in some countries. Annual per capita consumption of eggs often comes close to the annual laying capacity of the modern hybrid chicken which, in battery production, lays up to 280 eggs per year.

Chickens naturally enjoy moving around and flapping their wings, they love fresh air and fresh greenery, sand and sun, grain and worms, branches and nests, and above all their social structure, in which the rooster keeps things in order and bestows his favors on about ten hens. Their daily routine follows a strict ritual. The

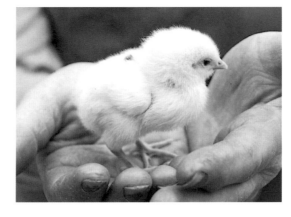

The chickens strut around freely in the farmyard and henhouse – an idyll which is reflected in meat of a quality rarely seen today.

importance to them of sunlight is proclaimed untiringly by the cockerels each morning. Once they have had their first meal, they see to their nest, pressing it into shape with their beaks and whole bodies or making it tidy before sitting down in it and – possibly – laying an egg. Then comes the midday period when they enjoy bathing in the sun and sand. After that, they set off in search of food again and socialize with their fellow chickens before settling down for the night on high perches. They should be in darkness for at least eight hours.

If the chickens lead a daily life similar to this, they are being looked after correctly. This natural pattern of behavior is used as a guide on organic farms.

High Outlay, Low Output

It seems that, of all the animal species farmed, chickens are the most difficult to keep under appropriate ecological conditions. The reason for this is simply that keeping chickens is only profitable for farmers if they keep hundreds, if not thousands, of laying hens. Certainly, once chicken runs are provided, their feathered friends can move around freely and scratch about as much as they like. However, as an experienced chicken keeper explains, "the constant contact with the earth and their own feces means they pick up germs much more easily when kept in organic conditions. Although free-range chickens are more resistant, their higher exposure to germs more than compensates for this."

The organic farmer therefore has to take other measures. The most important factor is to maintain very strict hygiene in the henhouse, which has to be thoroughly cleaned out and then whitewashed before it is occupied by each new set of birds.

When chicks can hatch out in the farmyard, the chicken world is as it should be.

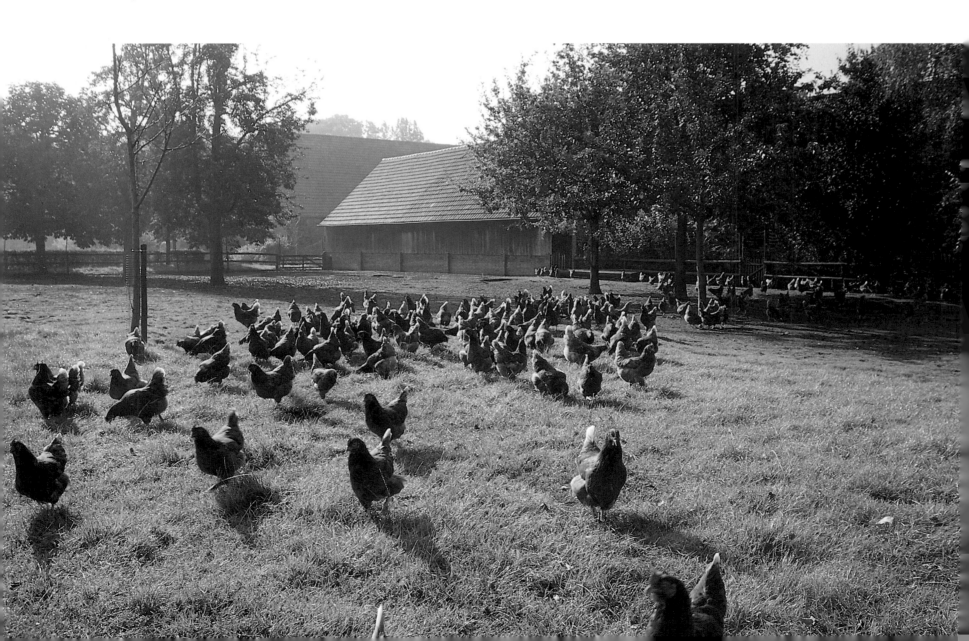

Quality Grades

These apply through the European Union.

Class A – fresh eggs

These eggs must meet the following criteria when they reach the end consumer:

- undamaged shell which has not been washed or cleaned
- air chamber not larger than $^1/_4$ inch (6 mm)
- transparent, jelly-like egg white
- yolk in the middle
- no foreign deposits
- no incubation
- no abnormal shapes

The "Extra" label must be removed on the seventh day after packing.

Class B – second quality or preserved eggs

These eggs, which are mostly supplied to small businesses and usually preserved by refrigeration, must meet the following criteria:

- red stamp
- undamaged shell
- air chamber not larger than $^3/_8$ inch (9 mm)
- no foreign deposits
- no incubation
- no abnormal shapes.

Class C – selected

Intended for the manufacture of pasteurised egg products or for industrial use

Size and Weight Ranges

XL	Very Large	73 g and above
L	Large	63 g up to 73 g
M	Medium	53 g up to 63 g
S	Small	under 53 g

Scrambled eggs

The eggs are beaten with a balloon whisk, poured into a pan containing melted butter and stirred with a wooden spoon until they start to set. Milk can be added for a lighter consistency and the eggs are then seasoned with salt and pepper.

Fried eggs

For perfect fried eggs cooked in hot butter, only the egg white is salted, and the yolk remains runny. Brown edges should be avoided as they are hard to digest.

Raw eggs

Otherwise known as Prairie Oysters these raw eggs are eaten simply with a pinch of coarse salt and pepper. Eggs should only be served in this way if you are quite sure of their origin and the date they were laid. Even then, they are still hard to digest.

Uses for Eggs

Whole egg:

as a binding agent for

- all types of bread doughs and cake mixtures, in which it also has a lightening effect
- noodles, pasta, dumplings
- ground meat

Egg white:

as a clarifying agent in

- clear soups
- jellies
- winemaking

Beaten egg white:

as a lightening agent for

- desserts and creams
- cake and cookie doughs
- vegetable, fish or meat mixtures

Egg yolk:

as a thickener in

- soups and sauces
- creams and mayonnaises

and as a shiny coating and adhesive agent for grains, seeds and spices on

- breads, cakes, cookies, and pastries.

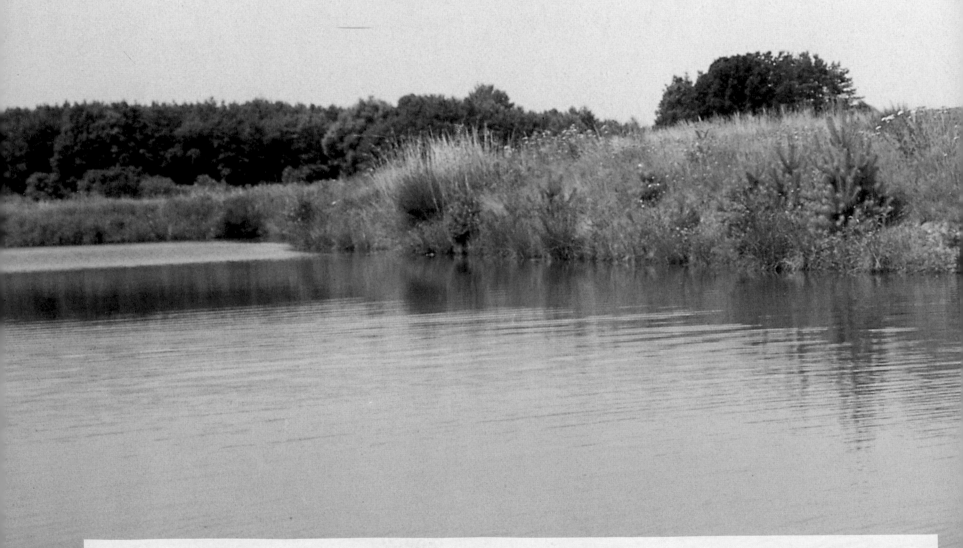

Fish

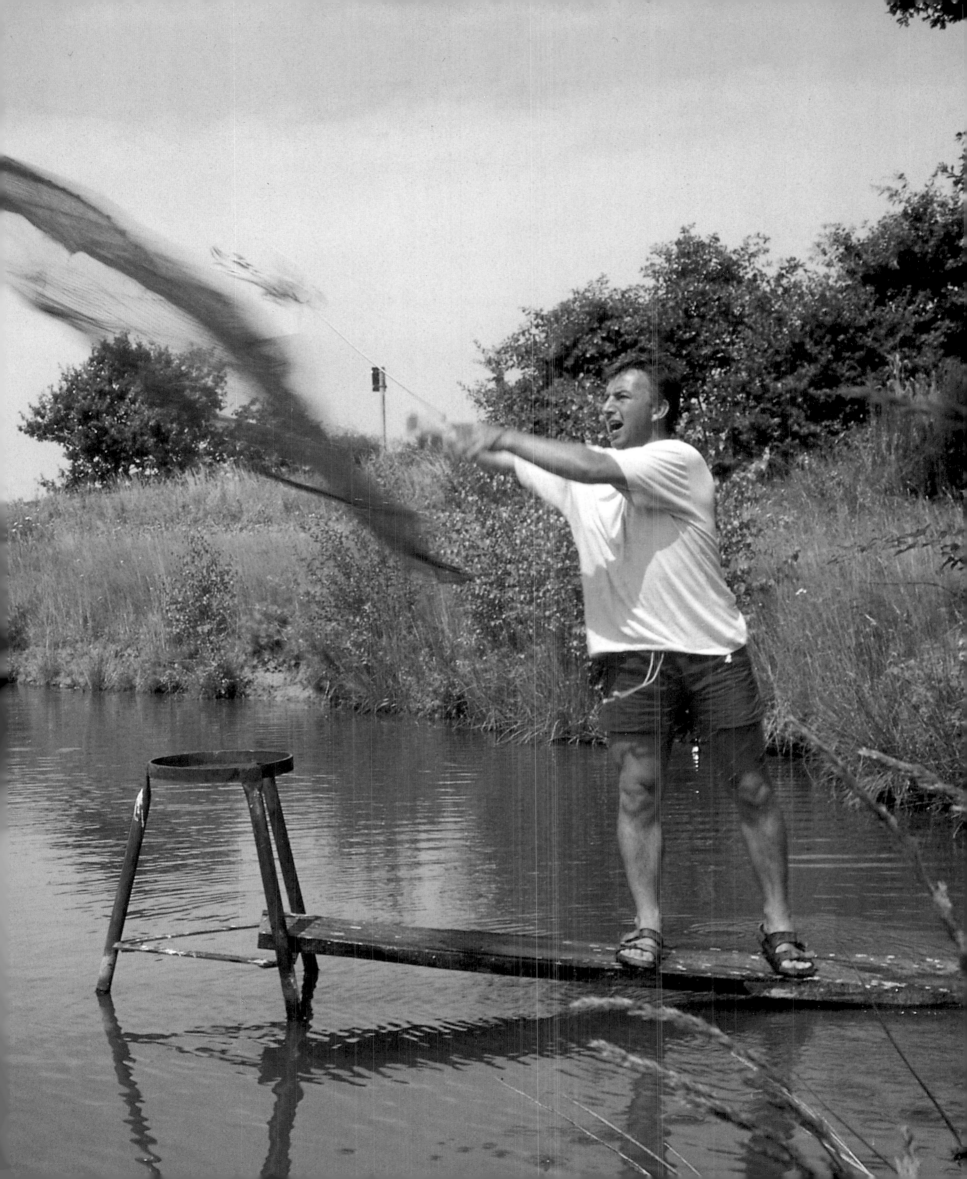

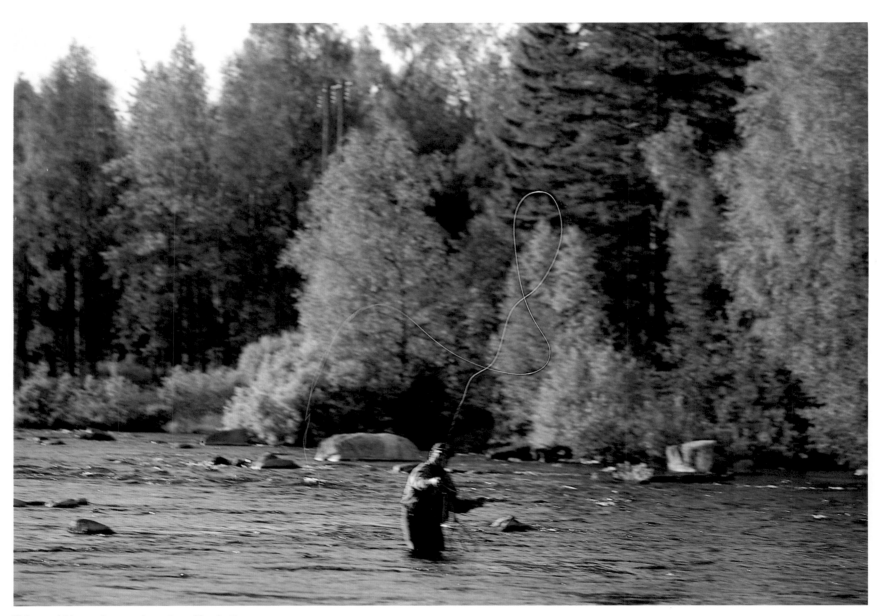

Fish caught by anglers can be eaten with a better
conscience than those caught by other methods.

Previous double page: Fish from biologically controlled
ponds are a particular delicacy as they are still a rarity.

The world of fish offers astonishing variety. While the butcher can only offer beef, veal, pork, lamb, some poultry and a little game, about forty species of fish, not to mention various shellfish and crustaceans, are commonly available. Not only is fish one of the most nutritional foods of any food type, but it also offers a far wider range of different flavors than meat does. There is a world of difference between, to name just a few examples, tuna and herring, turbot and mackerel, red mullet and carp, squid and blue mussels. But the idyllic times when riverside and coastal dwellers could catch high quality fish in clean waters now, sadly, belong to the past, as does the abundance of fish that once existed. Particularly in developing countries, fish is often an indispensable source of protein which is gradually being eroded away because of the great appetite of the western world for these delicate sea creatures. Nowadays, industrial factory ships cruise the coasts of many developing countries. A glance at the labels of conventional canned fish and frozen fish products reveals, for example, where the highly prized shrimp and crawfish originate from and from whose mouths they have been snatched. The highly damaging catch methods are responsible for the rich oceans being virtually fished empty in recent years.

Healthy freshwater fish left to live as nature intended can be obtained from the small number of organically controlled ponds. Organic food outlets therefore usually only sell saltwater fish, which have been caught humanely, without using driftnets, mostly off the coast of Greenland and in the North Atlantic. A proportion of each catch is preserved in cans using ingredients and edible oils from ecological cultivation. Some quality-minded fishermen have specialized in catching saltwater fish by angling only. Fish that are perfect in every respect have become a rare delicacy, which should be prepared with the utmost culinary care.

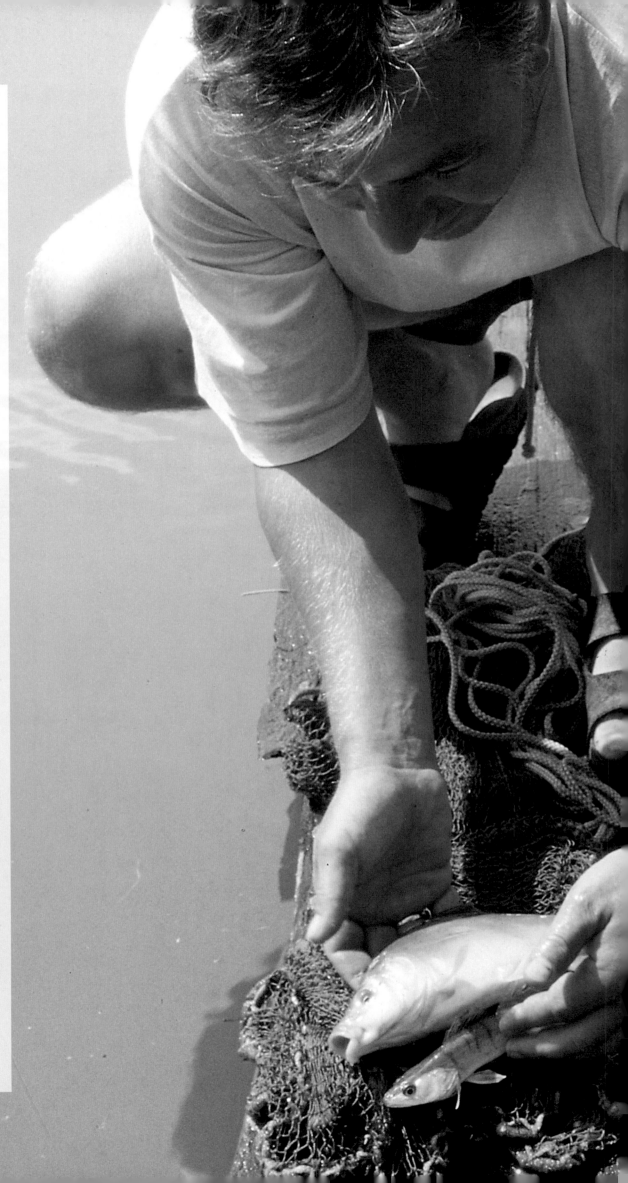

Carp in the Countryside

Organic pond systems apply the principles of correct animal rearing (see p. 257) to fish, taking account of their origin and patterns of behavior. In the delta of the Danube, for example, where carp live wild, there is regular flooding so the fish spawn in the adjacent fields. When the water subsides, the young fish – then about the thickness of a piece of string – find their way back to the river.

These conditions are artificially recreated by planting grass around the ponds and over-damming them. The pond farmer must be careful to plant robust grass blends which will not rot when flooded. When the weather and air pressure are right, and preferably when a storm is approaching, the carp mate and the female lays her eggs.

Once the young have found their way back to the ponds and are developing well, they are fished out. The parent fish return to their pond, while the young fish are placed in nursery ponds. Some of these ponds are sown with oats in the spring. Although oats rot quickly, they enable animal protein to be produced in the form of minute plankton which serve as food for the tiny carp. Larger, predatory plankton are kept at bay using sieves, as they would kill off the young fish. Once the fish are adult-sized, they are fed with bales of hay from green fields, as hay also generates a lot of plankton in the water. At the same time, cereal waste is used as a "high energy food."

Organic pond farmers like to maintain a closed development cycle. As with pig breeding and pig fattening, they keep the mother animals and do not buy any additional new fish. The carp grow to a weight of 20 to 25 pounds (9–11 kilograms) and can live to over 15 years, although three-year-old carp have the best taste.

Since organic farmers do not rate mono-culture very highly, other fish also live in the ponds; for example, the catfish. This predatory fish with a huge appetite is only introduced once the carp are too big to be attacked. But pond mussels, which are legally protected, also multiply in healthy ponds and testify to the good quality of the water.

The carp, which originally came from Asia, was introduced in Europe between the 13th and 15th century and became the most popular pond fish.

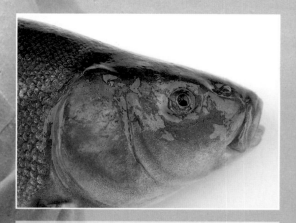

A fresh fish has clear, shining, bulging eyes.

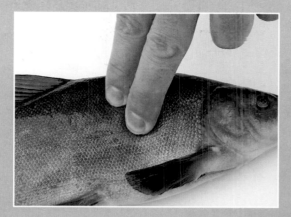

When finger pressure is applied, it should not leave an impression on the fish.

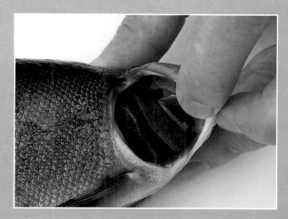

On a fresh fish, the gills are bright red and are firmly attached.

The Freshness Test

The freshness of the fish, whether of a freshwater or saltwater variety, depends on how long it has been stored and can be clearly ascertained by the five methods listed below. Fish caught by anglers generally have firmer flesh as they die out of water.

- **The eyes**
  must be clear, bright and protruding. If the fish is left on ice for too long, the eyes become dull and cloudy.

- **The gills**
  must be bright red and firmly attached. If the fish has been stored for too long, the gills become pale and look sticky.

- **The pressure point**
  only remains visible momentarily on fresh fish, when a finger is pressed into the skin. If the pressure point remains visible for some time, the fish is no longer fresh and the flesh no longer firm.

- **The entrails**
  of fresh fish have sharp contours and can be held apart easily. The longer the fish has been dead, the more unclear are the dividing lines.

- **The slime layer**
  on the skin of freshwater fish is a sign of freshness. If the skin looks dull, the fish is too old. Fish with scales do not have slime.

Industrial Fish Farming

As with cattle, pigs, and chickens, there is also large-scale fish breeding. In the ponds and pools where salmon, trout, carp, eels, and other fish are bred on an industrial scale, the same abnormal conditions are found as in the barns where the animals can only be kept alive with the aid of antibiotics and other medicines. The fish also suffer from a lack of space. They are given high-energy food consisting of entrails, slaughter waste, fishmeal or bonemeal, amongst other things, and consequently reach their slaughter weight in an unnaturally short time. Hormones are also used, and growth can be further accelerated by genetic engineering.

In the case of salmon, whose appetizing pink flesh is so prized by consumers, breeders use the coloring Canthaxanthin as a feed additive, despite the fact that it is known to cause visual disorders in humans. It speaks for itself that Norwegian salmon farmers use more medicines than the rest of the Norwegian population.

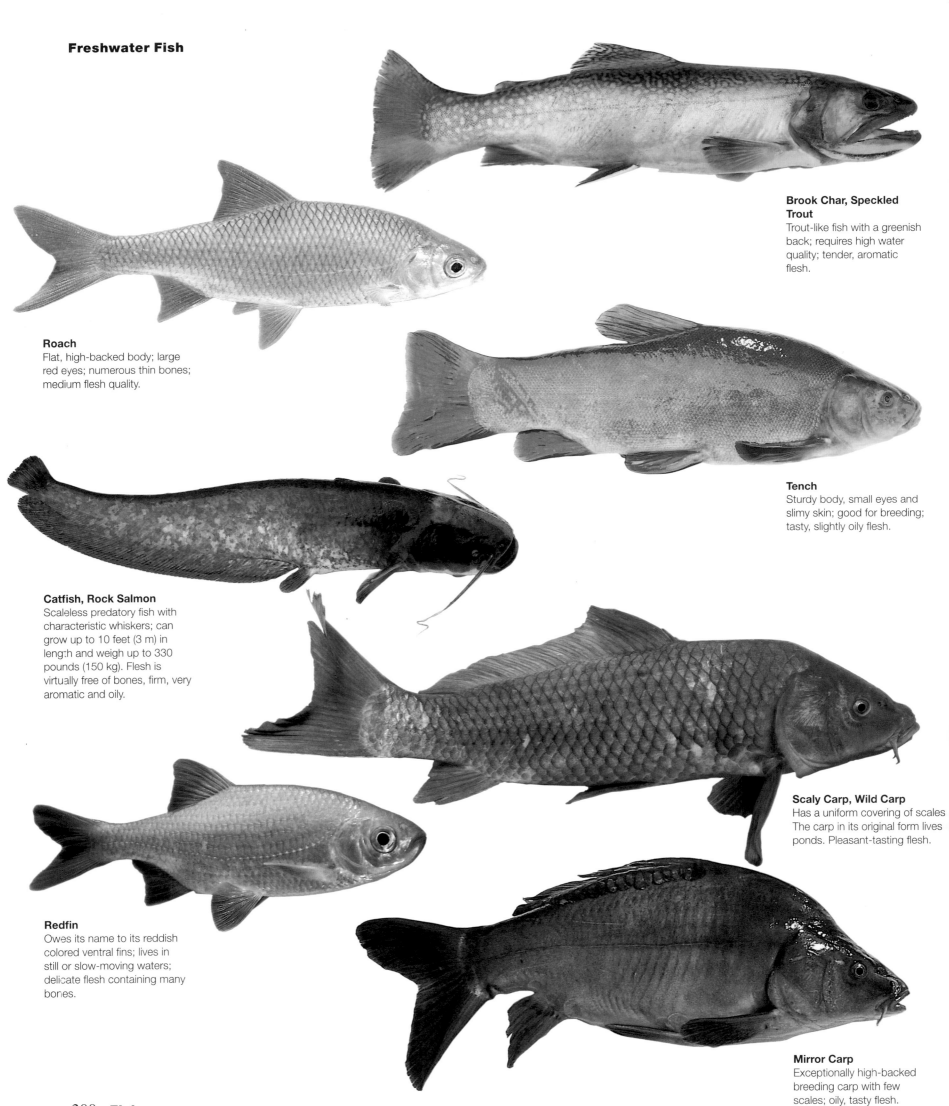

Freshwater Fish

Brook Char, Speckled Trout
Trout-like fish with a greenish back; requires high water quality; tender, aromatic flesh.

Roach
Flat, high-backed body; large red eyes; numerous thin bones; medium flesh quality.

Tench
Sturdy body, small eyes and slimy skin; good for breeding; tasty, slightly oily flesh.

Catfish, Rock Salmon
Scaleless predatory fish with characteristic whiskers; can grow up to 10 feet (3 m) in length and weigh up to 330 pounds (150 kg). Flesh is virtually free of bones, firm, very aromatic and oily.

Scaly Carp, Wild Carp
Has a uniform covering of scales The carp in its original form lives ponds. Pleasant-tasting flesh.

Redfin
Owes its name to its reddish colored ventral fins; lives in still or slow-moving waters; delicate flesh containing many bones.

Mirror Carp
Exceptionally high-backed breeding carp with few scales; oily, tasty flesh.

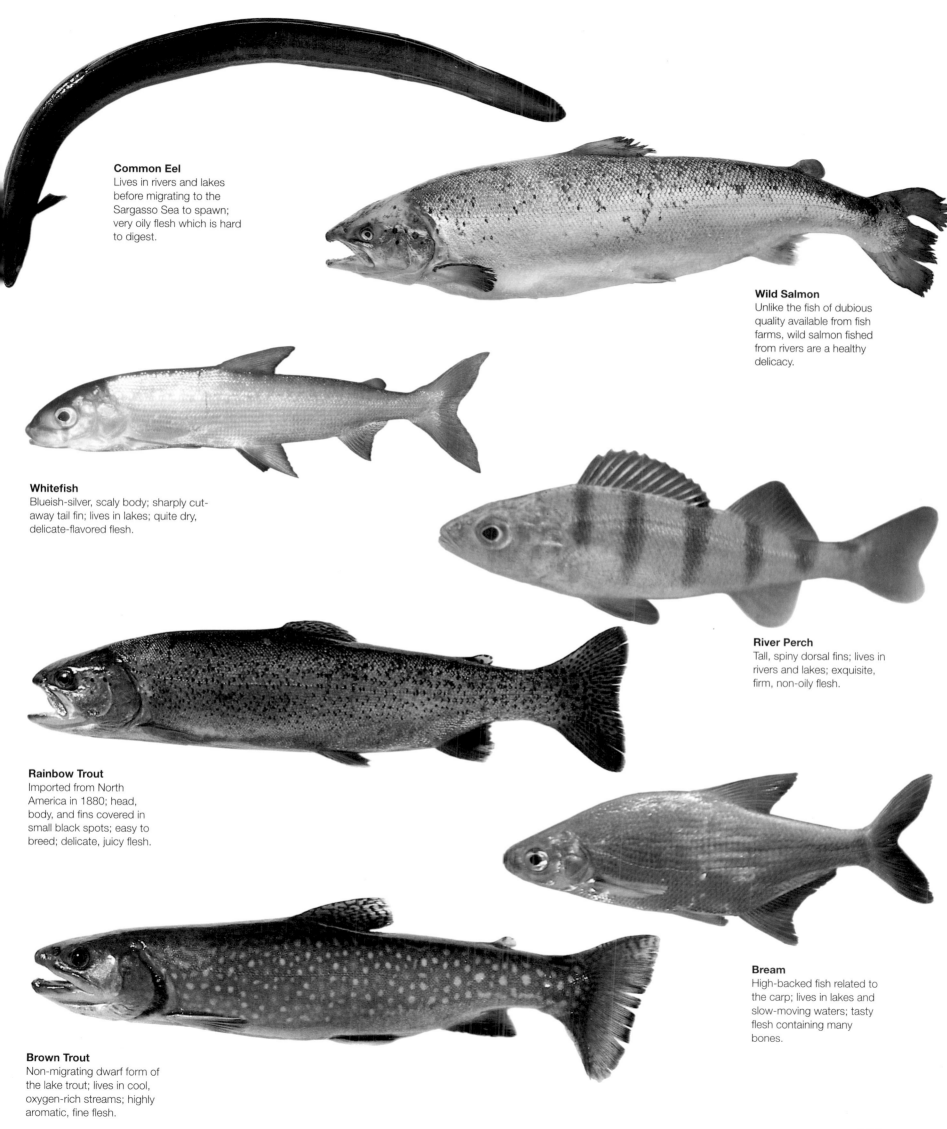

Common Eel
Lives in rivers and lakes before migrating to the Sargasso Sea to spawn; very oily flesh which is hard to digest.

Wild Salmon
Unlike the fish of dubious quality available from fish farms, wild salmon fished from rivers are a healthy delicacy.

Whitefish
Blueish-silver, scaly body; sharply cut-away tail fin; lives in lakes; quite dry, delicate-flavored flesh.

River Perch
Tall, spiny dorsal fins; lives in rivers and lakes; exquisite, firm, non-oily flesh.

Rainbow Trout
Imported from North America in 1880; head, body, and fins covered in small black spots; easy to breed; delicate, juicy flesh.

Bream
High-backed fish related to the carp; lives in lakes and slow-moving waters; tasty flesh containing many bones.

Brown Trout
Non-migrating dwarf form of the lake trout; lives in cool, oxygen-rich streams; highly aromatic, fine flesh.

301

Recipes with Freshwater Fish

Catfish on Red Beets in Ginger Sauce
(Illustration below)

11 oz (300 g) red beets
Pinch of caraway seeds
Coarse salt, pepper
1/2 cup (100 ml) vegetable stock
1 1/4 Tbs butter, cut into small pieces
1 carrot
1 small piece celery
3/4 cup (150 ml) fish stock
1 tsp coriander seeds
14 oz (400 g) catfish fillet with skin on

Ginger Sauce

1/5 cup (40 ml) dry white wine
1/8 cup (20 ml) dry sherry
2 cups (400 ml) fish stock
1 small carrot
1 small piece celery
1 finely chopped shallot
1/2 oz (10 g) root ginger
1 oz (30 g) cold butter
Coarse salt

Start by preparing the sauce. First substantially reduce the white wine and sherry. Pour in the fish stock. Cut the carrot and celery into pieces and add them along with

Char Fried in Paprika Paste

the shallot. Cut the ginger into thin slices and add it. Reduce the sauce to just under a third and strain it. Cut the butter into small pieces and mix it into the sauce. Add salt to taste. Clean the beets thoroughly, cut them into slices, put in an ovenproof dish with the caraway seeds, salt, pepper, and vegetable stock, and scatter the knobs of butter on top. Braise, covered, in a pre-heated oven at 350 °F (180 °C) for 10 minutes until firm. Cut the carrot and celery into pieces, place them in an ovenproof dish together with the fish stock, heat them, crush half the coriander seeds and add them. Cut the catfish fillet into four pieces. Lay them in the dish with the skin upwards, cover the dish, put it in the hot oven and cook for 7 minutes. Take out the dish and let it stand, covered, for 3 minutes. Carefully remove the fish skin with a fork.
Arrange a quarter of the beets on each plate, lay the fish fillet on top, scatter over the freshly crushed coriander seeds and pour over the ginger sauce.

Baked Tench with Mango Salad and Horseradish Mayonnaise
(Illustration on right-hand page)

Serves 2

1/2 mango
1 thumbnail-sized piece of ginger
1 finely chopped garlic clove
2 Tbs chopped mixed herbs: mint, basil and cilantro
1/2 tsp coriander seeds
2 tsp chopped leaves and grated zest of kaffir lime
6 drops chili oil
2 tench
3 oz (85 g) cornstarch
3 oz (85 g) fine whole-wheat flour
1/2 oz (10 g) baking soda
Coarse salt, pepper
3 saffron threads
Peanut oil for deep-frying

Mayonnaise

1 egg yolk
1/2 cup (100 ml) sunflower oil
Juice of 1 lime
Pinch of mustard
1 tsp freshly grated horseradish
Pinch of coarse salt
1/4 tsp honey
1/5 cup (40 ml) heavy cream

Catfish on Red Beets in Ginger Sauce

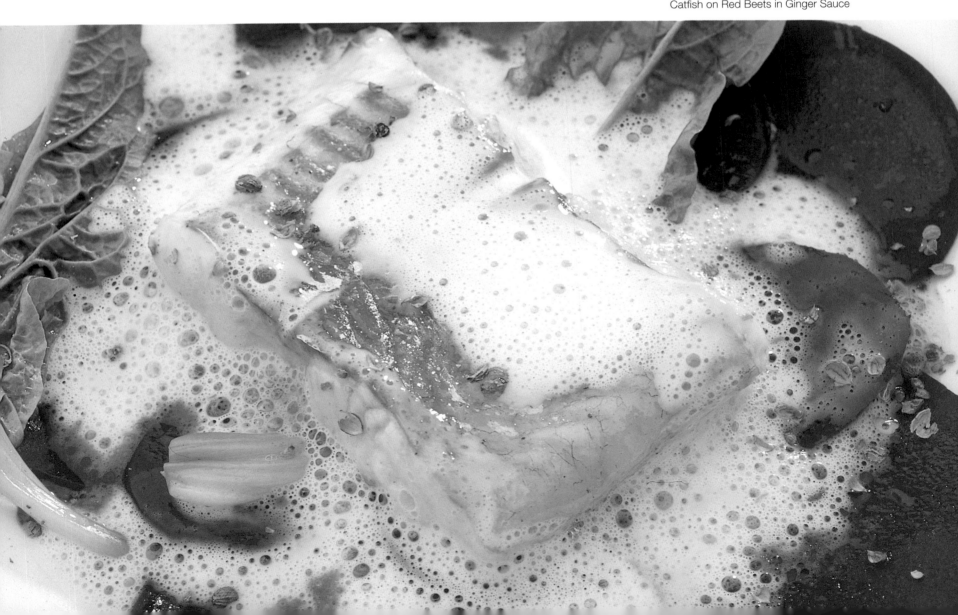

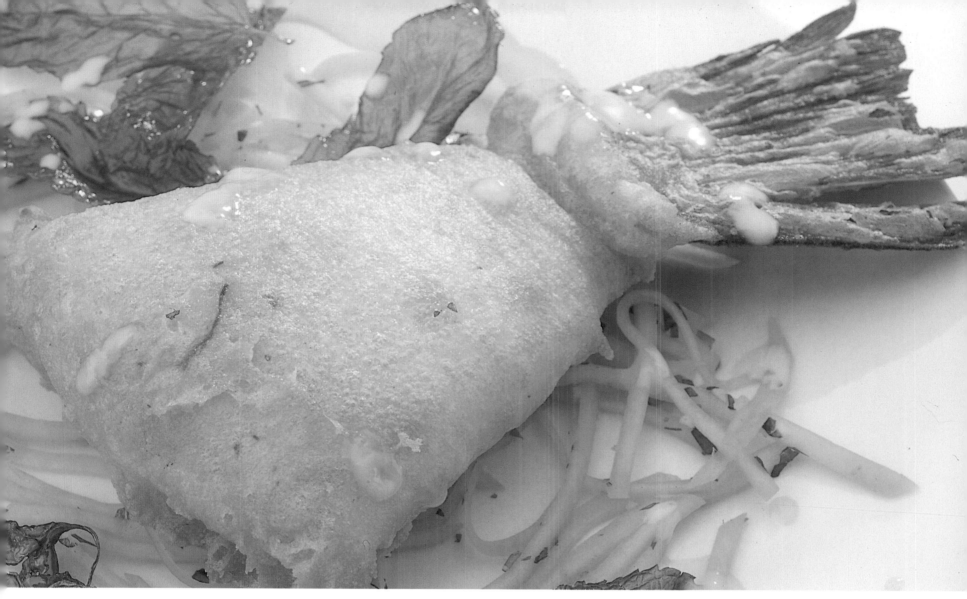

Baked Tench with Mango Salad and Horseradish Mayonnaise

Start by preparing the mayonnaise. Beat the egg yolk with a wooden spoon, then pour in the oil, first in a very thin trickle and then more quickly, stirring constantly. Next mix in the remaining ingredients, one at a time. Peel the half mango and cut into small cubes. Finely chop the ginger and add it to the mango together with the garlic, herbs, freshly crushed coriander seeds, lime zest and leaves (which have a very strong lime flavor), then add the drops of chili oil and mix well.

Gut the tench, rinse them and pat them dry. Mix the cornstarch, flour, baking soda, salt, pepper, and saffron threads together, pour over 1¼ cups (250 ml) lukewarm water and work into a very light batter. Dip the fish in the batter on both sides, so that they are coated all over. Heat the peanut oil in a large, high-sided pan until hot – 375 °F (190 °C). Add the fish so they float in the oil and deep-fry them for 3 minutes.

Arrange one tench on each plate with half the mango salad and half the mayonnaise and serve immediately.

Char Fried in Paprika Paste
(Illustration top left)

2 large carrots
1 large turnip-rooted parsley
2 Tbs olive oil
12 baby leeks
1 Tbs butter
Coarse salt
4 char
Flour for dusting
⅕ cup (40 ml) sunflower oil

Paste

1 red bell pepper
4 Tbs paprika paste
3 Tbs finely chopped ginger
3 Tbs finely chopped garlic
1 tsp honey
½ tsp chili oil
¼ tsp coarse salt
⅖ cup (80 ml) sunflower oil
1 Tbs (20 ml) sesame oil

For the paprika paste, which is prepared three days in advance, bake the red bell pepper in the oven until its skin blackens. Take it out, peel off the skin, remove the seeds and chop the bell pepper finely. Place the bell pepper with the paprika paste and all the other ingredients in a mixer and blend them together. Refrigerate for three days.

Peel the carrots and turnip-rooted parsley thinly and cut them into thin slices lengthwise. Heat the olive oil and fry the vegetables briefly so they are still crunchy. Clean the baby leeks and cook them in hot butter. Sprinkle the vegetables with a little salt.

Gut the fish, rinse them and pat them dry. Then coat them evenly with the paprika paste and dust with flour. Heat the sunflower oil in a large pan and fry the fish on both sides until crispy. Remove the fish, let any excess oil drip off, then arrange them on plates with the vegetables.

A Food of Great Variety

Fish in our Diet

The numerous species of fish can be grouped according to two criteria: depending on whether they originate in freshwater – which includes the migrating eels and salmon – or seawater, or whether they are oily or lean fish. In the case of oily fish such as salmon, herring, mackerel or tuna, the fat is contained in the meat and is eaten. In the case of lean fish such as pollack, cod or haddock, on the other hand, the fat reserve is in the stomach cavity and is removed prior to consumption. In cookery, a further distinction is often made between superior fish such as sole, turbot or salmon and everyday fish such as herring, cod or pollack, where not only the quality of the flesh, but also the price, is a factor. The depleted oceans make this latter distinction ever more meaningless, and in any case, salmon from today's mass farming can hardly be described as superior.

Fish can provide us with the following valuable nutrients:

- high-quality, easily digested protein with a high content of essential amino acids (see p. 21),
- several water-soluble vitamins of the B group and high levels of the fat-soluble vitamins A and D,
- minerals, particularly calcium and potassium,
- important trace elements, including, in particular, a high level of the rare element iodine, as well as iron, fluorine and others,
- mono- and polyunsaturated fatty acids, especially omega-3 fatty acids, which are closely related to linolenic acid, which occurs in plants. These are thought to help prevent arteriosclerosis when consumed in moderate quantities and concentrations.

However, freshly caught fish are becoming ever more of a rarity. A fish served up just hours after being caught is a special delicacy. One should never miss an opportunity to buy fish directly from the ship or the fisherman. "Fresh fish" describes fish which has not been preserved by deep freezing or other methods. The fish bought by the fish trade is kept cool on ice and is untreated. The same freshness criteria apply to saltwater fish as to freshwater fish. The simplest test is the smell: fresh fish never smells unpleasant or strongly fishy, but just smells of sea and water. Fish decays rapidly and should be consumed on the day of purchase. When fish starts to go off, microbial activity produces toxic concentrations of biogenic amines like histamine and tryptamine.

How Safe is it to Eat Saltwater Fish?

It is a sign of the times that industrial nations have developed at the expense of nature. Rivers and seas, and particularly the coastal regions, have been contaminated with pollutants contained in waste water. These dangerous substances, including, in particular, mercury, are taken up by fish as they feed on plankton, algae and micro-organisms and are thus able to enter the food chain which finishes with humans.

Mercury is highly toxic. Mercury poisoning causes embryos to develop severe deformities and leads to serious growth disorders in children. In cases of acute mercury poisoning, the kidneys, brain and nerves are always badly damaged. Fish contains the highest levels of mercury of any food in our diet. Fish living in polluted rivers and their estuaries are particularly at risk. However, mercury concentrations are also rising in predatory fish such as pike, tuna or halibut, in fish which live a particularly long time and in mussels. As animals are fed on fishmeal and the heavy metal is deposited in eggs, milk and meat, mercury can also enter our food chain in this way.

The chlorinated hydrocarbons contained in pesticides, which now pollute the sea water, and which cannot easily be broken down, are a further risk factor. Fatty fish such as eel, tuna, salmon, herring or mackerel are usually particularly badly affected by hazardous and toxic substances. In terms of the level of dangerous substances, the least harmful fish to eat are the deep sea fish such as pollack, turbot, plaice, cod or hake, as these fish are at the top of the food chain. However, the widespread use of driftnets for deep sea fishing today must be condemned in the strongest terms. As well as the fish caught intentionally in the nets, which can be up to 40 miles (60 kilometers) long, many larger sea creatures like dolphins, turtles, and whales get caught up in the nets, are unable to free themselves and come to a cruel end. What is more, with this fishing method, much of the fish is so badly damaged that it is only suitable for factory processing and cannot be sold as fresh fish. Good quality fish are only caught by smaller ships, and the best fish of all are those caught by anglers.

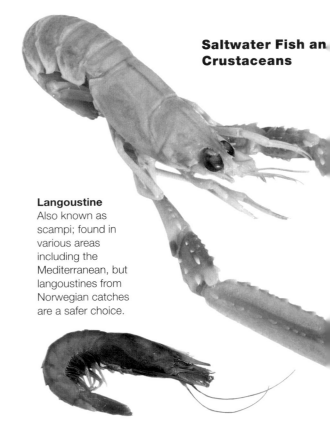

Saltwater Fish an Crustaceans

Langoustine
Also known as scampi; found in various areas including the Mediterranean, but langoustines from Norwegian catches are a safer choice.

Jumbo Shrimp
Larger than shrimp; rarely sold alive as they are usually cooked on board ship; the best come from Greenland.

Turbot
Disc-shaped body without scales; the most sought-after and valuable edible fish in the Atlantic.

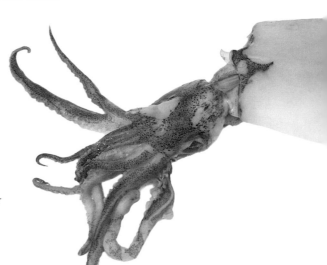

Squid
A type of mollusk, still plentiful in all oceans; popular in Mediterranean cooking.

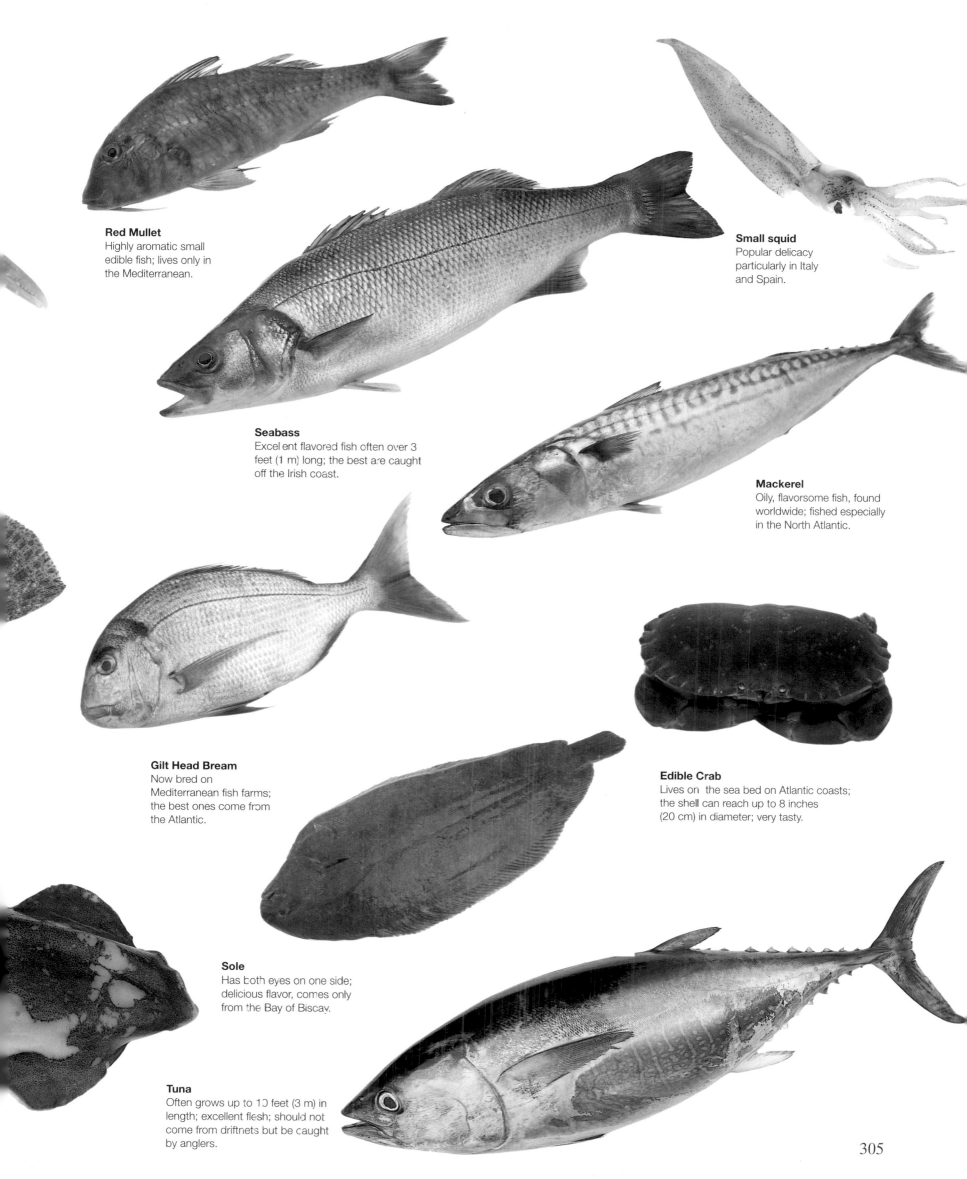

Red Mullet
Highly aromatic small edible fish; lives only in the Mediterranean.

Small squid
Popular delicacy particularly in Italy and Spain.

Seabass
Excellent flavored fish often over 3 feet (1 m) long; the best are caught off the Irish coast.

Mackerel
Oily, flavorsome fish, found worldwide; fished especially in the North Atlantic.

Gilt Head Bream
Now bred on Mediterranean fish farms; the best ones come from the Atlantic.

Edible Crab
Lives on the sea bed on Atlantic coasts; the shell can reach up to 8 inches (20 cm) in diameter; very tasty.

Sole
Has both eyes on one side; delicious flavor, comes only from the Bay of Biscay.

Tuna
Often grows up to 10 feet (3 m) in length; excellent flesh; should not come from driftnets but be caught by anglers.

A True Gem

The Gilt Head Bream

So-called because of the distinguishing gold band between its eyes, the gilt head bream is the queen of its family of many species. It is found not only in the Mediterranean, but also in the Atlantic, from the Azores to the waters off Brittany. Gilt head bream, also called dorade, love clear water and live above the sea bed at depths of up to 100 feet (30 meters). They can also be bred in warm saltwater pools. As they are so popular, more and more gilt head bream are being farmed on an industrial scale for the fish trade. You can only be sure of getting free-range fish if you buy them directly from the ship, have a reliable supplier, or can get hold of the rarely available large fish.

The dorade, which is often served in separate portions, has an adult body length of 20–30 inches (50–70 centimeters) and weighs between 11 and 15 pounds (5–7 kilograms). But it is rare to find gilt head bream weighing anything over 2 pounds (1 kilo) on sale. The white flesh, which contains few bones, is very tasty and is at its best from July through October.

Gilt head bream can be baked in the oven with tomatoes and Mediterranean herbs. They taste especially delicious baked in a salt crust – a method of preparation from the Andalusian coast of Spain.

Gutting and Filleting a Bream

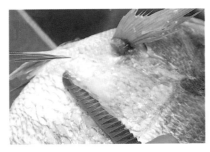

Scales
Cut off the fins with a pair of scissors, then scale the fish, preferably with a fluted butter knife.

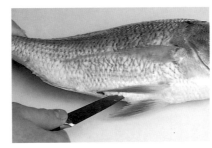

Belly cut
Carefully cut the belly open lengthwise, without damaging the innards.

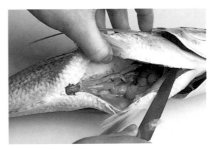

Gutting
Hold the belly sides apart, loosen the innards with your fingers and take them out.

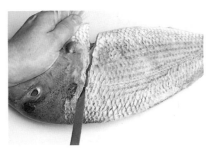

Head cut
Before filleting, make a cut diagonally to the head behind the gill opening.

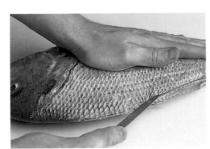

Filleting
Insert the knife under the large center bones.

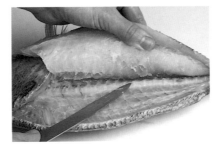

Dorsal cut
Slide the knife along the middle bones from bottom to top.

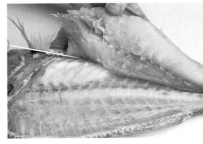

Separating
Lift up the fillet and separate it on the lower side. Pull out any bones.

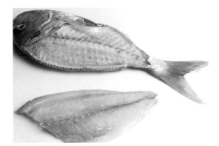

The fillet
For the second fillet, repeat the process on the other side of the fish.

Grilled Red Bream

1 red bream (dorade) weighing 3¹/₂ lbs (1.5 kg)
¹/₄ celeriac
1 small leek
2 finely chopped shallots
2 bay leaves
10 white peppercorns
³/₄ cup (150 ml) dry white wine
Coarse salt
¹/₂ bell pepper
1 large tomato
1 Tbs finely chopped marjoram
Black pepper
¹/₂ cup (100 ml) olive oil
1 tsp lime juice
1 sprig marjoram

Fillet the red bream and cut each fillet in half. Clean the celeriac and leek, chop them finely and put them in a pan with the shallots, bay leaves and peppercorns. Add the fish trimmings, except for the innards. Pour over the white wine and add 3 cups (600 ml) water. Boil for 30 minutes, then pass through a cloth to strain. Reduce the liquid to a fifth and add salt to taste.

Deseed the half bell pepper and peel it thinly with a low-waste peeler. Pour boiling water over the tomato, peel off the skin and remove the seeds. Chop the tomato into small dice and mix with the bell pepper, stir in the marjoram and set aside.

Season the skin side of the fillets with salt and pepper. Lay the fish on a preheated griddle with the skin side down, making sure it does not come into contact with any oil beforehand. Then brush the upper side with olive oil. When they are one-third cooked, carefully turn the fillets round on the griddle to make a criss-cross pattern on the skin. When the underside is crispy, turn the fish over and cook briefly on the other side.

Meanwhile, beat the remaining olive oil into the reduced stock, heat the liquid to bind it, but do not let it boil. Add lime juice, salt and pepper to taste, then stir in the tomato and pepper mixture.

Place the bream fillets on warmed plates and garnish with the sauce and small pieces of marjoram.

Right hand page: The skin of the bream must not come into contact with any grease before broiling as this prevents it getting crispy.

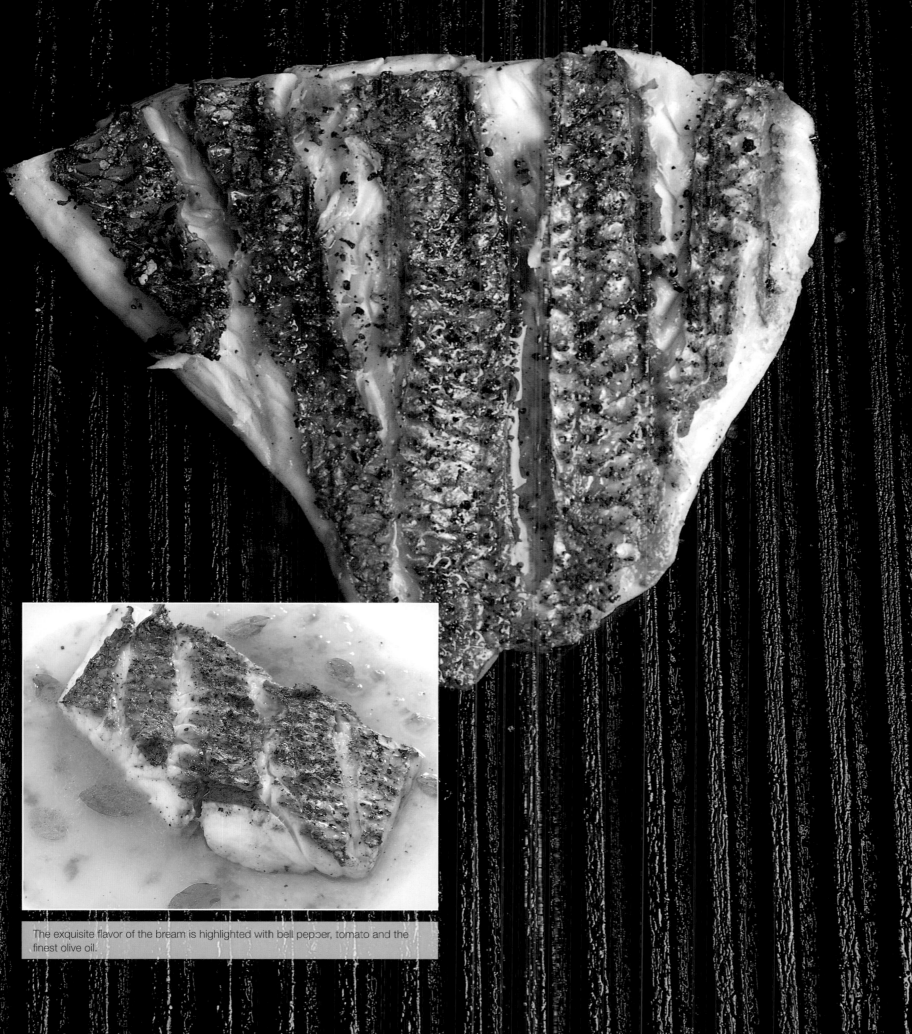

The exquisite flavor of the bream is highlighted with bell pepper, tomato and the finest olive oil.

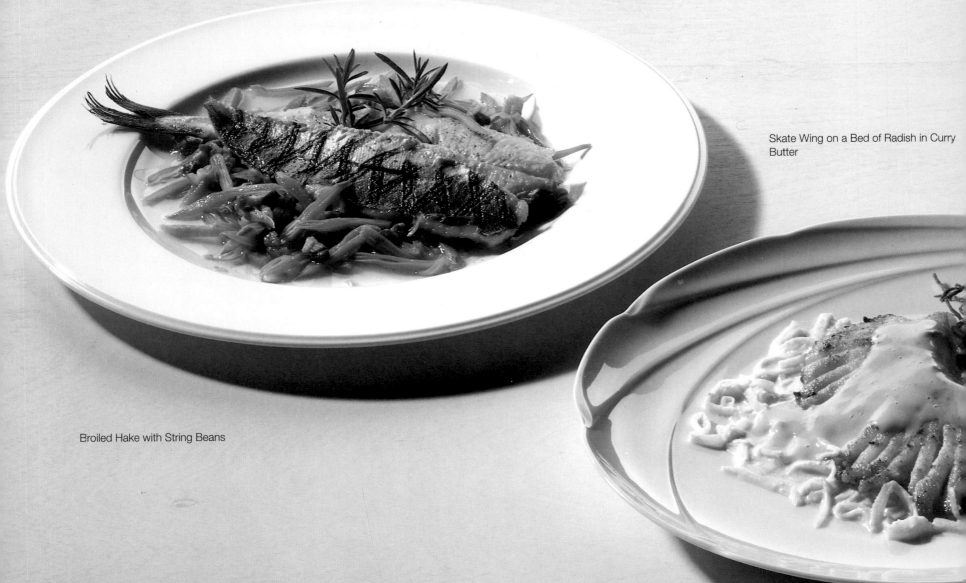

Skate Wing on a Bed of Radish in Curry Butter

Broiled Hake with String Beans

Recipes with Saltwater Fish

Broiled Hake with String Beans

11 oz (300 g) string beans
1 medium floury potato
1 finely chopped shallot
1/2 tsp finely chopped savory
2 oz (50 g) streaky bacon
2 oz (50 g) onions
1 tsp butter
Coarse salt, pepper
1 pinch nutmeg
4 hake fillets each weighing 4 oz (120 g)
1/4 cup (50 ml) olive oil

Wash the beans and cut them into thin strips. Blanch them briefly in boiling water, then rinse them with ice-cold water. Peel the potato and cut it into strips, place it in the bean juice, add the shallot and savory and boil for 15 minutes. Place the potato mixture in a blender, blend to a creamy purée, then pass through a sieve.
Finely dice the bacon and onions and fry them quickly in the butter, one after the other. Add the blanched beans and pour on the potato/bean stock. Season with salt, pepper, and a little nutmeg.
Season the fish fillets with salt and pepper and broil them briefly on both sides. Toss the beans in finest quality olive oil, arrange them on large plates and place the hake fillets on top.

Skate Wing on a Bed of Radish in Curry Butter

Five-spice powder

1 small piece of cinnamon
A few fennel seeds
1 Chinese anis
A few Szechuan peppercorns
A few cloves

Skate

12 oz (350 g) skate wing fillet
Coarse salt, white pepper
1/2 tsp five-spice powder
3/4 cup (150 ml) heavy cream
2 large carrots
Peanut oil for deep frying
1 tsp sunflower oil

Radish Sauce

7 oz (200 g) radishes
1/2 cup (100 ml) chicken stock
1/2 cup (100 ml) heavy cream
1/8 cup (20 ml) white wine
Coarse salt, white pepper
Pinch of five-spice powder

1 tsp crème fraîche
A little lime juice
1/2 tsp sesame oil

Curry Butter

1/5 cup (40 ml) white wine
1/8 cup (20 ml) Madeira
2 cups (400 ml) fish stock
1 carrot
1/4 celeriac
1 finely chopped shallot
1 tsp finely chopped ginger
2 Tbs cold butter
1/2 tsp curry powder
Coarse salt

For the five-spice powder, dry roast the spices and then grind them in an electric coffee grinder. It is best to make a slightly larger amount, as it will keep for a month in a screw-top jar. Divide the skate fillet into 4 evenly sized pieces, place them in a bowl, season with salt and pepper, pour over the five-spice powder and

Salad with Red Mullet and Cold
Ratatouille

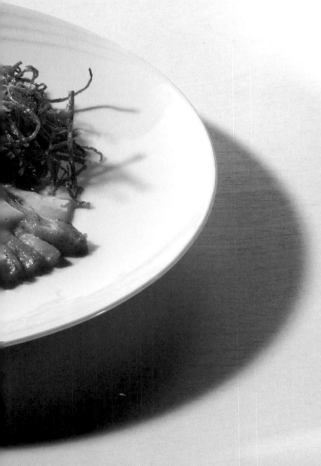

the cream and leave to marinate for a good hour.
For the radish sauce, wash the radishes, peel them and
cut them into thin strips. Boil up the radish trimmings
with the chicken stock, cream, and white wine, remove
from the stove and leave to stand for 1 hour. Strain the
mixture, heat it again, and let it boil until it thickens to a
creamy consistency. Season with salt and white pepper,
mix in a pinch of five-spice powder, the crème fraîche,
lime juice, and sesame oil. Then add the julienne-style
radishes and bring to the boil. The sauce is now ready
to serve.
For the curry butter, reduce the white wine and Madeira
substantially, then pour in the fish stock. Clean the
carrot and celeriac, chop them finely, add them to the
pan with the shallot and ginger and reduce the mixture
to a third. Strain the mixture through a cloth, cut the
butter into small pieces and beat it in. Flavor with the
curry powder and add salt to taste.
When the radish sauce and curry butter are ready,
remove the fish from the marinade and allow to drip for
a moment. Peel the carrots thinly, cut them into very
thin strips and deep-fry them in peanut oil.
Heat the sunflower oil in a skillet and fry the skate briefly

on both sides. Place the fish fillets on the warmed
plates, pour over the hot curry butter, add the radish
sauce and garnish with the fried shredded carrot.

Salad with Red Mullet and Cold
Ratatouille

1 egg yolk
2 Tbs (30 ml) balsamic vinegar
1/2 cup (100 ml) olive oil
1/2 cup (100 ml) mixed juice of tomatoes, bell peppers, cucumber
Coarse salt, black pepper
A few drops of chili oil
1/4 honeydew melon
1/2 eggplant
1/4 each of red, green and yellow bell peppers
2 baby leeks
1 garlic clove
1 Tbs finely chopped ginger
2 red mullet each weighing 11–14 oz (300–400 g)
1 tsp butter
1 tsp olive oil
1 tsp finely chopped thyme
A few arugula leaves

Beat the vinegar and olive oil into the egg yolk to form a
mayonnaise, then stir in the vegetable juice. Season
with salt, pepper and chili oil.
Wash and deseed the honeydew melon, eggplant and
bell peppers and dice them very finely. Chop the leeks
and garlic finely. Mix all the vegetables and the ginger
thoroughly with the salad dressing, check the
seasoning again and leave to stand in a refrigerator for
30 minutes. Fillet the red mullet. Heat the butter and
olive oil, add the fillets to the pan and fry them briefly on
both sides together with the thyme.
Arrange the ratatouille on 4 plates, place one fillet on
each and garnish with a few arugula leaves.

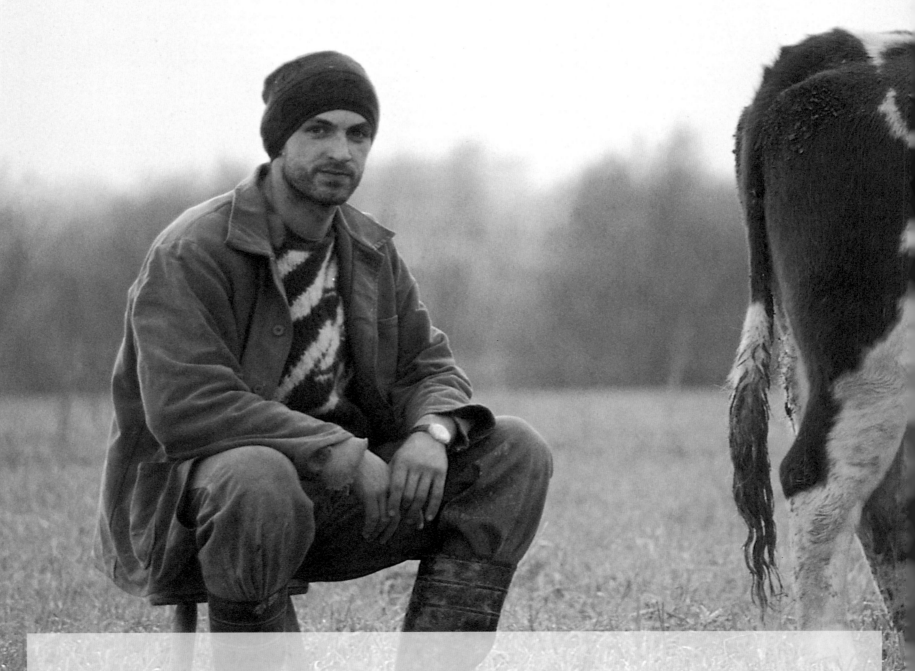

Milk and Dairy Products

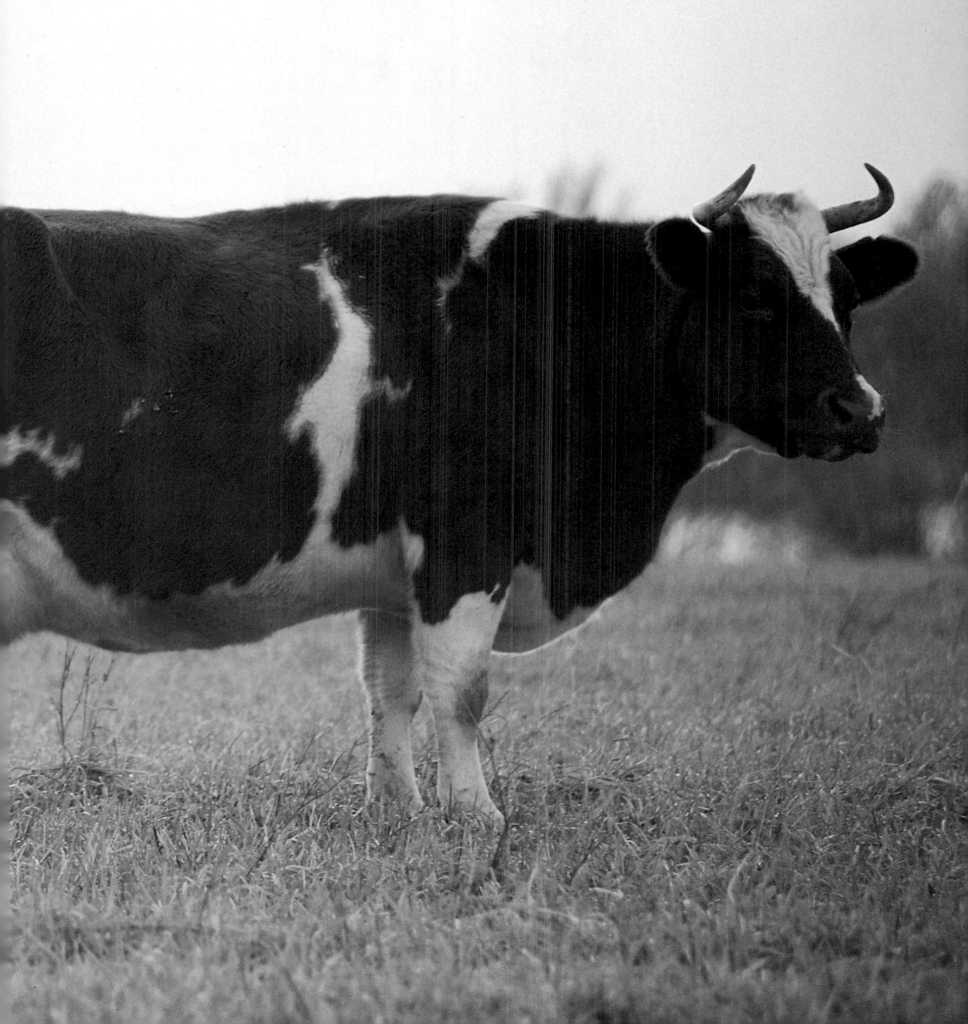

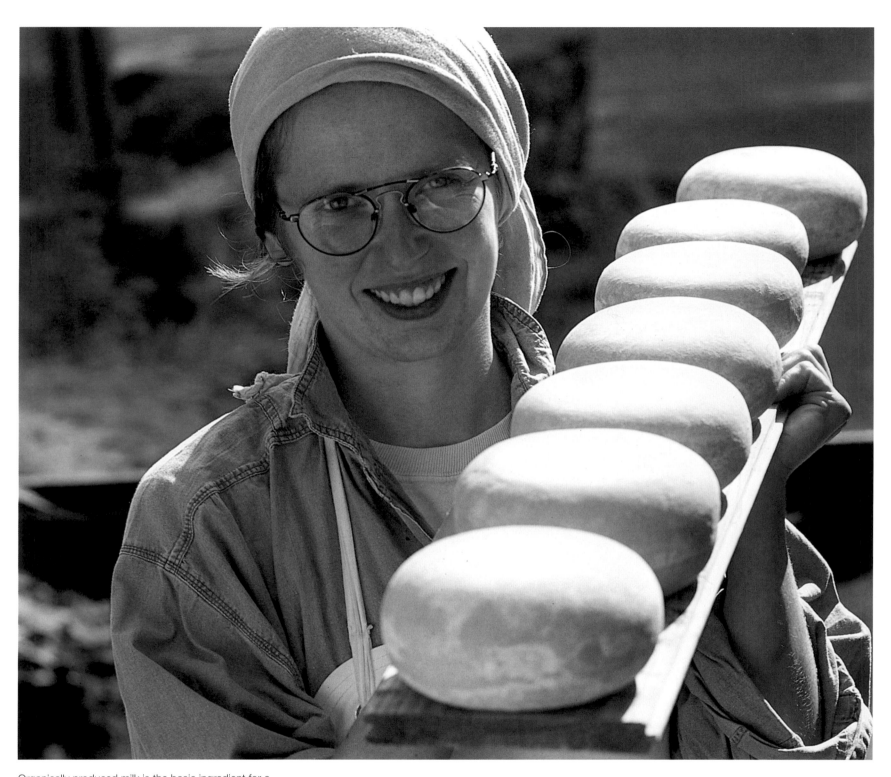

Organically produced milk is the basic ingredient for a wide range of cheese varieties which are a delicious source of protein.

Previous double page: Freshly collected milk from happy cows is a treat for the taste buds.

In central and northern Europe and in North America, milk plays a much more important part in the diet than on some other continents. Whole peoples in Africa, Asia, and South America do not produce the lactose-hydrolyzing enzyme lactase, without which milk cannot be digested. For this reason, but also because of climatic and environmental factors, dairy farming has remained limited in those areas. But even in Europe, where the Romans themselves made cheese and where, in the middle ages, monasteries practiced and passed on the art of butter and cheese-making, milk and milk products were relatively rare. It was not until the arrival of pasteurization and sterilization methods and modern refrigeration technology that new opportunities and markets opened up. Rapidly increasing demand was at the root of agricultural developments which were increasingly moving towards industrial-type production and which forced farmers into a strictly regulated system. Whilst many smaller dairies were no longer competitive, the milk industry boosted its sales of standardized products to unprecedented record levels. Hardly anybody knew the taste of raw milk any more. Thanks to organic farmers who sell raw milk on their farms or supply directly bottled certified milk to the retail trade, raw milk can now be enjoyed again, as can organically produced butter. Contrary to popular opinion, it is not harmful to eat butter, as cholesterol is not dangerous in itself. Denatured products such as long-life milk are much more harmful. When processed, cholesterol turns into oxycholesterol, which can actually cause arteriosclerosis. Choosing the least treated dairy products from good milk means you get not only the benefit of the highly valued vitamins and minerals, but also of the milk fat, which contains a high proportion of unsaturated fatty acids, which are so prized in olive oil. This is the only type of fat that can be absorbed by the body without first being converted in the liver. This should be reason enough not to reject butter and to prefer milk, yogurt, farmer's cheese, and other dairy products with their natural fat content.

Raw is Best

Milk from Organic Farms

Advertisements may promise consumers milk from happy cows, but there is not much of this happiness in evidence on conventional farms. Dairy cows are only rarely allowed out to pasture. Instead, they while away their lives chained up in sheds on split floors and metal grids. Concentrated feed imported from the developing world, which is often highly questionable in ecological and social terms, is frequently used to ensure the highest possible milk yield, which some people would like to increase still further by means of genetic manipulation.

On ecological farms, cattle are treated with respect and kindness from the start. They are an important, and for many organic farmers indispensable, link in the farm's production cycle. They are therefore kept under proper conditions, which means they spend plenty of time out grazing. Naturally tended pasture forms part of the animals' diet, which is supplemented with other types of feed such as hay and rutabagas. Each farm aims, as far as possible, to produce all its own fodder. If it cannot produce sufficient fodder, it buys extra from other organic farms. The use of biological concentrated feeds is kept to a minimum.

Chemicals which artificially increase milk production are, of course, avoided as is the preventive administration of antibiotics. Diseases are treated with homeopathic or other natural healing remedies, which have good success rates and do not leave traces in the milk.

In healthy cows, the milk is free of germs before it leaves the udder. But during milking, even with machines, it comes into contact with bacteria. Milking is often done by hand on organic farms, and with good reason, as studies have shown. Whilst milking machines transfer germs to the milk which target the fat and protein, the natural barn atmosphere puts lactic acid bacteria into the milk. Although these break down the lactose and cause the milk to turn sour quickly, they also prevent dangerous germs developing. One of the greatest advantages of organic milk is its natural bacterial content, as this tends to build up the body's defenses, particularly in children.

Correct animal keeping and biological methods of tending the pasture and fodder cultivation areas provide the ideal conditions for obtaining the best quality milk. Although, sadly, it is a fact that harmful substances are everywhere today and cannot be avoided, they are only present in minimal amounts, if at all, in ecological milk. For the milk to maintain its high quality, it must be manipulated as little as possible. For this reason it is only cooled, filtered, and bottled. It keeps for 3 to 5 days in the refrigerator, retains its natural fat content, is not homogenized and not heated. With milk of this kind, the cream floats to the surface, and the milk turns sour, in other words, it turns naturally into delicious sour milk. In several European countries it is sold as raw milk and as certified milk, with different legal requirements in each case.

- The untreated raw milk is only cooled and filtered and may only be sold directly to consumers by producers on their farms. The farm has to fulfill a whole range of special conditions relating to the health of the animals and dairy workers, the hygiene in the dairy and the quality of the milk itself. The milk must be free of salmonella, streptococci, and antibiotics. It has to be boiled to sterilize it before consumption.

- Certified milk is the only type of untreated raw milk available from retailers but even this is restricted to a few countries in Europe. As well as the conditions which apply to raw milk, other strict regulations apply: the milk and cows must be inspected monthly. There are strict guidelines on cooling and bottling on the farm, and the label has to give precise information on the fat content, perishability, quantity, and producer.

- Organic food retailers also sell non-homogenized bio-milk. It is pasteurized by a less damaging method in which hardly any of the vitamins are lost.

Is Milk Healthy?

The milk that humans and animals enjoy as their first food provided by their own mother is full milk in the truest sense. It contains all the substances which the newborn baby needs to survive this critical period of its life in good health, to grow rapidly and to boost its defenses.

The balance of nutrients in the milk is as varied as the different needs of each type of mammal. The carbohydrates, proteins, minerals, fats, vital substances, hormones, enzymes, and bacteria are contained in the combination most readily assimilated by the young of the particular species. Later, as the young animal becomes increasingly independent of the mother, the growing creature must not be denied the enzymes needed for breaking down lactoprotein.

Not all people can tolerate milk from other mammals containing proteins of a different species. Milk intolerance can lead to a whole range of allergies and disorders like neurodermatitis. Nowadays, conventional milk contains increasing levels of harmful substances, and the high tech processing methods destroy many of the beneficial constituents. Raw milk represents an excellent and very healthy alternative. Its lactoprotein is easily digestible, rich in the indispensable essential amino acids and ranks second only to chicken's egg white in terms of nutritional value. Nearly half the fat in cow's milk consists of monounsaturated, highly beneficial fatty acids, the milk contains only a small amount of cholesterol and is easy to digest. Apart from this, milk consists of lactose, numerous minerals, notably phosphorus, calcium, potassium, and magnesium, various trace elements and, above all, vitamins A, D, E, K, B1, B2, B3, B5, and B12. Milk and dairy products are an excellent complement to an otherwise vegetarian diet.

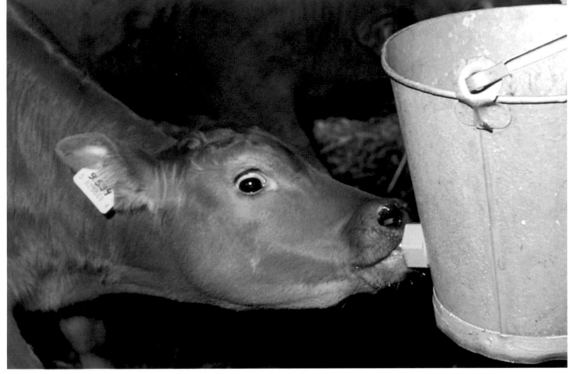
The calves love the taste of the milk too.

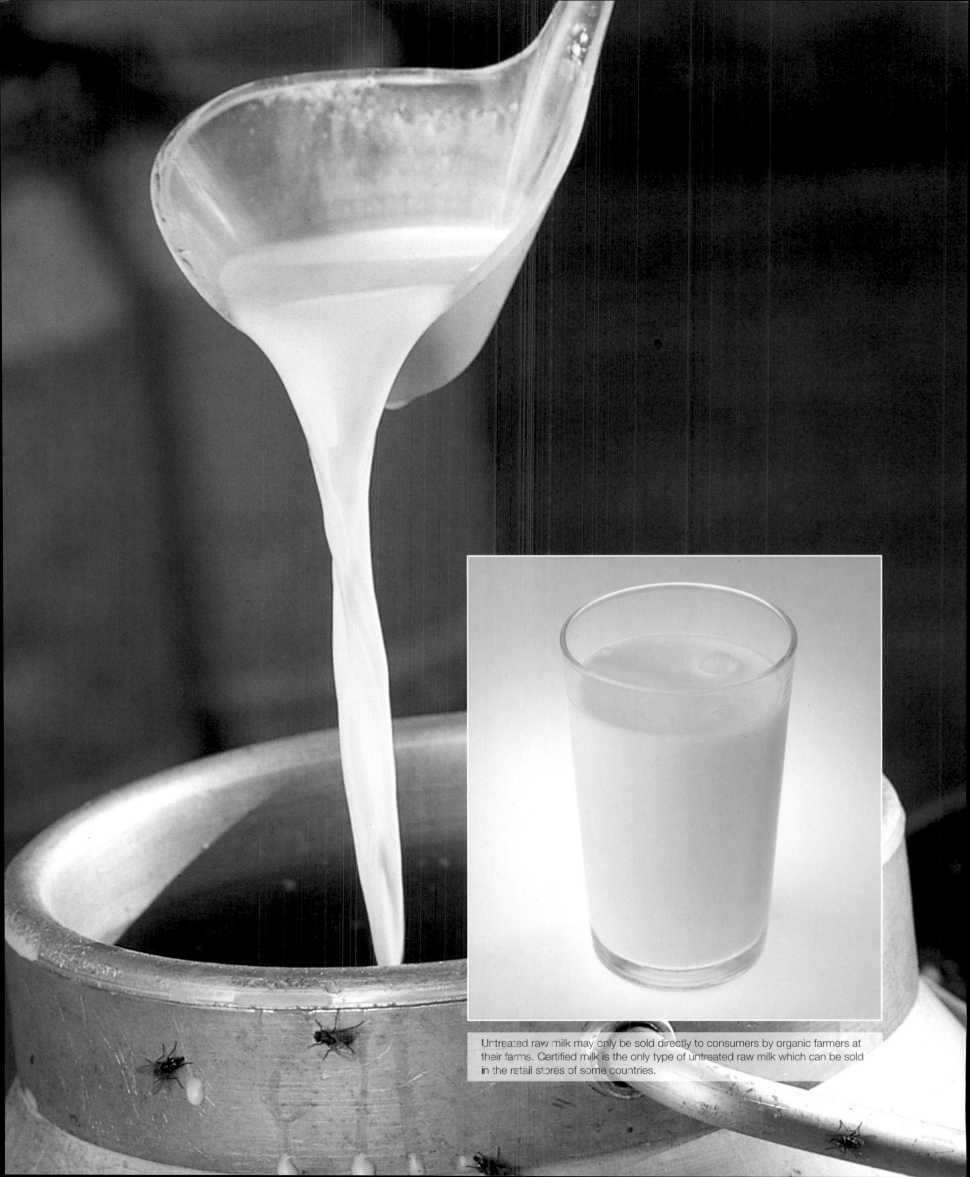

Untreated raw milk may only be sold directly to consumers by organic farmers at their farms. Certified milk is the only type of untreated raw milk which can be sold in the retail stores of some countries.

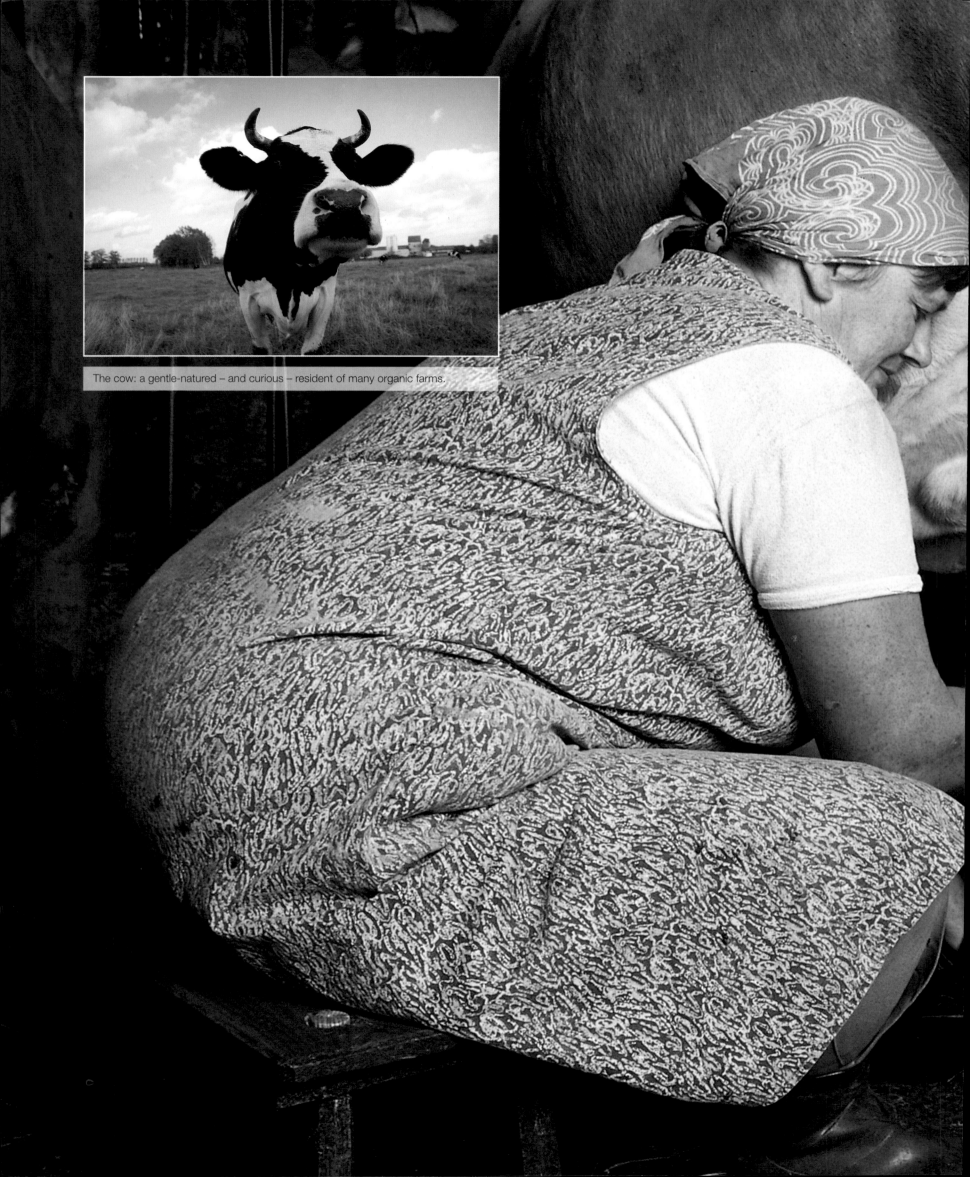

The cow: a gentle-natured – and curious – resident of many organic farms.

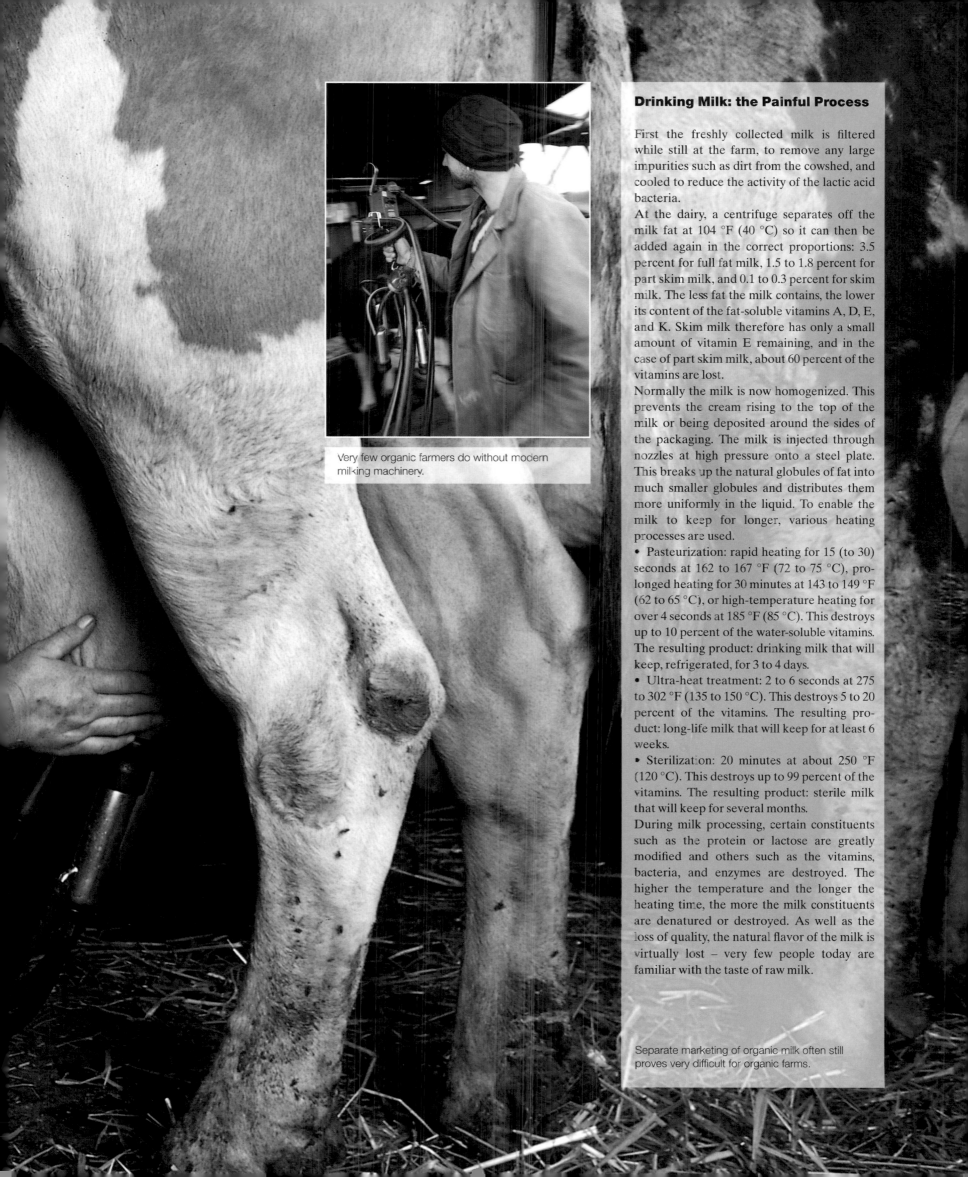

Very few organic farmers do without modern milking machinery.

Drinking Milk: the Painful Process

First the freshly collected milk is filtered while still at the farm, to remove any large impurities such as dirt from the cowshed, and cooled to reduce the activity of the lactic acid bacteria.

At the dairy, a centrifuge separates off the milk fat at 104 °F (40 °C) so it can then be added again in the correct proportions: 3.5 percent for full fat milk, 1.5 to 1.8 percent for part skim milk, and 0.1 to 0.3 percent for skim milk. The less fat the milk contains, the lower its content of the fat-soluble vitamins A, D, E, and K. Skim milk therefore has only a small amount of vitamin E remaining, and in the case of part skim milk, about 60 percent of the vitamins are lost.

Normally the milk is now homogenized. This prevents the cream rising to the top of the milk or being deposited around the sides of the packaging. The milk is injected through nozzles at high pressure onto a steel plate. This breaks up the natural globules of fat into much smaller globules and distributes them more uniformly in the liquid. To enable the milk to keep for longer, various heating processes are used.

• Pasteurization: rapid heating for 15 (to 30) seconds at 162 to 167 °F (72 to 75 °C), prolonged heating for 30 minutes at 143 to 149 °F (62 to 65 °C), or high-temperature heating for over 4 seconds at 185 °F (85 °C). This destroys up to 10 percent of the water-soluble vitamins. The resulting product: drinking milk that will keep, refrigerated, for 3 to 4 days.

• Ultra-heat treatment: 2 to 6 seconds at 275 to 302 °F (135 to 150 °C). This destroys 5 to 20 percent of the vitamins. The resulting product: long-life milk that will keep for at least 6 weeks.

• Sterilization: 20 minutes at about 250 °F (120 °C). This destroys up to 99 percent of the vitamins. The resulting product: sterile milk that will keep for several months.

During milk processing, certain constituents such as the protein or lactose are greatly modified and others such as the vitamins, bacteria, and enzymes are destroyed. The higher the temperature and the longer the heating time, the more the milk constituents are denatured or destroyed. As well as the loss of quality, the natural flavor of the milk is virtually lost – very few people today are familiar with the taste of raw milk.

Separate marketing of organic milk often still proves very difficult for organic farms.

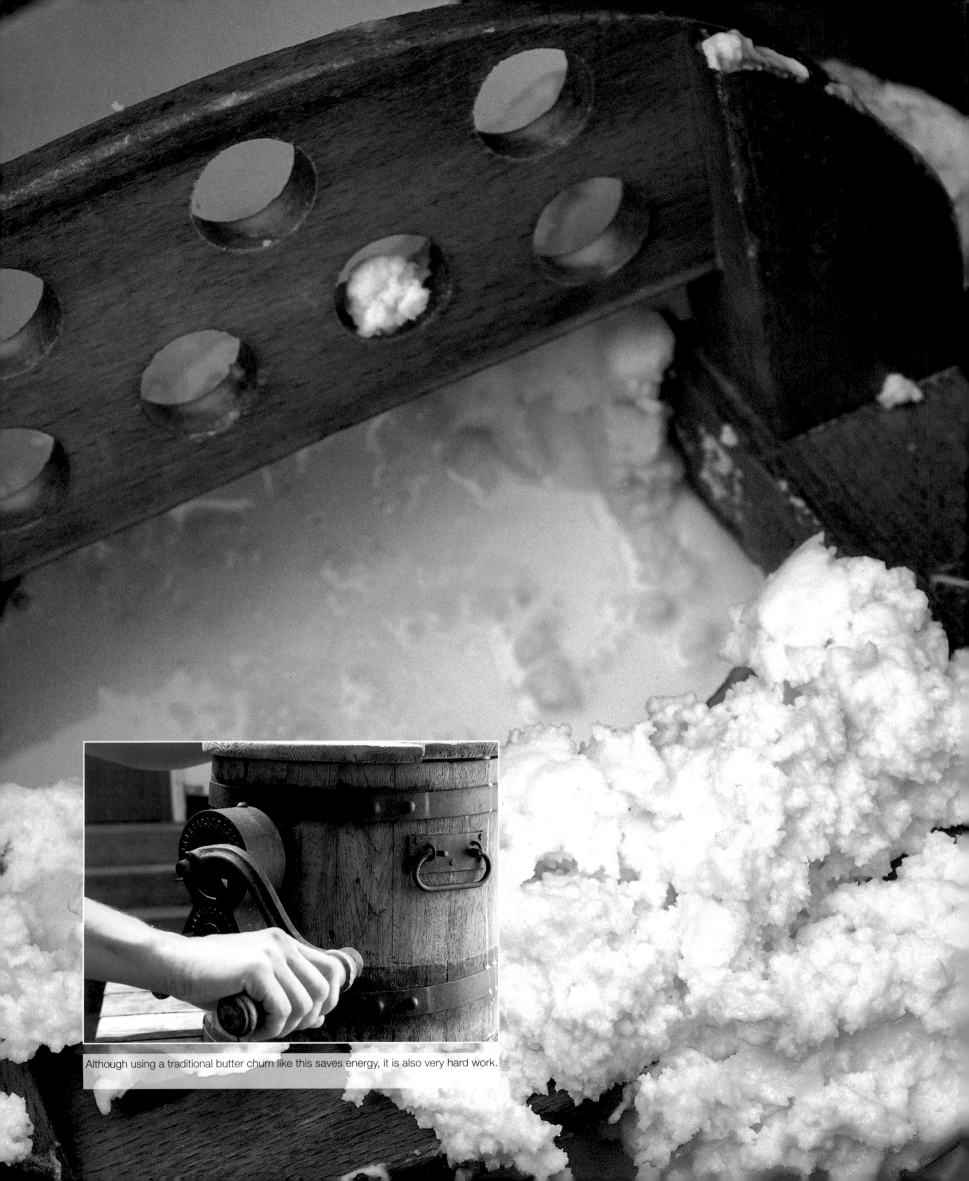

Although using a traditional butter churn like this saves energy, it is also very hard work.

Churning the Cream

Good Butter

In the past, butter was only made in summer, when the cows gave an especially large amount of milk. The surplus milk could be processed to provide a fat reserve for the lean seasons to come. Butter production is an arduous and expensive activity. 6 to 7 gallons (22 to 25 liters) of raw milk are needed for 2 pounds (about 1 kilogram) of butter. In addition, producers of milk and dairy products are required by law to comply with certain regulations, at considerable cost. It is for these reasons that butter from ecological farms is more than twice the price of conventional brand butter. However, its superb flavor more than justifies the price.

In an ideal situation, butter-making begins with freshly collected raw milk which is still warm. To remove the cream, it is put in a centrifuge to separate the cream from the low-fat milk. If the farm also produces farmer's cheese, for which the milk has to be stored in tubs, the old traditional method is used: the milk is left to stand for 12 to 18 hours, during which time the cream rises to the surface and can be skimmed off. During this time, the farmer has to keep the milk cool with water to prevent it going sour, as sour milk can no longer be separated. The resulting low-fat milk is used for making cheese. Farm cheese dairies often use part-skim milk for their hard cheese and can then also produce butter.

The cream, which has a fat content of about 20 percent, is immediately stored in a cool, dark place as light would cause the milk fat to spoil quicker. The cream can now be used to make sweet cream butter or sour cream butter. For the latter, buttermilk or another type of natural acid culture is added to the cream, which thickens in several hours. Souring of the butter enables it to develop a more distinct flavor and to keep for longer. Mild soured butter from dairies is produced by artificial souring, which organic farms reject.

For sweet cream butter, the cream is poured into a butter churn to about half full. The temperature is now a crucial factor on which the subsequent quality of the butter will depend. It may vary between 48 and 55 °F (9 and 13 °C) – the lower temperatures are necessary in summer. The temperature is directly related to the structure of the milk fat, which varies according to the animal's diet. If the temperature is too high, a high proportion of butter oil and consequently a greasy butter is produced, whereas if the temperature is too low, the butter becomes crumbly.

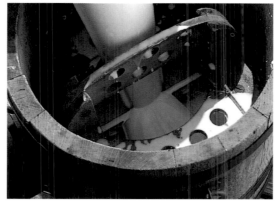
The skimmed-off cream is poured into the open butter churn.

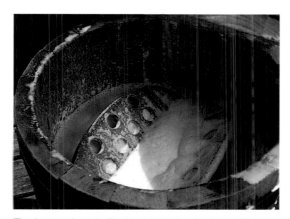
The butter churn is filled to just below the top of the beater, which nowadays is made of high-grade steel.

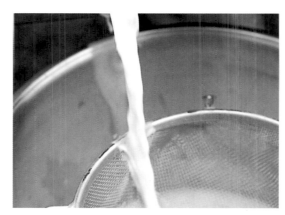
Once the butter grains have formed, the buttermilk is let out of the churn.

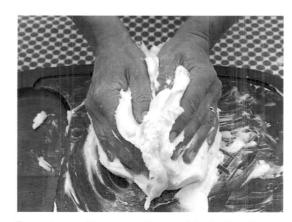
The water used to remove the remaining buttermilk must be reduced by vigorous kneading.

As the cream is churned, the butter fat is released and begins to stick together more and more.

With a traditional butter churn, the wooden beater is set in motion by turning the handle vigorously. Of course, modern machines of all sizes now perform this task. However, it remains important for the cream to churn quickly. First a froth forms, in which the fat globules are close together. Constant churning breaks down the bonds. The butter fat is freed and sticks together increasingly to form larger and larger lumps. Those in the trade call this the "butter grain." Once the lumps are larger than pea-sized, it is time to drain off the virtually fat-free buttermilk which has separated. There is a corked hole or tap at the bottom of the churn for this purpose.

Next, cold water is poured into the butter churn to wash away the remains of the buttermilk from between the butter grains. If any is left behind, the butter produced initially has a fresh and pleasant buttermilk aroma, but can soon smell and taste cheesy. For this reason, the butter grain is normally washed until the water no longer comes out cloudy – generally three or four times. The washed butter grain is then usually cooled again.

To remove some of the water and evenly distribute the rest – butter may contain up to 16 percent water – the butter has to be thoroughly kneaded. This is exhausting work when done by hand, but nowadays it can be done by kneading machines or, in larger-scale enterprises, by rollers. Whilst hand kneading preserves the lactic acid bacteria which provide a stronger flavor, forced processing lets the butter keep for longer.

The finished raw milk butter deserves an attractive shape. It can simply be rolled or pressed into traditional, well-wetted (otherwise it cannot be turned out very well) wooden molds. Its appearance is an important indicator that it has been produced by natural means and without cruelty. The difference speaks for itself.

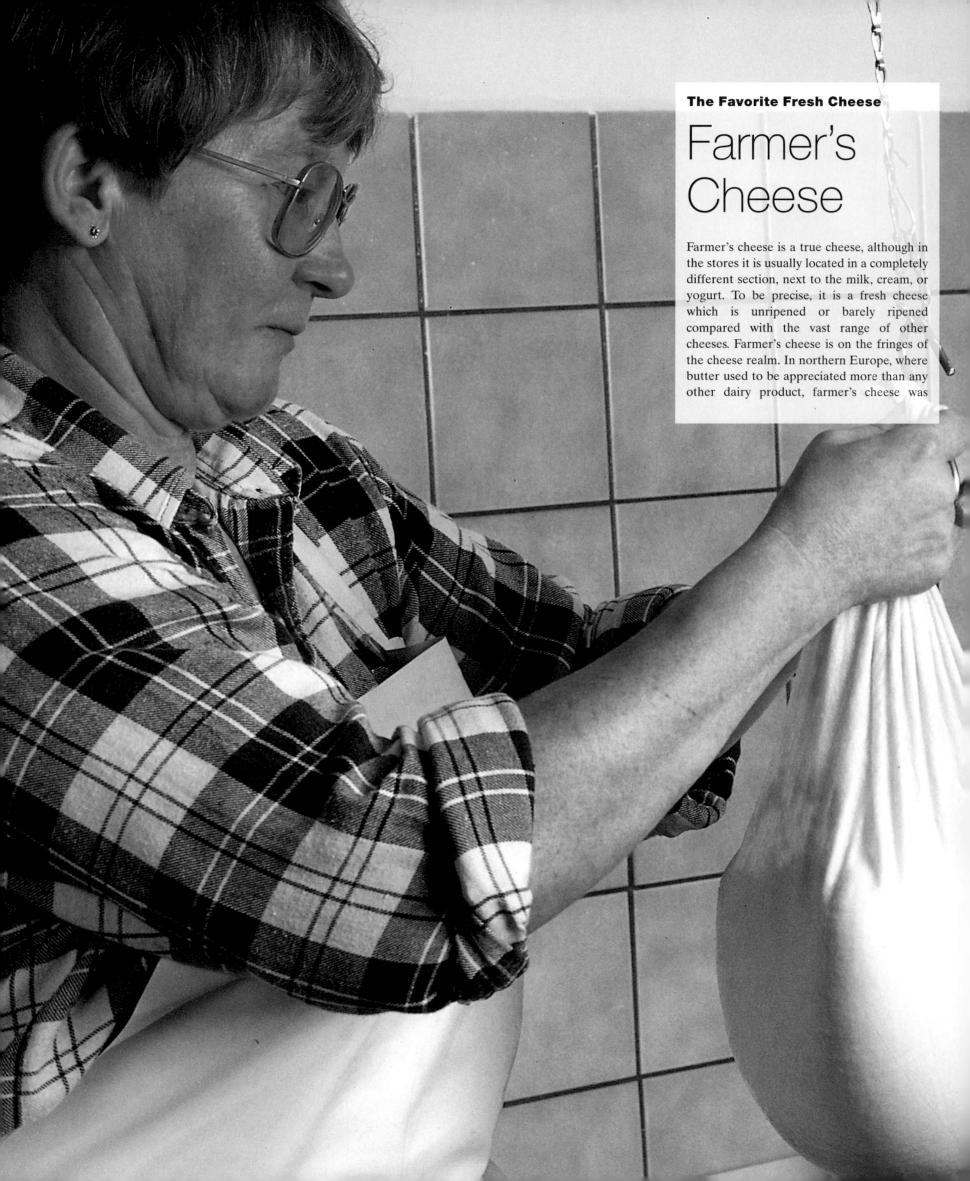

Farmer's Cheese

Farmer's cheese is a true cheese, although in the stores it is usually located in a completely different section, next to the milk, cream, or yogurt. To be precise, it is a fresh cheese which is unripened or barely ripened compared with the vast range of other cheeses. Farmer's cheese is on the fringes of the cheese realm. In northern Europe, where butter used to be appreciated more than any other dairy product, farmer's cheese was always made only from fairly fat-free milk. As it is easy to produce, it was made at home in major milk-producing regions up to the Second World War, and was often processed to make sour milk cheeses or scalded cheeses. In Europe's more southern countries, it was always produced using unskimmed full milk. In fact, it can just as easily be produced from sheep's or goat's milk as from cow's milk. Of all the cheese varieties, farmer's cheese is allowed to have the highest water content, with over 73 percent in the fat-free matter.

Fresh cheese has to be pasteurized. This process is carried out with great care in cheese dairies on organic farms. As well as the benefit in terms of hygiene, the advantage of heating is that the high-quality whey proteins albumin and globulin coagulate as a result. They are fully incorporated into the farmer's cheese,

whereas, when raw milk is used, they remain unprecipitated and run out with the whey. After heating, the milk is cooled to about 86 °F (30 °C).

If skim milk is used, it is sufficient to add a starter such as buttermilk or yogurt, as the lactic acid bacteria do the work by themselves. However, if full-fat milk is used, cheese-makers like to add a few drops of rennet, the protein-splitting enzyme obtained from a calf's stomach, or from bacteria. The precise amount is based on experience. Many natural factors affect the thickening of the milk, as its composition differs depending on the type of animal, pasture, feed, and season, and the bacteria are different in every region, and even from one farm to another.

The thickening takes time. At room temperature, it can easily take a whole day. If the

initial temperature of 86 °F (30 °C) is maintained, thickening is complete within five to ten hours. Once a coagulum has formed, it is cut into cubes of about an inch (2 to 3 centimeters) with a knife. It has to be firm enough for the cuts to remain visible and not merge together. The cheese is then left to stand for a while so the whey can run out.

Traditionally, the thickened mass is now transferred very carefully into a damp cloth and strained. Nowadays, it is often scooped into special plastic cups full of small holes. It takes six to eight hours for the whey to run off, depending on the temperature, consistency of the coagulum and desired result. For firmer farmer's cheese which keeps longer, the contents of the cloth are squeezed slightly. Otherwise the cheese is stirred to give it a creamy consistency and put into jars.

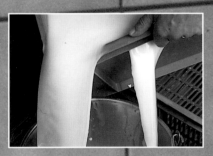
Carefully pasteurized milk is poured into the farmer's-cheese tub.

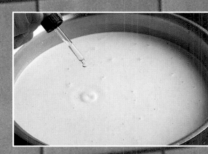
A few drops of rennet are added to the full-fat milk.

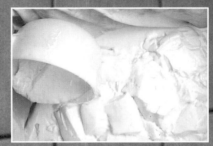
After thickening, the coagulum is cut into cubes.

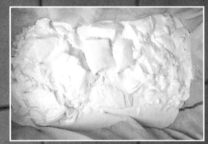
The pieces of coagulum are placed in a damp cloth.

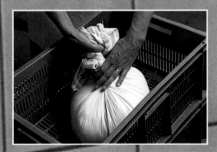
The whey takes six to eight hours to drain off.

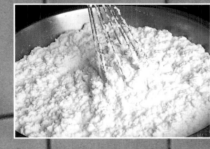
The contents of the cloth are put back in the tub and beaten.

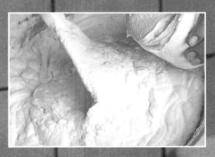
The farmer's cheese has reached the required creamy consistency.

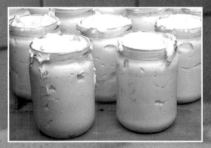
It is spooned into jars ready for sale.

Dairy Products in Cooking

The Dairy Essentials

Whole generations swore by the idea of enriching sauces with butter and using plenty of cream in their cooking. At that time, no one was worried about calories. Now people see things differently. In wholefood cookery particularly, it is undesirable to load dishes with excess energy by adding unnecessary helpings of butter or cream. However, butter and cream can improve dishes and they are indispensable to many delicious recipes. Butter mixtures flavored with olives, garlic, herbs, or mushrooms can transform plain boiled potatoes or lightly cooked vegetables into a surprisingly tasty treat. But farmer's cheese and other fresh cheeses make an excellent substitute for butter. They are best when used in combination with fresh, raw, and therefore particularly healthy ingredients. And, unlike ready-prepared products, the amounts of particular ingredients used can be varied according to taste. As a result, vitamin-rich foods are combined with readily digestible proteins, and fat intake is kept within reasonable limits. Yogurt, farmer's cheese, and fresh cheese are suitable not only as a base for sauces, dips, or creams, but also as fillings for vegetables or pastries, and give every dish a very distinctive touch of freshness and lightness.

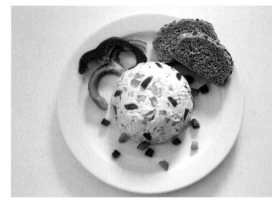

Fresh Cheese Terrine with Red and Green Bell Peppers

7 oz (200 g) fresh cheese
$^{1}/_{4}$ cup (50 g) sour cream
$^{1}/_{2}$ small red bell pepper
$^{1}/_{2}$ small green bell pepper
1 small bunch flat-leafed parsley, finely chopped
$^{1}/_{2}$ tsp coarse salt
$^{1}/_{4}$ tsp sweet paprika
Pinch of cayenne pepper

Blend together the fresh cheese and sour cream in a mixer. Dice the bell peppers finely and add them to the cheese together with the parsley and other flavoring ingredients. Mix well and season to give a spicy flavor. Line a small dish with aluminum foil, spoon in the cheese mixture, press it firmly into the dish and chill for at least 1 hour. Turn it out onto a plate and garnish with parsley, chopped bell pepper, or spices.

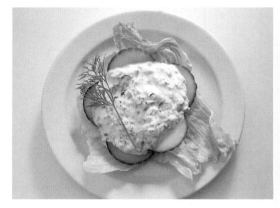

Tzatziki

5 oz (150 g) farmer's cheese
5 oz (150 g) yogurt
$^{1}/_{2}$ cup (100 ml) heavy cream
$^{1}/_{2}$ cucumber
2 garlic cloves
1 bunch parsley, chopped
1 Tbs olive oil
1 Tbs lemon juice
White pepper
$^{1}/_{2}$ tsp coarse salt

Put the farmer's cheese, yogurt, and cream in a bowl and stir until creamy. Peel the cucumber, halve it, remove the seeds, grate it finely and add it to the cheese mixture. Add the crushed garlic, finely chopped parsley, olive oil, and lemon juice and stir well to mix. Season with salt and pepper. Best served chilled.

Spanish Olive Butter

$3^{1}/_{2}$ oz (100 g) butter
1 Tbs low-fat farmer's cheese
1 tsp herb salt
2 tsp tomato paste
2 tsp lemon juice
$^{1}/_{4}$ tsp black pepper
1 tsp finely chopped thyme
1 crushed garlic clove
10 black olives

Mix together all the ingredients, except for the olives, with a whisk. Pit the olives, cut them into very small pieces and stir them into the butter mixture.
Olive butter is particularly suitable as a topping for canapés and also goes well with toasted whole wheat baguette.

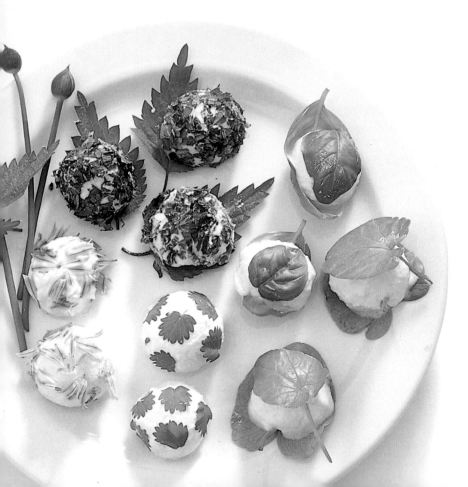

A refreshing variation – fresh cheese balls with herbs.

Pastries with a Herb and Pumpkin Seed Filling

Pastry
9 oz (250 g) fine whole wheat flour
2 eggs
$^1/_2$ tsp coarse salt
Flour for rolling out

Filling
3$^1/_2$ oz (100 g) farmer's cheese
$^1/_4$ cup (50 g) sour cream
2 eggs
$^1/_2$ tsp herb salt, pinch of pepper
2 Tbs finely chopped pumpkin seeds
1 small bunch chervil
1 small bunch parsley
1 small bunch dill
1 small bunch burnet saxifrage (optional)
Butter for greasing

Knead all the pastry ingredients into a firm, workable dough. Leave the dough to stand, covered, for about 30 minutes.

Mix together the farmer's cheese, sour cream, 1 egg, salt, and pepper until creamy. Add the pumpkin seeds. Chop the herbs finely and carefully mix them in. Check the seasoning of the filling.

Roll the dough out thinly. Cut out circles about 3 to 4 inches (8 to 10 cm) in diameter. Put half a tablespoon of filling onto the middle of each circle. Moisten the edges of the pastry, stick them together and press them together firmly with a fork. Place the pastries on a greased baking tray and brush them with the second beaten egg. Bake for 15 to 20 minutes in a preheated oven at 340 °F (170 °C).

Farmer's Cheese and Herb Quiche

Pastry
7 oz (200 g) fine spelt flour
3$^1/_2$ oz (100 g) cold butter
1 small egg
Butter for greasing dish

Filling
11 oz (300 g) farmer's cheese
3 eggs
5 oz (150 g) crème fraîche
2 Tbs corn meal
Coarse salt, pepper
2 scallions
1 small bunch basil, 1 bunch chives
2 tomatoes
5 oz (150 g) grated hard cheese

Sieve the flour, cut the butter into pieces and rub into the flour thoroughly. Mix the egg with 3 tablespoons of ice cold water, add to the mixture and work into a smooth dough. Chill for 30 minutes.

Roll the dough out and line a greased spring-release pie dish with it. Cover the dough with parchment paper, sprinkle with dried beans and bake blind for 15 minutes at 350 °F (180 °C).

Meanwhile, drain off the liquid from the farmer's cheese. Separate the eggs and mix the yolks with the farmer's cheese, crème fraîche, corn meal, salt, and pepper. Finely chop the scallions, basil and chives and add to the mixture. Pour into the pastry shell and decorate with slices of tomato lightly seasoned with salt and pepper. Sprinkle the grated cheese over the top and bake for 1 hour at 350 °F (180 °C).

Other Dairy Products

Delicious Milk Products

Buttermilk
Produced during butter-making, when the liquid is drained off after the fat coagulates. Virtually fat-free at only 0.5 percent, but rich in lecithin and minerals. As well as pure buttermilk, other forms are also available to which a maximum of 10 percent water or 15 percent skim milk may be added. Buttermilk is a healthy and very refreshing drink

Clarified Butter
Pure butter fat obtained by melting butter, contains nothing other than protein and water. It is similar to Indian ghee, can be kept for a long time, is easy to digest and can be heated to higher temperatures than normal butter.

Crème Fraîche
This sour milk product has a higher fat content than whipping cream and sour cream. It is used as a flavoring ingredient to provide a discreet sour flavor, but loses its fine taste when boiled.

Thick Milk
Produced naturally when raw milk, certified milk or gently pasteurized farm milk is left to stand at room temperature. Nowadays it is produced using starters, is dense and has a fat content of 3.5 percent. There are also low-fat varieties of thick milk, made from the skim milk produced during butter-making.

Cottage Cheese
Has a distinctive lumpy consistency, produced by pure acid-coagulation of the protein in skim milk. Cream is added to the resulting lumps of curd, and this is absorbed into the lumps and encloses them. Available salted, with added herbs or other flavorings.

Yogurt
Special lactic acid bacteria give yogurt, which originates from the Balkans and the Middle East, its flavor and consistency. The most well-known of these bacteria is the lactobacillus bulgaricus, which imparts a fresh, sour flavor. Yogurt always contains a mixture of dextro and levo rotatory lactic acids. In the case of organic yogurt, strains such as streptococcus thermophilus are increasingly being used, which generate the more readily digestible dextro rotatory lactic acids.
- Homemade yogurt: Bring the milk almost to the boil, then let it cool to 110 °F (45 °C). Mix in 2 tablespoons of ready-made (non heat-treated) yogurt per pint ($^1/_2$ liter). Pour into pots, cover and keep as warm as possible. The yogurt will set in a few hours.

Kefir
Sour milk drink originating from the Caucasus and the Middle East, produced by adding kefir lumps which consist of a combination of lactic acid bacteria and yeast fungi. As well as the lactic acid fermentation, there is also slight alcoholic fermentation. A low alcohol content of 0.2 to 0.8 percent is produced, along with some carbon dioxide, which gives kefir its sparkling taste. It is readily digestible thanks to its mainly dextro rotatory lactic acid.

Cream
Separated from the milk by skimming or centrifuging. Whipping cream has a fat content of at least 30 percent. It is heated to coagulate the proteins, which are essentially what forms the foam when whipped. It is then chilled and

The Adaptable Base: Fresh Cheese
In terms of quantity, the most important representative of this group of cheeses thickened by lactic acid bacteria and maybe a small amount of rennet is farmer's cheese. It is available with different fat contents, the level of fat being increased by adding cream. Various farmer's cheese products containing herbs and spices, which can constitute up to 15 percent of the total weight, or fruits, which can constitute up to 30 percent, are available. And the products listed as fresh cheese are even more multicolored and varied. In wholefood stores, too, we are spoilt for choice with all the new creations containing herbs, spices, all types of onions, vegetables, nuts, and other ingredients for added flavor. Different consistencies are achieved by more intensive pressing – the minimum water content of 73 percent is the only restriction. One rare specialty from some farm cheese dairies is layered cheese. It consists of layers of fresh cheese, each with a different fat content, and is made by hand.

allowed to mature for at least two days, during which the butter oil crystallizes into fat globules. This prevents the cream turning to butter too quickly when it is whipped. It can only be whipped up well when chilled.
Cream with a minimum fat content of 10 percent is described as light cream. This does not thicken when whipped.

Sour Milk
Sour milk, which is soured by so-called starters such as lactic acid bacteria or other bacteria, forms the basis of a whole range of sour milk products, such as sour cream, thick milk, crème fraîche, and others.
There are two forms of lactic acid – the dextro rotatory, mild flavored, easily digestible L(+) and the levo rotatory, sour flavored, slow-digesting D(−) lactic acid. The type is nowadays frequently stated on the labels of dairy products.
Sour milk for drinking contains 3.5 percent fat and has a creamy consistency. Cream sour milk has a fat content of 10 percent.

Sour Cream
Only differs from sour milk in that it has a higher fat content of over 10 percent and a slightly thicker consistency.

Sweden Milk
In Scandinavia, the containers used are rubbed with the common herb Butterwort, pinguicula vulgaris, to enable certain lactic acid bacteria to develop. These bacteria separate off slime and are responsible for the consistency of the sour milk. They also enable the milk to keep naturally for up to 10 months.

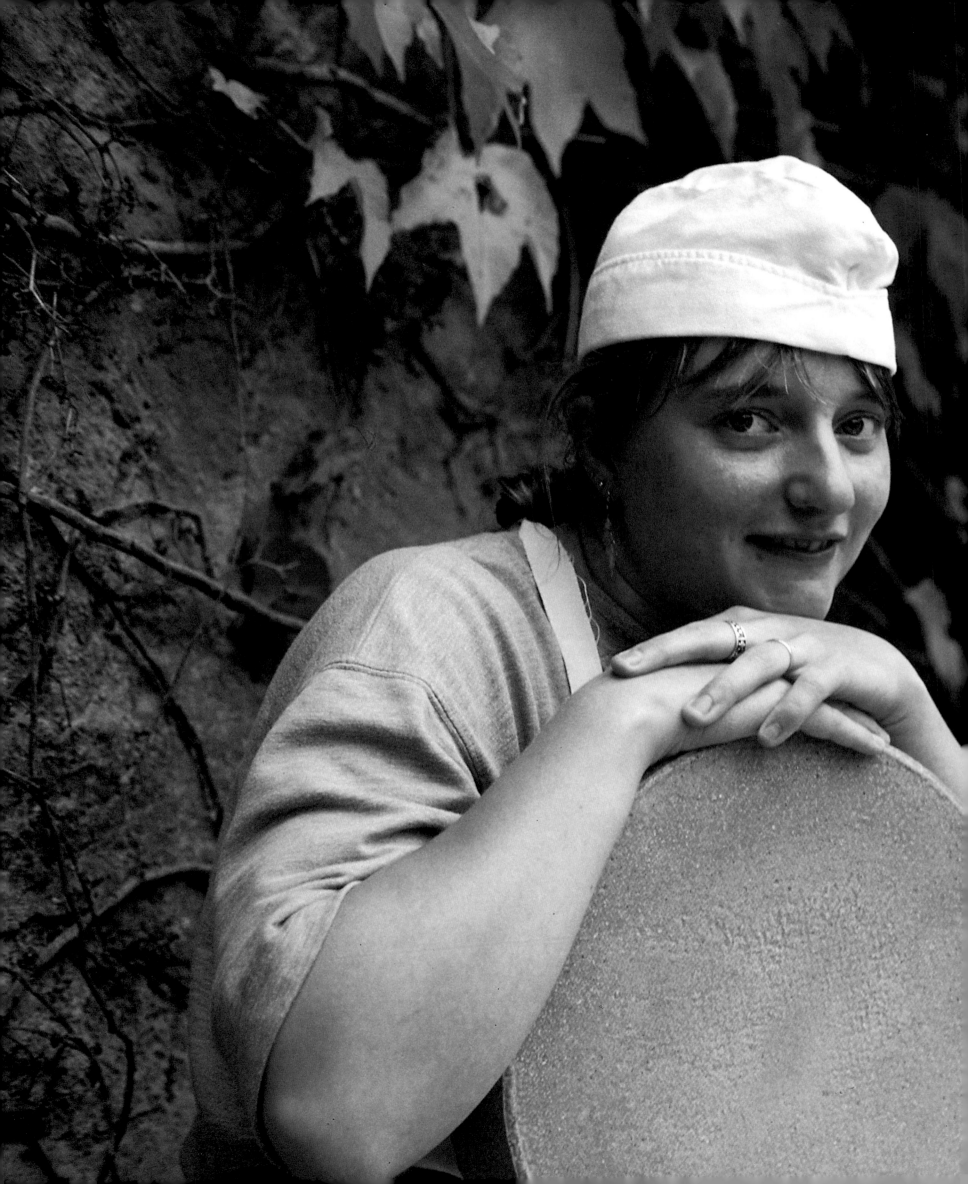

Spoilt for Choice

Cheeses: an Endless Variety

Our ancestors had hardly discovered milk as a foodstuff about 5,000 years ago when the first cheese came about. A container of milk only had to be left standing for a while for the phenomenon of coagulation to take place. Once the separated whey had drained away, the very first cheese emerged – the basis of every type of cheese. The methods which were subsequently developed for handling the cheese and mastering the thickening process, draining the curd and ripening in accordance with the animal type, feed or vegetation, climate, type of milk. and size of the premises resulted in the emergence of a vast number of different cheese varieties.

Six cheese categories can be identified. The first, fresh cheese, has already been described. The other categories are sour milk cheese, soft cheese, semi firm and firm cut cheese, and hard cheese (see page 329). Every type of cheese falls into one of these categories, but each also has its own characteristic properties and features which distinguish it to a greater or lesser extent from the other cheeses in that category.

Thanks to organic farming methods, new high-quality cheese varieties have come onto the market and others will no doubt follow, as organic cheese dairies multiply Cheese-making is an activity in which natural processes are clearly evident. The cheese gains a character all of its own. Organic milk with its natural germs and the external conditions that favor the growth of fungi and bacteria are responsible for the properties of a cheese. The most well-known examples of micro-organisms affecting the cheese while it is maturing are from the southern French village of Roquefort, where the *penicillium roqueforti* mold developed in the Berges Combalou caves; Emmental, whose charac-

teristic holes are formed by propionic acid bacteria; the Belgian Herve, where the air of the whole surrounding region is populated by red mold bacteria; or Camembert, whose surface becomes covered with white mold due to ambient conditions.

Nowadays, practically all countries produce organic cheeses. Many of the well-known varieties are also available from organic production. The cheese counters of good whole-food retailers put many delicatessens to shame. Not all cheeses come from farm cheese dairies: some also come from cooperatives. The high costs associated with cheese production mean that many organic farmers prefer to join large cooperatives, some of which have now started processing organic milk. There are now also firms which take over the often expensive task of ripening the cheese from the organic farmers. These firms can then supply special varieties in larger quantities. This is why Gouda and Tilsit, Emmental and Comté, Camembert and Brie, Roquefort and Manchego, Pecorino and Pencarreg are available from wholefood retailers. Many organic cheese dairies only produce small quantities of cheese which can often only be bought directly or in regional stores. Fortunately, the number of cheese connoisseurs with a nose for a good product is steadily growing.

Background: Such a magnificent slab of hard cheese with its superb rind whets the appetite – for all the countless other cheese varieties too.

General fat grades for all cheese varieties based on fat in dry matter in percent

Fat grade	Fat in dry matter
Low-fat	0–9.9%
Quarter-fat	10–19.9%
Half-fat	20–29.9%
Three-quarters-fat	30–39.9%
Fat	40–44.9%
Full-fat	45–49.9%
Cream	50–59%
Double cream	60–85%

Note: The dry matter is obtained by deducting the water content from the total weight of a cheese.

Making Cut Cheese

In the Organic Cheese Dairy

Organic cheese production uses the shortest method. The freshly collected milk is brought to the farm's own cheese dairy. For fresh or sour milk cheese, the milk is allowed to thicken naturally or home-cultured lactic acid bacteria are added. In the case of soft, semi firm, or firm cut cheeses, and hard cheese, rennet is mainly used for thickening.

Rennet comes from calves' stomachs and contains the enzyme chymosin, which splits lactoprotein. Today, microbial rennet is often used, which contains laboratory-cultivated enzymes for coagulation and for breaking down the protein. In some countries, rennet from genetically engineered bacteria is already being used. Organic cheese dairies strongly reject this practice.

The farm cheese dairies consider it important to retain the germ content of the raw milk. For this reason, the milk is not cooled to the usual 39 °F (4 °C) – a temperature which inhibits lactic acid bacteria to a greater extent than other types – and

is not pasteurized. When adding the rennet, the raw milk is warmed to about 90 °F (32 °C). The highly effective enzyme – just a few drops are sufficient for several gallons of milk – acts very rapidly. The milk is thickened after just 30 to 60 minutes.

The reason for this process being so quick and easy is the casein content of the milk. The action of the rennet (and/or lactic acid bacteria) causes the casein to coagulate and be deposited. The jelly-like curds are formed, while the whey proteins albumin and globulin remain in the whey. The gel or coagulum is separated from the whey by cutting it into pieces. This process is what decides the type of cheese produced:

• The larger the cut pieces are, the more whey remains in the cheese mass and the softer the consistency of the cheese.

• The smaller the pieces are, the more whey drains off and the harder the cheese becomes.

• The more uniformly the coagulum is cut, the smoother the cheese will be.

In the case of firm cut cheese and hard cheese, the cubes are only $1/4$ to $1/2$ inch (0.5 to 1 centimeter) wide and are cut using a cheese harp. In organic cheese dairies this process is done by hand.

It takes time for the curd to collect and the whey to drain off. With unheated cut cheese, this part often takes place in stages: the coagulum is first

cut into fairly large pieces and then weighed down and left for the first whey to drain off. After this, the curd is cut into smaller pieces, may now be salted, and is lifted out of the vat with a cloth. Traditionally a cloth is pulled through under the curd and held together above it. Lifting up the cloth containing the curd enables the whey to drain off well.

The cheese is pushed into a mold, then pressed for about 24 to 48 hours, during which it is turned several times. Usually the salting is not done until this stage. The firm cut cheese and hard cheese are laid in a salt bath for their outermost layer to harden. Salt is not only important for preserving the cheese – it also plays an important part in developing the flavor.

During the ripening, which can take weeks or months, the cheeses are turned regularly and rubbed with salt to help a rind form and make the cheese mature evenly. The atmosphere, i.e. the temperature and air humidity, in the maturing cellar affects the further development of the cheese. As it ages, the cheese takes on a darker color, it gains a stronger aroma, and its protein content becomes increasingly digestible – it has reached its peak quality.

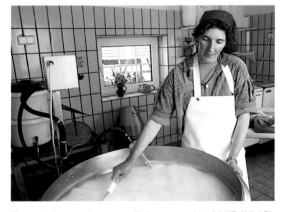
For cut cheese, the raw milk is warmed to 90 °F (32 °C) and a few drops of rennet are added. Enzymes cause the milk to coagulate within a short time.

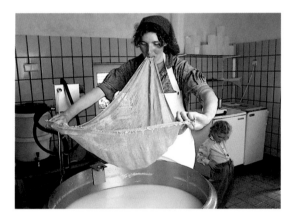
The coagulum is cut into small pieces to enable most of the whey to drain out. Then a cloth is folded into a triangle and held at the three corners.

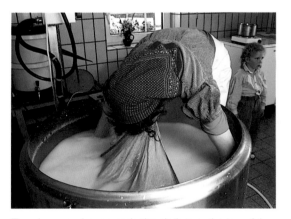
The cheesemaker spreads the cloth over the top of the curd, then skillfully pulls the ends through under the cheese mass.

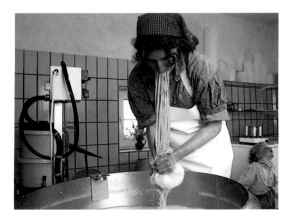
The curd can now be lifted out of the vat and pressed out hard with the aid of the cloth to rid it of as much of the remaining whey as possible.

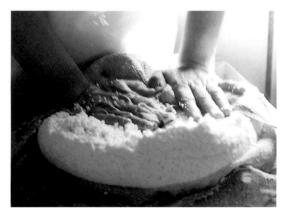
The relatively dry cheese mass is pressed firmly into a wooden mold and the surface smoothed.

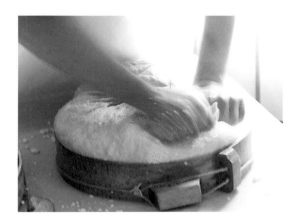
The clamped mold is put in a press for one to two days and turned several times during this period. Then the rind is brushed down with salt (right).

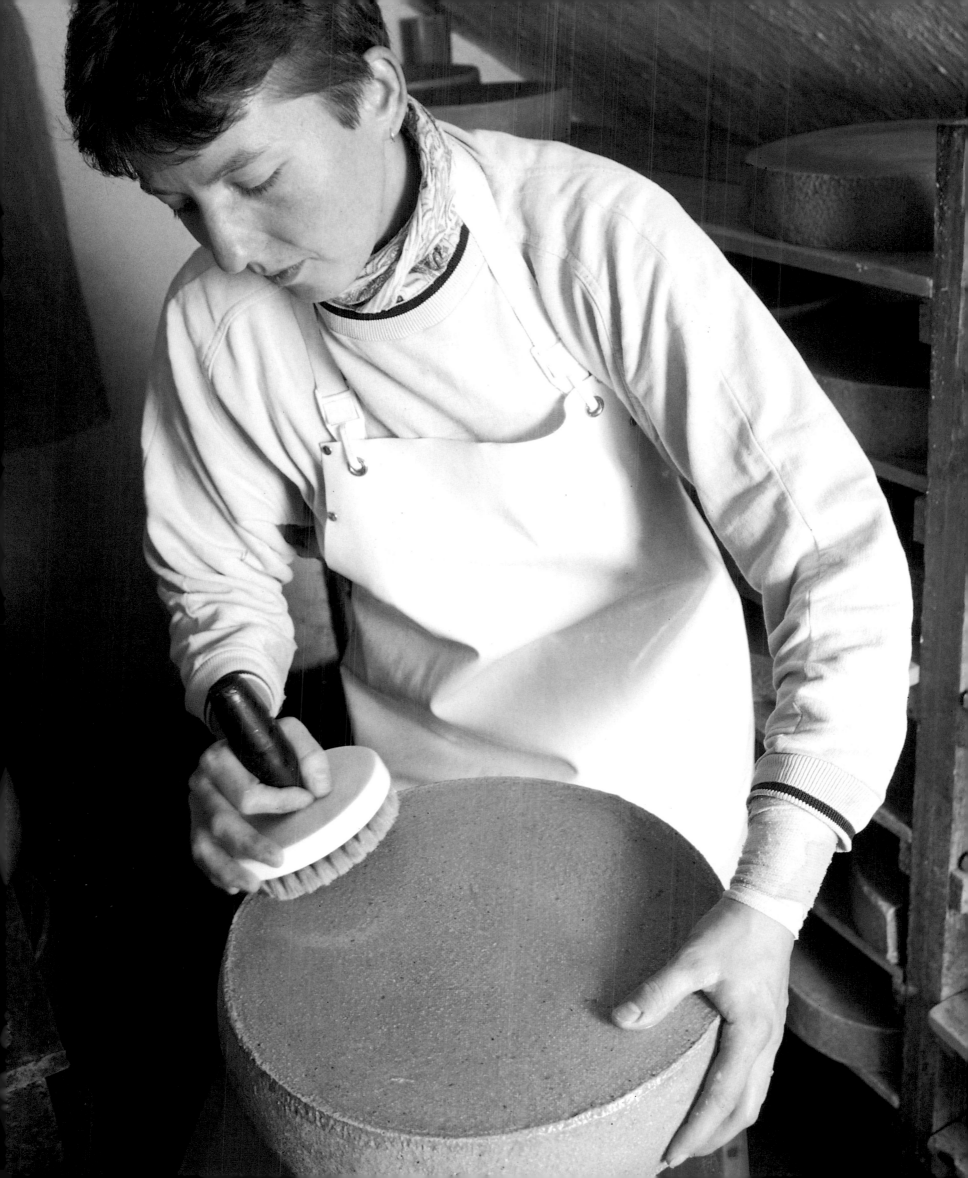

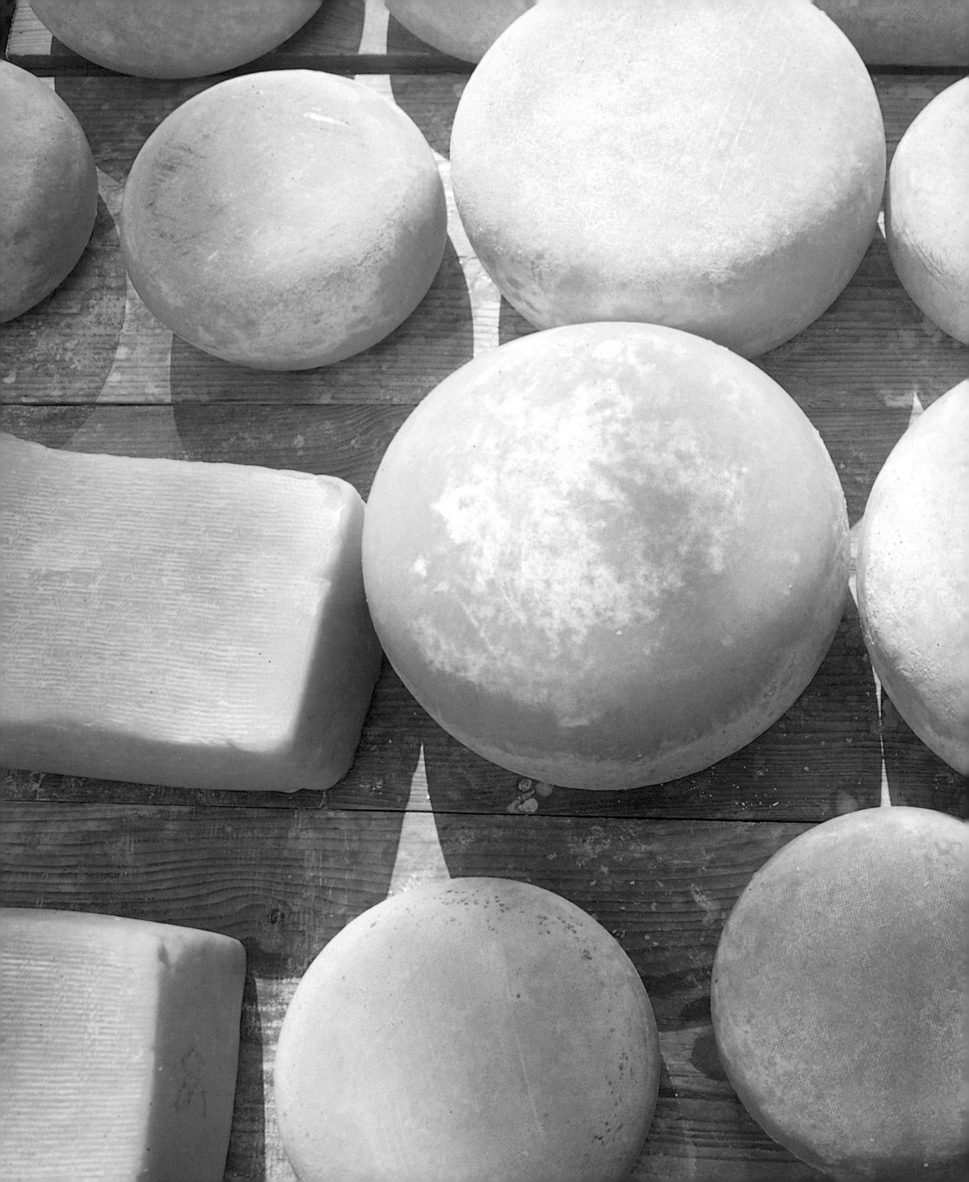

How a Soft Cheese is Made

Camembert is the most famous of the soft cheeses. It is thought to have been "invented" by the farmer Marie Harel from the Normandy village of Camembert. During the French Revolution, she hid a priest from the Brie region on her farm, and he passed on to her everything he knew about cheese-making. Madame Harel created half-pound cheeses which she left for three weeks in damp cellars to allow the natural white mold to form on the surface. This produced an exceptionally delicate thick yellow cheese with a distinctive aroma.

Since then, Camembert production has become common throughout Europe, including, of course, organic cheese dairies. However, the maturing period of three weeks, which produces a very intense flavor, is now only observed in exceptional cases. Instead, it is sold, at a slightly younger age, with a pure white downy skin and in rounds weighing from 3 to 14 ounces (80 to 400 grams).

How a Camembert is made

5.30 am   The fresh milk, which has only been filtered, is warmed to 93 °F (34 °C) – the ideal temperature for adding a dose of cheese dairy culture, the starter. This homegrown strain of lactic acid bacteria cultured by each individual cheese dairy can be compared with the sour dough additive for bread. It triggers a souring process which continues constantly and powerfully throughout every stage of the cheese-making. If the milk were not soured in this way, there could be faults in the ripening.

6.15 am   Calves' rennet is added. At the same time, a mold culture specific to Camembert is added to the milk. This ensures that the desired white mold, rather than any unwanted competing variety, develops on the cheese at a later stage.

7.00 am   The milk has coagulated and has taken on a semi solid structure. Using a cheese harp, the coagulum is cut into evenly sized pieces which must be no larger than walnuts and no smaller than hazelnuts. Whey immediately starts to run out from the curd. To encourage the whey to separate out, the curd is stirred several times.

8.00 am   The curd has solidified in the vat, and as it is heavier, has settled at the bottom. On top is the whey, and as much of this as possible is now scooped off. Then the curd and remaining whey are thoroughly mixed.

9.00 am   The curd is scooped out of the vat with a cheese-sized ladle and transferred into molds with small perforations all over. As more whey trickles

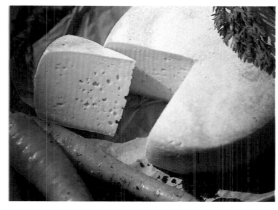
Semi firm cut cheeses colored with carrot juice – often called carrot loaves – have become a sought-after specialty amongst organic cheeses.

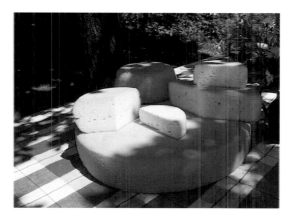
From fine Camembert to the firm slab of hard cheese – the selection from an excellent organic cheese dairy.

out gradually, the cheese becomes progressively firmer. To aid the draining process, the molds are turned five or six times between now and the afternoon.

5.00 pm   The cheeses are laid in a salt bath consisting of a 17 percent salt solution. As well as improving the flavor, the salt also has a preserving effect. Like the souring, the salt component keeps the continued development of the cheese under control so that it does not go off, but instead begins the actual maturing process. This is when the cheese gains all its characteristic properties.

5.30 pm   The cheeses are taken out of the salt bath and left to stand overnight.

The next morning they are taken to the maturing room, which has a temperature of 61 to 63 °F (16 to 17 °C) and 85 percent air humidity. They are turned every day and after four or five days, the Camembert mold has formed, covering the small rounds with a fine white down. The cheeses are then allowed to stand for a further one to two days to enable the mold to become firmer. Once the cheese has been packaged, it is placed in a cool cellar for about a week. The cheeses continue to mature – a process which, with soft cheeses, happens from the outside inwards. After no more than 14 days, the Camembert has reached the required consistency and flavor and is ready to go on sale.

Cheese Categories at a Glance

Fresh Cheese
Thickening: after pasteurization, souring with sour milk or buttermilk, some rennet may be used
Maturing: none
Maturing time: none
Fat in dry matter: all fat grades
Water content of the fat-free cheese matter: more than 73%
Varieties: farmer's cheese, layer cheese, creamed fresh cheese, mascarpone

Soft Cheese
Thickening: a little starter and rennet
Maturing: formation of white mold or red smear-coating by means of special fungal cultures
Maturing time: 1–4 weeks
Fat in dry matter: 38–52%
Water content of the fat-free cheese matter: more than 67%
Varieties: Camembert, Brie, Saint-Marcellin, Münster, Herve, Romadur, various goat's and sheep's milk cheeses and others

Sour Milk Cheese
Thickening: starter and rennet, skim milk only
Maturing: by means of various mold cultures, but mostly yellow smear-coating bacteria
Maturing time: 1–3 weeks
Fat in dry matter: less than 15%
Water content of the fat-free cheese matter: 60–73%
Varieties: Harz cheese, farmer's round cheese and others

Semi firm Cut Cheese
Thickening: only with rennet or a starter
Maturing: either by natural rind formation or by means of a wide range of mold cultures, including blue molds like *penicillium roqueforti*
Maturing time: varies considerably – can be a few weeks, 3 to 4 months, or even in some cases up to 2 years
Fat in dry matter: about 45–55%
Water content of the fat-free cheese matter: 61–69%
Varieties: Caciotta, Reblochon, Saint-Nectaire, Roquefort and other blue vein cheeses, Butterkäse and others

Firm Cut Cheese
Thickening: only with rennet or a starter
Maturing: natural rind formation
Maturing time: from 4 weeks to over a year
Fat in dry matter: about 48–60%
Water content of the fat-free cheese matter: 54–63%
Varieties: Edam, Gouda, Tilsit, Havarti, Tomme de Savoie, Brebis and others

Hard Cheese
Thickening: only with rennet or a starter
Maturing: curd is first heated to 52 °C, then a natural rind forms after pressing
Maturing time: 3 months to 2 years
Fat in dry matter: around 60%
Water content of the fat-free cheese matter: up to 56%
Varieties: mountain cheese, Emmental, Gruyère, Comté, Cheddar, Manchego, Pecorino, Parmigiano-Reggiano
Note: The data refers to ecologically produced cheeses. Only the main cheese varieties are mentioned, and special cheeses like Feta, Filata or Ricotta are not taken into account. In some countries, there are separate categories for blue vein cheeses or extra hard cheeses, for example.

Mare's Milk and Koumiss

Right back in ancient times, Homer, Hesiod, and Herodotus wrote about peoples who drank mare's milk. They described the Scythians, a nomadic people who traveled across the steppes of southern Russia on horseback. More recently, horseriding peoples like the Mongol, Tartar, and Kirgiz peoples became experts at milking mares and using the milk or the products obtained from it such as a dry paste or fermented koumiss to fortify themselves. The frequently proven extraordinary stamina and resistance of these peoples was attributed to this unique form of nutrition. It was also said to have various healing properties, which doctors in 19th century Russia were able to use, often to great effect. The most notable successes were with cases of ordinary tuberculosis.

Although there are numerous stud farms in Europe today, very few of them specialize in mare's milk. Horse breeds suitable for milk production include the Haflinger breed. It originates from the Sarntal Alps in the South Tyrol, where these small animals were only able to survive thanks to their great sturdiness, modest requirements, and stamina. The fox-colored mountain horses are relatively easy to milk, and the lactation period can be extended for longer than with other breeds. They are kept outdoors and are so robust and healthy that they are able to give birth to their foals without assistance. They are fed on organically cultivated alfalfa, a basic forage consisting of grass, clover grass and hay, and some oats as a high-energy food.

At night, when the foals are together and sleeping apart from the mother animals, the mares are milked. Milking requires great skill and the horses must be treated with the utmost sensitivity. The mares are led into the milking stand, which is separate from the main stable. Once their udders have been cleaned with cotton wool, the milking machines are attached. The udder is better protected and located higher up on mares than on cows, which means that infection is much rarer. The milking time is also considerably shorter.

Mare's milk, which is still used as a natural remedy, must be handled extremely carefully and hygienically. In the dairy, which is

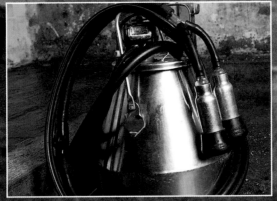

The milking equipment is specially designed for use on mares.

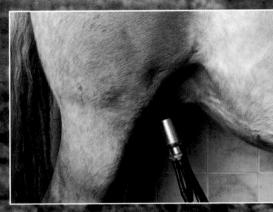

The mares are led to the milking stand at night and milked while it is very quiet.

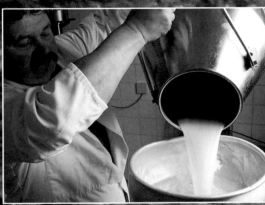

The freshly collected milk is poured straight into the filling container without further processing.

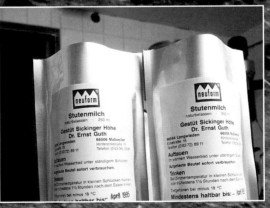

The natural healing milk, heat-sealed in special bags, is intended for immediate consumption.

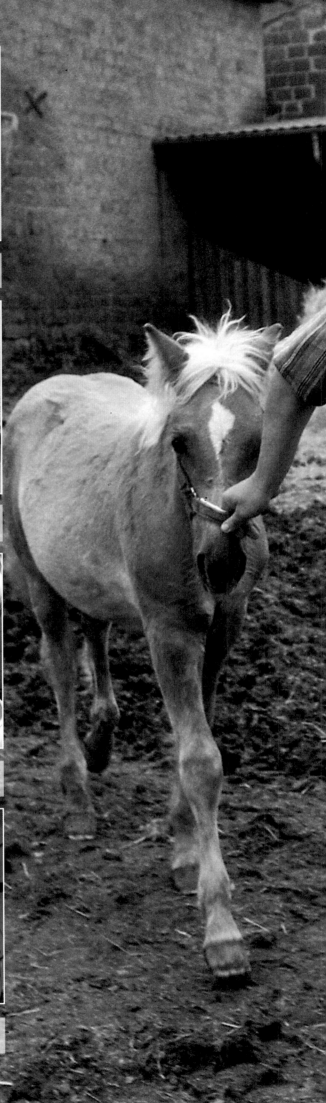

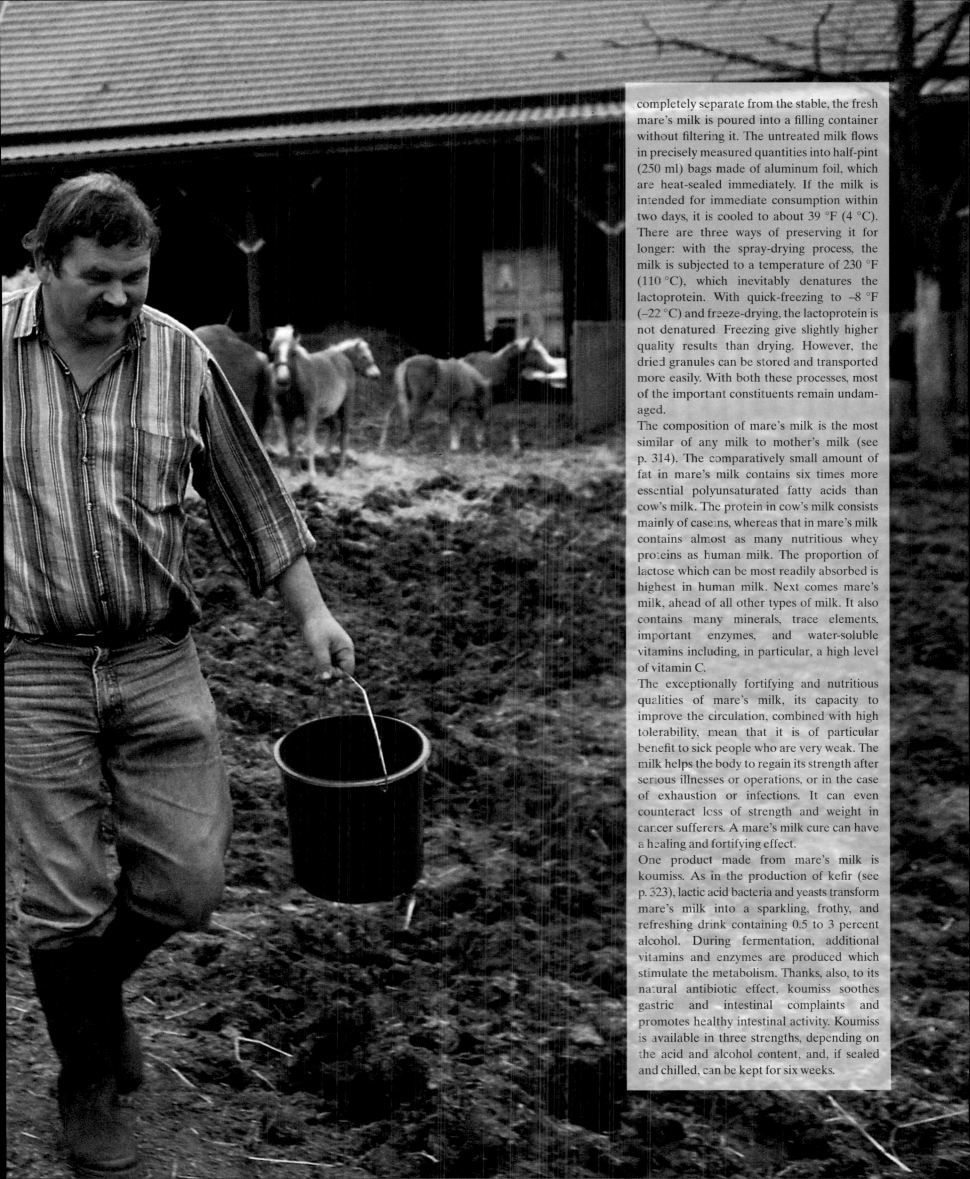

completely separate from the stable, the fresh mare's milk is poured into a filling container without filtering it. The untreated milk flows in precisely measured quantities into half-pint (250 ml) bags made of aluminum foil, which are heat-sealed immediately. If the milk is intended for immediate consumption within two days, it is cooled to about 39 °F (4 °C). There are three ways of preserving it for longer: with the spray-drying process, the milk is subjected to a temperature of 230 °F (110 °C), which inevitably denatures the lactoprotein. With quick-freezing to –8 °F (–22 °C) and freeze-drying, the lactoprotein is not denatured. Freezing give slightly higher quality results than drying. However, the dried granules can be stored and transported more easily. With both these processes, most of the important constituents remain undamaged.

The composition of mare's milk is the most similar of any milk to mother's milk (see p. 314). The comparatively small amount of fat in mare's milk contains six times more essential polyunsaturated fatty acids than cow's milk. The protein in cow's milk consists mainly of caseins, whereas that in mare's milk contains almost as many nutritious whey proteins as human milk. The proportion of lactose which can be most readily absorbed is highest in human milk. Next comes mare's milk, ahead of all other types of milk. It also contains many minerals, trace elements, important enzymes, and water-soluble vitamins including, in particular, a high level of vitamin C.

The exceptionally fortifying and nutritious qualities of mare's milk, its capacity to improve the circulation, combined with high tolerability, mean that it is of particular benefit to sick people who are very weak. The milk helps the body to regain its strength after serious illnesses or operations, or in the case of exhaustion or infections. It can even counteract loss of strength and weight in cancer sufferers. A mare's milk cure can have a healing and fortifying effect.

One product made from mare's milk is koumiss. As in the production of kefir (see p. 323), lactic acid bacteria and yeasts transform mare's milk into a sparkling, frothy, and refreshing drink containing 0.5 to 3 percent alcohol. During fermentation, additional vitamins and enzymes are produced which stimulate the metabolism. Thanks, also, to its natural antibiotic effect, koumiss soothes gastric and intestinal complaints and promotes healthy intestinal activity. Koumiss is available in three strengths, depending on the acid and alcohol content, and, if sealed and chilled, can be kept for six weeks.

Four-legged Frolics

Goat Keeping

Traits such as boisterousness, stubbornness, and wildness are typical of goats which, historically, can be regarded as the oldest domestic animals. This only seems to be a contradiction at first glance. Even the poorest families were able to keep these undemanding animals, as goats do not need expensive feed or lush pasture. They feel more at home in rough, mountainous, and dry terrains, in a world where food is not all that easy to come by.

Even the domestic goat has retained the climbing urge which is natural to wild goats and ibexes, and it would rather eat leaves from bushes or trees and weeds than grass from a sown meadow. Goats are particularly content when the surroundings cater for their natural preferences.

Goat-keeping under natural conditions is possible wherever the animals can run around freely in the countryside. They should have the opportunity to climb and have access to stony ground to smooth down their hard hoofs. If they are then able to nibble wild grasses and weeds, flowers, leaves, and bark at will, they will remain in peak health and their milk and the cheese made from it will gain a delicious flavor. Their milk is especially digestible for children and people with allergies.

Man's first domesticated animal, which does not mind the dry cold and only suffers in wet weather, still prefers being out in the wilds. Although almost none of our natural environment has remained untouched, there are large regions, particularly in southern Europe – whether in southern France, Spain, Portugal, the Balkans, or Greece – which are still ideal from a goat's point of view. In the more northern countries, mountainous landscapes offer goats the best environment.

If the external conditions for goat keeping are not ideal, extra measures must be taken to ensure the goats can roam around sufficiently. As goats do not require high-grade farmland and take up less space than cows, it has become possible for many new starters in organic farming to keep milk-producing animals. Organic farmers often have a greater understanding of the character of the animal. This is why goats with horns are now becoming increasingly common again. If the shed is large enough and the eating and sleeping quarters are separate, the horns and any associated risk of injury do not pose a problem. Clearly, goats feel better with their natural head attire and, instead of giving birth to hermaphrodites, bear healthy, fertile young.

In the barren landscapes of southern Europe – like here in the mountains of Andalusia — goat herds are a relic of the traditional and natural way of life.

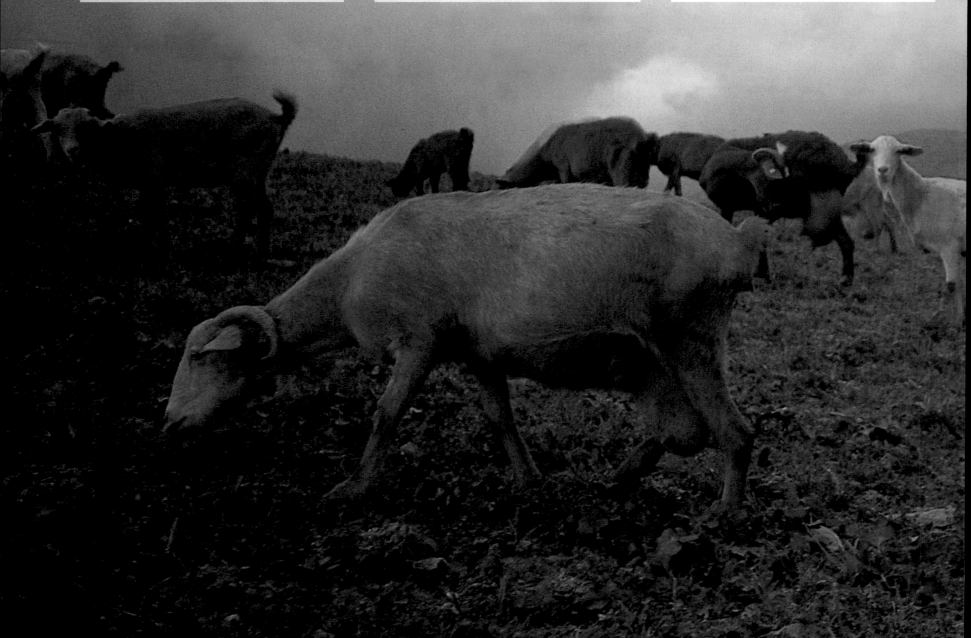

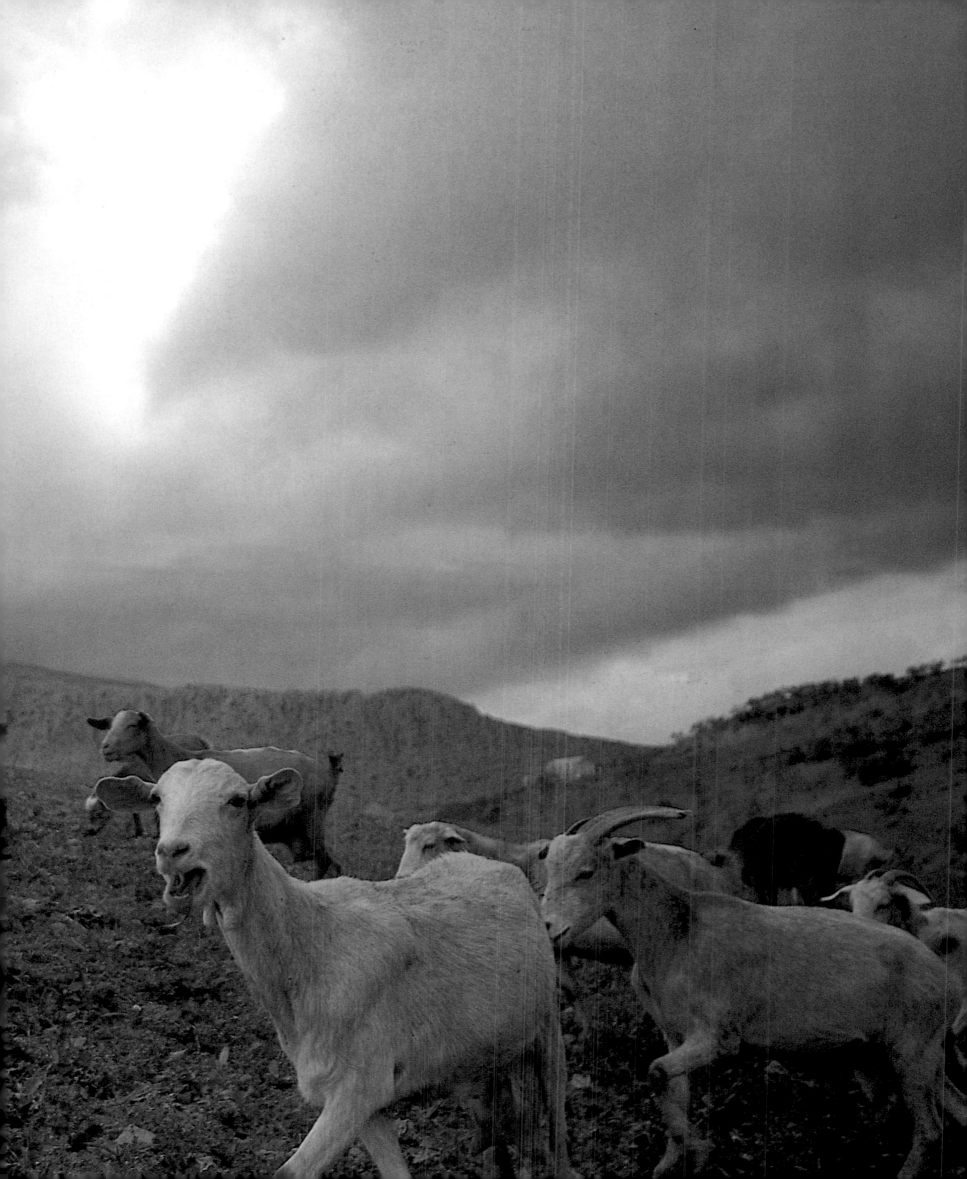

Milk and Cheese from Goats

Goat's Cheese

Once the goat has given birth to her young, she produces the first milk, known as colostrum, for the first five or six days. This contains the immune substances for the young and is not suitable for human consumption. Milk production then increases rapidly, reaching its peak after a month. From then on, less and less milk is produced. The milking period ends after nine months, before the goats mate again.

The fat content of the milk is relatively constant during these nine months. In the spring, from April through the beginning of July, when there is plenty of grass, it rises slightly. It only rises significantly in the last month. Goat's milk contains on average between 3.5 and 4.5 percent fat. This means its fat content is slightly higher than that of cow's milk. Sheep's milk has the highest fat content at over 6 percent.

The most important prerequisite for a high milk fat content is healthy food, such as goats find in the wild in meadows and pastures, on mountain slopes or on moorland. At the same time, the variety of flavors of the plants eaten by the goats is reflected in the milk and also gives the goat's cheese a distinctive taste.

The milk constituent which is the crucial element in cheese-making is the dry extract, which only makes up 10 to 12 percent of the total, as almost 90 percent is water. Two pints (1 liter) of goat's milk on average contains 1½ to 2 ounces (40 to 50 grams) of lactose, 1 to 1½ ounces (28 to 35 grams) of casein, 1 to 1¾ ounces (35 to 45 grams) of fat and ¼ ounce (7 to 9 grams) of mineral salts, including vitamins, enzymes, and trace elements. On average, 26 gallons (100 liters) of milk yield 24 pounds (11 kilograms) of goat's cheese.

The quality of the milk is the most important factor when making the cheese. Goat's cheese from organic cheese dairies is made from freshly collected raw milk which has not been pasteurized, treated in other ways or stored for any length of time. To produce goat's cheese by the French method, the first step is to filter the milk by pouring it through a muslin cloth. The coagulation is usually simply left to the natural bacteria in the air, which convert the lactose into lactic acid.

To accelerate the coagulation process, rennet is added in a ratio of 2 teaspoonfuls (10 milliliters) for every 26 gallons (100 liters). If it is being added to freshly collected milk in summer, it is necessary to wait for the milk to cool to about 68 °F (20 °C).

To ensure the curd reaches the right consistency, it is left to stand for 24 hours. The curd is now scooped out from the vat using a ladle into molds with a perforated base which allows the whey to drain off. The cheese dries in the molds for 15 to 36 hours. This process can be hastened by turning the molds one or more times.

Next the cheese is taken out of the mold, salted, and dried in the air for one to three days. Then comes the finishing stage – the cheese is allowed to mature in a cool, damp cellar. Usually, goat's cheese does not ripen for longer than 10 days. The ripening period determines the appearance of the cheese and the intensity of flavor. The longer it matures, the harder, drier, and sharper it becomes. Goat's cheese is commonly available in the form of rounds, but it is also sold in the shape of pyramids, rolls, or cylinders. Some varieties are coated with powdered charcoal, others with herbs or spices whilst still other varieties come wrapped in vine leaves.

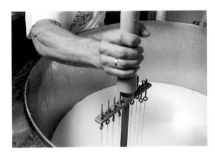
Once acid bacteria and rennet have coagulated the milk, the coagulum is cut up with a cheese harp.

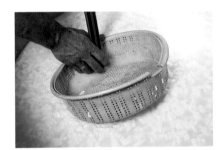
The curd collects at the bottom of the vat. The whey which lies above it is extracted with a hose through a strainer.

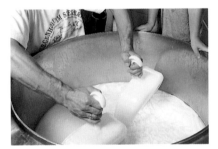
With the aid of the scoop, the curd is rotated, turned, and scooped out of the vat.

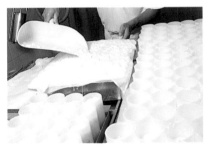
The curd is now placed in the funnel used for filling the molds.

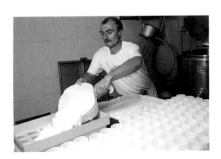
In this way, each mold is filled with an equal sized portion of curd sufficient to produce a 4½ ounce (125 gram) cheese.

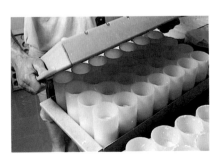
The molds are turned eight to ten times with the aid of turning trays to help the whey to drain off better.

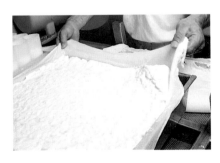
To make blocks of cheese which, in the case of Feta, are kept in brine, the curd is placed in a lined mold.

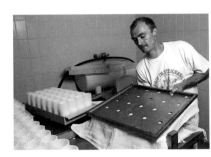
Again, the turning trays help in draining the whey. The cheese can now achieve the desired firmness and structure.

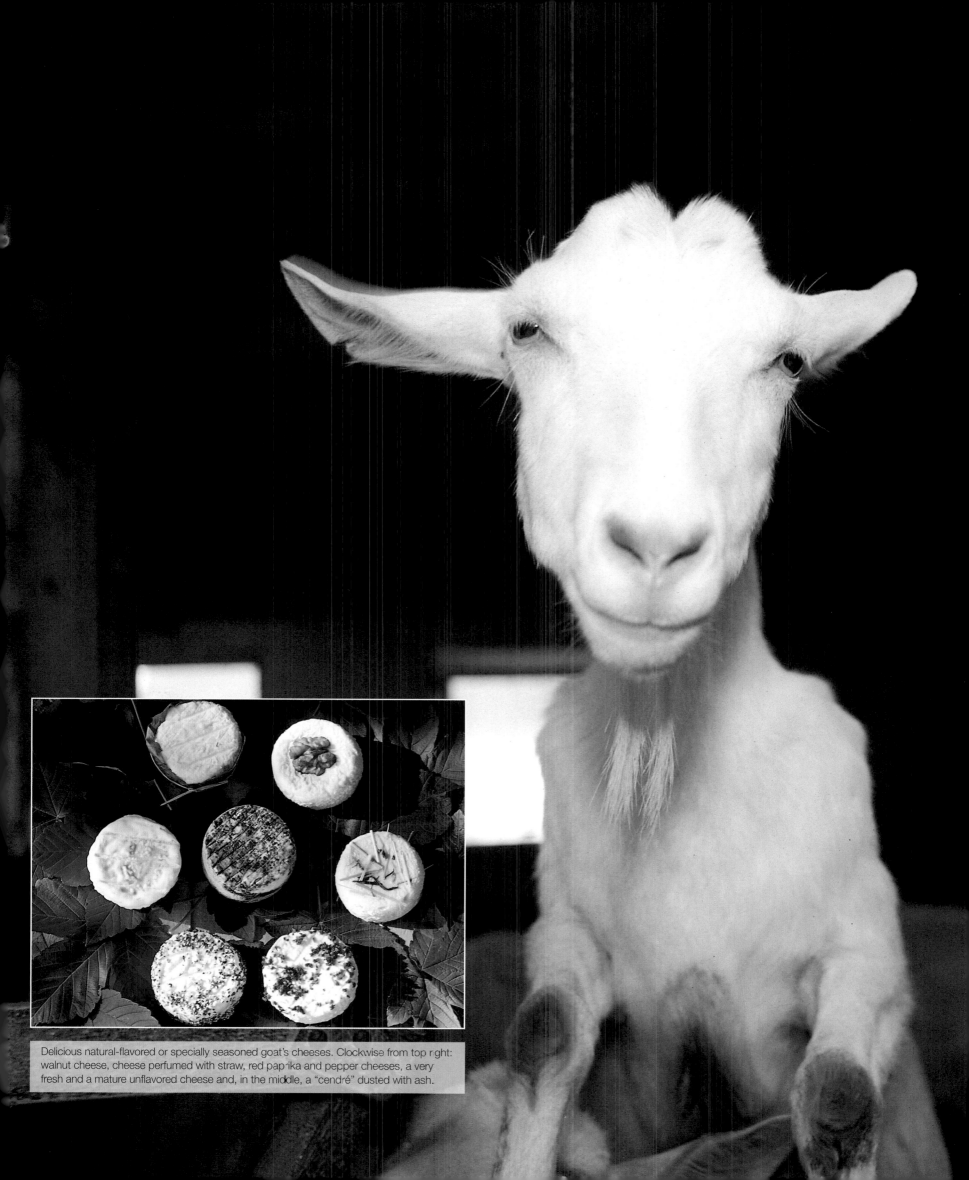

Delicious natural-flavored or specially seasoned goat's cheeses. Clockwise from top right: walnut cheese, cheese perfumed with straw, red paprika and pepper cheeses, a very fresh and a mature unflavored cheese and, in the middle, a "cendré" dusted with ash.

Recipes with Goat's Cheese

Trout and Goat's Cheese Pâté
(Illustration below)

3 finely chopped shallots
3 Tbs olive oil
9 oz (250 g) smoked trout fillet
9 oz (250 g) fresh goat's cheese
4 1/2 oz (125 g) creamy fresh cheese
3 oz (80 g) butter
1 tsp lemon juice
A few drops of Tabasco sauce
2 Tbs chopped parsley
A few sprigs of flat-leafed parsley
Wafer-thin slices of lemon
Toasted whole wheat bread

Fry the shallots in the olive oil until they become transparent. Add 2 tablespoons of water, bring to the boil and leave to cool. Place all the ingredients except for the parsley sprigs, lemon slices, and toast in a mixer and beat them to a smooth cream on the medium setting. Transfer the trout and cheese mixture into an oiled mold and chill for 2 hours.
Turn out the pâté and garnish with the parsley leaves and lemon slices. This is good served with lightly browned whole wheat toast.

Marinated Goat's Cheese
(Illustration below)

4 garlic cloves
8 small firm goat's cheeses
4 bay leaves
1 cup (200 ml) white wine
1 cup (200 ml) olive oil
1 tsp mustard
2 dried bell peppers

Peel and quarter the garlic cloves and place them in layers in a jar with the goat's cheeses and the bay leaves, torn in half. Beat together the white wine, olive oil, mustard, and chopped bell peppers with a mixer. Pour the marinade over the cheese so that the cheese is completely covered. Leave to marinate for at least a week in a cool, dark place.
The cheese can keep for up to 6 weeks in a refrigerator, where it only ripens very slowly.
The cheese tastes superb with a slice of coarse rye bread. It can also be broiled briefly and served with a mixed leaf salad with a wine vinegar and olive oil dressing.

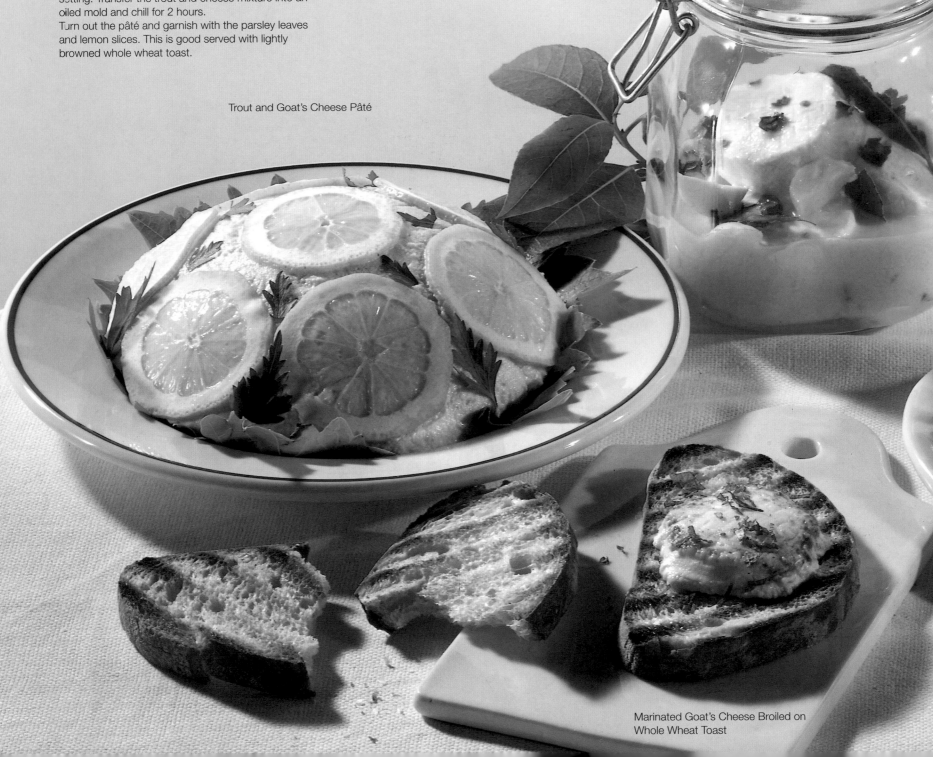

Marinated Goat's Cheese

Trout and Goat's Cheese Pâté

Marinated Goat's Cheese Broiled on Whole Wheat Toast

Bell Pepper Strips with Goat's Cheese Cream

1 red, 1 green and 1 yellow bell pepper
9 oz (250 g) fresh goat's cheese
3¹/₂ oz (100 g) Roquefort
3–4 Tbs heavy cream
Black pepper

Wash and deseed the bell peppers and cut them into thin strips lengthways.
Mix the goat's cheese and Roquefort with enough cream to form a smooth paste. Then season with coarsely ground pepper.
Put the cheese cream in the middle of a large plate and arrange the strips of bell pepper around it.

Tasty Goat's Cheese Balls

9 oz (250 g) fresh goat's cheese
Coarse salt, black pepper
1 tsp sweet paprika
1 tsp poppy seeds
1 tsp sesame seeds
2 Tbs finely chopped dill
2 Tbs finely chopped chives
2 Tbs finely chopped arugula
2 Tbs finely chopped parsley

Season the goat's cheese with salt and pepper and shape it into small balls. Then roll them in the various herbs and/or spices.
Can be served on cocktail sticks with an aperitif.

Green Goat's Cheese

10 celery heart leaves
1 bunch flat-leafed parsley
1 bunch basil
4 garlic cloves
4 Tbs olive oil
1 lb 2 oz (500 g) fresh goat's cheese
1 Tbs lemon juice
Coarse salt
White pepper
Celery sticks with leaves attached

Chop the celery heart leaves, parsley, basil, and garlic very finely. Mix the chopped herbs and olive oil into the fresh goat's cheese. Season with lemon juice, salt, and pepper.
Put the cheese mixture in an oiled mold and leave to stand in the refrigerator for a good hour. Turn out the cheese mixture and garnish with celery leaves.
Serve as a dip with the celery sticks.

Broiled Goat's Cheese
(Illustration below left)

1 slice white bread
2 chopped garlic cloves
7 Tbs olive oil
1 head of lettuce
2 Tbs red wine vinegar
Coarse salt
Black pepper
4 young, firm, small goat's cheeses

Cut the bread into small cubes and fry with the garlic in 1 tablespoon of olive oil.
Wash the lettuce, let the water drip off, tear into small pieces and arrange on four plates. Mix the remaining oil, the vinegar, salt, and coarsely ground pepper together to make a vinaigrette.
Put the goat's cheeses in a flame-proof dish and broil them until they start to brown slightly. Lift them carefully out of the dish and place them on the lettuce.
Scatter the fried bread on top and pour over the vinaigrette. Serve immediately.

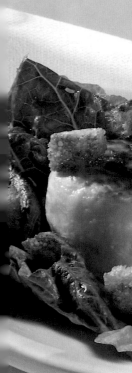

Broiled Goat's Cheese

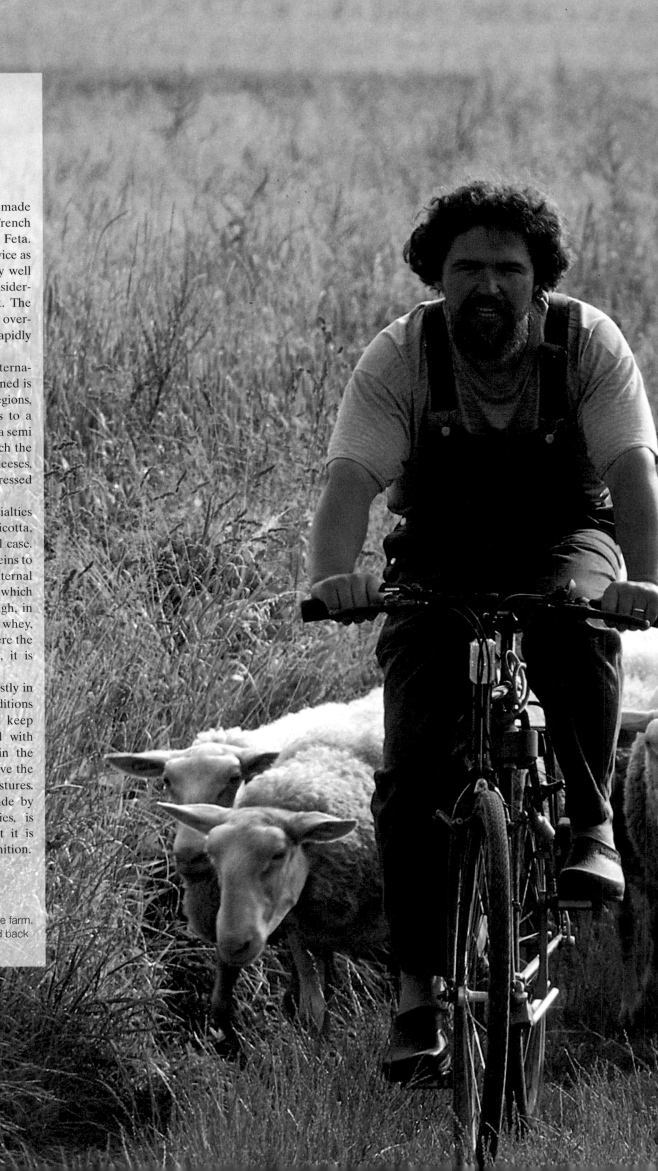

Sheep's Cheese

Some of the most exquisite cheeses are made from sheep's milk, for example, French Roquefort, Italian Pecorino, or Greek Feta. The creamy sheep's milk – it contains twice as much fat as cow's milk – is particularly well suited to cheese-making. It is also considerably richer in protein than cow's milk. The readily digestible protein consists overwhelmingly of caseins. It coagulates rapidly and gives a comparatively high yield.

What is noticeable about the three internationally known cheese varieties mentioned is firstly that they all come from hot, dry regions, and secondly that each cheese belongs to a different cheese category: Roquefort is a semi firm blue vein cheese, Pecorino, in which the curd is cooked, belongs to the hard cheeses, and Feta is a fresh cheese which is pressed and stored in brine.

There are also many other cheese specialties based on sheep's milk. Of these, Ricotta, obtained from whey, is a rather special case. Prolonged boiling causes the whey proteins to separate. The result, in terms of its external appearance, is a type of fresh cheese which has a slightly sour milk flavor. Although, in the north of Italy, it is made from cow's whey, in the south, on Sicily and Sardinia, where the famous Pecorino cheese comes from, it is produced using sheep's whey.

The largest dairy sheep regions are mostly in dry, barren areas – wherever the conditions mean there is insufficient pasture to keep cows. Shepherds often move around with their undemanding flocks of sheep in the traditional way or, in summer, they drive the animals up onto the high mountain pastures. Much of the best sheep's cheese, made by shepherds or in small cheese dairies, is therefore intrinsically organic so that it is often only a small step to organic recognition.

The pastures are not always very close to the farm. The dairy sheep willingly follow the shepherd back to the farm for milking.

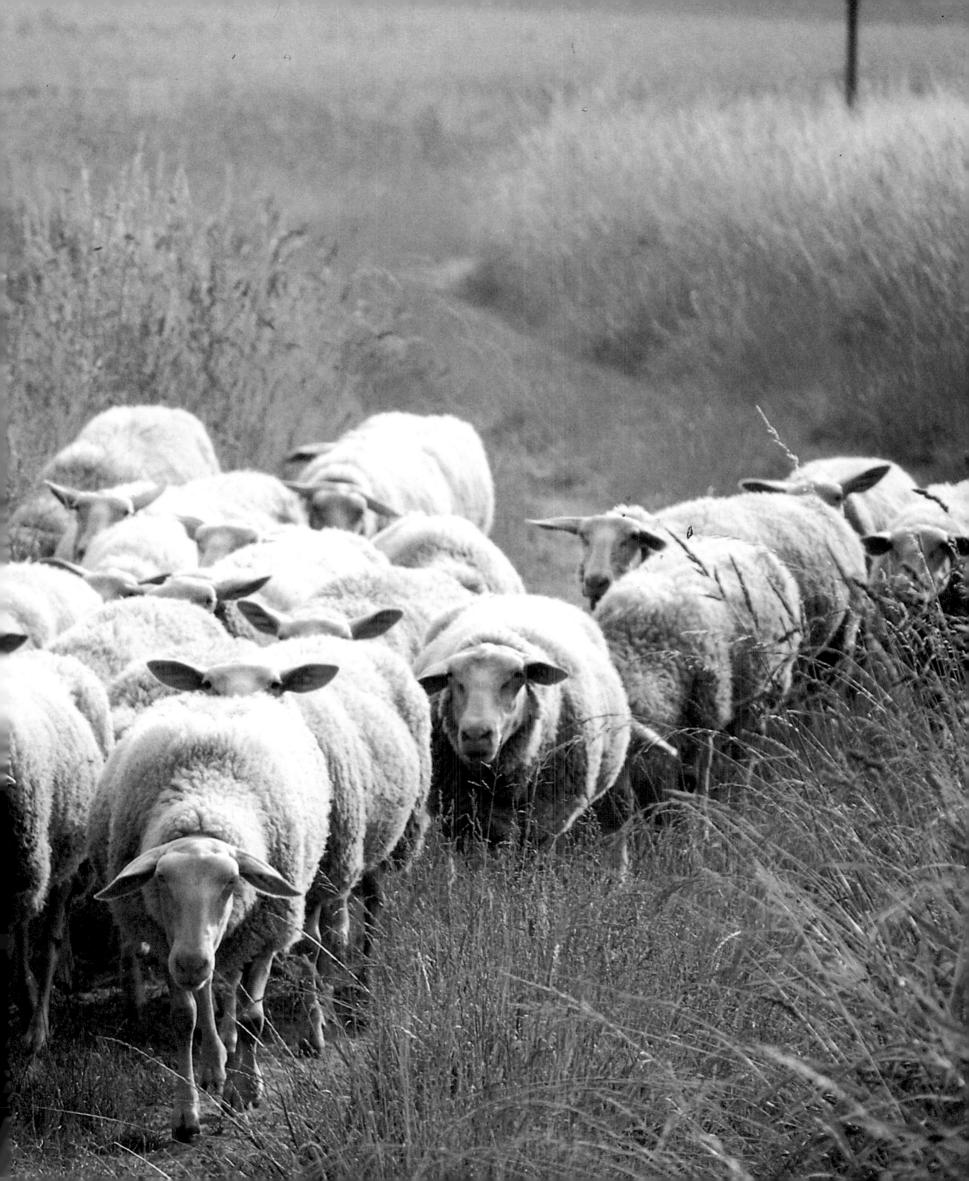

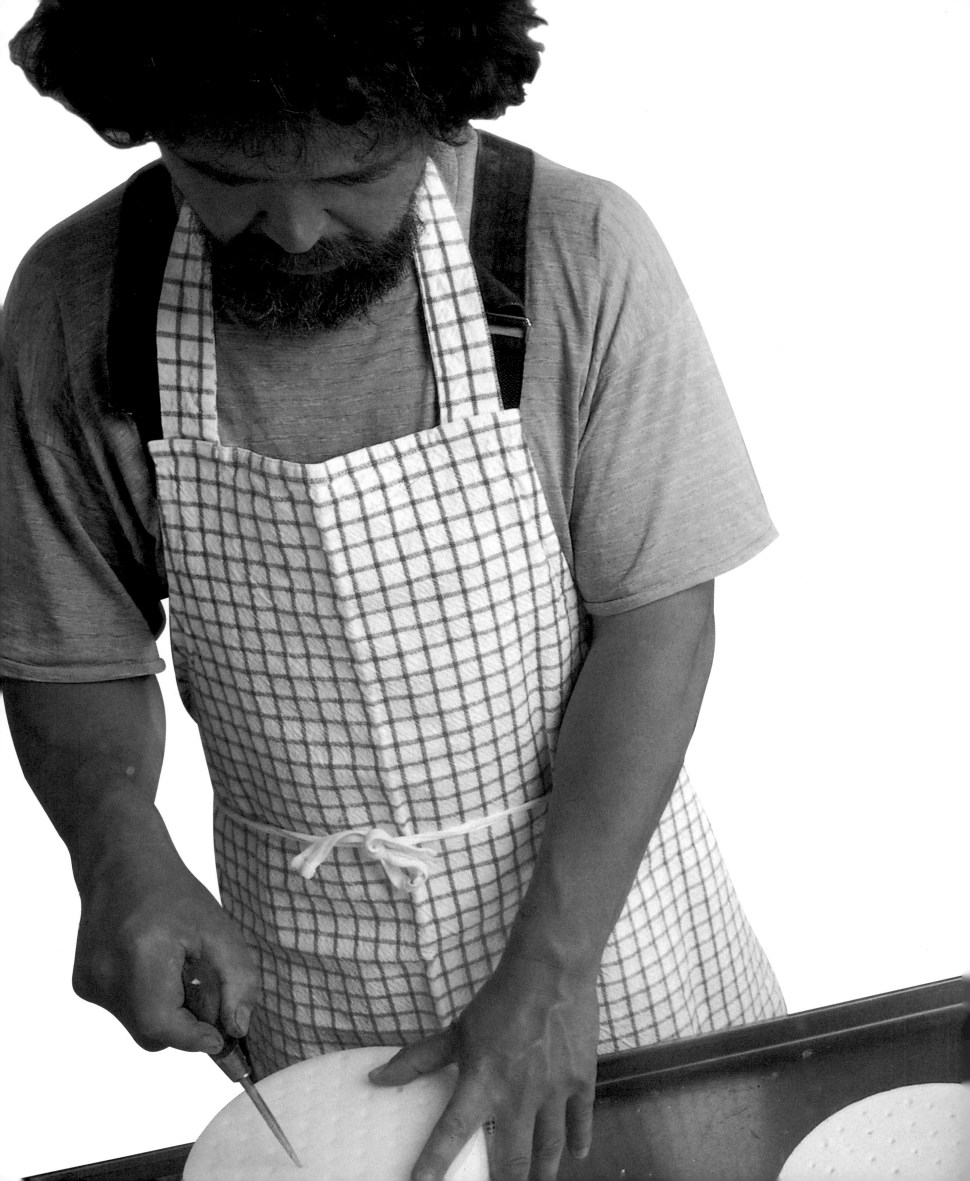

Sheep's Cheese

Varieties	Type	Character
Agrino, Robiola, Niolo, Broccio, Brousse, and other fresh cheeses	Fresh cheese; lactic acid bacteria play a crucial part in the production.	Creamy, slightly sour, with little flavor of its own, therefore often seasoned with pepper, herbs, garlic, etc.
Feta	Fresh cheese, whose curd – usually pressed – is shaped into blocks.	Stored in whey with brine; completely white, firm, crumbly, salty but not very sour.
Camembert style, Pérail and other soft cheeses	Sweet milk cheese with a downy outer layer produced by white mold cultures.	After ripening for 3 weeks, inside is creamy with a melting consistency; tastes nutty and of mushrooms; potent smell.
Roquefort and other veined cheeses	Unpressed, semi firm, cylindrical cheese, coagulated with rennet, inoculated with blue mold bacteria.	Slightly porous, only just semi firm consistency, very light in color, patterned with mold; tangy, spicy flavor.
Tomme, Ossau-Iraty, Ardi gasna, Fiore sardo, and other semi firm or firm cut cheeses	The curd is pressed but not cooked; natural rind produced by rubbing down and 2–3 months' aging.	Younger cut cheese with a mild, nutty aroma rind is not too hard; cheese becomes harder and drier as it continues to mature.
Hard cheese such as Pecorino, Manchego, Kefalotiri, Kaskaval	The curd is reheated, then pressed (wrapped in a cloth), salted, and matured over several months by rubbing down.	Firm cut cheese, with distinctive spicy, tangy aromas which intensify as the cheese ages.

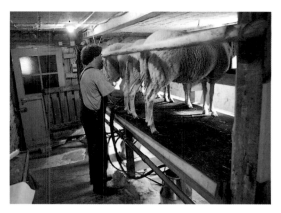

This homemade milking stand is practical and hygienic.

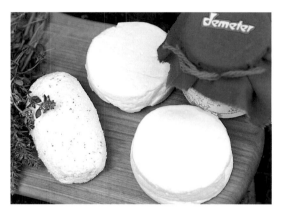

Fresh cheese made from sheep's milk in the style of Swiss Agrino and Italian Robiola.

Orotic Acid

This vitamin-like substance – formerly known as vitamin B13 – helps in the formation of protein in the cell nucleus and thereby promotes cell growth. Orotic acid also plays a part in protein exchanges, most particularly in the brain, and increases thought and memory capacity. As it is taken up directly by the liver cells, the liver is protected and regenerated by it. In infants and small children, it helps establish healthy microbial activity in the intestine. It is present in substantially larger amounts in mare's and sheep's milk than in cow's milk.

Blue Vein Cheese

Two factors determine the character of southern French Roquefort: the tasty sheep's milk of the Aveyron region, which, with its high fat content, gives the cheese an incomparable smoothness, and the caves of the Combalou mountains where the *penicillium roqueforti* mold responsible for the tangy flavor develops best.

But suitable conditions can also be provided elsewhere, if sheep's milk, mold, and a good cellar are available. The mold culture is produced quite naturally when rye bread turns moldy. The milk is usually inoculated with tiny amounts of the mold right at the start of the process. Once rennet has been added to coagulate the milk and the curd has been cut into small pieces, the whey is allowed to drain off without reheating the curd or pressing it. Before the cheese mass is put into the molds, a little salt is added and now – if this has not already been done – a dose of *penicillium roqueforti* is introduced. To enable the mold to spread throughout the cheese it needs to be treated in a particular way. In a few days, when the cheese is firm enough to take out of the mold, steel nails are used to punch holes in each cheese in several places. This creates passages through which oxygen, which encourages mold, can enter the cheese. As the cheeses in any case have a not too solid, slightly porous structure, the mold finds many ways of circulating throughout the cheese and giving it its fine flavor. However, the cheese dairy and connoisseurs need to exercise patience, as the whole process takes three to four months.

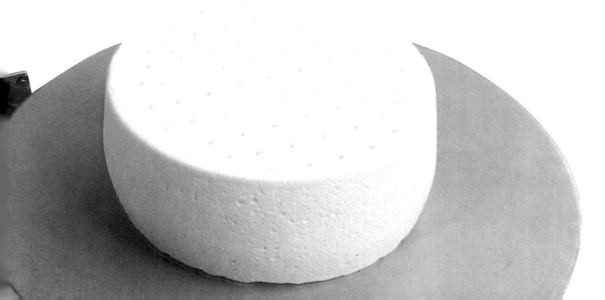

Overview of Cheese Varieties

Soft Cheeses

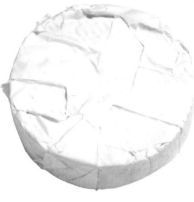

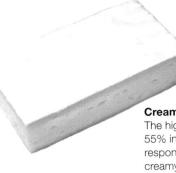

Cream Brie
The high fat content of over 55% in dry matter is responsible for the mild, creamy flavor.

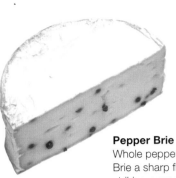

Pepper Brie
Whole peppercorns give the Brie a sharp flavor and striking aroma.

Camembert
This famous Normandy classic with the delicate white mold is at its best in summer and fall.

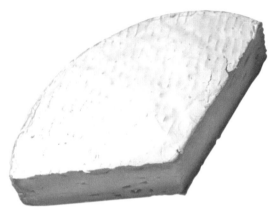

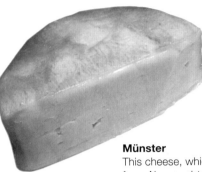

Fresh Cheeses

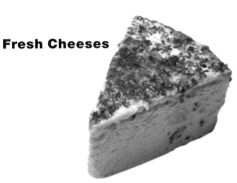

Münster
This cheese, which originates from Alsace, obtains its characteristic reddish appearance by frequent rubbing down.

Fresh Cheese with Herbs
Finely chopped herbs provide flavor and seasoning.

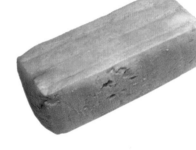
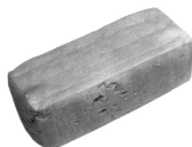

Limburger
The tangy red smear-coated cheese is always sold in rectangular blocks.

Traditional Brie
This French soft cheese is sold in large flat rounds with a white down and yellow center.

Hard Cheeses

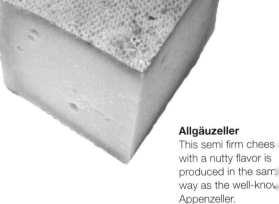

Allgäuzeller
This semi firm chees with a nutty flavor is produced in the sam way as the well-kno Appenzeller.

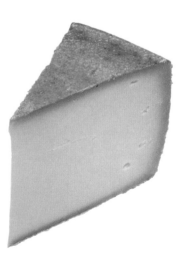

Pecorino
This scalded sheep's cheese from Italy is good for grating.

Mountain Cheese
Following Alpine tradition, this typical hard cheese is made from heated curd and then pressed.

Feta

Sheep's Cheese
Greek-style block che stored in brine.

Gruyère
The classic Swiss cheese with a very fruity, well-matured flavor.

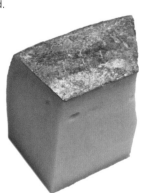

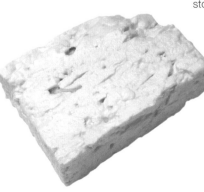

342

Semi-firm and Firm Cut Cheeses

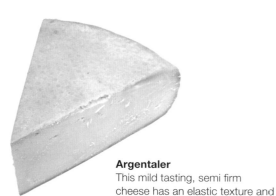

Argentaler
This mild tasting, semi firm cheese has an elastic texture and a slightly orange rind.

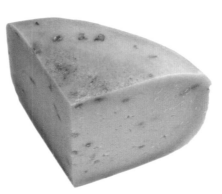

Bockshorn Cheese
The fine caraway flavor of the bockshorn clover characterizes this firm cheese.

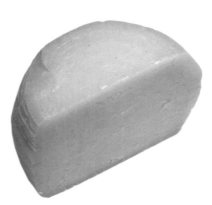

Sheep's Gouda
This Dutch cheese made from sheep's milk has a very discreet, mild flavor of hazelnuts.

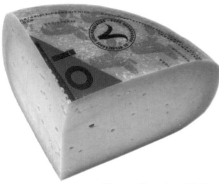

Young Gouda with Carrot
Carrot juice gives the heated and pressed Gouda its slightly sweet flavor and bright orange color.

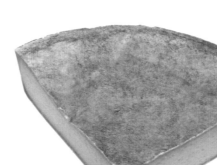

Tomme c'Auvergne
This cheese made from unheated part skim milk comes from France's volcanic region.

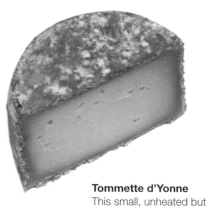

Golosella Piccola
This exquisite semi firm cheese is – as the Italian name suggests – something for a *goloso* or someone with a sweet tooth.

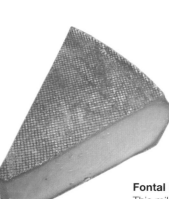

Fontal (Fontina)
This mild northern Italian cut cheese made from cow's milk is characterized by its smooth, melting texture.

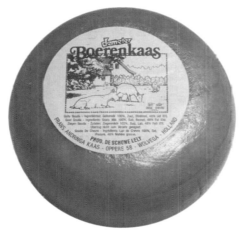

Goat's Gouda
This light, mild Gouda is obtained from goat's milk and pressed in a small mold.

Tommette d'Yonne
This small, unheated but pressed cow's cheese comes from northern Burgundy.

Blue Vein Cheese

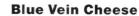

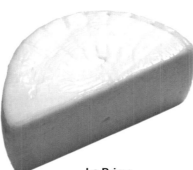

La Prima
This mild to slightly piquant semi firm sheep's cheese comes from Italy.

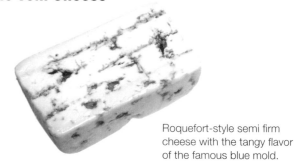

Roquefort-style semi firm cheese with the tangy flavor of the famous blue mold.

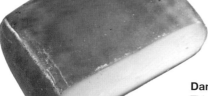

Danbø
This Danish cut cheese tastes buttery and very mild.

343

Recipes with cheese

The cheese fondue – as sociable as it is nutritious – originated in Switzerland. To serve a fondue, it is necessary to have a Caquelon, an earthenware fondue dish with a handle and a spirit burner, to keep the prepared fondue bubbling slowly.

Each person is given a plate of cubed white or light-textured whole wheat bread. Using a long-handled fork, a piece of bread is dipped into the cheese and lifted out while turning, to prevent the cheese dripping. If all the guests are garlic fans, several whole cloves can be added to the dish, and these then cook in the cheese, giving a delicious flavor.

According to a Swiss custom, anyone who lets a piece of bread fall into the cheese has to buy a round of kirsch for everyone. The liquor also aids digestion, as a cheese fondue is hardly a light dish. Drinking hot, black tea with it is also recommended. Another possibility, although not as good for the digestion, is a dry white wine. One of the tastiest treats only appears at the end: the delicious cheese crust stuck to the base of the fondue dish.

Hard cheeses such as Emmental are good for using as gratin-style toppings. Extra hard cheeses such as Parmigiano or Pecorino can be used as a fine flavoring, grated over pasta and in the form of shavings on salads and meat, particularly served with carpaccio. Blue vein cheeses are an excellent addition to creamy sauces.

While cheese fondue is something for the colder seasons, the other recipes show how summery, light, and varied cheese dishes can be.

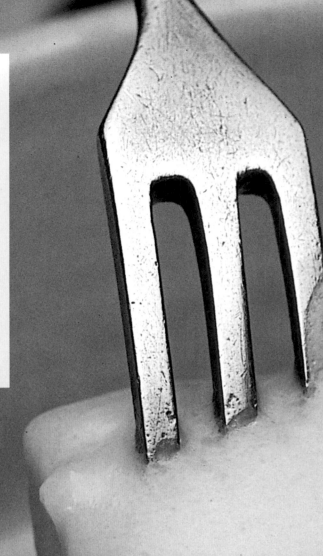

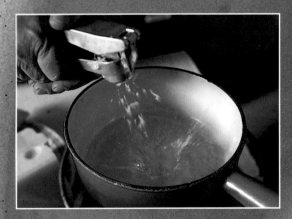

Pour the white wine into the dish. Crush the garlic cloves and add them.

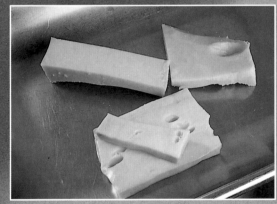

Mild Emmental and tangy Gruyère complement one another perfectly.

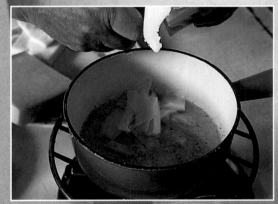

Slice the cheese as thinly as possible and put it in the dish. Slowly bring to the boil.

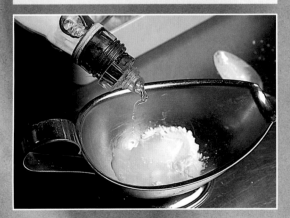

Meanwhile, mix the cornstarch with the kirsch.

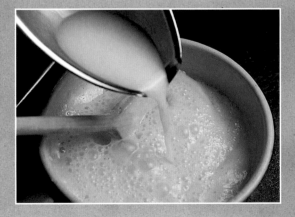

Slowly pour the cornstarch mixture into the bubbling cheese mixture, stirring constantly.

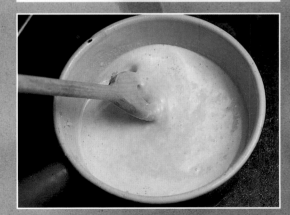

Finally season the fondue with lemon juice, salt, and pepper.

Swiss Cheese Fondue

1 loaf of pale, light-textured whole wheat bread
3 garlic cloves
1¹⁄₂ cups (300 ml) dry white wine
11 oz (300 g) Emmental
11 oz (300 g) Gruyère
2 tsp cornstarch
¹⁄₄ cup (50 ml) kirsch
Lemon juice
Coarse salt, white pepper

Cut the bread into large, bite-sized cubes. Rub the inside of the fondue dish with one of the cloves of garlic. Pour the white wine – preferably a Fendant from an organic vineyard in the Swiss Valais region – into the dish. Crush the remaining garlic and add it to the wine. Cut both types of cheese into thin slices and put them in the dish. Slowly bring the wine and cheese to the boil, stirring continuously. Mix together the cornstarch and kirsch and stir them into the mixture in the dish. Add lemon juice, salt, and pepper to taste. When the cheese mixture is smooth and creamy and no longer producing any small bubbles, stand the dish on the burner and place it on the table.

Greek Salad

3 slicing tomatoes
1 cucumber
1 green and 1 yellow bell pepper
1 large red onion
1 Tbs finely chopped oregano
7 oz (200 g) cubed Feta
6 Tbs olive oil
2 Tbs red wine vinegar
Black pepper
Coarse salt according to taste
3¹⁄₂ oz (100 g) large black olives
2 oz (50 g) mild chilies

Wash and dry the vegetables. Cut the tomatoes into eighths, cut the unpeeled cucumber into cubes, remove the seeds from the peppers and cut them into thin strips, peel the onion and slice it into rings. Place the vegetables in a salad bowl. Add the oregano and half the Feta and mix them into the vegetables.
Carefully mix together the oil and vinegar with some pepper and a small pinch of salt. Pour the dressing over the salad, and gently toss the ingredients together. Scatter the remaining Feta over the top and sprinkle with freshly ground black pepper. Garnish with the olives and chilies.

Roquefort Pâté

1 shallot
2 sprigs thyme
7 oz (200 g) Roquefort
7 oz (200 g) crème fraîche
7 oz (200 g) fresh cheese
2 ripe Williams pears
A little lemon juice
3 Tbs olive oil
1 Tbs balsamic vinegar
Black pepper, coarse salt
A few lettuce leaves
4 tsp cranberries

Finely chop the shallot and the thyme, mash the Roquefort and mix these with the crème fraîche and fresh cheese. Divide the cheese mixture between 4 small oiled molds and chill for 2 hours. Halve the pears, remove the core and cut them into a fan shape and sprinkle with lemon juice. Make a dressing with the oil, vinegar, pepper and salt and dip the lettuce leaves into it.
Arrange the lettuce on plates. Place one pear fan on the edge of each plate and decorate with the cranberries. Carefully slide the cheese out of the mold and place it in the middle of the plate. Serve with a whole wheat baguette.

Arugula Salad with Mango and Mozzarella

4 Mozzarella (each weighing 5 oz/150 g)
1 red and 1 green bell pepper
7 Tbs olive oil
2 Tbs balsamic vinegar
5 oz (150 g) arugula
1 ripe mango
¹⁄₂ tsp mustard
¹⁄₄ cup (50 ml) vegetable stock

Cut each Mozzarella into 4 slices. Deseed the bell peppers and cut them into rings. Mix 4 tablespoons of olive oil with 1 tablespoon of vinegar, add to the bell pepper rings and pour over the Mozzarella. Marinate for at least 30 minutes. Wash the arugula and dry it in a salad spinner. Peel the mango and cut the flesh from the stone in thin slices. Beat together the remaining oil and vinegar, mustard and vegetable stock, and briefly marinate the arugula in it. Put the arugula in a sieve to drain off the dressing and arrange it on plates. Arrange the mango slices on the arugula. Place four slices of Mozzarella on top on each plate and sprinkle the marinade over it.

Bell Peppers Stuffed with Robiola

3¹⁄₂ oz (100 g) each of cleaned red, green, and yellow bell pepper
3¹⁄₂ oz (100 g) carrots
Skin of 1 small zucchini
1 crushed garlic clove
1 Tbs each finely chopped parsley and chives
14 oz (400 g) Robiola (or alternatively fresh goat's cheese)
1 red and 1 yellow bell pepper
4 Tbs olive oil
1 tsp mustard
Juice of 1 lemon
Black pepper, coarse salt
7 oz (200 g) mixed green salad

Finely dice the cleaned bell peppers, carrots, and zucchini skin. Put the carrot and zucchini cubes into a pan of boiling salted water and blanch for 2 minutes, rinse with cold water and pat them dry. Mix the vegetables, garlic, and herbs with the Robiola. Wash the bell peppers, halve and deseed them and pat them dry. Divide the cheese mixture between the 4 bell pepper halves.
Combine the oil, mustard, lemon juice, salt, and pepper to make a smooth dressing toss the salad in it. Arrange it on 4 plates and place a stuffed bell pepper half in the middle of each plate.

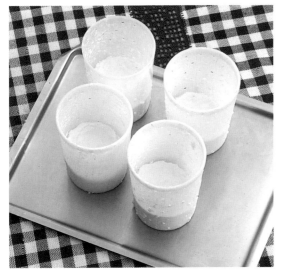

The life of a goat's cheese begins with 2 pints (1 liter) of milk, which coagulates due to the action of acid bacteria and rennet. Once the whey has drained off, the curd is put in small molds.

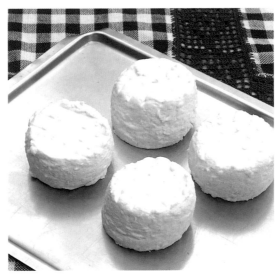

If the cheese is sold still in its mold, it has the consistency of farmer's cheese. After a short drying time, the pure white, creamy cheese can be taken out.

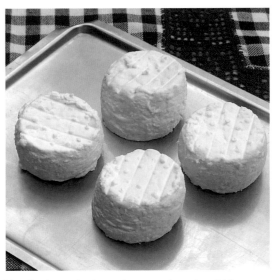

Very fresh goat's cheese has an extremely mild flavor. The cheese literally melts in the mouth.

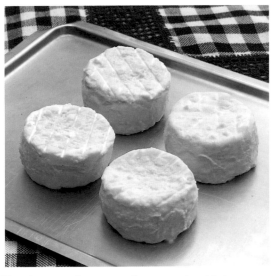

The cheese undergoes continuous and rapid changes. It starts to turn light yellow after just two to three days.

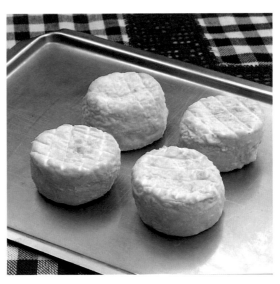

Its outer layer dries and it and the cheese inside become a little firmer. The mild flavor begins to gain more character.

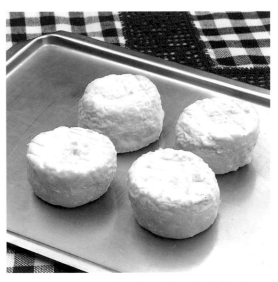

After four to five days, the cheese has shrunk by almost a third. It now has a firmer, but still moist consistency and a more distinctive flavor.

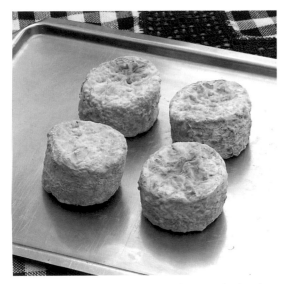

After about a week, the natural mold present in the air begins to appear on the cheese and adds – still discreetly – to the complexity of the flavor.

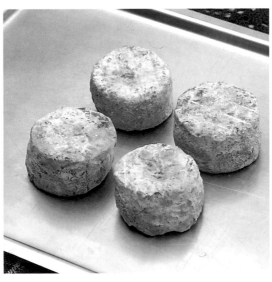

After ten days, the cheese has become even drier. The now bluish mold gives it its tangy character.

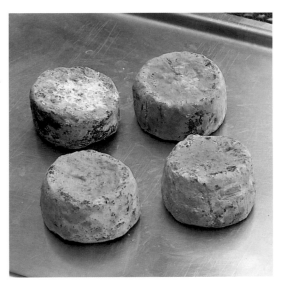

After two weeks, the mold has formed a complete covering. Inside, the dry cheese mass begins to crack and the cheese is dominated by a sharp flavor.

Storing Cheese

Cheese is a natural product which, with the exception of fresh cheese, goes through various ripening stages between the start of its life and consumption. Optimum ripening can only take place in rooms or cellars with the correct temperature and air humidity. Cheese should generally be kept in a cool, dark place such as in the vegetable compartment of the refrigerator. In winter, provided the temperature does not fall too low, it keeps very well in the open air under a cheese cover or, better still, in a wire-mesh cupboard, for example on the balcony. Cheese continues to ripen if stored at not too low a temperature – the higher the temperature, the quicker it ripens.

• Ripening is accelerated at 59 to 64 °F (15 to 18 °C).

• Normal ripening takes place between 54 and 59 °F (12 and 15 °C).

• Below 54 °F (12 °C), ripening takes place at a slower than normal rate. However, the temperature should never be allowed to fall below 39 °F (4 °C) as this would damage the structure of the cheese and harm the useful cheese bacteria.

• The relative air humidity should ideally be between 85 and 95 percent.

Cheeses behave differently depending on the type, and have to be handled differently.

• Soft cheeses are mostly sold when at the initial ripening stage, as they then have the preferred degree of mildness and firmness. Moreover, this also gives stores time flexibility. Soft cheeses should be stored in their original packaging. With a little practice, it is possible to assess the ripeness of a soft cheese by pressing on the middle of it with a finger. If the cheese gives a little, it is ripe, as soft cheese ripens from the outside inwards. Soft cheeses are best ripened at 57 to 59 °F (14 to 15 °C), and can be stored for a few more days at 43 to 46 °F (6 to 8 °C).

• Semi firm cut cheeses can be divided into several types which have to be treated differently:
Butter cheeses (Butterkäse) appeal because of their fatty freshness. They are not supposed to ripen. They are only sold in small pieces which should be wrapped in parchment paper or aluminum foil and stored in the refrigerator at 50 to 54 °F (10 to 12 °C).
Red mold cheese like Reblochon must be left to ripen whole, wrapped either in its original paper or in a clean, damp cloth, preferably unenclosed and open to the air in a damp room at 54 to 59 °F (12 to 15 °C).
For blue mold cheese to continue ripening without its rind, it is best stored whole and in its original packaging or in large pieces wrapped in

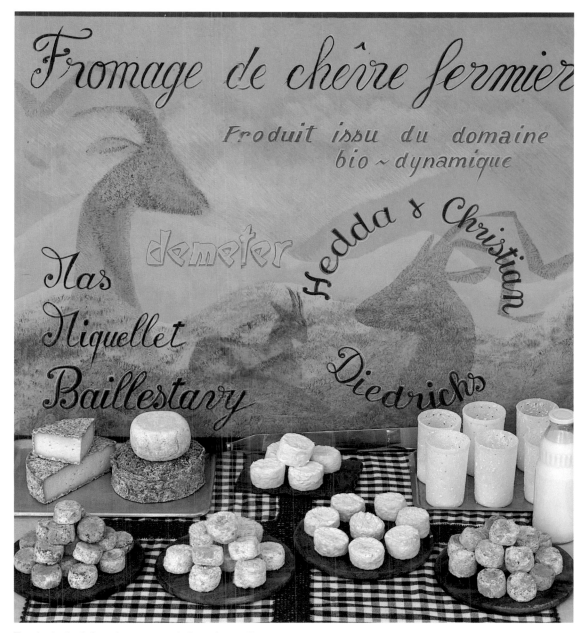

Thanks to the influx of young people from the north, production of organic goat's cheese has become established in the French Pyrenees.

aluminum foil at 54 °F (12 °C). Cheeses with a rind layer such as Fourme d'Ambert mature better.

Semi firm cut cheeses with a rind such as Saint-Nectaire ripen well for several weeks if whole and unwrapped or wrapped in a cloth in a damp cellar at 54 to 59 °F (12 to 15 °C). They have to be turned regularly. Cut segments can be stored in a damp cloth.

• Firm cut cheese with a waxed or oiled rind keeps whole for several weeks, becoming increasingly dry. Cheeses with a natural rind mature whole for a long time when left unwrapped or wrapped in a damp cloth in a cellar, but have to be brushed down with salt water and turned regularly. Segments wrapped in a damp cloth also keep well.

• Pieces of hard cheese are stored in the same way as firm cut cheeses. Extra hard cheeses should be wrapped in aluminum foil and kept in the refrigerator.

If the cheese has already been cut, the cut edges must be protected with aluminum foil to prevent them drying out. Cheeses must always be wrapped individually. If cloths are used, they must be washed regularly.

If a cheese's own type of mold spreads, this is a good sign and the mold can be eaten without concern. Blackish, foreign mold, on the other hand, is harmful to health and must be removed. Bluish mold growing on the rind of cut cheeses or hard cheeses can be washed off with salt water. If it is growing on the cut edges, a generous slice should be cut off the side to remove it.

Connoisseurs disagree over whether natural rinds with white, red, or blue mold should be eaten with the cheese. Some regard it as a great delicacy, while others trim it off. Either way, all cheeses must be taken out of the cool cellar or refrigerator at least 30 minutes before eating to enable them to develop their full flavor.

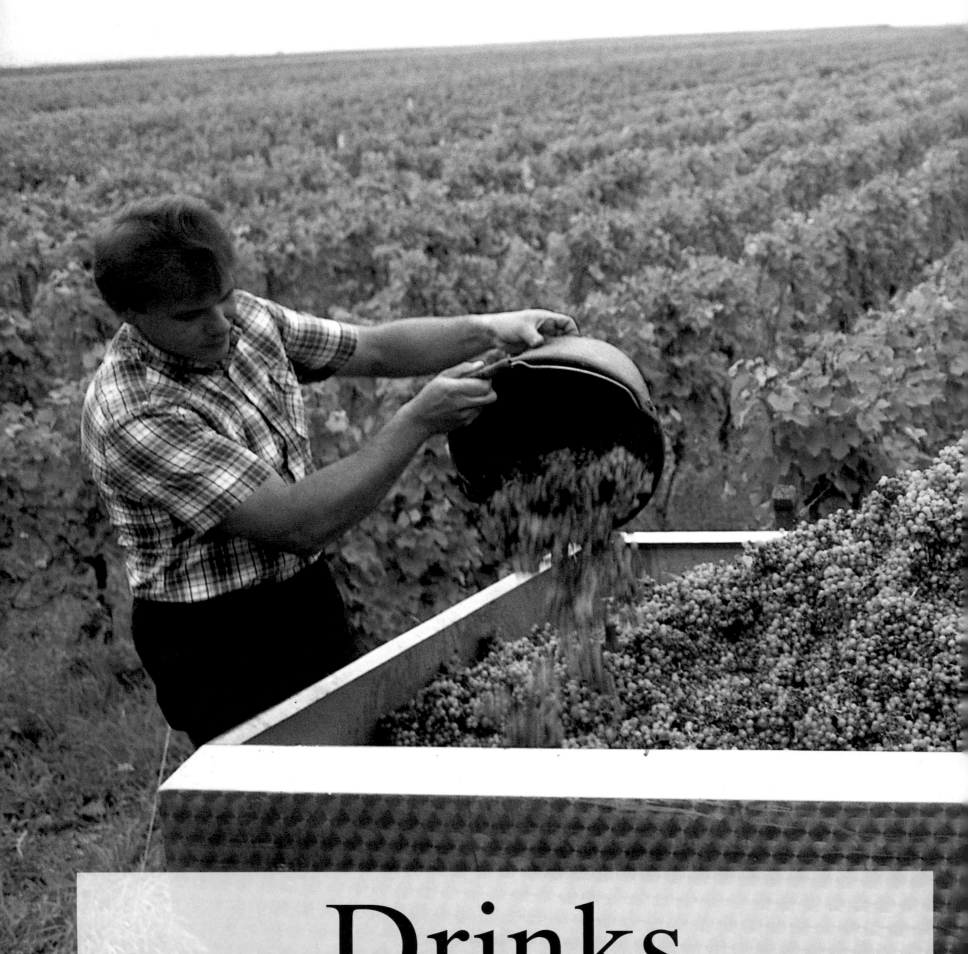

Drinks

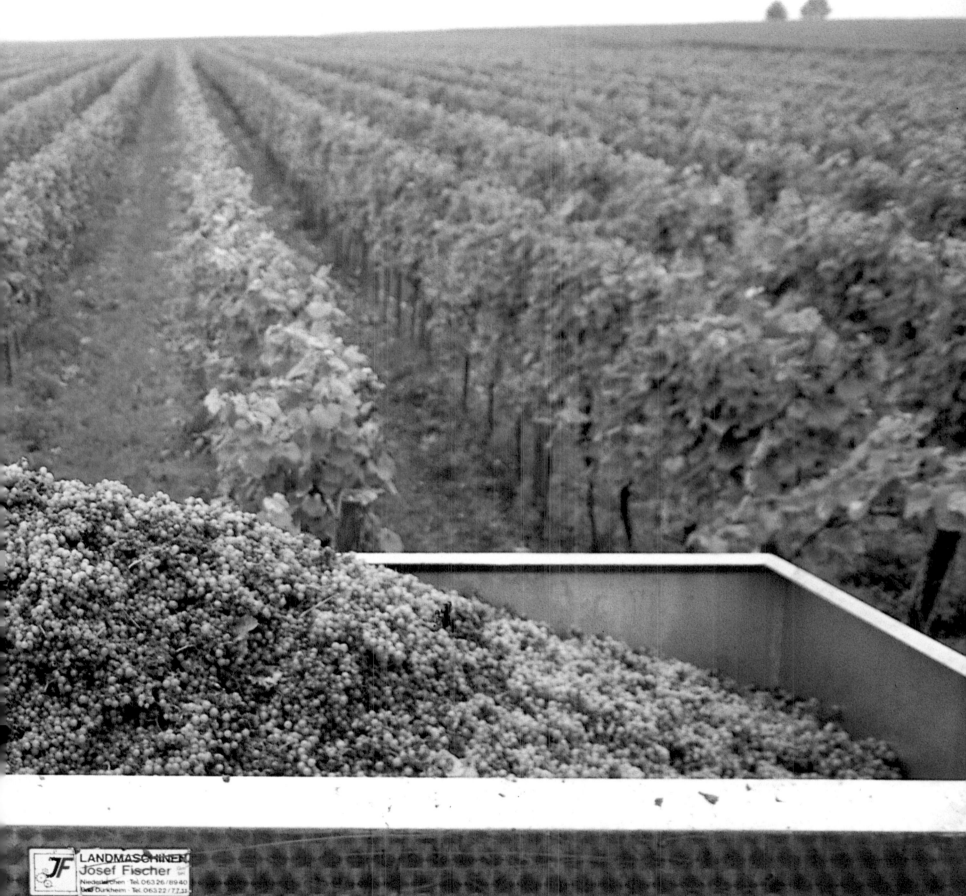

LANDMASCHINEN
Josef Fischer GmbH
Niederkirchen · Tel. 06326/8940
Bad Dürkheim · Tel. 06322/7733

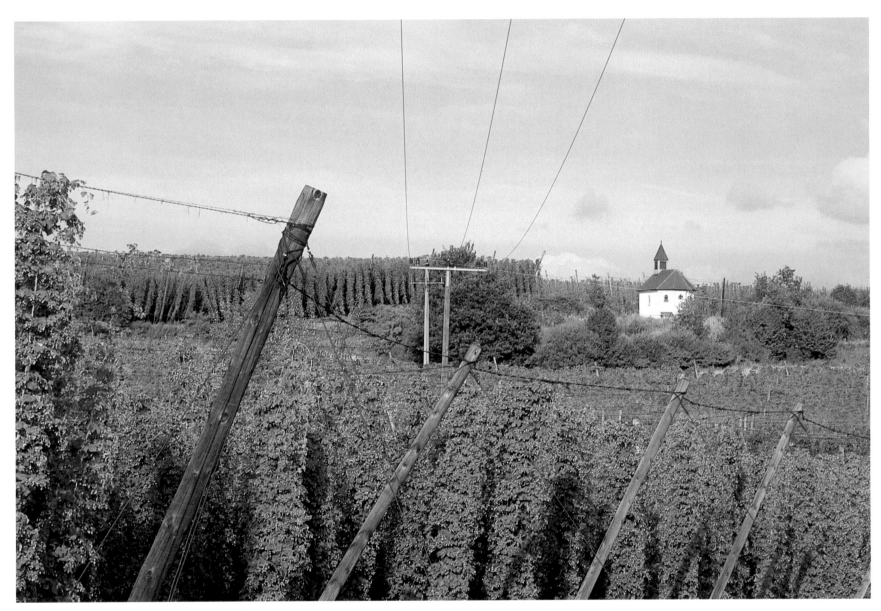

Hops are one of the most delicate crops and cultivating
them organically is a real art.

Previous double page: Grape harvest in the Palatinate
region of Germany – a small trailer is used to avoid
damage to the grapes and transport them quickly.

ater: the most ancient of all thirst quenchers and, many believe, the most healthy. Water supplements and maintains the body's mineral levels with various substances, depending on the source from which it originates, and its valuable qualities are especially highly appreciated by whole food lovers. A lifestyle like ours, in which health is the number one concern, makes a pure, natural drink a necessity.

In fact, more and more people are turning to commercial mineral waters because, in many places, the drinking water is hardly drinkable any more – a result of pollution of the ground water by industry and chemical-dependent agriculture. This essential nutrient is gradually becoming a valuable, even expensive, commodity.

But water and juice, beer and wine, coffee and tea do more than just quench thirst. Drinking, much more than eating, is surrounded by a whole culture of pleasure, conviviality and contemplation. For centuries, Far Eastern cultures have regarded tea as the drink of the wise. Coffee houses in Vienna, Berlin and Prague became famous for their literary gatherings. Wine has always shaped the landscape in which it grows but, more than that, it has also shaped the lives, history, and myths of many peoples. On the subject of wine: Wine is not only a superior intoxicating drink, but also, when consumed in moderation, is beneficial to health. Science has shown that the phenols it contains have an anti oxidizing effect and therefore help prevent heart and circulatory illnesses and supposedly even cancer. This may well be so, but we have to remember that, like any other drink, wine can only be as healthy as the raw materials from which it is made. So when ever more top-quality wine growers in the most prestigious (and also the less well-known) wine growing regions decide to go back to producing their exquisite wines in harmony with nature, we can once again experience the pure pleasure afforded by this magical drink.

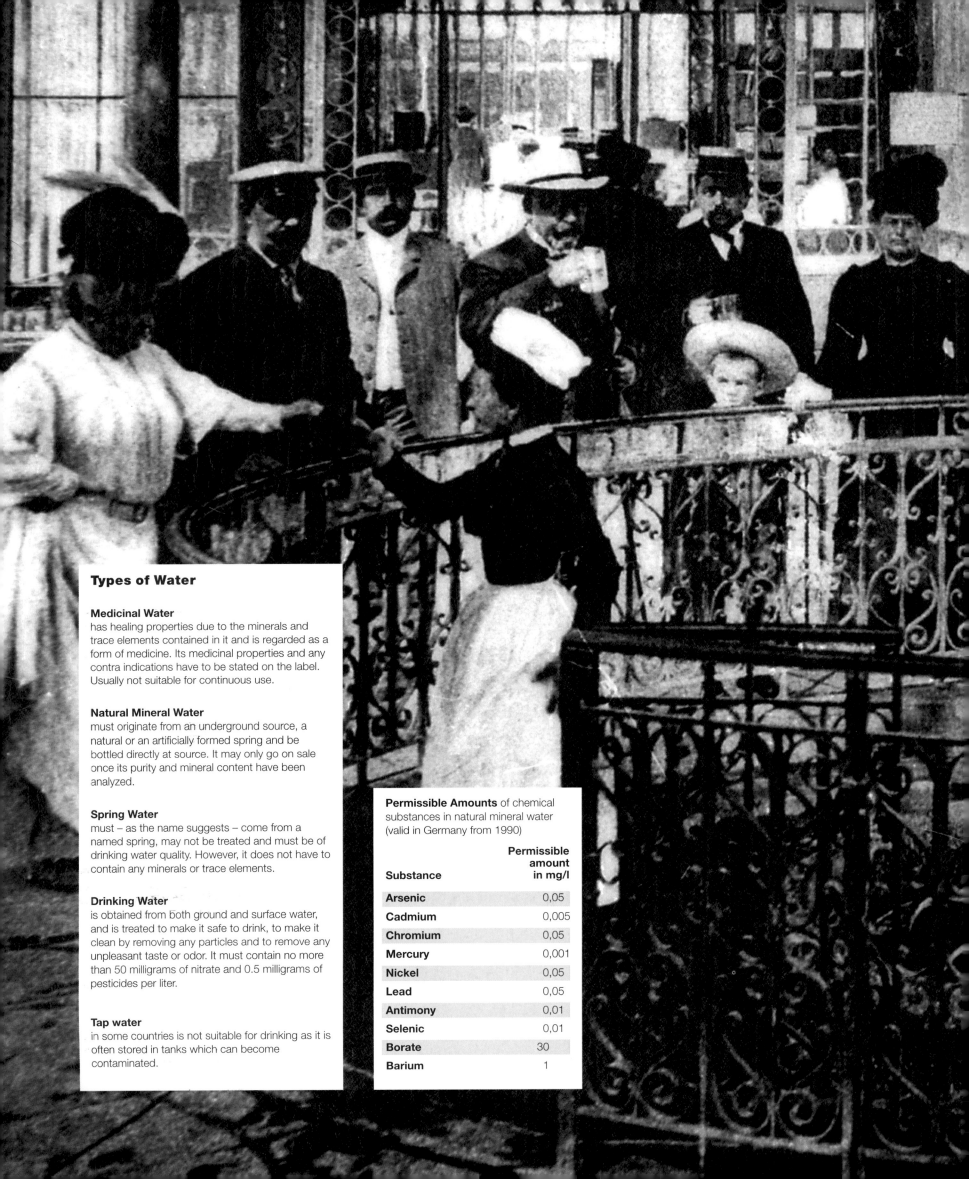

Types of Water

Medicinal Water
has healing properties due to the minerals and trace elements contained in it and is regarded as a form of medicine. Its medicinal properties and any contra indications have to be stated on the label. Usually not suitable for continuous use.

Natural Mineral Water
must originate from an underground source, a natural or an artificially formed spring and be bottled directly at source. It may only go on sale once its purity and mineral content have been analyzed.

Spring Water
must – as the name suggests – come from a named spring, may not be treated and must be of drinking water quality. However, it does not have to contain any minerals or trace elements.

Drinking Water
is obtained from both ground and surface water, and is treated to make it safe to drink, to make it clean by removing any particles and to remove any unpleasant taste or odor. It must contain no more than 50 milligrams of nitrate and 0.5 milligrams of pesticides per liter.

Tap water
in some countries is not suitable for drinking as it is often stored in tanks which can become contaminated.

Permissible Amounts of chemical substances in natural mineral water (valid in Germany from 1990)

Substance	Permissible amount in mg/l
Arsenic	0,05
Cadmium	0,005
Chromium	0,05
Mercury	0,001
Nickel	0,05
Lead	0,05
Antimony	0,01
Selenic	0,01
Borate	30
Barium	1

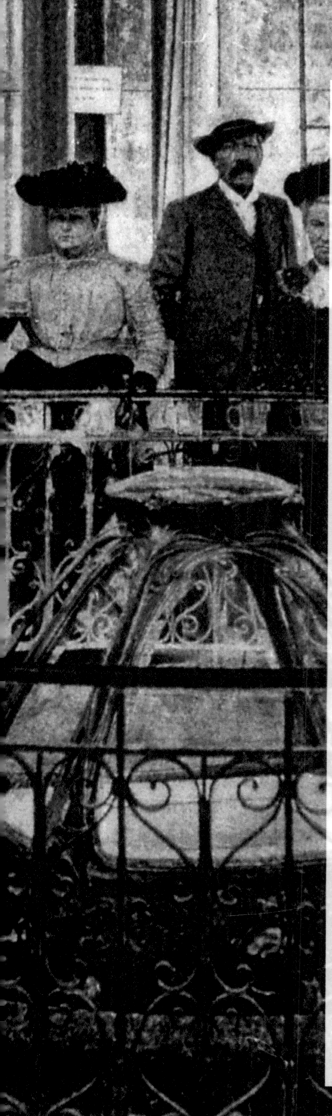

The Liquid of Life

Mineral Water

Our bodies are made up of about 60 percent water. The proportion is even higher in small children and starts to decrease in older adults. Without water, our metabolism would cease to function. Water plays a crucial role in transporting important substances into the body and flushing out waste materials and toxins.

The body works in such a way that it requires varying amounts of water to be able to function properly, depending on the situation. The reason is that it does not have a reserve supply. The body's water requirement can rise sharply, especially as a result of heat, exertion, excessive salt consumption, and also illness. Under normal circumstances, an adult should consume about 4½ pints (2.5 liters) of water per day in the form of liquids and in solid foods, as this corresponds to the average amount of water expelled from the body. If water intake falls to zero, death will result within a few days. Water is therefore our most essential nutrient.

This is why drinking water is considered to be so important. In the past, epidemics were transmitted through drinking water in Europe, and this is still the case today in Third World countries. Chlorine and ozone treatments have enabled us to control the risk. Nowadays, impurities are caused by other factors. Industry, emissions and agriculture cause substances to get into the ground water which are potentially damaging to health. The substances in question are, in particular:

• nitrates and nitrites, which can lead to the formation of carcinogenic nitrosamines in the body and

• pesticides, meaning the various highly toxic plant protection compounds.

Although there are strict guidelines specifying the maximum quantities of particular health-threatening substances which may be contained in drinking water, in reality these values are often exceeded. As a result only a small percentage of mains drinking water is used for drinking or food preparation in European households. More and more consumers are switching to bottled water, which is even being used increasingly frequently for making tea and coffee.

Mineral Water: Health in a Bottle

Consumption of mineral water is growing year by year in Europe. This boom is due partly to reports of contamination of the ground water, rivers and lakes, and partly to the fact that the water is so heavily chlorinated in some areas that it is not always drinkable. Natural mineral water is underground water originating from subterranean sources. Over dozens of years, the upper layers of earth and rock filter the rain water seeping down and enrich it with minerals and trace elements. Its health-giving properties are the result of this richness and vary from one type of water to another.

Natural mineral waters must be bottled directly at source. It is forbidden by law to transport the water to a different location for bottling. No treatments are permitted, except:

• if the water contains too much iron or sulfur which affects the flavor, the content can be reduced by filtering or oxidation;

• and the carbon dioxide content may also be altered. The following varieties are available:

• Natural sparkling mineral water contains the same level of natural carbon dioxide in the bottle as is present at the spring.

• Natural mineral water with added natural carbon dioxide from the same spring often has a higher carbon dioxide content than the original water.

• Natural mineral water with added carbon dioxide indicates that carbon dioxide from a different origin has been added.

• Still water is a natural mineral water containing less than 0·175 ounce (5 grams) of carbon dioxide per 2 pints (1 liter).

• Flat water is a natural mineral water containing less than 0·035 ounce (1 gram) of carbon dioxide per liter.

Although mineral waters are thoroughly filtered by nature, this is not an absolute guarantee that they are totally free of harmful substances. Increased concentrations of nitrates and nitrites at some springs testify to this. Anyone wishing to be quite sure that a mineral water contains as few unhealthy additives as possible should choose a type labeled "suitable for infants."

Background: The mineral spring at Contréxville around the turn of the century, when it was popular amongst high society to visit the spas regularly for a health cure.

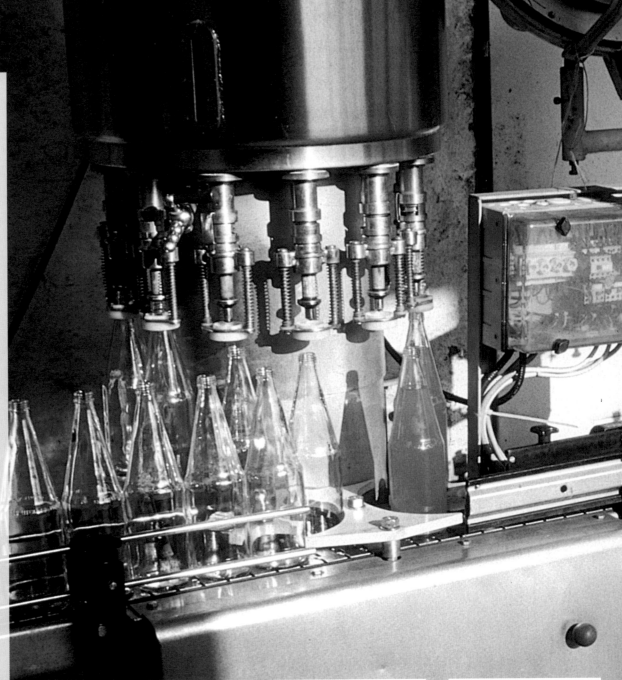

Fruit and Vegetable Juices

Liquid Vitamins

To come straight to the point, the best juices are homemade ones made from home-pressed fresh fruit or vegetables and drunk immediately, before any of the vital constituents can be destroyed by oxidation or warmth. Fresh juices offer the advantage that they contain considerably higher quantities of minerals, enzymes, essential oils, and vitamins in concentrated form than solid food. You only need to count the number of oranges used to make one large glass of fresh juice to understand why this is so.

In contrast, all commercially produced juices lose many of their essential ingredients due to the requirements of pasteurization and storage. The reason why juices produced from biologically grown fruits and vegetables are nevertheless important in whole food retail is quite simply convenience. People who are thirsty or fancy a fruit juice are not always prepared to go to the trouble of getting the press going and cleaning it thoroughly afterwards.

Furthermore, consumers often do not have access to the raw materials needed for making juices, for example in the case of red and blackcurrants, sloes, rosehips, or sea buckthorn, or they do not have suitable equipment. And even with apple juice which, in all the more northern European countries at least, is the clear favorite amongst organic juices, it is impossible to achieve the same result at home as on a fruit farm, where several varieties are usually combined to produce a juice with a well-balanced flavor. It is also important to read the label carefully when buying organic juices. It will tell you:

- whether the juice really consists wholly of fruits and vegetables with no added sugar;
- whether fruit nectars have a 50 percent or only 25 percent fruit content, and how much sugar has been used for sweetening;
- whether, in fruit drinks, the strong natural acid has been balanced out with concentrated fruit juices, honey or maple syrup.

Background: A fruit farmer bottles the juice from the fallen fruit on his own farm.

An Example: Organic Apple Juice

The apples are checked for blemishes and rotten areas, sorted and washed. They are then put in a mill where they are crushed. The crushed fruit is laid on the platform of the packing press in a layer about 2½ inches (6 centimeters) thick then covered with a cloth. In all, the press holds six or seven such layers of apple mash. The platform is pressed upwards by the lifting force. Pressing is finished when the juice just comes out in droplets.

The freshly pressed juice then spends six to ten days in a cooling room. Afterwards, when the preliminary sedimentation has taken place, the juice can be drawn off. To stabilize the juice, it is subjected to rapid heating immediately before bottling. A water bath and additional washing down ensures that the bottles cool rapidly and are clean. They can then be labeled as appropriate.

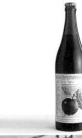

Apple juice is number one amongst organic juices.

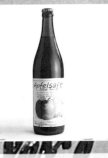

Fruit juice made from apples and redcurrants.

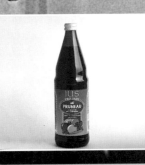

Plum juice from south west France.

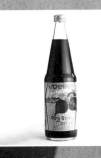

Red beet juice, an extremely healthy drink.

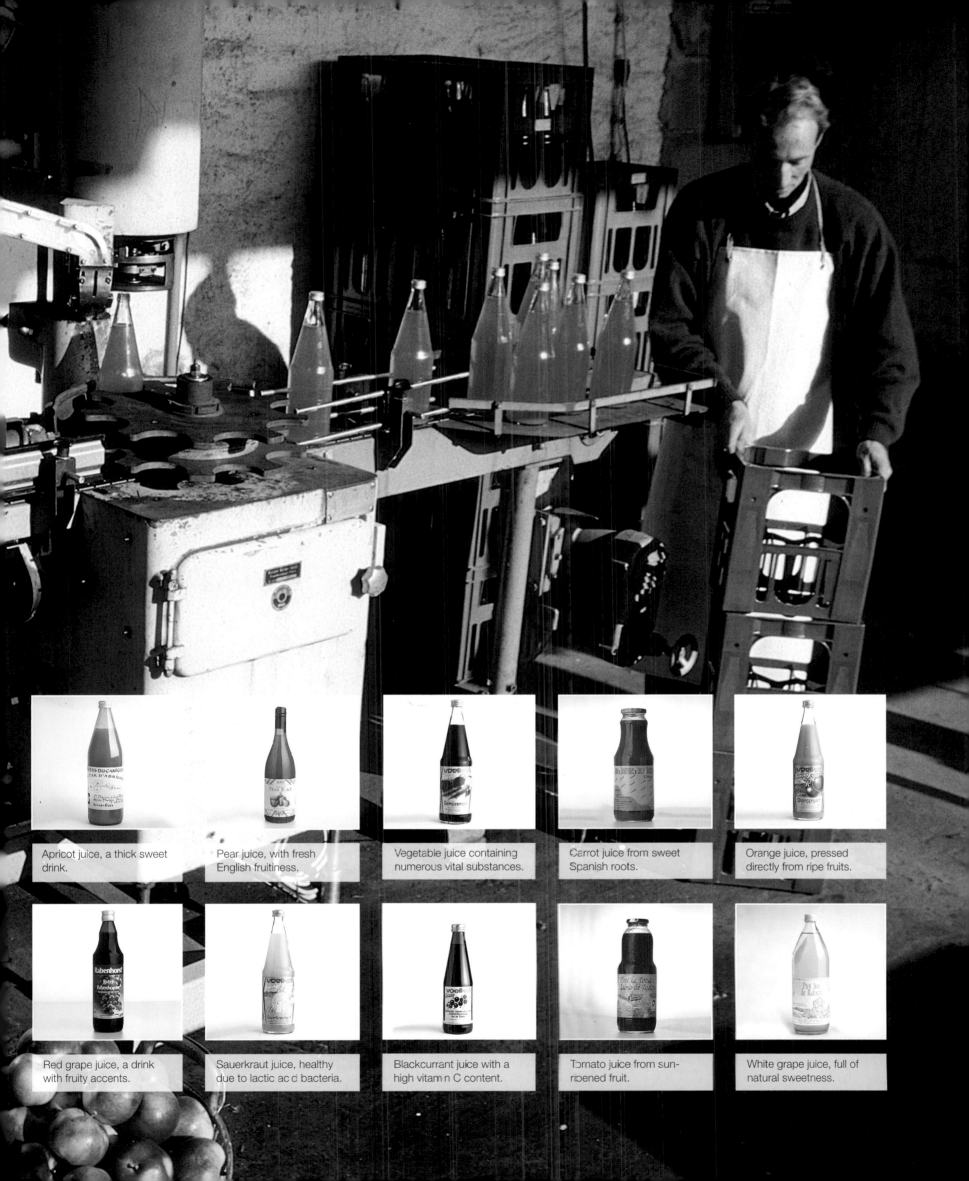

Apricot juice, a thick sweet drink.

Pear juice, with fresh English fruitiness.

Vegetable juice containing numerous vital substances.

Carrot juice from sweet Spanish roots.

Orange juice, pressed directly from ripe fruits.

Red grape juice, a drink with fruity accents.

Sauerkraut juice, healthy due to lactic acid bacteria.

Blackcurrant juice with a high vitamin C content.

Tomato juice from sun-ripened fruit.

White grape juice, full of natural sweetness.

Cider

Cider, cidre, sidra, or Apfelwein is a lightly alcoholic drink which is still produced on many farms in Britain, France, Spain, Germany, and other countries. Surprisingly, the tradition survives to this day, despite the fact that sparkling and still, sweet and dry cider has long been widely available from industrial production. In Britain, where winemaking is a popular hobby, orchard owners like to ferment their own cider or crab apple wine. Organic farmers also cultivate this tradition, which gives them a further opportunity for using cider apples and selected eating apples to make a refreshing drink.

The character of the cider varies from one region to another. The first reason for this is the various, mainly local, varieties of crab apple and cider apple. In areas like Normandy, in northern France, which has been famous for its cider for centuries, the varieties are divided into sweet, bitter and sour. All three types are necessary to give the tangy cider its typical character and balanced taste. The rule of thumb is that one sour apple should be added for every two sweet and two bitter apples used. In other places – and particularly with home production – different fruit such as pears or grapes are added to the apples.

Although it is common practice everywhere for the apples to be shaken from the trees and collected on the ground, the rest of the process varies considerably depending on the region. In the Hesse region of Germany, where the local cider or "Ebbelwoi" is a popular choice, the apples are processed straight after the harvest so that fresh cider can be had as early as December. The later it is left, the more carbon dioxide is lost from the sharp, dry cider. In the Basque region and in Asturias, the sidra strongholds of Spain, production does not start until the end of November, when cool temperatures mean the initial fermentation can take up to two months.

Before the juice is completely fermented out, it is drawn off and transferred to wooden casks. While the remaining sugar is being converted into alcohol, much of the carbon dioxide produced is retained. The new sidra is ready for drinking in May. Sparkling cider is preferred in Britain too, so the cider with its high carbon dioxide content has to be put in extra strong bottles.

However, cider production takes longest in Normandy. Although the earliest apples are ripe in September and are also gathered then, producers wait patiently until the latest variety also drops from the tree in November and the first frost has come. Only then is the fruit washed, the rotten apples discarded and the fruit pressed. Because of the cold, fermentation in the vats now takes place at reduced speed. Cider farmers bottle the unfiltered cider, with varying amounts of

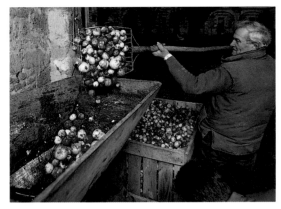

Cider production starts after the first frost with the chopping of the fruit.

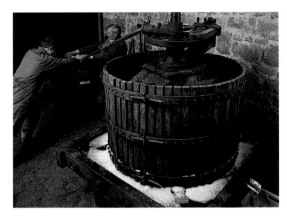

The chopped apples are pressed hydraulically in the hand-operated press.

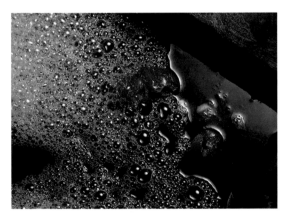

The apples are crushed under the increasing pressure and the juice begins to flow.

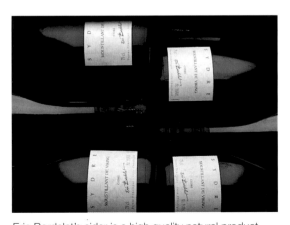

Eric Bordelet's cider is a high quality natural product, beautifully presented.

sugar remaining, in thick glass bottles and secure the cork with wire around the neck of the bottle, as, is done with Champagne. This is because the fermentation continues in the bottle, converting some or all of the fructose into alcohol and generating carbon dioxide. This is how cider, which contains only 3 to 4.5 percent alcohol, gets its fizz. Genuine *cidre fermier* does not have the sediment removed and therefore retains natural yeast residues which are rich in vital substances.

The Secret of Cider

Crab apples and cider apples are the main types of apple used, and every region has its own particular varieties. Damaged apples, apples which have not fully ripened or excessively small eating apples are also added. With homemade cider, pears or grapes are sometimes also used in the mixture. These give the cider a milder flavor, raise the alcohol content and thus lengthen its shelf life. First the apples are placed in a barrel or vat and washed to get rid of earth and large particles of dirt. They then have to be cut up, which can be done using a shredder. The pieces or strips of apple are then loaded into the press in layers. Presses vary greatly in capacity, depending on the size. Smaller, hand-operated presses can hold about two hundredweight of apples, giving a yield of only 13 to 16 gallons (50 to 60 liters), whereas hydraulic presses can squeeze out 20 to 21 gallons (75 to 80 liters). The freshly pressed, unfermented, sweet-tasting fruit juice is now poured into the fermentation container. This can be a barrel, but glass demi johns, which are easier to clean, are advisable for use at home.

The containers are put outside in a shady place, in a shed or in the cellar. Each one is sealed with a plug to prevent air, dust, insects, and microbes from entering. Fermentation yeast can now be added, to achieve a uniform quality. It is more ecological to leave the fermentation to chance. The cider will develop its own unmistakable flavor, depending on which natural yeast gains the upper hand. The fermentation, the vigor of which can vary, takes a few weeks. It is worthwhile to separate the young cider from the yeast lying on the bottom by pouring the liquid into different demi johns.

After a few days' settling, the new cider is ready for drinking. It can keep for up to eighteen months in a cool cellar, but loses some of its flavor after a year, although of course by that time, the next year's cider will be ready for consumption.

Horst Nagel

Opposite page: When, after a few hours, the apples have been pressed into a cake, the press is opened.

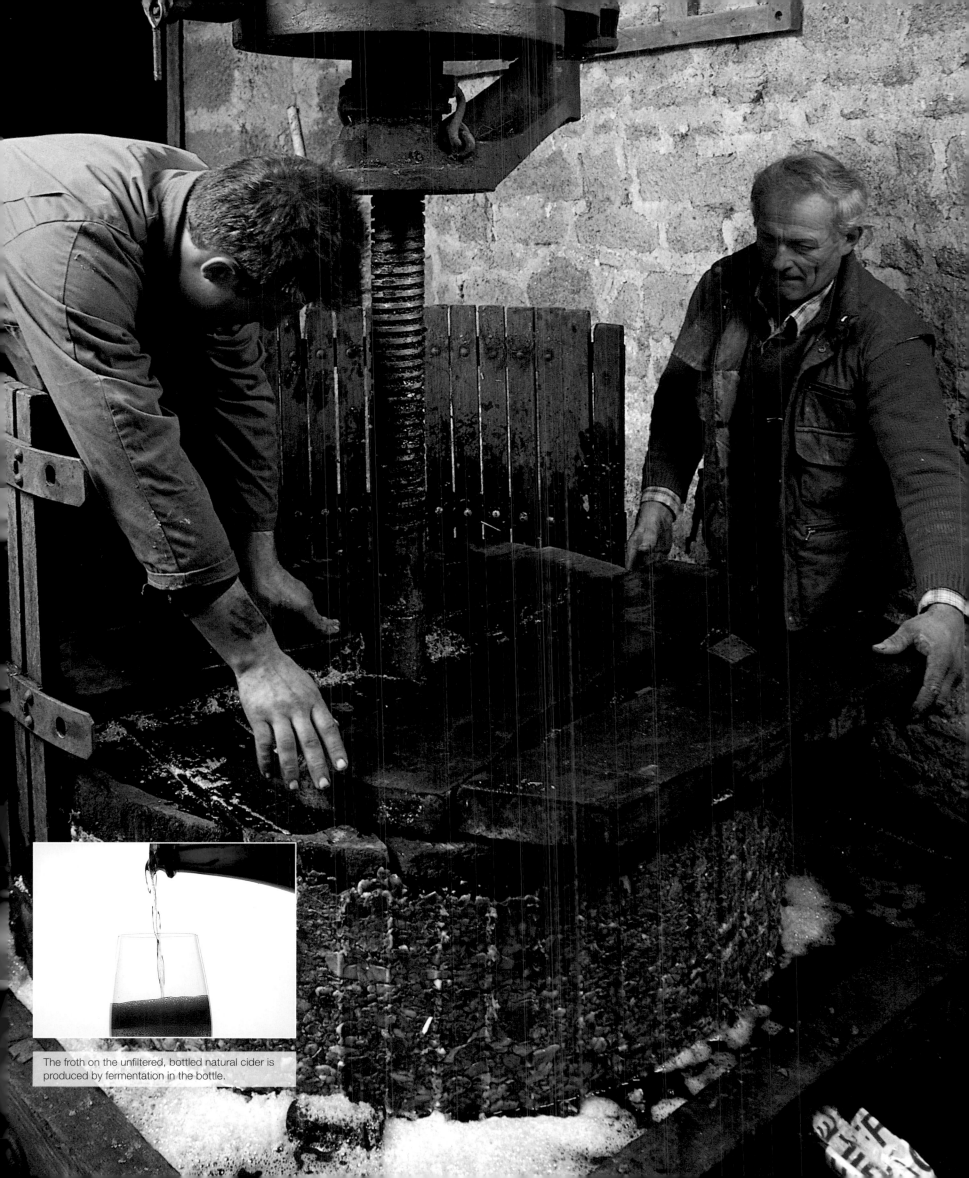

The froth on the unfiltered, bottled natural cider is produced by fermentation in the bottle.

An Organic Climbing Feat

Hops

One of the most famous, if also one of the smallest, cultivation areas for flavoring hops in Europe is near the south German town of Tettnang, where nearby Lake Constance influences the climate.

The hop plant is a climbing plant related to hemp and belonging to the Cannabaceae (hemp) family. Only the female plants of the diecious hop species are cultivated. Inside their umbels are the lupulin glands which produce the "green gold," the hop flour, a greenish yellow sticky powder. Its active ingredient is what gives beer – and especially Pils – its full bodied, bitter flavor. It also substantially prolongs its life as it helps to precipitate the proteins which stop the beer, including the froth, from keeping for long. Hops, which have been grown widely in Europe since the 16th century, are used extremely sparingly: just 7 ounces (200 grams) are sufficient to flavor 26 gallons (100 liters) of beer.

Hop cultivation puts its own unmistakable stamp on every landscape, as the clockwise winding creeper needs huge frames towering 26 feet (8 meters) high. The hop plant manages to grow 26 feet in six weeks. The main work involved is therefore in guiding this rocketing growth in the right direction. Running wires are strung up between the posts, and each year new climbing wires have to be attached to them. They give the shoots something to hold on to, and although the stalks cling on to them by their tendrils, they still have to be tied on in several places.

To achieve this immense growth, hops need a warm clay or marly (carbonate-rich) soil and a lot of strength. Whilst conventional growers assist with chemical nitrogen, organic farmers use composted manure, natural preparations and green fertilizers to provide sufficient humus. Providing a healthy, living soil is the only way of building up resistance in this plant which is otherwise extremely susceptible to attack by fungi and pests. In conventional cultivation, hops are one of the crops requiring the highest use of pesticides.

Once the umbels have developed a pronounced aroma, the tractor tows the harvesting machine along between the tall green walls formed by the rows of plants. It cuts off the climbing wires with the shoots wound around them and loads them onto the trailer, to take them back to the farm, where the picking machine is installed. One wire at a time is fed in, so that the machine can pick off the unpollinated female fruit clusters, umbel by umbel. The hop grower also needs a dry storage area as the umbels have to be dried immediately at 86 °F (30 °C) or so. This is the only way in which they can maintain their intense flavor.

Background: Hops are incredibly intense flavor providers – a tiny dose is all that is needed to give Pils its refreshing tanginess.

Brewer's Barley

Compared with the now more widespread winter barley, summer barley, which is used in brewing, produces lower yields. However, it is less fussy about its location. Although summer barley can also be used as a fodder crop, it has to meet strict requirements when produced for breweries, which makes it more difficult to cultivate it organically. The most important criterion is a low protein content. Too much protein makes the beer spoil more quickly. As organic breweries do not use any stabilizers, they have to keep the protein under control. The protein content of barley can be up to 16 percent. For beer, 9.5 to 10.5 percent is ideal, and over 11.5 percent will not be accepted. As protein levels tend to rise when there is a good yield, organic growers not only avoid using pesticides, but also often avoid organic fertilizers too. However, brewing barley likes fields which were spread with a small amount of farmyard manure the previous winter. It can be incorporated into virtually any crop rotation system and can also be sown in successive crops, another reason why it is popular. Purity is another of the requirements it has to fulfill. It may only contain very small amounts of other grains and weed seeds. In addition, full germination capacity and big, fat grains are required for the malting.

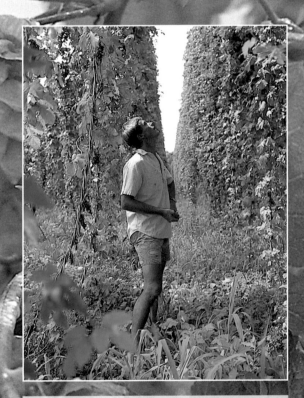

The rapid growth of the hops is regulated by 26 foot (8 meter) high frames.

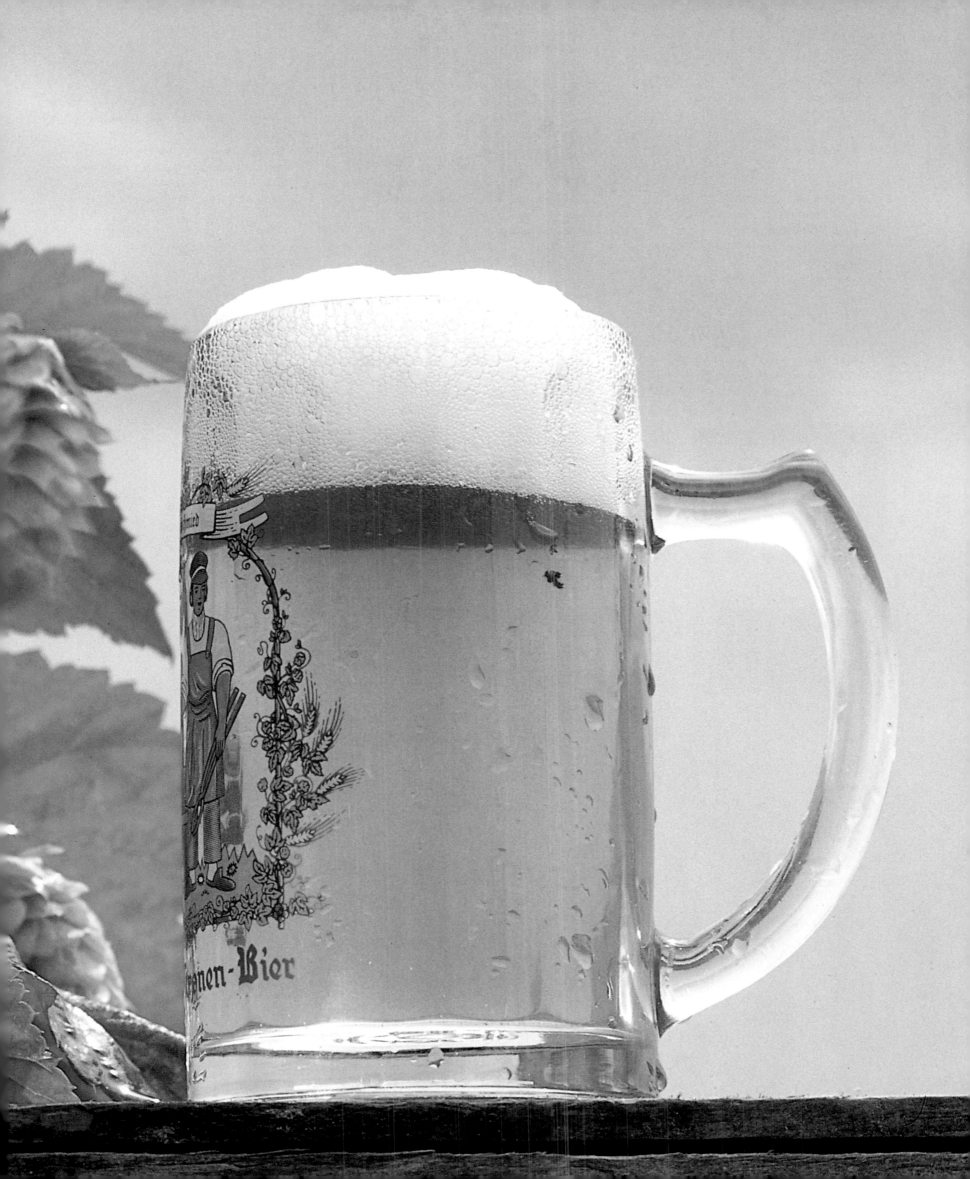

Beer: Deliciously Organic

The purity of beer was a subject of heated debate in the European Community. The international drinks giants wanted to gain access to the German market, where annual per capita consumption of beer is as high as 246 pints (140 liters). But in Germany, beers have to comply with a purity law introduced by Duke Wilhelm IV in Bavaria in 1516. It specified that beer must be made of barley, hops, and water only. Yeast, the fourth essential ingredient, was unknown at that time. But it was added when, in 1872, the Bavarian purity law came into effect for all the German states. However, the European Court of Justice refused to allow such a restriction and since 1987, beers which do not meet the regulation can be sold in Germany. In other countries, the beer industry had long ago adopted the practice of adding chemicals and using cheaper grain such as maize, millet and rice to produce longer-lasting and more profitable mass-produced beers.

But German beer, too, had for a long time not been all that pure. In top fermented beers, other types of grain such as wheat and spelt, as well as caramel and starch were permitted. And many brewers were reluctant to reject the highly practical use of protein stabilizers and prepared hop products. Nevertheless, in Germany, as in other countries, there are still traditional breweries which produce beer in compliance with the purity law.

In the case of organic beers, the following criteria also apply:
• Grain and hops are grown organically.
• The grain is not preserved with gases during storage.
• Hops are added to the beer in the form of umbels and not as extract.
• The water comes from a spring or natural source.
• The yeasts are natural pure strains.
• No flavoring, coloring or preserving substances are used.
• Organic beer is not pasteurized.
• Filtration is carried out with extra care or not at all.
• The packaging meets ecological requirements: the beer is sold in deposit bottles and delivered in deposit crates.

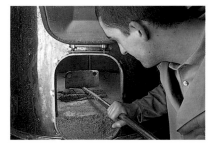

Malt extracted from dried barley is put into the vat.

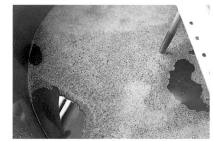

It is mixed with hot water to produce the mash.

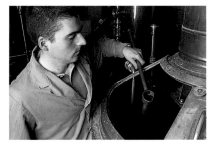

The mash is stirred for up to two hours, during which time samples are taken.

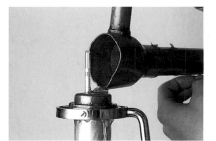

The master brewer checks the temperature with a thermometer.

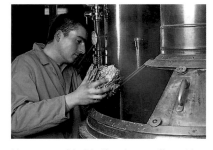

Hops are added to the drawn off wort in the brewing pan.

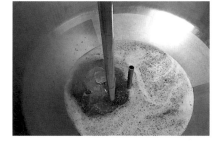

The wort then bubbles for two to four hours.

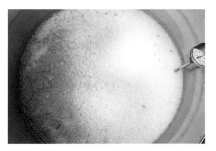

The bullseye allows visual checking of the fermentation process.

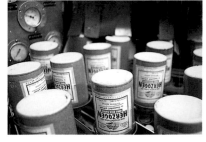

Before filling, the steins are rinsed out with water.

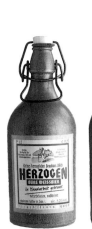
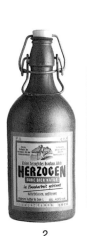
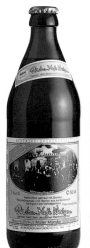
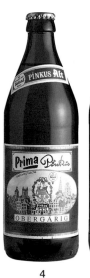
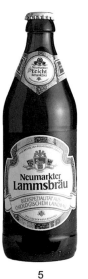
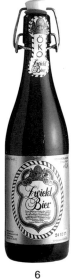
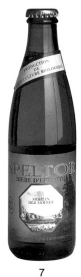
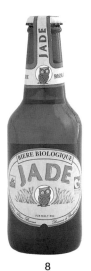
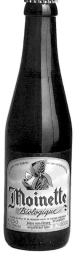
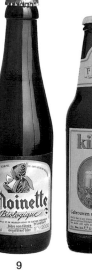
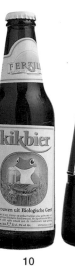
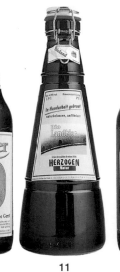

1   2   3   4   5   6   7   8   9   10   11

Beer Brewing

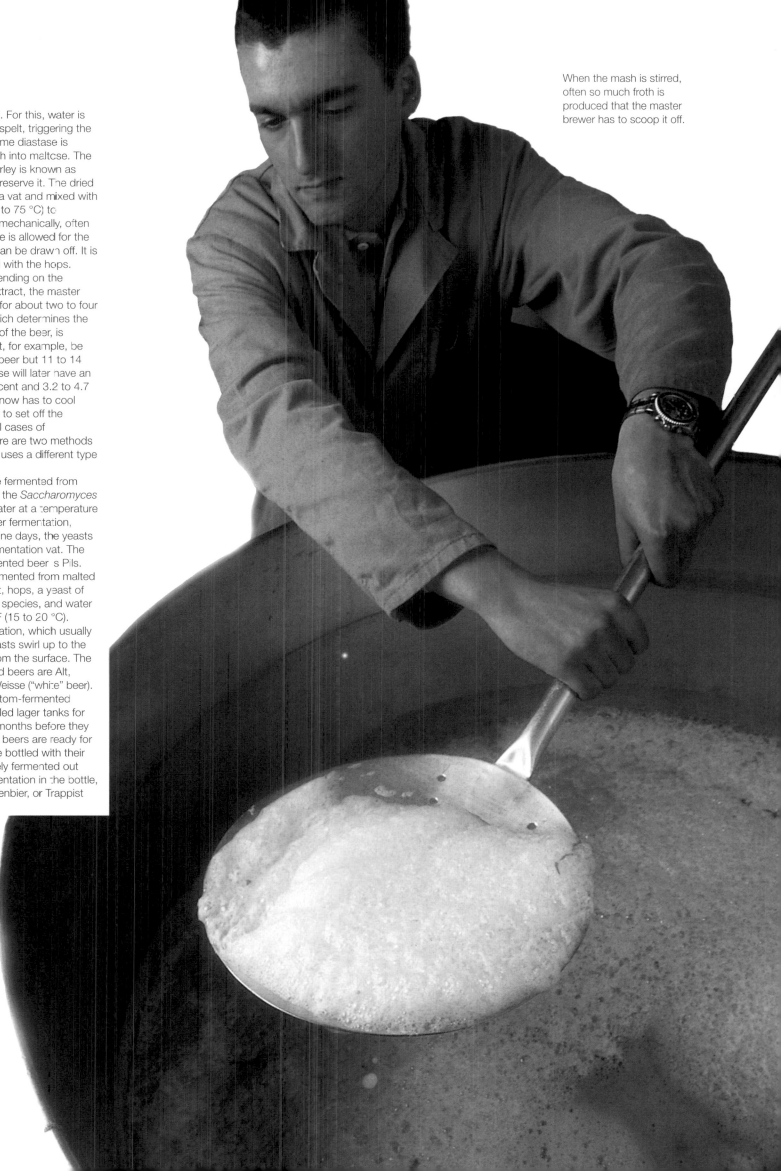

Brewing starts with the malting. For this, water is added to the barley, wheat, or spelt, triggering the germination process. The enzyme diastase is produced, converting the starch into maltose. The germinated, highly sensitive barley is known as green malt. It is then dried to preserve it. The dried malt is ground coarsely, put in a vat and mixed with hot water at 122 to 167 °F (50 to 75 °C) to produce the mash. It is stirred mechanically, often for a good two hours. Now time is allowed for the solids to settle, then the wort can be drawn off. It is put in brewing pans and mixed with the hops. Based on experience and depending on the desired concentration of the extract, the master brewer will let the wort bubble for about two to four hours. The extract content, which determines the character and alcohol content of the beer, is known as original wort. It might, for example, be 7 to 8 degrees for a light draft beer but 11 to 14 degrees for a full beer, and these will later have an alcohol content of 2 to 2.7 percent and 3.2 to 4.7 percent respectively. The wort now has to cool before the yeast can be added to set off the fermentation. Excluding special cases of spontaneous fermentation, there are two methods of fermentation, each of which uses a different type of yeast:

• Bottom-fermented beers are fermented from malted barley, hops, a yeast of the *Saccharomyces cerisbergensis* species, and water at a temperature of 41 to 50 °F (5 to 10 °C). After fermentation, which usually takes seven to nine days, the yeasts settle on the bottom of the fermentation vat. The most well known bottom-fermented beer s Pils.

• Top-fermented beers are fermented from malted barley or malted wheat or spelt, hops, a yeast of the *Saccharomyces cerevisaie* species, and water at a temperature of 59 to 68 °F (15 to 20 °C). During the tumultuous fermentation, which usually takes three to six days, the yeasts swirl up to the top and can be scooped off from the surface. The most well known top fermented beers are Alt, Weizenbier (wheat beer), and Weisse ("white" beer). Even the aging is different. Bottom-fermented beers have to be stored in cooled lager tanks for between four weeks and four months before they can be bottled. Top-fermented beers are ready for drinking sooner unless they are bottled with their yeast before they are completely fermented out and then undergo further fermentation in the bottle, as in the case of Weisse, Weizenbier, or Trappist beer.

1 Herzogen Bure Weissbier
2 Herzogen Bure Bier Natur
3 Pinkus Hefe Weizen
4 Pinkus Alt
5 Neumarkter Lammsbräu
6 Zwickl Bier
7 Speltor Bière d'Epautre
8 Jade
9 Moinette
10 Kikbier
11 Herzogen Natur
12 Eko Bier

When the mash is stirred, often so much froth is produced that the master brewer has to scoop it off.

Essence of the Soil and Climate

Organic Wine

Wine occupies a special place amongst drinks. Neither water nor juice, beer nor spirits can offer such a broad spectrum of bouquets and flavors. Even in antiquity, wine lovers recognized the differences and prized the wines of some regions more highly than others. Each region had not only its own particular climate and soil, but also its own varieties of vine. The reputation of a particular area, demand for the wine, and price were based on these factors. The reputation of particular locations was confirmed over centuries. In the meantime, European wine growing nations have precisely demarcated their traditional cultivation regions, defined and specified their properties and now meticulously supervise the production.

But wine was and is a delicate product. The further vine plantations spread, the more they were afflicted by fungal diseases which, in the past, drastically reduced the harvest or destroyed it altogether. None of the vine varieties common in Europe has much or any resistance to the two dominant forms of mildew. In addition, infested grapes cause considerable problems when preparing the wine. In any case, for a long time people did not really know what happened in the cellar. Using their experience, many wine-growers and vintners nevertheless succeeded in producing outstanding vintages. However, the bulk remained crude and often had defects. But in the last two decades, a real revolution has taken place. Huge investments have been made to introduce modern hygiene measures and install hot and cold technology in wine cellars to control the fermentation processes.

In the vineyard, people believed that great progress had been made with the introduction of chemicals which could be used to control diseases, kill weeds, destroy insects, and boost yields with nitrate fertilizers. Arduous tasks like plowing and hoeing thus became superfluous. However, they did not anticipate the consequences: contamination of the ground water and environment, damage to flora and fauna, and devitalization and erosion of the soil. These developments inevitably have a negative effect on the wine.

Thanks to advances in cellar technology, more and more wines are now being vinified and bottled under clean conditions. At the same time, there has been a huge flood of completely bland wines onto the market. In contrast to this, there has been an increase in the number of wines from all regions produced with care and in moderate quantities, which, with the good vintages at least, have excellent fruit flavors and an acceptable degree of concentration. However, what they often lack is the specific character of the region, on which their reputation and the criteria for the description of origin depend. But how can grapes reflect the unique characteristics of their location when they are growing in dead soil, their roots only penetrate the top layers, and they are fed with chemical fertilizers?

For this reason, some of the most famous wine estates in the world have for some years been trying a different approach, inspired primarily by the organic sector. By adopting the same respect for nature and life and the same measures as in ecological agriculture, vineyards can get back a healthy soil full of vitality and a living environment. Then the vines can once again push their roots several feet deep into the soil and benefit from its mineral structure, passing on the unique flavoring ingredients into the grapes. Provided the other conditions exist that characterize the location, and wine growers show conscientiousness and ambition, wines can be produced which contain the true essence of their location – wines which are hard to resist.

Background: When the grapes are as well ripened as these Riesling grapes, the harvest is just around the corner.

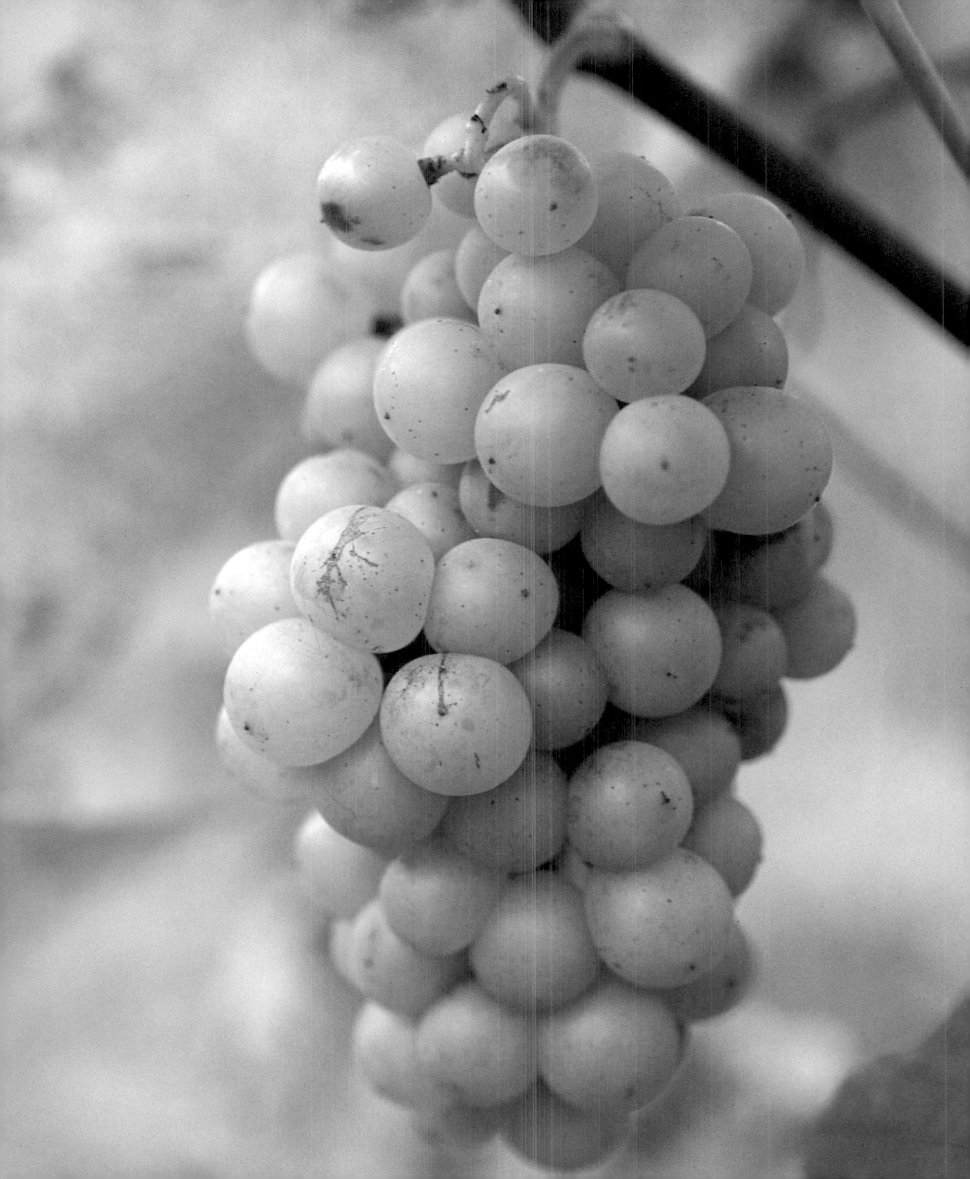

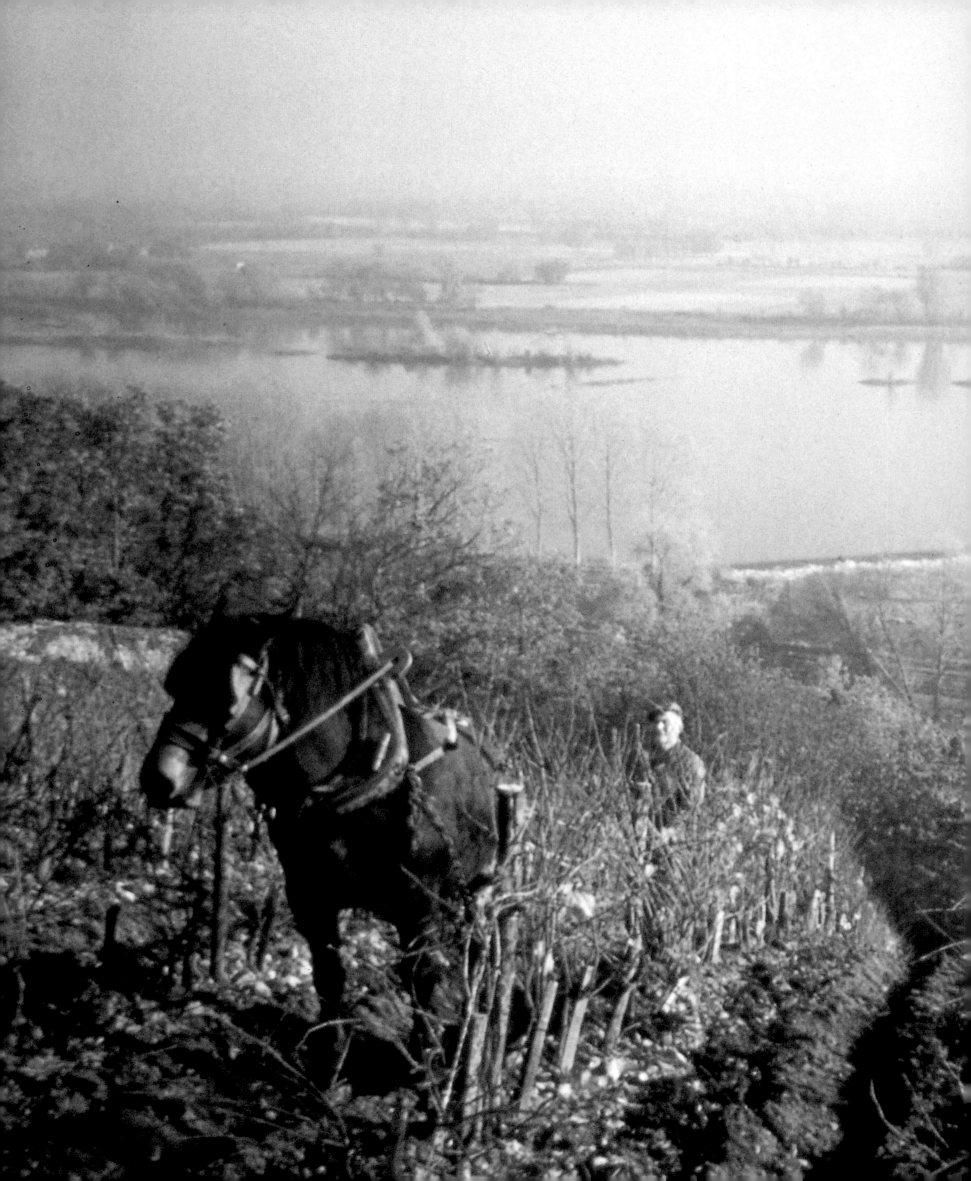

Where the Differences Lie

In the Vineyard

Like every field of organic production, ecological wine growing avoids the use of synthetic chemical fertilizers, weedkillers, insecticides, fungicides, and acaricides. But organic viniculture involves a much more comprehensive approach which aims to preserve the soil and clean ground water, to protect nature and tend the countryside, and to supply the raw ingredients and dispose of waste in ecologically acceptable ways.

The life of the soil in the vineyard is the basis for this. Wine growers use organic material to activate, promote and nourish soil life. Compost plays a major role here. It is produced from the leftover grape skins, manure, chaff, straw, and vegetable waste. Wine estates often have to buy the raw material from outside, as only very few vineyards are able to establish a closed farm cycle. However, there are also examples of estates branching out into organic animal rearing in order to produce their own valuable manure.

Of particular importance in organic wine growing is grassing, which replaces crop rotation on organic farms. The resulting thick network of roots in the soil has a permanent positive effect on the population of microorganisms. The diverse mixtures of leguminous plants, clovers, cereals, grasses, and weeds, which are mown and composted two or three times, also serve as an excellent green fertilizer and promote humus formation. The flowers bring insects back to the vineyards, useful in keeping down the populations of red spider and grape moth. Grassing prevents the vineyards from eroding and also helps to balance the water content of the soil. However, it has to be carefully matched to the conditions of the particular location. A full, permanent grass covering is not suitable everywhere – grassing for part of the time can sometimes be more useful.

The main difference from conventional wine growing enterprises lies in the fundamentally different approach and totally different objectives. This relates not only to care of the soil, but applies equally to tending the vines and protecting them from disease. European wine growers have to contend with the ubiquitous "true mildew" (*Oidium*) and "false mildew" (*Peronospera*). Whilst conventional growers always rely on chemicals, ecological growers concern themselves with reducing the risk of infection. Every single factor has to be checked and examined with this in mind. It starts with the choice of

- a suitable location,
- a suitable grape variety,
- the right distance between the plants and rows,
- the best form of cultivation,

and continues with

- limiting the number of shoots which are left when the vines are pruned back in winter,
- careful tending of the foliage which has to ensure good air circulation during the vegetation period,
- the cutting back in spring, when the number of shoots per vine is reduced to the optimum number,
- any thinning out of the grapes or leaf-stripping.

These measures must be coordinated with each other and carried out in good time to enable this biological system to work successfully.

Most of these measures are not employed in conventional vineyards, except on estates which specialize in producing top quality grapes and use partly organic methods. Organic growers need to avoid awkward locations and particularly susceptible grape varieties. Plant juices, plant preparations, stone powders etc. are used to strengthen the vines.

Compared with their conventional counterparts, organic growers have to put much more care and thought into their work. More constant yields and uniform quality, and often higher weights of juice, even in a bad year, are an indication of their success. This naturally puts organic wine estates on a lower yield level in line with high-quality conventional growers.

But as far as the wine quality is concerned, wine growers have always agreed that the way the grape is cultivated in the vineyard is what makes all the difference.

Background: On the steep slope of the Coulée de Serrant overlooking the Loire, Nicolas Joy piles up the earth at the base of the vines with the aid of a horse.

Biodynamism and Appellation

When people talk about controlled description of origin, it must be clear that although the soil is only the last link in a chain, at the same time it is the control center of a more subtle, less accessible sphere situated above the earth's surface. This control center keeps in contact with everything that surrounds us, primarily with the atmosphere, which consists of air, light, and warmth. It is important to realize that the earth's influence does not stop at its surface, which we inhabit. It stretches several hundred miles over our heads, right out to that hydrogen-saturated band of heat which we call the heliosphere. And this sphere above our earth acts as the control station of a more subtle cosmic system clearly dominated by the sun.

For centuries those who farmed the land worshipped the sun because they sensed that its energy penetrated deep into the ground. The latest scientific findings have shown that the soil contains an extraordinary assortment of life forms, uniquely combined not only in accordance with the geological composition of the soil, but particularly in accordance with the characteristic microclimate in the broadest sense, which determines the unique properties of the soil.

To understand this is to rediscover the deep meaning of the controlled description of origin. In other words, the varieties of microorganisms vary depending on various criteria like the prevailing wind directions, temperature fluctuations, length of the seasons, orientation of the sloping sites, local forms of vegetation, and so on. When one realizes that the roots of a vine can form a close bond with the soil only with the aid of these microorganisms, one has also understood how the controlled description of origin (Appellation d'Origine Controlée – AOC) came about.

Our apparently progressive agriculture has largely destroyed the soil as a living entity. As a result, the soil is now hardly capable of sustaining growth. It has consequently become dependent on chemical fertilizers, which are inevitably absorbed into the vine itself. But these growth stimulants are as foreign to our vineyards as their use in vineyards from South America to Europe is common. In the past, wine growers enriched the soil whereas nowadays, they feed the vines directly. This amply explains the ever-increasing uniformity of wines available from retailers.

The uniqueness of bio dynamic forms of cultivation lies not only in supporting the infinitely varied life forms in the soil by adding plant and animal compost, but also by using a wide range of preparations which enable the plants to provide themselves with sufficient light and warmth or, in short, to intensify photosynthesis. When we look at a flower or a fruit it becomes perfectly clear that they owe their beauty, their color, their fragrance, their variety of shapes and flavors to the sun. And it is precisely this power of expression, which manifests itself in constantly new variations, that must again be allowed to flourish in wine – and in every foodstuff.

Nicolas Joly, Clos de la Coulée de Serrant

Flavor From the Soil

It is astonishing that mankind has concerned itself so little with investigating its nearest resource, namely the soil. Some amazing discoveries were made only recently by the microbiologist Claude Bourguignon from Burgundy in France. In the late 1980s, he caught the attention of some wine-growers in this region by pointing out that the Sahara had more soil life than their vineyards. He made them think about the fact that vines nourished only via surface roots were not capable of expressing the "terroir" (see right) in which they were growing. And Bourguignon was able to explain why a grape can be an expression of the soil at all, and what the preconditions for this are.

In simple terms, there are three families of microorganisms in the soil. There are those which live on the organic material on the surface. They are very active as they have to deal with an enormous workload. They have to convert all the organic material which falls to the ground and make it usable again. Others exist only in the mineral layers, attacking stones and layers of rock and breaking them down to produce soil. The third group lives along the roots, feeds on the plant and dead roots, but in return provides the plant with minerals which it could not absorb by itself.

"The soil can only function when it is able to breathe," Claude Bourguignon explained. "The microbes produce oxides to nourish the plants: nitrates, sulfates, and phosphates. This is necessary as roots do not give off any oxygen, but consume it. The only way for oxygen to enter the soil is from the atmosphere. To enable it to penetrate, there needs to be very high porosity on the surface of the soil. Who produces this porosity? The fauna. And for the fauna to exist, firstly it must not be killed off by pesticides, and secondly it needs something to feed on. What does it feed on? On organic material that falls to the ground." Preferably in the form of compost.

Deep under the ground, another family of microorganisms feeds on dead roots. This also creates porosity. "This produces what one could call a draft of air, which enables oxygen to circulate in the soil. The more aerated the surface soil is, the deeper the plant can grow into the ground." These are the conditions that vines need if they are to optimally reflect the characteristics of their location and soil.

Terroir

In wine terms, terroir is a magic word. Although the quality of a wine is also influenced by other factors such as the variety of grape, the processing, and the attitude and commitment of the wine-grower, in all the traditional wine producing regions, the system for describing the wine's origin uses the terroir as a basis. This French word refers not only to the soil or ground, as the dictionary suggests, but to the whole combination of factors which affect the vine on a particular site and determine the nature of the wine. The mineral composition of the soil is only one of the factors. The altitude and slope and the angle of the sun in relation to the site are judged to be as important as the natural level of moisture, for example, from a nearby river and or rainfall. The microclimate with its temperatures and dry periods which mark the changing seasons to a greater or lesser extent has just as much influence as the frequency and direction of the wind. All these factors taken together define the terroir and thus its range of flavors, the "goût du terroir," or flavor of the soil. But the vine can only transmit this to the wine if it is healthy itself and is rooted in a living soil. However, the soil is able to change and gain particularly intensive powers of transmission if it has been tended using natural means for a long period of time. It is not by chance that the most famous terroirs are those sites which were first cultivated back in Roman times or by monks in the Middle Ages.

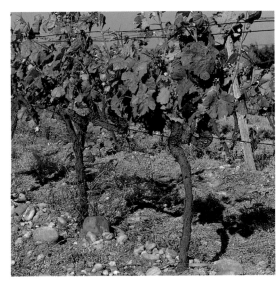
The soil of a vineyard treated with weedkillers is hard and lifeless. One can see how these useful plants have been burnt and withered by the chemicals.

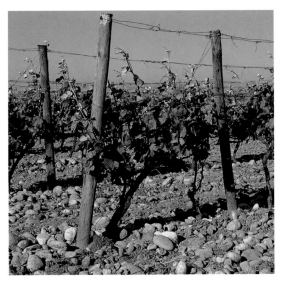
The soil of this organically tended vineyard was loosened despite the stony surface to encourage soil life and enable the vines to get more oxygen and moisture.

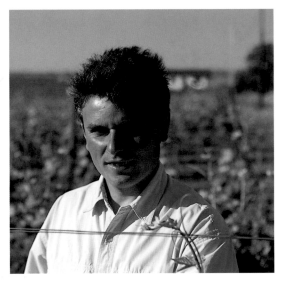
Laurent Combier is one of the most experienced organic wine growers in France. Even in difficult years, his Crozes-Hermitage has the optimum concentration.

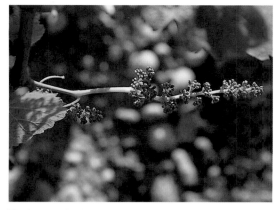

The harvest is already partly determined during the blossoming of the vine and formation of buds.

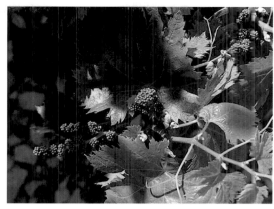

The Carignan grape which is widely found in southern France gives low yields, producing distinctive red wines.

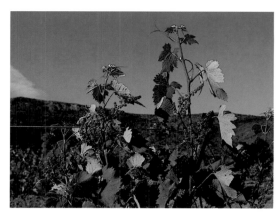

Young Syrah vine in Languedoc-Roussillon, the largest growing region in France for organic wines.

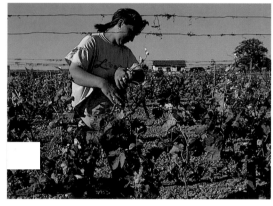

If the vines are grown on wire frames, the stems have to be carefully tied up.

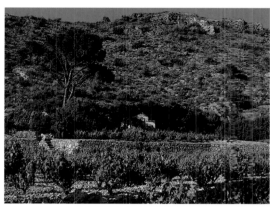

The barren countryside and dry, windy weather are a hindrance to natural wine growing in the South of France.

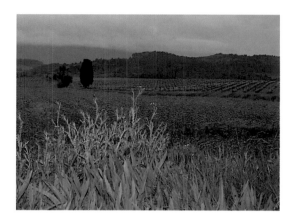

Vineyard of the Château de Caraguilhes in the Corbières region near Narbonne.

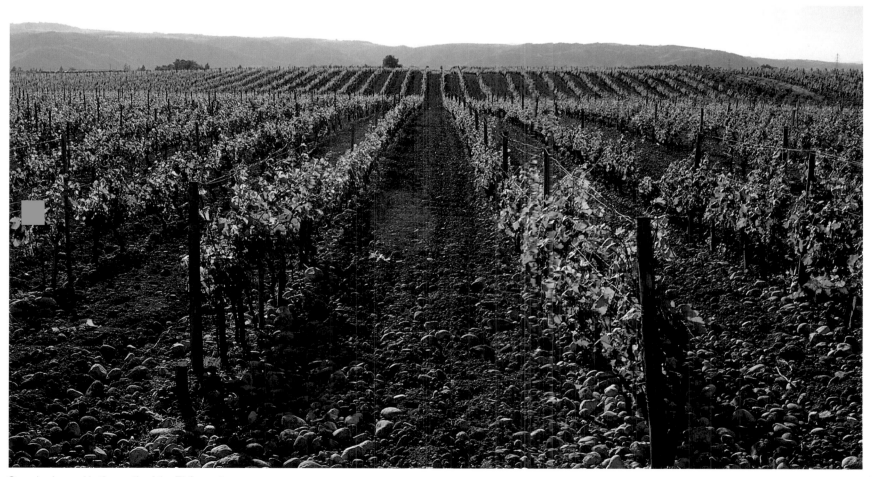

Organic vineyard in the north of the Rhône valley.

367

Climax and Decision-time

The Harvest

For every wine grower, the harvest is the most critical time of the year. It is only possible to be certain of the quality of the grapes once they have been gathered in. The size of the vintage when it comes to bottling is another matter. All the same, the harvest gives the producer cause for satisfaction or concern.

Even before the growth period begins, the weather has an effect on the grapes to be produced later on. A wet or dry winter is the first determining factor. The flowering season is a particularly delicate stage: unfavorable conditions can cause the flowers to be destroyed. And some of the latent fungal diseases and insect infestation can be encouraged or hindered, depending on the weather. Rain and dryness can accelerate or retard development, as can heat and cold. The more extreme the conditions, the more they leave their mark. Of course, biological management of the vineyards does have a moderating influence. A grassy vineyard necessarily has completely different water resources than one treated with weedkillers.

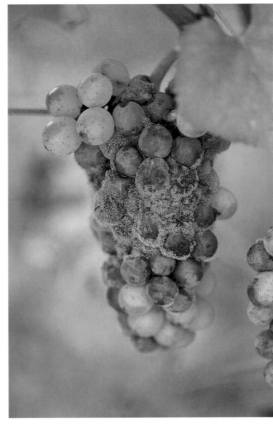

Riesling grapes with noble rot, which concentrates the natural sugar content and strengthens the flavor.

The more the grapes ripen, the more critical the situation becomes. The last few weeks have the greatest effect on the final quality. The aim is to bring in the grapes when they are at their optimum stage of ripeness. But what this means depends on the variety of grape and the type of wine the grower wants to produce. The higher the quality of wine he wants to make, the more is expected of nature and the greater the risk facing the producer. As the weather is changeable and creates the conditions for a good vintage more rarely or more frequently, depending on the region, the earlier work in the vineyard now pays off. A vine rooted deep in the living soil is less at risk from sudden weather extremes. If it only bears a moderate quantity of grapes, these will ripen better under adverse conditions than if they were on an overloaded vine nourished only by artificial fertilizers and planted in dead soil. Correct tending of the foliage also helps.

During ripening, the sugar content of the grapes gradually increases, and the acid decreases correspondingly. For every type of vine and every site there is an ideal balance to be struck, in order later to create balanced and intense-flavored wines. A high, aggressive acid content is to be avoided, as are juices with an excessive alcohol potential but only minimal acid levels. Even the

Below: What is the point of the grape harvest if you can't raise a glass to the quality of the new vintage?

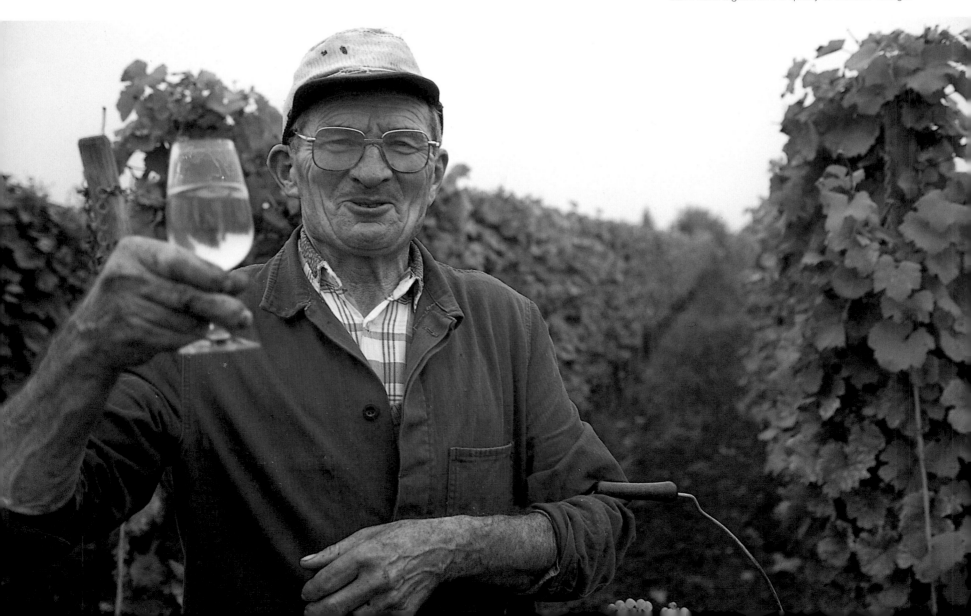

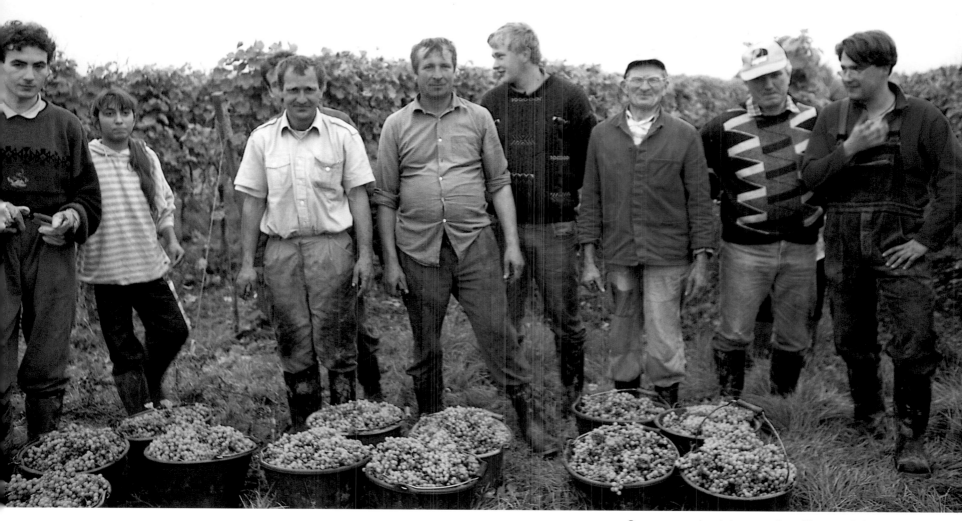

On many organic estates, a number of the same helpers gather together for the harvest almost every year.

extract plays a part and with red wines, the tannins have an effect. Some white grape varieties can be struck by noble rot, which draws water out of them and concentrates the sugar and flavoring substances. Although the grower can analyze these values and adapt his procedures accordingly, the timing of the harvest is still dependent on his objectives and intuition.

If he is lucky, the harvest will take place during dry weather. If a wine producer has gone to the trouble of cultivating active soil life, has tended the vines by tying, leaf-stripping or thinning out during the growth period, and is aiming to produce a wine of as high a quality as possible, he will want the grapes to be harvested by hand.

This is tiring work, and many people, preferably with plenty of experience, are needed. Picking by hand means it is possible to be selective in this final, all-important stage. Unripe grapes can be left on the vine, rotten grapes or ones affected by gray mold can be thrown out and any fruit not of the highest standard can be separated from the healthy, fully-ripened grapes. The grapes are therefore collected whole and undamaged in buckets and always transported to the cellar in small containers to prevent them being crushed and starting to oxidize. If the wine has to come up to a particularly high standard, the harvested fruit

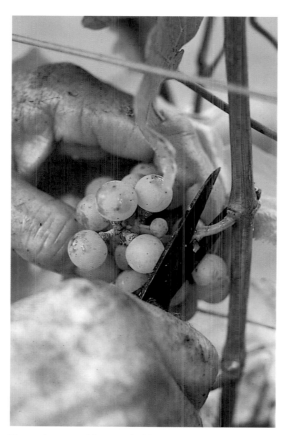

The cutters must be used with care, to avoid damage to either the vine or fingers.

is emptied out onto sorting tables before or in the producer's cellar. There, a team of people – on larger estates eight or ten people are often needed – carries out an additional, more rigorous selection to separate the best grapes from the less good ones.

In many wine producing regions nowadays, picking machines are used. It is true that they bring the grapes in quicker and that this can be of practical, and above all economic, benefit. However, picking machines cannot make the same careful selection the grape pickers can. And they certainly do not treat the grapes very gently. A vineyard which has been harvested by machine afterwards looks as if it has had a good beating. This is why quality-conscious and, in particular, organic wine growers keep to the more laborious but gentler manual method. It takes more time and labor and raises the cost of production, but it also guarantees a pure, unspoilt wine.

New Beginnings in Burgundy

The foundations for wine growing in the Burgundy region were laid by Cistercian monks in the Middle Ages. They discovered that the slopes between Dijon and Chalon, ideally suited to wine-growing, possessed an astonishing variety of soils wherever they looked – a result of their location in the foothills of the Alps, the edge of which had collapsed and been altered by the most varied influences such as erosion and melting ice. By taking account of other factors such as the altitude and microclimate, the monks developed a unique classification system: every hill slope which lent the wine growing there its special flavors was separated off, named, and its grapes pressed separately. This system of classification has been handed down to the present day. The wines based on this classification have fascinated wine lovers the world over, especially since the broad spectrum of flavors is achieved with just one black grape and one white grape variety: Pinot Noir and Chardonnay.

But in recent decades, even the Burgundy wine growers kept up with developments in the industry, sprayed pesticides, stopped plowing their vineyards, and employed large amounts of artificial fertilizers. At the same time, the Chardonnay grape and, to a lesser extent also the

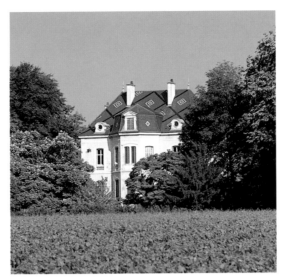

The Château of Comtes Lafon with its vineyard Clos de la Barre is the most famous estate in Meursault.

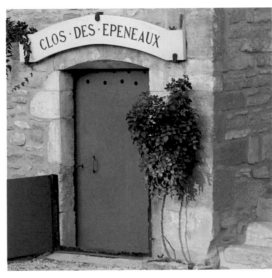

The Clos des Epeneaux in Pommard owes its rapid growth not least to its organic methods.

Pinot Noir, started to dominate the wine regions of the world. However, as these large, expensive plants were starting to fall out of favor on cost grounds, the Burgundy wine growers began to see things in a new light. And thanks to their vivid memories of traditional methods, thanks to old vintages still in existence, thanks to pioneering organic wine-growers like Jean-Claude Rateau, Alain Verdet and Emmanuel Giboulot and thanks to the discoveries of soil scientists like Claude Bourguignon and Yves Hérody, an astonishing new way of thinking developed. More and more wine producers understood the link between soil life and terroir flavor. Since then, they have made every effort to improve their soils again by gentle, considered means.

Amongst the first wine estates to switch to organic methods was Domaine de la Romanée-Conti, which produces the most famous red Burgundy of all. The changeover of the top estate, Domaine Leroy in Vosne-Romanée, to biological cultivation in 1988 caused a sensation. At the same time, the extensive experiments with the same method by the no less well-known Domaine Leflaive in Puligny-Montrachet aroused great interest.

And eventually, after such respected estates as Clos des Epeneaux in Pommard and Domaine des Comtes de Lafon in Meursault also introduced measures for revitalizing the soil by the use of compost, an association for compost production of which more than 80 of the most famous estates were members was formed in 1995. The estates mentioned above exemplify the changing trend in wine production in the Burgundy region. As is now generally accepted, a successful future for the great Burgundy wines lies with the organic vineyards.

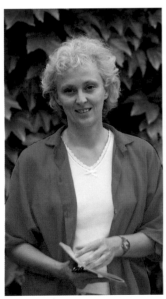

Anne-Claude Leflaive, Domaine Leflaive, Puligny-Montrachet, has been experimenting successfully with organic methods for years.

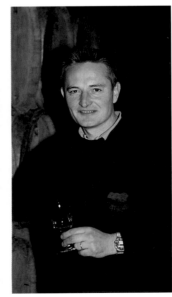

Dominique Lafon, Domaines des Comtes Lafon, Meursault, has brought the estate wines up to a superb quality.

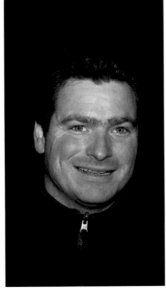

Pascal Marchand, director of Clos des Epeneaux, a Canadian by birth, creates top wines by organic cultivation.

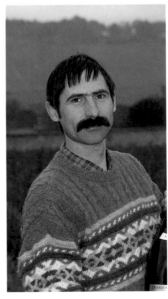

Jean-Claude Rateau, Beaune, sets an encouraging example as the pioneer of organic cultivation in Burgundy.

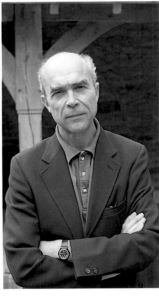

Aubert de Villaine, head of the world-famous Domaine de la Romanée-Conti, has been using organic methods for ten years.

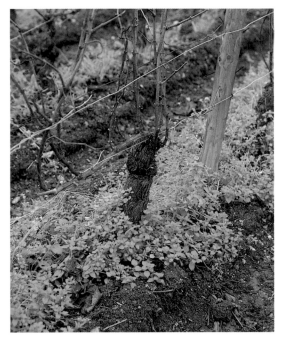

Clos des Mariages, Beaune: organic cultivation.

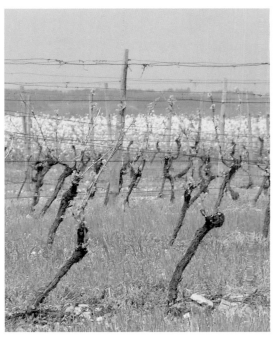

Grassing of a vineyard in the Hautes-Côtes.

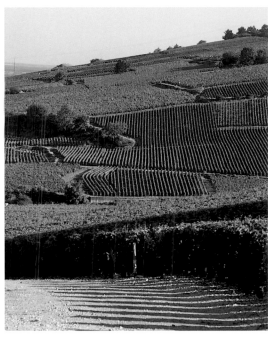

Vineyards near Vosne-Romanée.

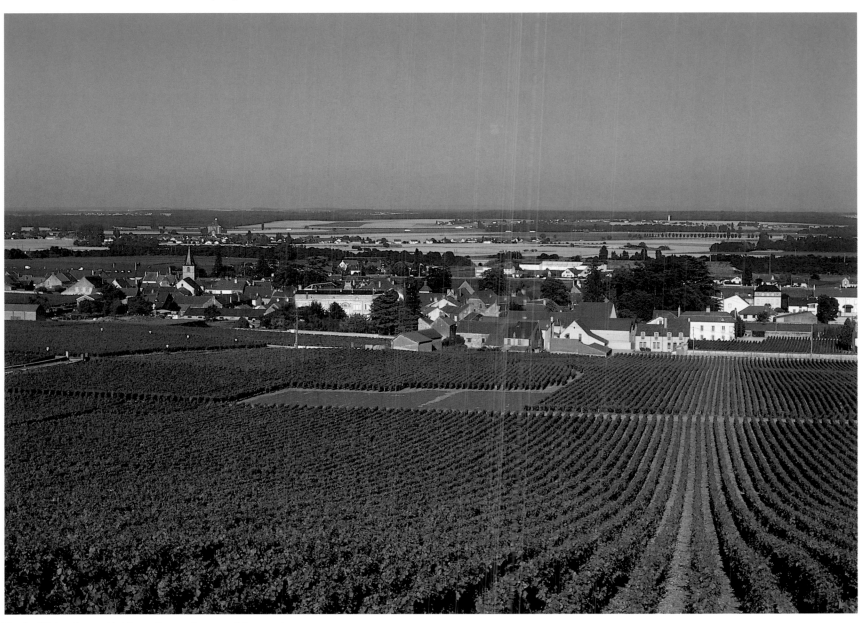

The La Tâche vineyard in Vosne-Romanée, one of the most famous organic vineyards in the world.

Mysterious Transformation

In the Wine Cellar

The quicker the freshly harvested grapes reach the cellar, the better. Now, the main aim is to preserve their quality of flavor undiminished. Oxygen is the greatest enemy. It immediately starts to affect the juice of any burst fruit by oxidizing it and high temperatures accelerate this process. Good wine producers and vintners do all they can to prevent this. Establishments, whether conventional or organic, which are aiming for high quality proceed very similarly in this respect. The differences in the cellar are much smaller than in outdoor cultivation.

White grapes are usually immediately separated from the stems and stalks, crushed and put in the press. The majority of the juice trickles out now, without any additional pressure, just from the sheer weight of the grapes. This free-run juice, as it is called, is the highest quality juice and is therefore stored in separate tanks. Next, during the pressing, stronger flavors from the skin and flesh of the grapes are incorporated in the juice, which are not very suitable for fine white wines.

With wine, most of the flavors develop during fermentation. Because of this, it is in the producer's interest for the juice to be as clean and pure in tone as possible. It is always better to take action at the juice stage than at the wine stage, for if unwanted nuances develop during the fermentation, they are often impossible to correct. Many producers therefore turn their whole attention to the juice, an approach which demands quick decisions and rapid action. It means, above all, that they have to continuously assess the sensory qualities of the juice from the moment it runs out of the press right up until fermentation. This means repeated smelling and sampling and continual testing, on the basis of their experience of past years, to ensure that the aromas are clean, clear, and free of bad overtones.

After pressing, the first step is the preliminary sedimentation. This can be achieved simply by leaving the juice to settle overnight and drawing it off in the morning. Settling of the solids on the bottom of the tank is encouraged by cold temperatures, which is why producers specializing in white wine are usually equipped with the appropriate technology. A further method of clarification used also by organic producers is fining, in which small quantities of gelatin are added to the juice. It binds the coarser particles and then sinks to the bottom. To soften the flavor of a juice strongly characterized by the flavor-dominating *Botrytis* (noble rot), carbon granules are used.

Many growers then start the fermentation with pure culture yeasts. Many ecological producers, as well as some top conventional producers, prefer the natural yeast found on grape skins and allow fermentation to take place spontaneously. However, this requires very healthy fruit. If, on the contrary, the fruit has been severely affected by rot, making a sharp preliminary sedimentation necessary, pure culture yeasts minimize the risk of the fermentation going wrong.

Nowadays, most producers are in a position to monitor the fermentation temperature and keep it at the desired level. With temperatures of between 64–72 °F (18–22 °C) for white wine, it is possible to achieve a longer fermentation period, which is of great significance for the ultimate quality of the wine. The longer the fermentation lasts, the more aromas develop and the more complex the wine becomes. Three weeks is a good fermentation period. Afterwards, young wines remain on yeast for a little longer. Here, careful preliminary sedimentation pays off again as the wine can now be kept in yeast storage for longer, which will improve the flavor. The producer again has to monitor the sensory qualities of the wine, using the most important tool in his cellar: the tasting glass.

If the wine was not fermented in small 60 gallon (225 liter) oak casks or "barriques," or if it does not have to be matured any further, it is drawn off from the fine yeast in November or December and filtered. It is then usually ready for bottling. Ecological producers avoid using clarifying agents. But even they use some sulfur to complete the production, as sulfur protects the wine during the critical phases. However, much smaller amounts are permitted in organic wines than in conventional wines. After bottling, which puts the wine under stress, it is allowed a rest period to ensure that it has a good flavor when it goes on sale.

Nevertheless, some of the highest quality wines in particular tend to be rather reserved to start with. But they make up for it by having the structure and strength to be able to mature and improve over several years.

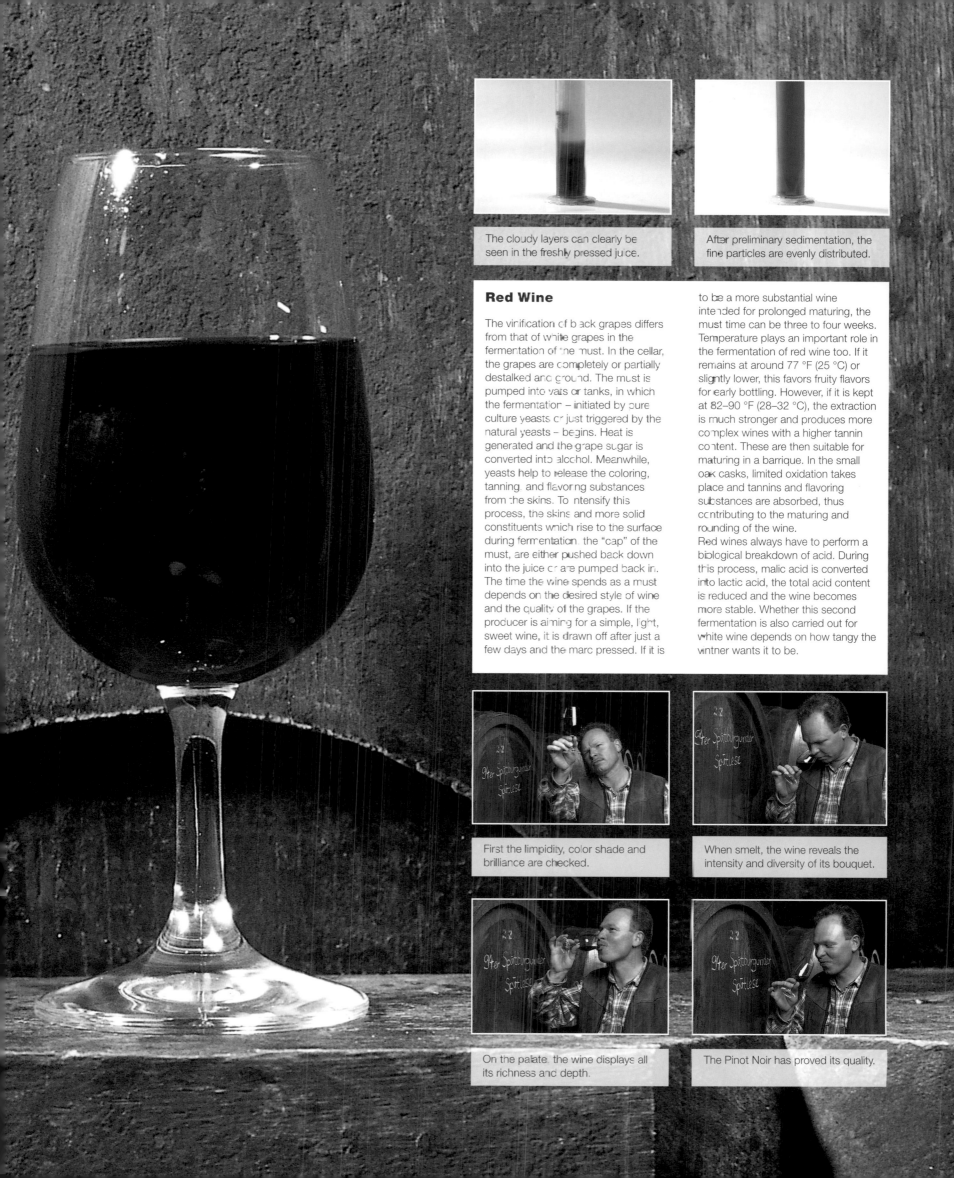

The cloudy layers can clearly be seen in the freshly pressed juice.

After preliminary sedimentation, the fine particles are evenly distributed.

Red Wine

The vinification of black grapes differs from that of white grapes in the fermentation of the must. In the cellar, the grapes are completely or partially destalked and ground. The must is pumped into vats or tanks, in which the fermentation – initiated by pure culture yeasts or just triggered by the natural yeasts – begins. Heat is generated and the grape sugar is converted into alcohol. Meanwhile, yeasts help to release the coloring, tanning, and flavoring substances from the skins. To intensify this process, the skins and more solid constituents which rise to the surface during fermentation, the "cap" of the must, are either pushed back down into the juice or are pumped back in. The time the wine spends as a must depends on the desired style of wine and the quality of the grapes. If the producer is aiming for a simple, light, sweet wine, it is drawn off after just a few days and the marc pressed. If it is to be a more substantial wine intended for prolonged maturing, the must time can be three to four weeks. Temperature plays an important role in the fermentation of red wine too. If it remains at around 77 °F (25 °C) or slightly lower, this favors fruity flavors for early bottling. However, if it is kept at 82–90 °F (28–32 °C), the extraction is much stronger and produces more complex wines with a higher tannin content. These are then suitable for maturing in a barrique. In the small oak casks, limited oxidation takes place and tannins and flavoring substances are absorbed, thus contributing to the maturing and rounding of the wine.

Red wines always have to perform a biological breakdown of acid. During this process, malic acid is converted into lactic acid, the total acid content is reduced and the wine becomes more stable. Whether this second fermentation is also carried out for white wine depends on how tangy the vintner wants it to be.

First the limpidity, color shade and brilliance are checked.

When smelt, the wine reveals the intensity and diversity of its bouquet.

On the palate, the wine displays all its richness and depth.

The Pinot Noir has proved its quality.

White Wines

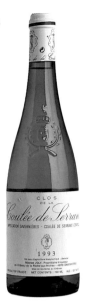

Nicolas Joly: Coulée de Serrant
Legendary, long-maturing Loire wine from the organically cultivated Chenin variety; extraordinary structure and complexity – one of France's greatest white wines.

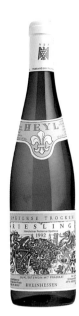

Heyl zu Herrnsheim: Rheinhessen Nierstein Spätlese
Isa and Peter von Weymarn, amongst the organic wine growing pioneers since 1978; great wines from famous sites. This is an exceptionally potent Riesling with a long finish, produced on red slate slopes.

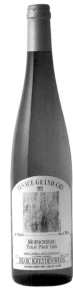

Marc Kreydenweiss: Alsace Grand Cru Moenchberg
Art-loving organic wine grower in Andlau, Alsace; this Tokay Pinot Gris impresses with its superb balance between sugar and acid, its elegance and exceptionally long finish.

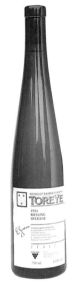

Rainer Eymann: Pfalz Riesling Spätlese
Exemplary organic grower from Gönnheim with a wide selection of convincing red and white wines such as this top Riesling: intense, ripe fruitiness, balanced, with a fine lingering sweetness.

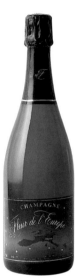

Fleury: Champagne Fleur de l'Europe
Hundred-year-old wine business switched over to organic methods by Jean-Pierre Fleury in 1989. First organic champagne produced in 1993; ripe, diverse bouquet, full flavor with elegant bouquet and long finish.

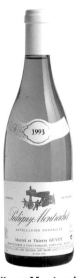

Thierry Guyot: Puligny-Montrachet
One of the pioneers of organic wine growing in Burgundy, Chardonnay wines only. This renowned village site gives a typically nutty, buttery, spicy nose and an excellent structure.

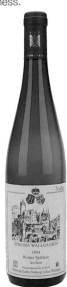

Graf von Kanitz: Rheingau Riesling Spätlese
Estate with slate slopes, has been using natural methods since the 14th century, organic since 1991, now run by Ralf Bengel. Fine fruity wine with discreetly lingering sweetness and elegant acidity.

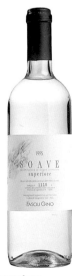

Fasoli: Soave Superiore
The Amadio brothers and Natalino Fasoli work with modern, ecological methods in Veneto; Soave based mainly on the Garganega variety: floral, with peach overtones, balanced and finely fruity.

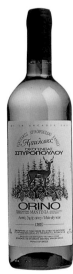

Spiropoulos: Orino
Important, ultra modern family estate in Mantineia, in the Peloponnese, turned to organic cultivation in 1993; single-variety Moshofilero: fresh, pleasant aromas of Granny Smith and aniseed.

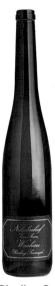

Nikolaihof: Wachau Riesling Smaragd
Christine and Nikolaus Saahs run this fascinating,
historic estate in Mautern, employing organic methods
in the vineyard and consciously traditional techniques in
the cellar; Smaragd is an outstanding example.

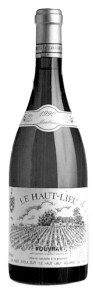

Domaine Huet: Vouvray Haut Lieu
Top ecological estate on the Loire run by Noël Finguet;
outstanding Chenin wines, both dry and sweet, like this
highly aromatic and elegant Vouvray.

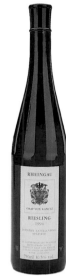

Schloss Wallhausen: Nahe Kerner Spätlese
The fact that Michael, Prince of Salm-Salm, President of
the Association of German Quality Wine Estates, has
gone over to ecological methods was a boost to
organic cultivation. This is an intensely fruity, full Kerner.

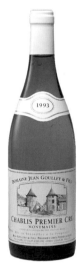

Jean Goulley: Chablis Premier Cru
Philippe Goulley and his wife Dominique use organic
methods on a fifth of the estate; this Montmain with a
complex, fruity mineral bouquet is well structured and
balanced.

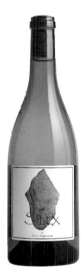

Didier Dagueneau: Pouilly Fumé Silex
Revolutionary wine grower from the Loire; he plows
plants very close together, thins out, and picks in three
or more stages. Silex is a landmark, one of the most
distinctive Sauvignon Blancs in the world.

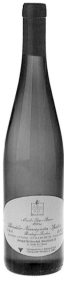

Steffens-Kess: Mosel Riesling Auslese Trocken
Harald Steffens and Marita Kess from the small town of
Reil specialize in Riesling; their Reil Goldlay is a dense,
concentrated, harmonious wine with a long finish and
good body.

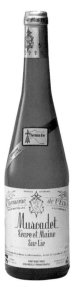

Domaine de l'Ecu: Muscadet Sèvre et Maine
The 42 acre (17 hectare) estate run by Guy Bossard
has been cultivating by organic means since 1975; its
excellent Muscadet is piquant, fresh, has fine yeast
tones and astonishing volume.

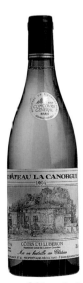

Château la Canorgue: Côtes du Luberon
Jean-Pierre and Martine Margan have worked
organically on their 185 acre (75 hectare) estate for
20 years; its rare, very successful white wine tastes
of lemon, fennel and Provence.

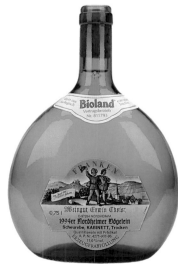

Erwin Christ: Franken Scheurebe Kabinett
The first wine estate in Franconia to produce organic
wine in 1964, now run by Ludwig Christ; very distinctive
wines; this one has an explosive black currant flavor and
earthy, mineral overtones.

Red Wines

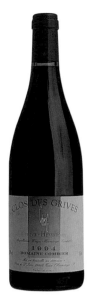

Laurent Combier: Crozes-Hermitage
With his Clos des Grives, a single variety Syrah, Laurent Combier works a miracle of aromatic diversity and depth each year; his parents were amongst the first organic fruit farmers.

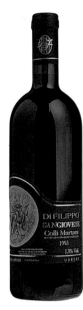

Di Filippo: Sangiovese Colli Martani
Roberto di Filippo, a qualified enologist, converted the Tuscan family estate to organic methods; this wine mixed with some Merlot and Barbera is exquisite, fruity, piquant, and elegant.

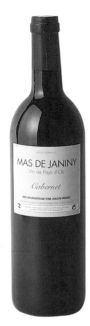

Mas de Janiny: Vin de Pays d'Oc Cabernet
The Julien brothers, organic growers also working on Domaine de Beau Séjour and Mas de Chinon, achieved great success with their Cabernet, which has a low yield: a mature, potent wine with attractive tannins.

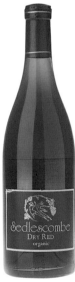

Sedlescombe Vineyard: Dry Red
Ray Cook and his wife Irma Hartmann produce ecological wines such as Rivaner and Bacchus in Sussex, England – but their dry red is also light, clean and fruity.

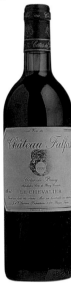

Château Falfas: Côtes de Bourg, Le Chevalier
John and Véronique Cochran have been cultivating their 54 acre (22 hectare) vineyard organically since 1988 and produce some convincing wines; this complex, marvelously structured 1990 vintage is simply outstanding.

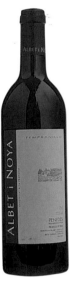

Albet i Noya: Penedès Tempranillo Col-lecció
Josep Albet i Noya, pioneer of organic wine growing in Spain, switched the Catalan family estate over to organic methods in 1980; strong vanilla and roasted tones from the barrique maturation with ripe berries.

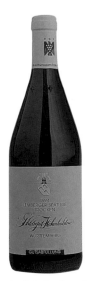

Schlossgut Hohenbeilstein: Lemberger Spätlese
Amongst his Württemberg white and red wines, Hartmann Dippon's dry Lemberger is a star; bouquet with fruity accents, fine aroma, elegant tannins, and long finish on the palate.

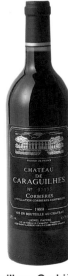

Château de Caraguilhes: Corbières
Castle estate out in the wilds; converted to organic methods by Lionel Faivre 35 years ago; 308 acres (125 hectares) of vineyards, good rosés and red wines; rounded, velvety and quite typical of Corbières after six years' aging.

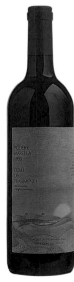

Podere Marella: Colli del Trasimeno
Fiammetta Inga produces very individual wines on her Umbrian estate near Lago Trasimeno; her exciting, challenging, profound, quality wine is based on Sangiovese and old Gamay.

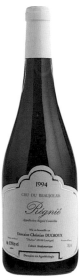

Christian Ducroux: Régnié
A pioneer in organic cultivation in the Beaujolais region; bottles some Beaujolais Nouveau, but the highly successful Cru Régnié is much rounder and juicier with a longer finish and fresh red berry aromas.

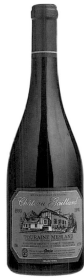

Château Gaillard: Touraine-Mesland
Vincent and Béatrice Girault use organic methods on their 69 acre (28 hectare) estate; in addition to aromatic white wines, they produce this typical red, fruity-accented Loire wine with a light character.

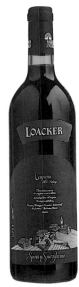

Rainer Loacker: Alto Adige Lagrein
Rainer Loacker produces Chardonnay, Sauvignon, Cabernet, and also Vernatsch and the typical South Tyrolean Lagrein organically on his estate near Bozen; fruity with a very fine bouquet.

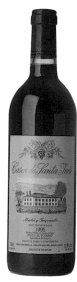

Casar de Santa Inès: Merlot y Tempranillo
Péres Caramés's red wine from Finca El Toleiro in the El Bierzo region of north west Spain surprises you with its clear, clean cherry tones, lovely harmony and good length of finish; an uncomplicated drink.

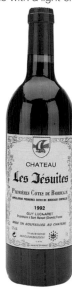

Château les Jésuites: Premières Côtes de Bordeaux
Guy Lucmaret tends 12 acres (5 hectares) of vineyards to the south east of Bordeaux, where Jesuits planted the first vines in the 17th century; plenty of Merlot; can be drunk early; ripe, clean fruit and typical character.

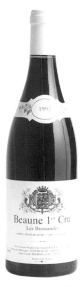

Jean-Claude Rateau: Beaune Premier Cru
This pioneer of organic wine cultivation has influenced many estates in Burgundy; Les Bressandes is his top wine, full of exquisite fruit, fine aroma, amazing finesse, and long finish.

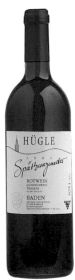

Kirchberghof: Baden Spätburgunder
The Hügle family converted their 30 acre (12 hectare) estate in 1986; specializes in Burgundy varieties; very attractive, intense, pure-toned Pinot Noir nose, clear fruit, discreet aroma, good structure, and finesse.

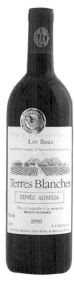

Terres Blanches: Les Baux-de-Provence
Noël Michelin has been cultivating his 86 acre (35 hectare) estate at the foot of the Alpilles organically since 1970; Cuvée Aurélia is a splendid, ripe, multi-layered wine with a powerful character.

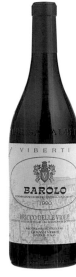

Viberti: Barolo Riserva
While his father Giovanni takes care of the trattoria, his enologist son Gian Luca is in charge of the organic work in the vineyard and producing fine wines; Barolo is smoky, mature, soft, sensual, and voluminous.

Traditions

When the mules loosen the soil between the old gnarled vines and the laborer uses his skill and strength to make sure that the plowshare turns the furrows correctly, it feels as if one has been transported back to a different age.

In fact it is true that nothing has actually changed in the vineyards of the mountain village of Villaviciosa de Córdoba for many years – apart from the opinions of the bodeguero. He has recognized that the only chance of safeguarding the future of the wine region situated in the wild Sierra Morena, one-and-a-half hours by car from Córdoba, lies in organic cultivation. For this region was too insignificant and too remote for it to be allocated one of the official descriptions of origin or even to be given one of its own.

The vines planted decades ago still stand higgledy-piggledy, as in earlier times the producer determined the grape blend by the mix of varieties in the vineyard. Three-fifths of the vines are of the Airén variety, also known as Lairén. It originates from La Mancha and dominates one third of the entire Spanish wine-growing area. It likes the chalky soil of the Sierra and tolerates the sometimes extreme heat and dryness well.

Combined with the Airén grapes are equal parts of Palomino Fino and Pedro Ximinez. The first is known as the sherry variety. It likes chalky ground and gives fairly high yields. The second is predominant in Montilla-Moriles, sherry's rival in the southern part of the province of Córdoba, but it is also used in sweet Málaga and is very reliable. So the vineyards of Villaviciosa bring together the three most important varieties in southern Spain.

In the extreme climate of the high-altitude Sierra, where it is bitterly cold in winter but can be over 104 °F (40 °C) in summer and where it seldom rains even once during the vine's growth period, the vines virtually never suffer from disease. The vineyards nestle between woods of holm oaks and pine trees and barren slopes where large herds used to be kept. Few of these remain today, although flocks of sheep graze between the vines in winter and provide natural manure. Alternatively, the ground is sown with lupins to improve the soil, following the old tradition. They accumulate nitrogen and are plowed into the soil as fertilizer in the spring.

The wine growers here recognized that traditional wine cultivation with its old processing methods was actually ecologically sound – they just had to continue in the traditional way.

The old vines bear only small amounts of healthy, golden grapes with very high sugar levels, from which a unique wine is produced. Modern chemistry could, no doubt, improve yields in the short term, but in the long term would actually destroy the special richness of this wine region.

In organic wine growing, producers often have to deny their instincts as far as quantity is concerned. But they are amply rewarded by the quality of the wine, and only this can guarantee continued business success in the long term too.

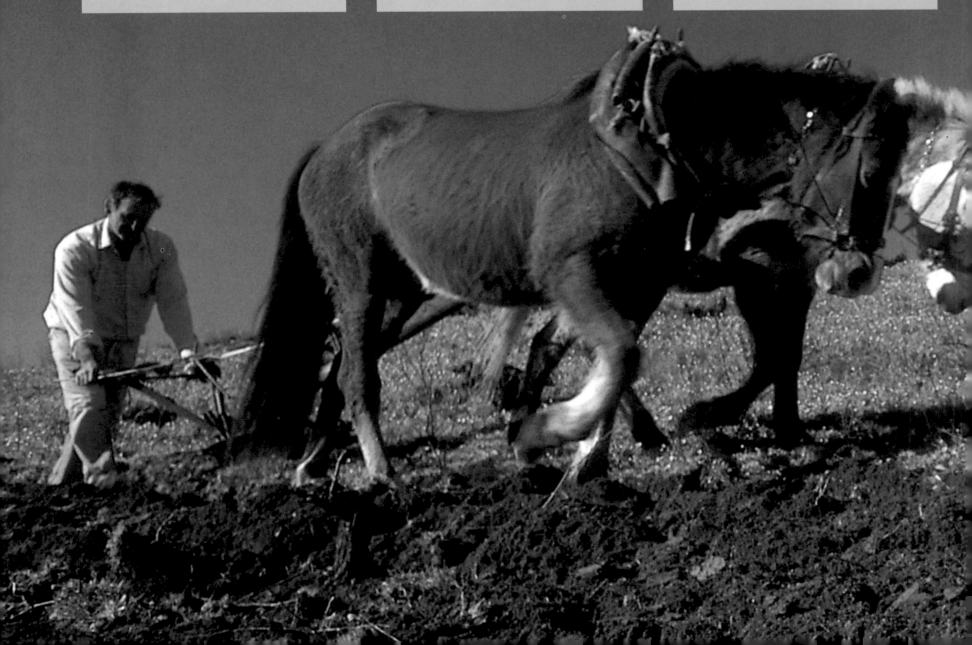

Fine Flor in Amphoras

Sweet Wine

The harvest falls in September. The hand-picked grapes are carted to the bodega and tipped through the funnel into a continuous press. They then go into large high-grade steel tanks where they ferment right out over about 20 days at a maximum temperature of 72 °F (22 °C). Even in Villaviciosa, producers know how to take advantage of modern technology. Until the early summer, the young wines remain in the steel tanks, well protected against oxidation. The wines of the Sierra Morena differ from sherry in that they achieve the necessary 15 percent proof thanks to their natural grape sugar content and do not have to have additional distilled alcohol added. For the next stage, the young wines are transferred to tinajas. These amphoras made of clay or, nowadays, often concrete with a narrow opening at the top, are large enough to hold 800 gallons (3,000 liters). They stand in a drafty cellar which is kept cool and damp.

During the summer, the miracle now occurs by which Fino, the finest sherry, is also produced. The flor, a layer of cotton wool-like yeast mold, grows on the surface of the wine. The bodeguero carefully watches it develop, as this determines the classification of the wines. He will only let the wine stay in the tinajas for a further one to two years if there is a large amount of flor forming a dense, protective layer on the surface.

The wine is then poured into the solera. Unlike table wines, this southern Spanish system of maturing strong or fortified wines does not aim to preserve the particular character of the vintage, but to cancel it out in favor of the overall character of the wine. The solera for Pálido, as the Sierra Morena Fino variety is called, consists of four rows of 126 gallon (480 liter) casks containing wines of different ages. Twice a year, some of the wine is drawn off only from the oldest cask which stands on the suelo, the ground. The amount removed is made up with wine from the next oldest row or criadera. So the casks are topped up row by row and the young wine from the tinajas is poured into the youngest, uppermost row. The older wines can there-

fore influence the younger wines, and the solera retains its character.

With Pálido, the flor remains the decisive factor, as it gives the wine an exquisite flavor of yeast and nuts and a wonderful freshness. This is why it tastes best direct from the cask. Once it is bottled, usually after four years in the solera, it loses its extra special something within several months, just as Fino does. For this reason, it should not be stored for long and, once opened, should be kept cool and consumed within a short time.

However, if the wine has less flor and stronger accents in the cask, the cellarer transfers it to a second cask, the Dorado solera, which has one criadera more. Dorado is similar to dry Amontillado, which is based on matured and developed Finos. After a further five years' maturing, the wine comes shimmering out of the bottle, the color of old gold, a multi-layered, hugely aromatic drink with hints of walnut and hazelnut, dried fruits and pepper. It can be served as an aperitif, sipped with rich tapas, or enjoyed as a digestive.

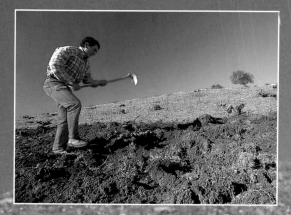

The vines are weeded with the hoe and by hand after plowing.

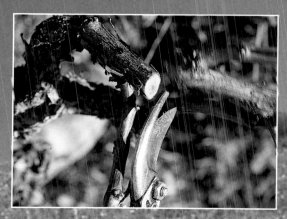

in winter, the vines have to be pruned. This requires considerable experience and precision.

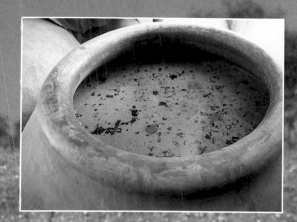

The protective, flavor-generating yeast flor forms on the young wine in tinajas or huge amphoras.

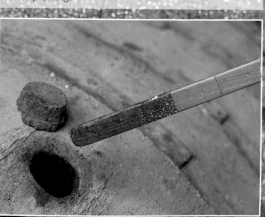

An ancient and proven method: the bodeguero tests the liquid level in the cask with a stick.

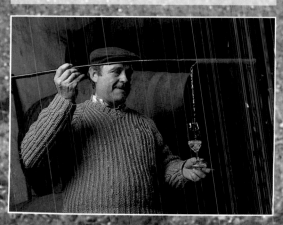

Samples are drawn from the casks and poured into glasses using a special instrument called a venencia.

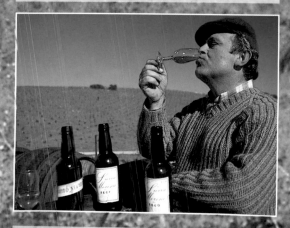

Gabriel Gómez enjoys tasting his superb, dry aperitif wines.

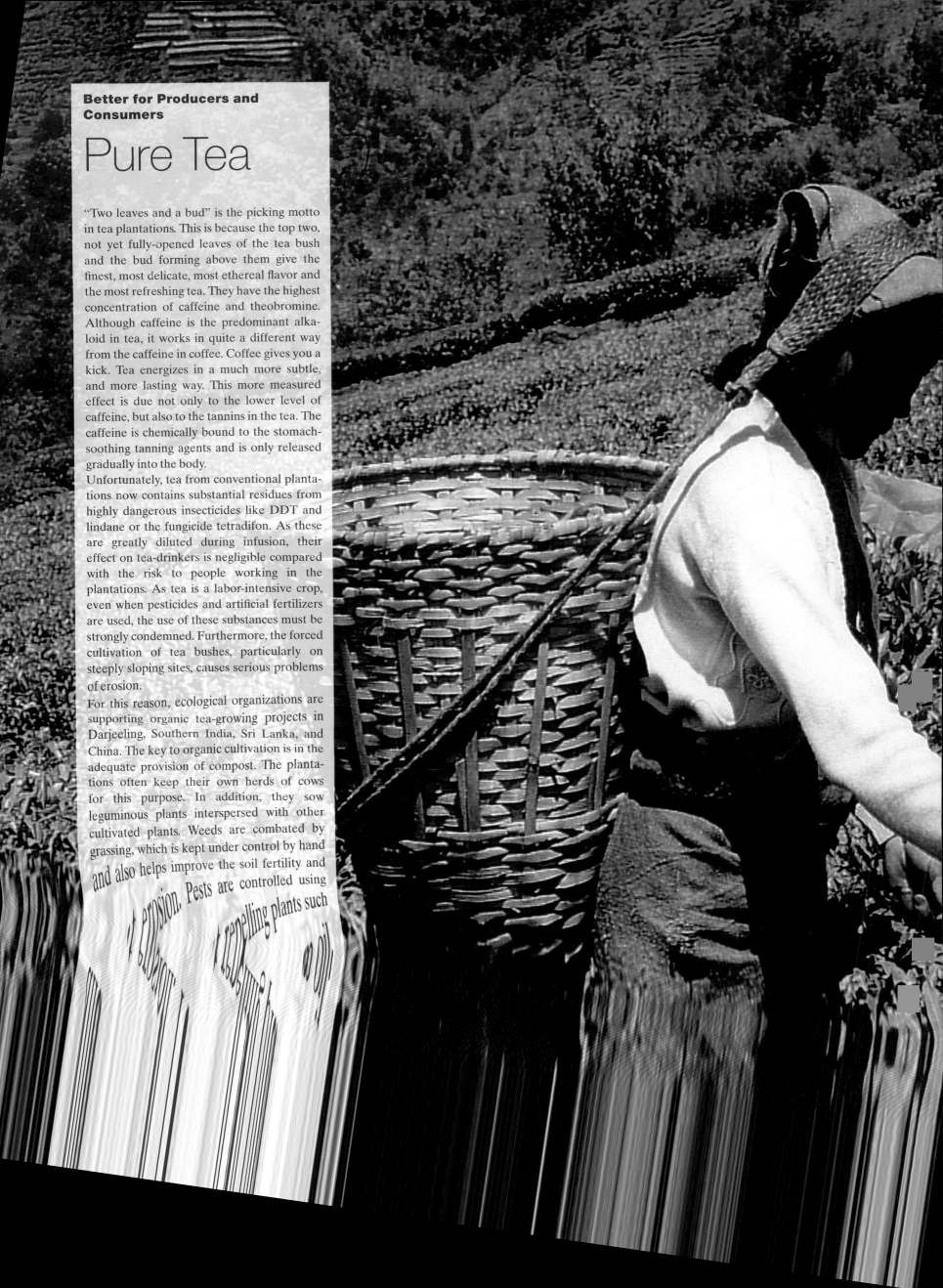

Better for Producers and Consumers

Pure Tea

"Two leaves and a bud" is the picking motto in tea plantations. This is because the top two, not yet fully-opened leaves of the tea bush and the bud forming above them give the finest, most delicate, most ethereal flavor and the most refreshing tea. They have the highest concentration of caffeine and theobromine. Although caffeine is the predominant alkaloid in tea, it works in quite a different way from the caffeine in coffee. Coffee gives you a kick. Tea energizes in a much more subtle, and more lasting way. This more measured effect is due not only to the lower level of caffeine, but also to the tannins in the tea. The caffeine is chemically bound to the stomach-soothing tanning agents and is only released gradually into the body.

Unfortunately, tea from conventional plantations now contains substantial residues from highly dangerous insecticides like DDT and lindane or the fungicide tetradifon. As these are greatly diluted during infusion, their effect on tea-drinkers is negligible compared with the risk to people working in the plantations. As tea is a labor-intensive crop, even when pesticides and artificial fertilizers are used, the use of these substances must be strongly condemned. Furthermore, the forced cultivation of tea bushes, particularly on steeply sloping sites, causes serious problems of erosion.

For this reason, ecological organizations are supporting organic tea-growing projects in Darjeeling, Southern India, Sri Lanka, and China. The key to organic cultivation is in the adequate provision of compost. The plantations often keep their own herds of cows for this purpose. In addition, they sow leguminous plants interspersed with other cultivated plants. Weeds are combated by grassing, which is kept under control by hand and also helps improve the soil fertility and ... erosion. Pests are controlled using ... repelling plants such ...

Fine Flor in Amphoras

Sweet Wine

The harvest falls in September. The hand-picked grapes are carted to the bodega and tipped through the funnel into a continuous press. They then go into large high-grade steel tanks where they ferment right out over about 20 days at a maximum temperature of 72 °F (22 °C). Even in Villaviciosa, producers know how to take advantage of modern technology. Until the early summer, the young wines remain in the steel tanks, well protected against oxidation. The wines of the Sierra Morena differ from sherry in that they achieve the necessary 15 percent proof thanks to their natural grape sugar content and do not have to have additional distilled alcohol added. For the next stage, the young wines are transferred to tinajas. These amphoras made of clay or, nowadays, often concrete with a narrow opening at the top, are large enough to hold 800 gallons (3,000 liters). They stand in a drafty cellar which is kept cool and damp.

During the summer, the miracle now occurs by which Fino, the finest sherry, is also produced. The flor, a layer of cotton wool-like yeast mold, grows on the surface of the wine. The bodeguero carefully watches it develop, as this determines the classification of the wines. He will only let the wine stay in the tinajas for a further one to two years if there is a large amount of flor forming a dense, protective layer on the surface.

The wine is then poured into the solera. Unlike table wines, this southern Spanish system of maturing strong or fortified wines does not aim to preserve the particular character of the vintage, but to cancel it out in favor of the overall character of the wine. The solera for Pálido, as the Sierra Morena Fino variety is called, consists of four rows of 126 gallon (480 liter) casks containing wines of different ages. Twice a year, some of the wine is drawn off only from the oldest cask which stands on the suelo, the ground. The amount removed is made up with wine from the next oldest row or criadera. So the casks are topped up row by row and the young wine from the tinajas is poured into the youngest, uppermost row. The older wines can there-

fore influence the younger wines, and the solera retains its character.

With Pálido, the flor remains the decisive factor, as it gives the wine an exquisite flavor of yeast and nuts and a wonderful freshness. This is why it tastes best direct from the cask. Once it is bottled, usually after four years in the solera, it loses its extra special something within several months, just as Fino does. For this reason, it should not be stored for long and, once opened, should be kept cool and consumed within a short time.

However, if the wine has less flor and stronger accents in the cask, the cellarer transfers it to a second cask, the Dorado solera, which has one criadera more. Dorado is similar to dry Amontillado, which is based on matured and developed Finos. After a further five years' maturing, the wine comes shimmering out of the bottle, the color of old gold, a multi-layered, hugely aromatic drink with hints of walnut and hazelnut, dried fruits and pepper. It can be served as an aperitif, sipped with rich tapas, or enjoyed as a digestive.

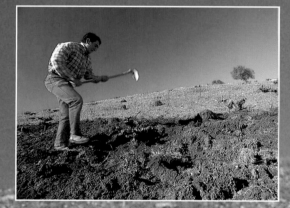
The vines are weeded with the hoe and by hand after plowing.

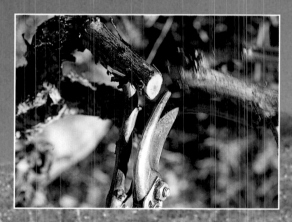
In winter, the vines have to be pruned. This requires considerable experience and precision.

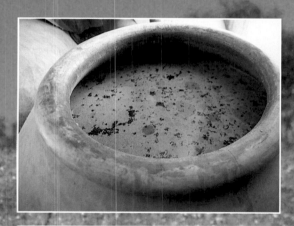
The protective, flavor-generating yeast flor forms on the young wine in tinajas or huge amphoras.

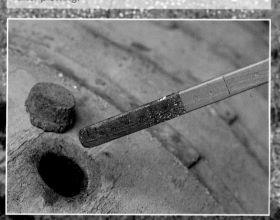
An ancient and proven method: the bodeguero tests the liquid level in the cask with a stick.

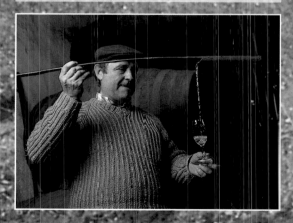
Samples are drawn from the casks and poured into glasses using a special instrument called a venencia.

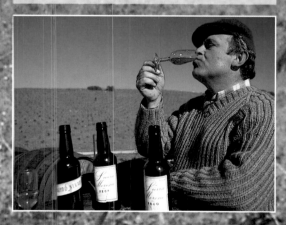
Gabriel Gómez enjoys tasting his superb, dry aperitif wines.

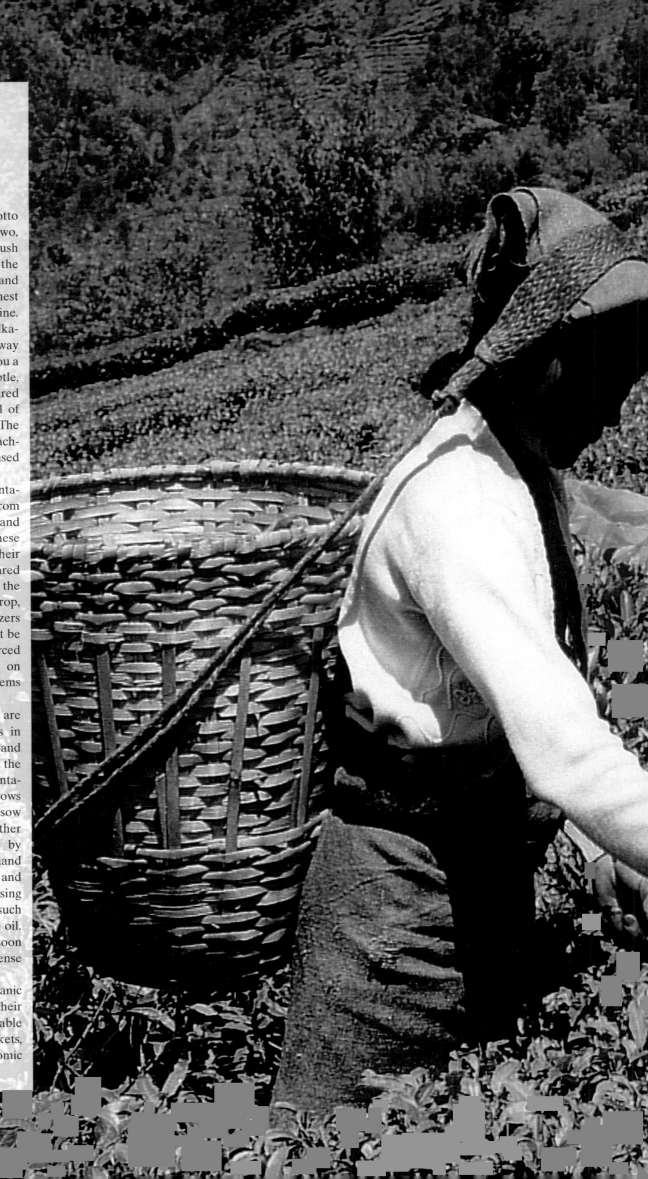

Better for Producers and Consumers

Pure Tea

"Two leaves and a bud" is the picking motto in tea plantations. This is because the top two, not yet fully-opened leaves of the tea bush and the bud forming above them give the finest, most delicate, most ethereal flavor and the most refreshing tea. They have the highest concentration of caffeine and theobromine. Although caffeine is the predominant alkaloid in tea, it works in quite a different way from the caffeine in coffee. Coffee gives you a kick. Tea energizes in a much more subtle, and more lasting way. This more measured effect is due not only to the lower level of caffeine, but also to the tannins in the tea. The caffeine is chemically bound to the stomach-soothing tanning agents and is only released gradually into the body.

Unfortunately, tea from conventional plantations now contains substantial residues from highly dangerous insecticides like DDT and lindane or the fungicide tetradifon. As these are greatly diluted during infusion, their effect on tea-drinkers is negligible compared with the risk to people working in the plantations. As tea is a labor-intensive crop, even when pesticides and artificial fertilizers are used, the use of these substances must be strongly condemned. Furthermore, the forced cultivation of tea bushes, particularly on steeply sloping sites, causes serious problems of erosion.

For this reason, ecological organizations are supporting organic tea-growing projects in Darjeeling, Southern India, Sri Lanka, and China. The key to organic cultivation is in the adequate provision of compost. The plantations often keep their own herds of cows for this purpose. In addition, they sow leguminous plants interspersed with other cultivated plants. Weeds are combated by grassing, which is kept under control by hand and also helps improve the soil fertility and prevent erosion. Pests are controlled using beneficial insects, insect-repelling plants such as lemon grass or, in India, organic neem oil. After the switchover phase, the tea very soon gains a higher quality and more intense flavors.

The sales structure also differs. Organic plantations usually deliver direct to their customers. This avoids the often considerable price fluctuations on the official tea markets, which significantly improves the economic and social situation of the producers.

Coffee Substitutes

Ersatz coffee and the like were used as a substitute even back in the last century by all those coffee lovers who could not afford, obtain, or tolerate the black drink. In order to avoid the caffeine, but not the taste, healthy eating fans have turned to the burnt substitute. Apart from chicory, which is produced from the roots of a chicory plant, and substitute coffee made from dandelion roots, ersatz coffees are mainly cereal-based. The most well known of these is malt coffee from malted, roasted barley. Other cereal

coffees are based on barley and rye, but are smoothed with chicory, dandelion, acorn meal figs, and other plant additives. To reproduce the flavor of the original stimulant drink as exactly as possible, the basic ingredients are strongly roasted, usually more strongly than coffee beans. And, even with organic production, this is the heart of the problem, as roasting, like broiling, can result in benzpyrene being produced which is known to be carcinogenic.

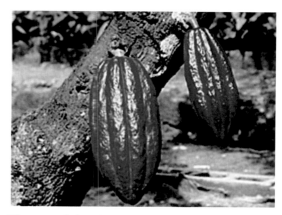

The cacao fruits, which are often the size of melons, grow directly out of the trunk or the main branches of the cacao tree.

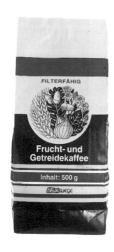

A coffee substitute made from fruits and cereals, suitable for filter use.

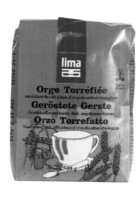

Roasted barley – the basis of many coffee substitutes.

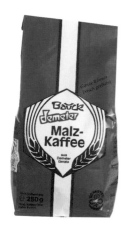

Malted barley forms the basis of this malt coffee.

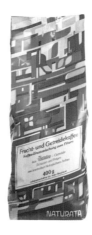

Chicory, figs, and cereal – another fruit and cereal coffee.

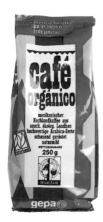

High-quality, naturally mild Arabica coffee cultivated organically.

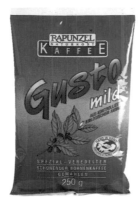

A refined, gently roasted bean coffee produced by controlled cultivation.

Tropical Powder: Cocoa

Organic cocoa is still a rarity. The most interesting project was carried out in the lowlands of Bolivia, on the banks of the Alto Beni. 800 families were relocated there from the Andean highlands, to give them a better chance of supporting themselves. They started by planting cacao and in 1977 formed a cooperative. From 1987 onwards, members began switching over to organic cultivation. Now the cocoa is produced in the growers' own factory in La Paz. This is an enormous advantage, not only from a financial, but also from an ecological point of view. Apart from the pesticides which are used in large quantities in conventional cultivation, the reason cocoa is so harmful is that the beans, which can easily go moldy or attract insects, are gassed with highly toxic chemicals for the long journey to Europe, and these can leave traces in the cocoa powder. Cocoa drinks available as instant powders – and mainly intended for consumption by children, are also a potential risk to health, as they mostly consist of factory sugar (see p. 242).

The evergreen cacao tree can grow up to 26 feet (8 meters) in height. Its reddish flowers are surprisingly small compared with the large melon or cucumber-like red to yellow fruits which grow directly from the trunk or main branches of the tree. Although the trees like hot temperatures and plenty of moisture, which is why they only thrive in the hottest tropical regions, they are damaged by direct sunlight, particularly when young. At that time, they need the shade provided by surrounding trees. A tree has to be almost ten years old before it really starts to bear fruit. The fruit ripen at different rates and are picked at six week intervals. Below the tough, semi hard, ribbed shell is the sugary flesh which surrounds the cocoa beans. After picking, the fruits are smashed open, the seeds removed and put into boxes, where the fruit pulp surrounding them ferments. The heat of fermentation causes the first flavoring substances to form. The beans are then dried to produce the raw cocoa. To make it into cocoa powder, it is first roasted. After shelling and grinding, a paste-like cocoa mass is produced. The cocoa butter is pressed, then the press cake is ground and sieved. The dark but mild lightly oil-extracted cocoa powder with at least 20 percent fat is used for drinks, whilst the strongly oil-extracted lighter colored powder with a minimum of 8 percent fat is used for cakes and desserts.

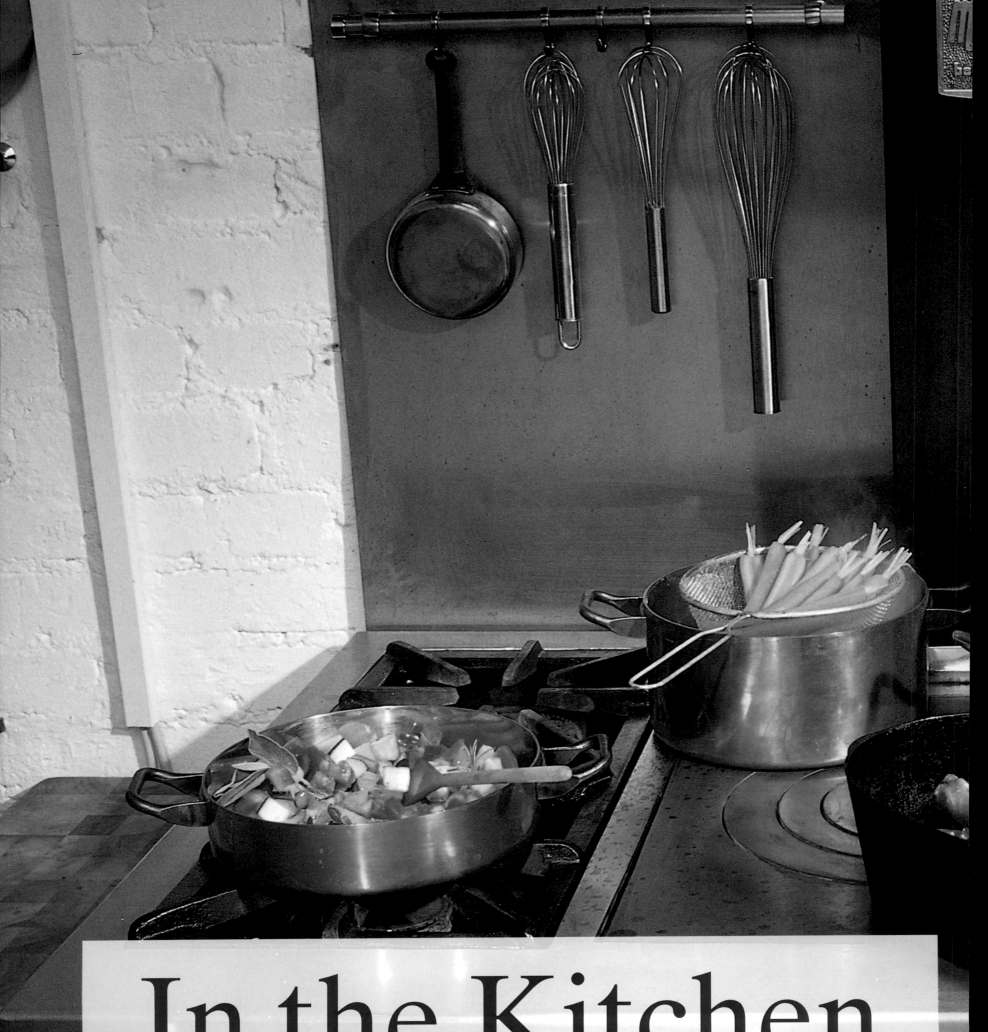

In the Kitchen

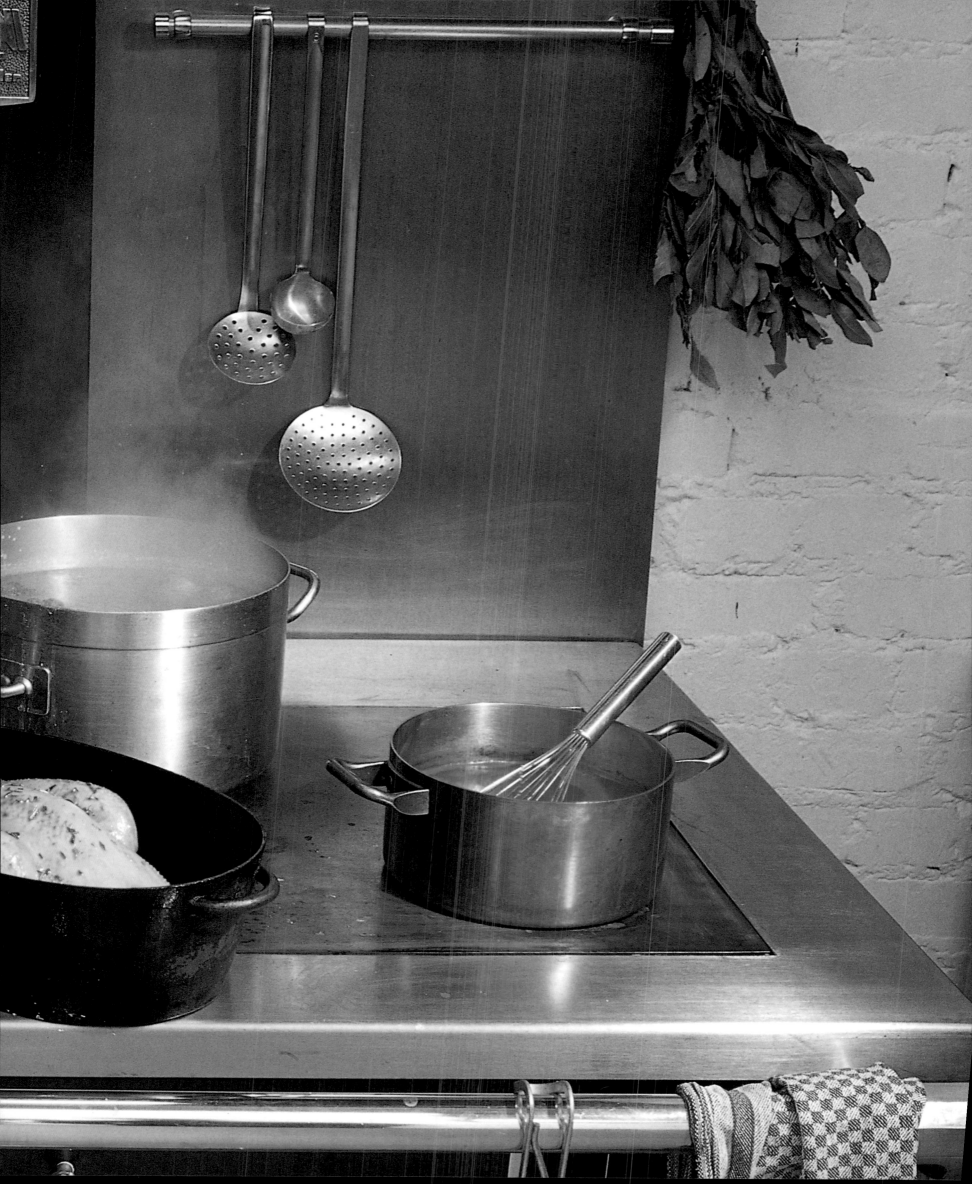

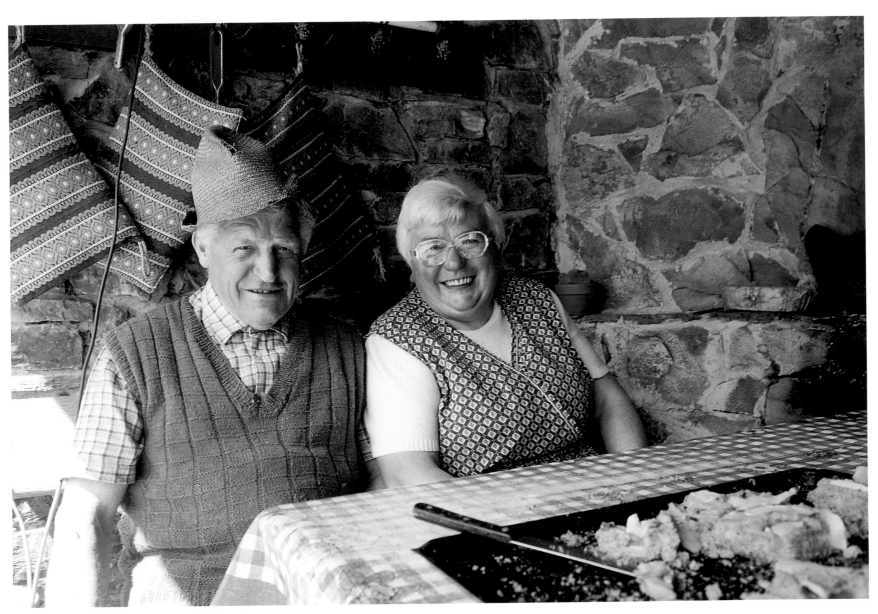

Mealtimes around the kitchen table have always been at the center of family life.

Previous double page: Numerous utensils are needed when working at the stove – the focal point of any kitchen.

What is the point in using organically produced foods if they are not stored or handled correctly? Fresh fruits and vegetables can lose a large proportion of their vital constituents if they are even washed wrongly, and excessively high cooking temperatures can produce drastic changes in the most important nutrients. It is advisable to find out about the different cooking methods and their effect on foodstuffs. Simple implements which do not run on electricity can be used for preparing and processing foods. They also transform raw foods into attractive and decorative shapes, as it is well known that the enjoyment of food also depends greatly on its appearance.

In the kitchen viewed as a living space, the organic way of thinking is starting to become accepted on various different levels. People are beginning to sort their waste material and compost a lot of it. Kitchen furniture is increasingly made from ecologically sound materials. Plastic-coated chipboard, once so popular, is becoming a thing of the past. It has long been recognized that it contains and gives off the allergenic and allegedly carcinogenic formaldehyde. More and more carpenters and furniture stores are offering furniture which is environmentally friendly in terms of the method of manufacture and in everyday use, since no dangerous solvents or pesticides have been used. "Sustainable" is the new catchphrase. In order to earn this description, a product has to meet seven criteria: it must be produced with the minimum resources and minimum emissions, must be durable, must not produce emissions during use, must be repairable, spare parts/accessories must be available, it must be recyclable after use, and must be able to be disposed of without harming the environment. Anyone concerned about quality in general and quality of life in particular will welcome the fact that durability is included as an important criterion. The home atmosphere will ultimately be one of wholeness, and the kitchen will gain character thanks to its enduring and reliable furniture and equipment.

Kitchen Utensils

The significance of the kitchen and the amount of time spent there are greater for some people than for others. However, anyone who is interested in food, whether for reasons of health or taste or both, sees the kitchen as being of great importance. The focal point of the kitchen is the stove which, in the past, was at the center of every household. Numerous useful implements are needed for working in the kitchen. When choosing utensils it makes sense to look at them from an ecological point of view. Whether it is a question of the oven itself, or whether you are choosing devices like mixers or beaters, grinders (see p. 34) or slicers (see p. 33), food processors or stirrers, juice and garlic presses, pots and pans, kettles, knives, forks, spoons, brushes, graters, or other implements, it is worthwhile thinking about the material used, the surface treatment, the method of production, the amount of energy required for the manufacture, and, in everyday use, the place of manufacture, the durability, the repairability, and recyclability. Professional cooks rightly prefer to use high-grade steel equipment as there is no shortage of resources, unlike non ferrous metals. Steel is easy to clean and look after and, unlike aluminum, is produced using little energy and with little waste. Steel does not wear thin like enamel, does not rust like cast iron, does not break like glass or ceramics, and is extremely long-lasting.

Careful Preparation

Fruits and vegetables should be consumed raw whenever possible in order to benefit from the important vital substances rather than destroying them. But even with raw food, some substances are lost just by washing, particularly the very delicate vitamins C, B1, E, and folic acid. As water is the main enemy of these vital substances, fruit and vegetables should be cleaned with a vegetable brush or
• rinsed as rapidly and as cold as possible under running water;
• washed before peeling and chopping;
• never be left in a water bath.
More vital substances are lost when fruit and vegetables are peeled. Foods should not be chopped until just before cooking or consumption, to prevent oxidation by the oxygen in the air. It is also important not to chop them smaller than is absolutely necessary, since the smaller the fruit and vegetables are chopped, the greater the loss during cooking.

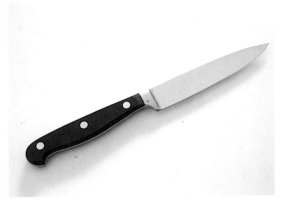
Kitchen knife

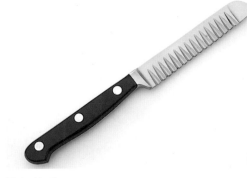
Fluted knife

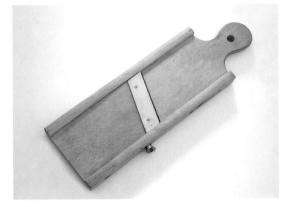
Vegetable slicer

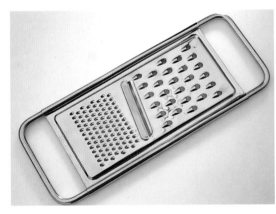
Multi purpose grater

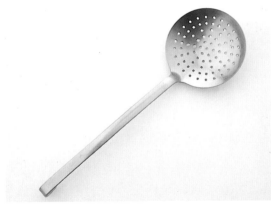
Skimmer

Plastic chopping board

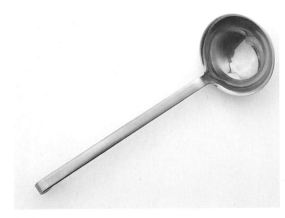
Ladle

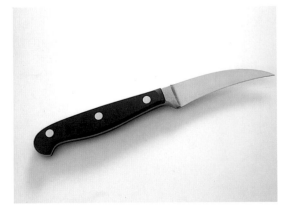
Paring knife

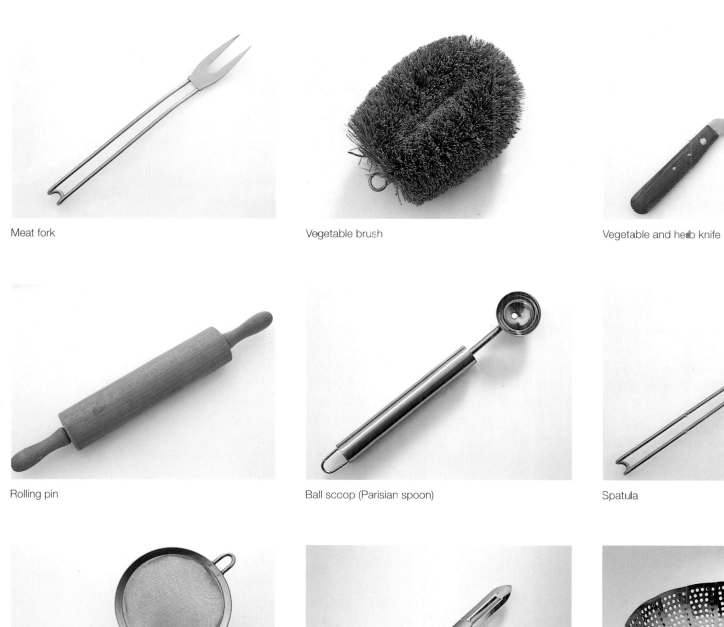

Meat fork

Vegetable brush

Vegetable and herb knife

Rolling pin

Ball scoop (Parisian spoon)

Spatula

Sieve

Thin-cutting peeler

Steamer

Chopping board

Carving knife

Zester or Julienne shredder

Basic Methods

It is a pleasure to prepare fresh, healthy fruit and vegetables full of vital substances ready for use in a chosen recipe. Anyone interested in organic nutrition will want to pay particular attention to the preparation and put a little more effort into it. As the skin contains a lot of goodness, fruit and vegetables should only be peeled very thinly, if at all. Attractively presented raw products appeal to the eye and whet the appetite.

Ecological Kitchen Furniture

Anyone who uses organic foods, which have to meet high environmental standards, should also pay attention to the materials used in the kitchen furnishings. An excellent raw material for kitchens is solid wood, which should come from sustainable forests. More and more forests planted and tended by organic methods are being established. Local woods are preferable because they do not have to travel such a distance. Apart from the soft woods, pine and spruce, other woods now gaining in popularity for kitchen furnishings are beech, birch, and cherry. Tropical woods should be avoided at all costs.

The wood itself must have been treated organically, in other words, without using wood preservatives, which may contain formaldehyde, pentachloro-phenol, or heavy metal compounds. The surface treatment should only use solvent-free natural substances which let the wood breathe, and synthetic paints and lacquers which contain harmful chemicals should be avoided. But wood is not the only material suitable for using in kitchens. Polished natural stone is also possible for the work surfaces. As far as plastics are concerned, PE (polyethylene) and PP (polypropylene) are acceptable, but PVC (polyvinyl chloride) is not. Furniture should, if possible, only contain one type of plastic, to make it easier to recycle. Coatings which are hard to separate are undesirable for that reason. Kitchen fittings should be made up of components which are solidly fixed together, but which can easily be detached by hand or using tools. This makes it easier to carry out repairs or replace individual parts, and also facilitates recycling. Gluing should only be done between like materials, and only using adhesives which are free of damaging solvents, formaldehyde and so on. It is also important to choose materials carefully when painting in the kitchen. The standard artificial resin dispersions are produced by environmentally damaging methods, many of their constituents are unsuited for interior use and they prevent walls and building materials from being able to breathe. The best alternatives, apart from whitewash for new buildings, are casein paints, which are durable and provide a good covering, and can easily be painted over.

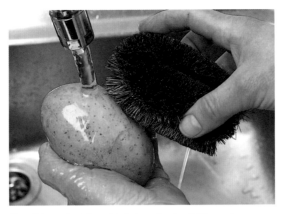

Brushing: Just the skin is brushed quickly under running cold water to get rid of earth and other dirt.

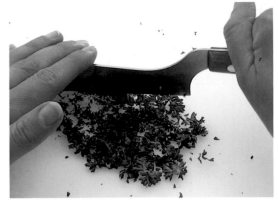

Chopping: Herbs and onions can be chopped with a herb or chopping knife using a see saw action.

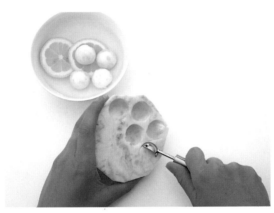

Ball cutting: Attractive fruit and vegetable balls can be cut out using a ball scoop.

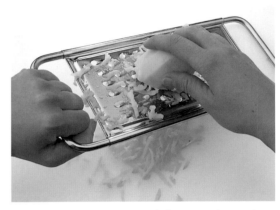

Grating: Potatoes, carrots, celeriac, or apples can be prepared with a grater.

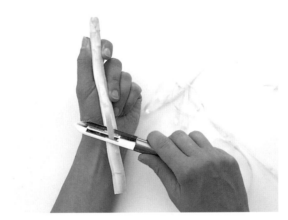

Peeling: The skin can be removed evenly, thinly, and quickly with a thin-cutting peeler.

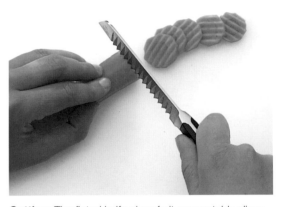

Cutting: The fluted knife gives fruit or vegetable slices an attractive crinkled surface.

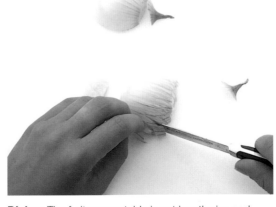

Dicing: The fruit or vegetable is cut lengthwise and then crosswise to produce cubes.

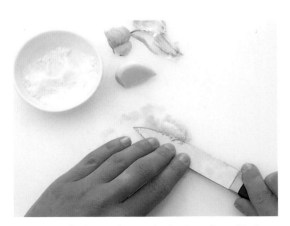

Crushing: Garlic can be crushed using a broad knife blade.

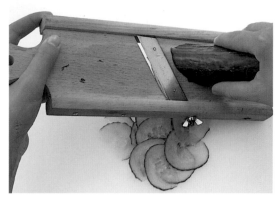

Slicing: Cucumbers can be sliced thinly by sliding them back and forth over the slicer blade.

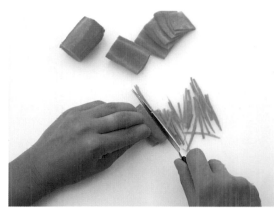

Cutting Julienne strips: The vegetables are cut into very fine, decorative strips.

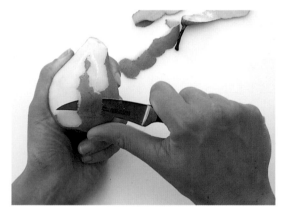

Peeling: The slightly curved blade of the paring knife peels fruit very thinly.

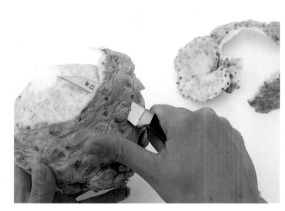

Peeling: Vegetables can be peeled very thinly by sliding the knife towards the thumb.

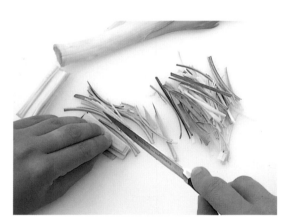

Cutting: Vegetable strips as thin as this can be produced with well sharpened kitchen knives.

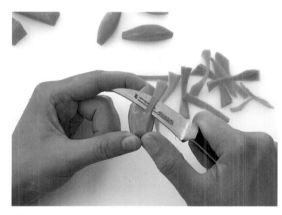

Trimming: Vegetables can be cut into decorative shapes using a paring knife.

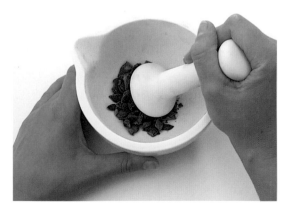

Crushing: Spices can be crushed and mixed using a pestle and mortar.

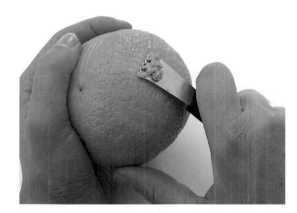

Zesting: The zest of citrus fruits can be shredded with a zester.

Cooking Methods

Boiling
Most of the vital substances are lost with this method of preparation. The food is immersed in hot water which washes out its valuable constituents. As a result, the vital substances are transferred to the water, which is poured away.

Steaming
With this gentler method, the food cooks in steam, separated from the boiling liquid by a sieve. Comparatively few of the vital substances are lost, provided it is not done under pressure and consequently at excessive temperatures.

Vapor cooking
In this, the least damaging cooking method, the food cooks at a low temperature in only a little liquid, so that most of the vital substances are retained.

Poaching
With this gentle, often long cooking method usually carried out at between 150 and 175 °F (65 and 80 °C), the vitamins and minerals are released, as with boiling. This preparation method is therefore only a good idea if the cooking liquid is also going to be used in the meal.

Frying
This method of cooking ingredients in a hot fat, which is bad for the digestion, overloads dishes with excessively high levels of low-quality fat. High-quality cooking oils containing a high proportion of polyunsaturated fatty acids are unsuitable for frying.

Broiling
Because of the high temperature, losses of vital substances are very high with this low-fat cooking method. Fatty foods should never be grilled directly over burning embers as burning fat produces carcinogenic benzpyrenes.

Roasting
This fairly damaging cooking method involves cooking with added fat at very high temperatures, so losses of vitamins and polyunsaturated fatty acids are correspondingly high. The roasting aromas enhance the flavor. The best fat for roasting is olive oil, as it can tolerate the high temperatures.

Braising
This preparation method involves brief browning in hot fat, with accompanying losses of heat-sensitive vitamins followed by long, gentle cooking at a low temperature. Vital substances are dissolved in the sauce, which is eaten with the food.

Baking
This cooking method with its many uses involves cooking in a dry heat. The amount of vital substances lost depends on the temperature and cooking time. At low temperatures, this can be a very gentle method.

Microwaving
This cooking method which is being viewed with increasing criticism causes the food molecules to vibrate by exposing them to electromagnetic radiation at 2450 megahertz. This damages some of the cells, in particular destroys the important B vitamins and indirectly encourages consumption of mass-produced ready meals.

Clever Storage Ideas

The Store Cupboard

Every year, there comes a time when the harvest reaches its peak, as anyone with a garden of their own will know. Suddenly the yield exceeds one's own needs and the surplus can be processed immediately for storage. As the vitamins are gradually lost from fresh fruit and vegetables day by day, the method of storage or preservation should be decided on as quickly as possible. It is only worth making the effort to preserve or store the produce if healthy, unblemished, and extremely fresh fruit and vegetables are used. Even for those who do not have a garden of their own, there are ample opportunities to buy large quantities of fruit and vegetables from organic market gardens or farms at a reasonable price at harvest time. This is a good way of being prepared for the months when not as much fresh produce is available – instead of having to buy expensive fresh goods or preserves, one can fall back on one's own reserves. Various methods of storage and preservation can be used for different types of fruit and vegetable.

Storing

Certain types of fruit and vegetable can be kept for months in a dark, ventilated cellar ideally at a temperature of 39 °F (4 °C) and with 90 percent air humidity. It is important to sort out any rotten items regularly. Late apples and pears, potatoes and cabbage, red beet, carrots, and other root vegetables (ideally in a sandbox) are particularly suitable.

Drying

Fruit, vegetables, mushrooms, and herbs can be dried at 86 °F (30 °C) or higher. It is important to have good ventilation to prevent mold from forming. Some fruits can only be dried in the sun and air in the attic or on the balcony, in which case they have to be protected from insects, for example with gauze. Ovens or special drying equipment can be used for this traditional method of preservation. Very high temperatures cause increased losses of vitamins. Dried produce – apples, pears, plums, apricots, peaches, grapes, soup vegetables, tomatoes, onions, ceps, and herbs are especially suitable – should always be kept tightly sealed in cans or jars in the dark.

Pickling

The acid in the vinegar has a preserving effect. Wine vinegar is usually diluted with an equal quantity of water and heated, after adding spices, kosher salt, and a little cane sugar. The fruit or vegetables are then brought to the boil in the vinegar mixture or put straight into jars and the hot liquid poured over them. The jars must be sterilized if the contents are to be kept for a long time, although this is not necessary if they are to be eaten almost straight away. Gherkins, cauliflower, carrots, bell peppers, onions, small corn, tomatoes, capers, white cabbage, mushrooms, plums, and cherries can be pickled.

Boiling

Sterilization is a widely used conventional method of preserving fruit and vegetables using heat. The sterilization time and temperature vary depending on the type of fruit or vegetable. The often prolonged heating produces significant losses of vital substances, and changes in the protein and flavor. For this reason, sterilized produce is not of great importance in a wholefood diet. The high consumption of energy is also environmentally damaging. This method is most suitable for preserving mirabelles, apricots, peaches, pears, and cherries.

Fermented Vegetables

This natural preservation method makes use of spontaneous lactic acid fermentation and is achieved without heat. The vital substances are preserved and no energy is used. As well as the most famous fermented vegetable, sauerkraut, other vegetables can be fermented and stored for up to one year. White cabbage, bell peppers, onions, olives, eggplants, celery, cucumber, carrots, and green tomatoes are suitable.

Deep Freezing

With this modern preservation method, the vital substances in the fruit and vegetables are conserved. It is advisable to blanch vegetables briefly in steam to inhibit enzyme activity. Vegetables can be cooked without defrosting. Berries are particularly suitable for deep freezing. It is important for the produce to freeze through quickly, so flat containers should be used in preference. Peas, beans, Brussels sprouts, kale, broccoli, cauliflower, artichokes, bell peppers, tomatoes for sauces, mushrooms, and herbs are especially suitable.

Bottling fruits is a traditional, although not ideal, way of preserving them.

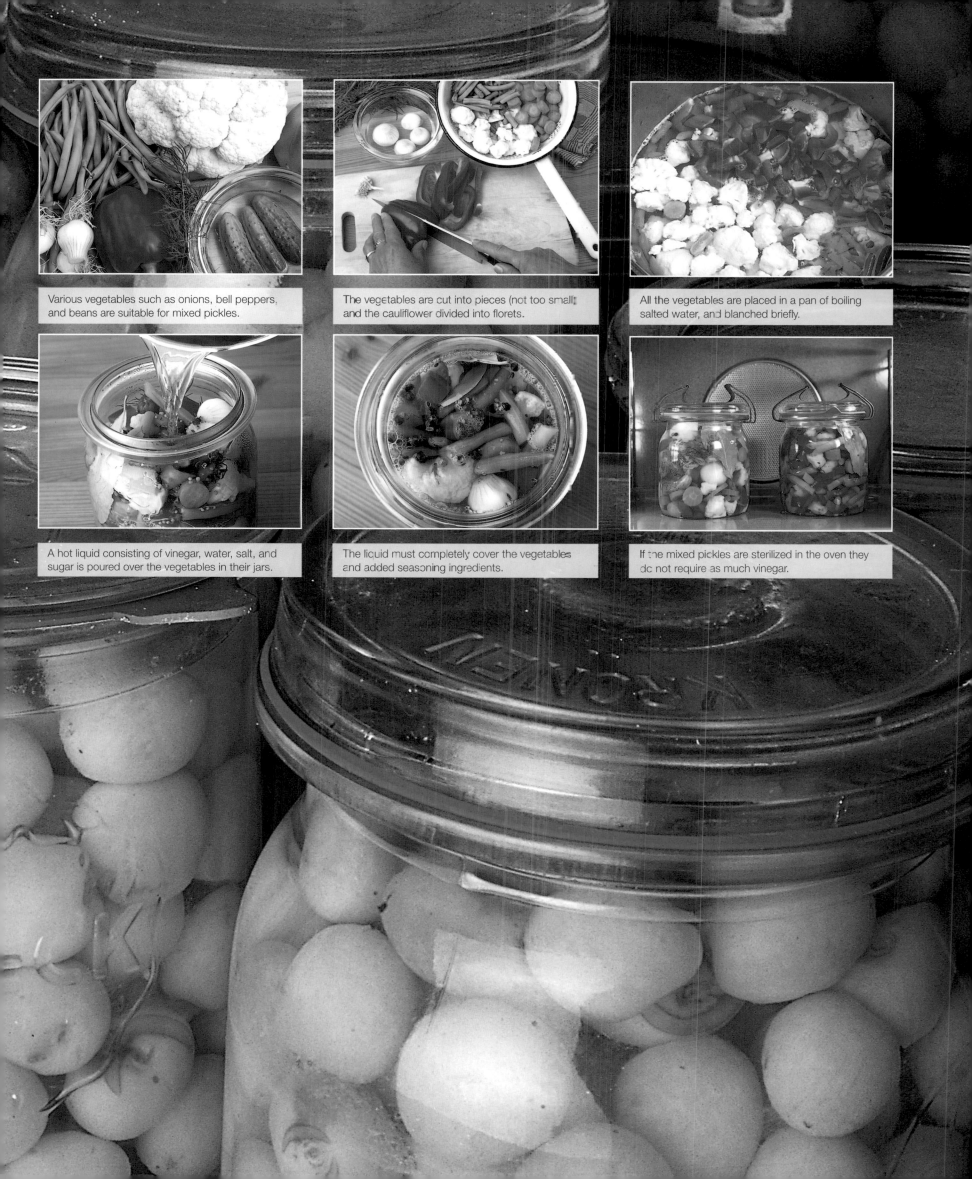

Various vegetables such as onions, bell peppers, and beans are suitable for mixed pickles.

The vegetables are cut into pieces (not too small) and the cauliflower divided into florets.

All the vegetables are placed in a pan of boiling salted water, and blanched briefly.

A hot liquid consisting of vinegar, water, salt, and sugar is poured over the vegetables in their jars.

The liquid must completely cover the vegetables and added seasoning ingredients.

If the mixed pickles are sterilized in the oven they do not require as much vinegar.

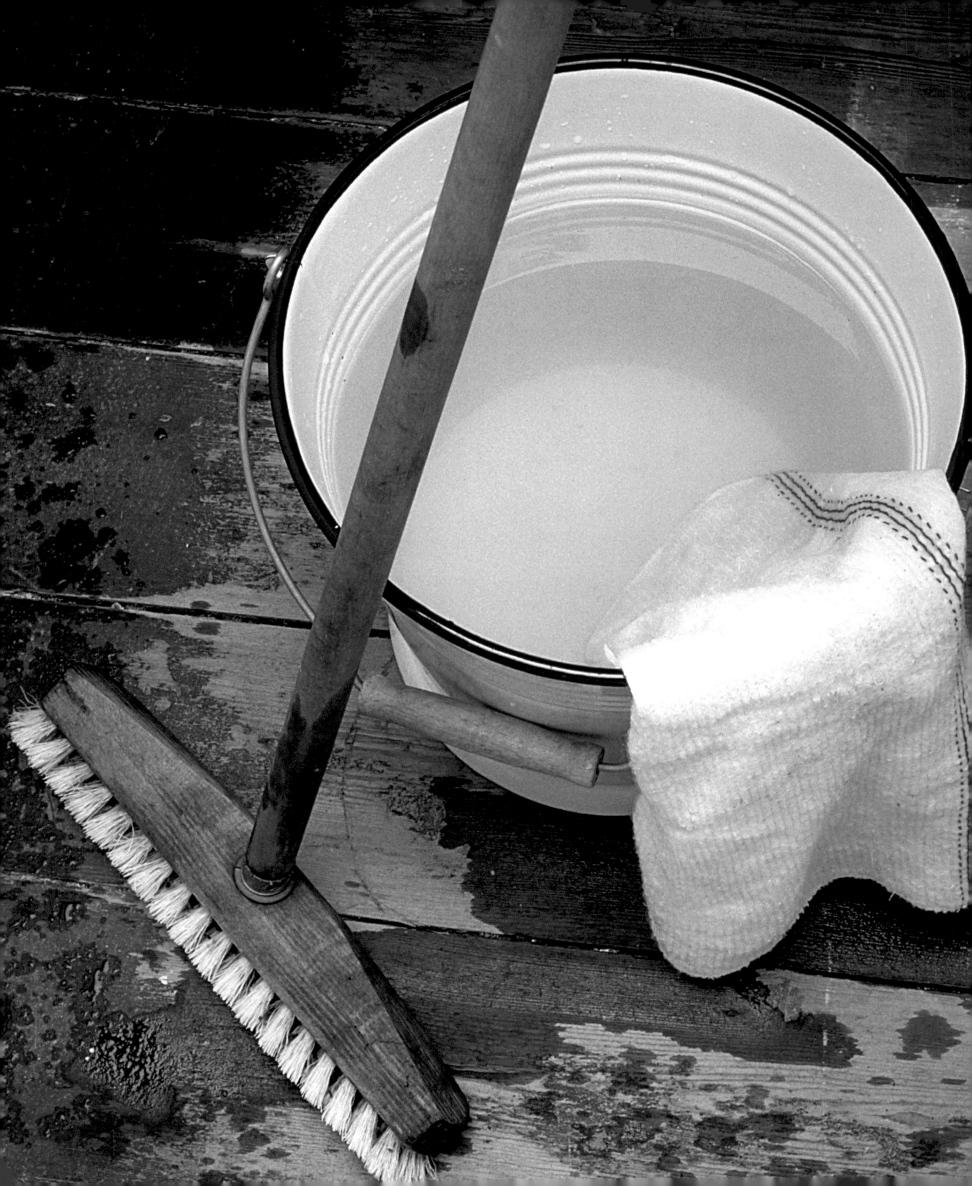

Ecological Cleaning

Unfortunately, the kitchen does not stay clean by itself. As well as dust and dirt brought in from outside, there is also dirt from food preparation and cooking, of which grease is the most stubborn. None of this would be a problem if there existed a completely environmentally friendly cleaning method. However, to get things perfectly clean with the minimum effort, it is hard to do without chemical agents, as an effective, but nonpolluting cleaning or washing agent has not yet been discovered.

However, some progress has been made in the cleaning and washing detergent market. The disastrous consequences of pollution by phosphates, which are not, in fact, harmful, provided the incentive. Used as water softeners, they had been an important constituent of all washing and many cleaning products since the 1960s, as the active washing ingredients only give satisfactory results in soft water. The phosphates drained away with the waste washing-water into the sewage system and into the inland waters, where they caused over-fertilization and, as a consequence, excessive vegetation growth. Decay processes which polluted the water then followed. Since the 1980s, phosphates have mostly been replaced with other substances, mainly the harmless zeolite A. But washing and cleaning agents still contain substances which cannot easily be broken down naturally. Cleaning agents, particularly special cleaners, are often based on corrosive agents and solvents, not to mention disinfectants, anti bacterial and anti fungal poisons like formaldehyde, which are a severe hazard to health and the environment.

Alternative solutions start by questioning the need for the various substances contained in dishwashing, cleaning and washing agents. Synthetic colorings and fragrances are avoided, as are disinfectants and enzymes. But even in alternative products, surfactants are used in general purpose cleaners and dishwashing products, but they are based on cooking oils. Apart from these, traditional domestic cleaners such as washing soap and soft soap or scouring powder are now seeing a new rise in popularity. The best way of helping the environment is to do without cleaning products altogether, for example, glasses and non-greasy items can be washed with water only, windows can be cleaned with water and newspaper, natural fibers can be dried in fresh air and fabric conditioners can be avoided.

Left-hand page: A scrubbing brush, a cloth and a bucket of clean water are the most environmentally friendly cleaning aids.

Main Constituents of Cleaning and Washing Detergents

Surfactants

These active washing substances – linear alkylbenzenesulfonates (LAS) made from crude oil are usually used – are largely, but not completely, broken down at sewage treatment works. Even in concentrations of below 0.6 mg/l, they are lethal to fish and can cause inflammation of the skin. Other surfactants – fatty alcohol sulfates (FAS) – are obtained from renewable plant oils like coconut, palm, or rapeseed oil which are readily degradable, but which are generally cultivated using high levels of pesticides.

Softeners

Technically described as builders. They include zeolites and other phosphate substitutes which improve washing performance, as well as polycarboxylates, which, although not toxic, are not very degradable. Citrates or citric acid salts, on the other hand, are kinder to the environment, but only react optimally between 86 and 140 °F (30 and 60 °C) and no hotter. Other salts such as soda are used to increase the alkalinity of the suds, but can also damage fibers, glass, and metals. Floor cleaners contain corrosive ammonia.

Bleaching Agents

Used in washing or scouring agents for removing stains by oxidation, for example, chlorine, which is toxic in large quantities. Perborate, a commonly used, ecologically damaging substance, is only effective at over 140 °F (60 °C). Because of this, more harmless bleach activators like TAED are added. Added stabilizers, on the other hand, like phosphonates, are harmful.

Enzymes

Biological catalysts like lipases, proteases, amylases, or cellulase, which are being used increasingly, dissolve grease, protein, starch, or cellulose at 86 to 122 °F (30 to 50 °C). They are ineffective at higher temperatures. Although they are readily degradable, they can cause allergies and are partly or wholly produced by genetic engineering, the consequences of which are totally unknown at present.

Texturing Agents

Sodium sulfate (Glauber's Salt), which puts extra salt into waste water, is usually added to improve the consistency and pourability. It is always contained in scouring agents, but no longer contained in compact washing agents.

Perfumes

Produced synthetically, do not degrade easily in waste water, irritate fish and can trigger allergies.

A Different Way of Washing

Environmentalists recommend the modular system for washing clothes.
It consists of a

• basic washing compound made of soap with or without added surfactants,

• softener precisely matched to the hardness of the mains water, which can be omitted altogether in areas of soft water,

• bleaching agent, which is only added very rarely for heavily soiled whites which need to be washed at over 140 °F (60 °C).

In addition, various steps can be taken to avoid unnecessary pollution of the environment.

Colorings

Produced synthetically, some are harmless, some are suspected of being carcinogenic.

Abrasive Substances

Ground curds, marble or chalk in general purpose cleaners and scouring agents.

Washing Detergents: Compact Versus Modular System

Nowadays every manufacturer on the washing detergent market wants to be seen to be environmentally friendly. So now a war is being waged between the two more environmentally compatible product concepts, compact washing detergent and the modular system. The compact detergents benefit the environment by the simple fact of their smaller volume, achieved by omitting the texturing agents which are superfluous in any case. Glauber's Salt, the most commonly used texturing agent, accounts for a third of the volume of conventional detergents. Omitting it can hugely reduce the volume of environmentally damaging material by tens of thousands of tons, provided the consumer realizes that the proportions have changed and does not continue to use the same quantity of detergent as with conventional detergents. As far as active washing substances are concerned there is practically no difference between compact detergents and full detergents. However, no detergent is completely harmless to the environment. This is why the most important objective is to reduce consumption, which in any case is lower with the modular system, provided the consumer adjusts the proportions correctly. Modular washing agents do not contain any texturing agent either. Since, moreover, the softener and bleaching agent are only added as required, the reduction in chemicals used is significantly greater – and actually twice as much as compared with compact detergents. The careful selection of the components produces other benefits: the actual active washing substance is not based on synthetic surfactants but on soaps which are made with renewable raw materials, ideally fats or oils from organically cultivated crops like palms, flax, or sunflowers. They are boiled together with caustic soda for powders or caustic potash for liquid detergents to produce alkaline salts of fatty acids. Soaps made in this way are fully biodegradable.

• The prewash can usually be omitted and dirty washing soaked instead.

• Instead of selecting boil wash, soak the dirty washing beforehand and then wash it at just 100 or 140 °F (40 or 60 °C).

• Only set the machine going when it is full and avoid using the so-called economy program with the machine half empty. However, do not overfill the machine either.

• Particularly noticeable stains should preferably be removed immediately, and always before washing. Marks containing protein can be removed with soap and cold water, greasy marks with soap and hot water.

• Do not use fabric conditioners as they are unnecessary.

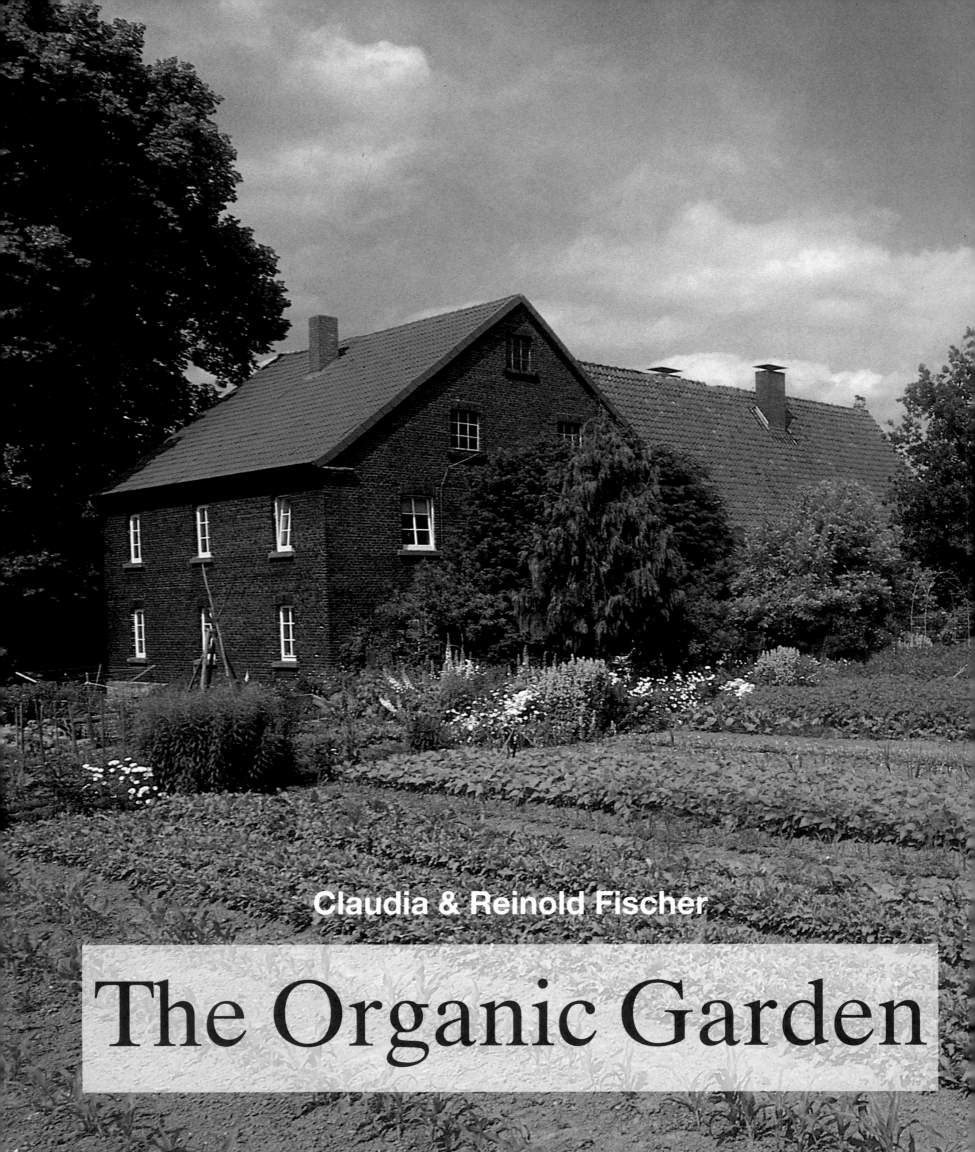

Claudia & Reinold Fischer

The Organic Garden

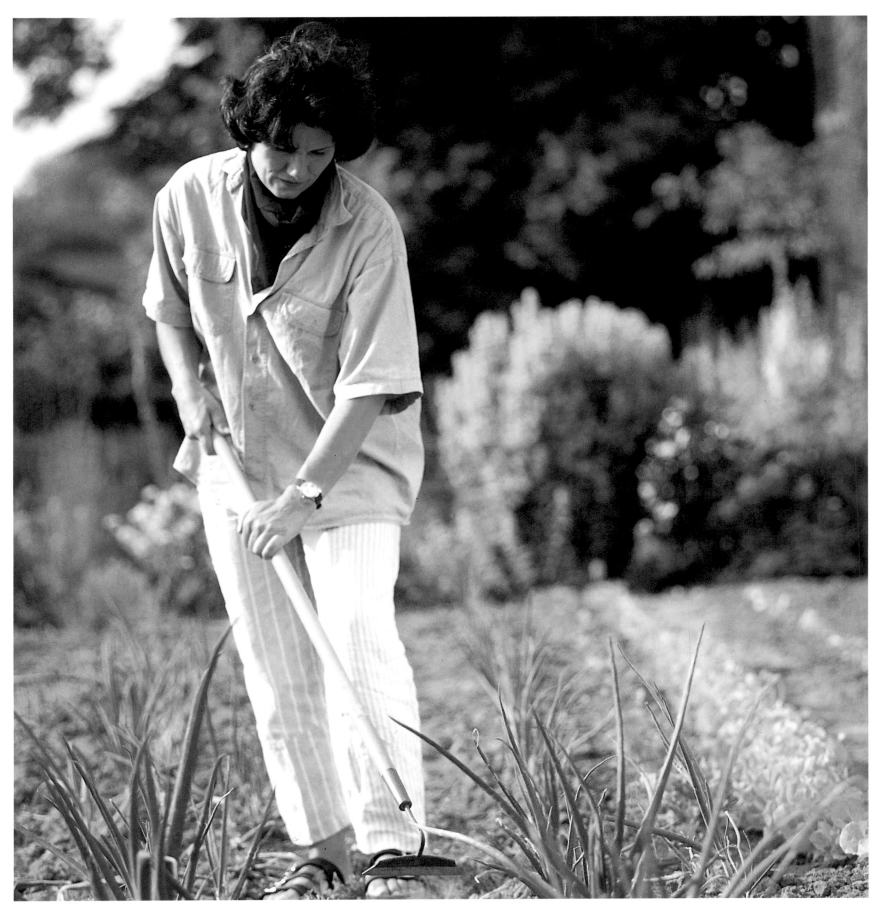

In an organically cultivated garden, unwanted plants are removed with a hoe.

Previous double page: A large farm garden – more than enough vegetables for all the family.

Gardens are amongst the oldest forms of cultivation. Whether they are planted for their decorative appeal or for a practical use, they are always oases of pleasure, arousing all the senses with bright flowers and fragrant herbs, sweet berries and crispy vegetables. The loveliest gardens are those which are allowed to develop as naturally as possible, and modern organic gardeners always have this objective in mind. Organic gardening means more than just abandoning the use of artificial fertilizers and pesticides. It is, in fact, based on recent findings by ecologists, supported by centuries of experience, on lessons learnt from nature itself and on the relationships between living organisms and between them and their environment.

Every garden is a biological community and habitat for countless species which all influence one another. If one species is driven out, the whole system is affected. However, this does not mean that gardeners should simply allow nature to take its course. Gardens are always living spaces created and designed by people. This applies both to gardens kept for pleasure and market gardens producing fruit, vegetables and herbs on a larger scale. For hundreds of years, good gardeners have succeeded in maintaining the equilibrium of these microcosms and thinking and acting ecologically. The rules and methods of organic gardening help gardeners to develop a sense of the importance of even the smallest life forms and to be aware of the harmonious interaction of the living species within the boundaries of a garden.

These rules are easy to follow. And they guarantee the best results: a blooming garden and magnificent, healthy yields.

Environment, Climate, Soil

Whether a garden is to be planted from scratch or an existing garden is to be converted to an organic one, good preparation always pays off. The very first step is to find out the specific properties of the particular piece of land, as not all plants can grow in any location and under any conditions. By finding out about the local climate and wind conditions and the type of soil, you can make the right choice when it comes to deciding whether and where to plant fruit trees and hedges, wind shields and vegetable patches. Gardeners who work by organic methods on principle only choose plants which are well suited to the particular location. A plant in the wrong location may become chronically ill or so badly infested with pests that it cannot be cured by gentle, organic means.

Climate and Microclimate

Meteorological offices can provide information on the local average figures for precipitation, temperature and hours of sunshine. They can also tell you about any climatic peculiarities, for example, whether the garden lies in a natural frost valley. Even the altitude is important. Someone with a garden in a low mountain area will be more likely to opt for a greenhouse in order to produce ripe tomatoes than a gardener in the warm, wine-growing climate of a lowland plain. Town gardens are generally warmer and more protected, whereas gardens in the country often require additional wind protection with hedges and trees. Gardens near the sea are exposed to salty winds, but enjoy a more moderate climate than inland.

To get an accurate picture of the microclimate, it is useful to produce a scale drawing of the house and garden showing all the fixed objects like trees, paths and so on. You then have to observe:

• Which parts of the garden are in shadow for most of the time, e.g. shaded by the house or the neighbor's fence?
• Where is there dark shadow only in summer, e.g. beneath a deciduous tree?
• Which is the strongest wind direction?
• Which areas are protected from the wind?
• Which areas are especially at risk from frost?
• Are individual areas of the garden particularly wet or dry?

Such information about the natural characteristics of the site can be put to good use, for example, by locating a pond in the wettest hollow of the garden. Or the characteristics can be changed for the better in the long term, for example by planting wind barriers, trees and hedges.

Vegetable Cultivation Areas for a Four-person Household

Plant	Annual requirement in lbs (kg)	Cultivation area in sq. yds (sq. m)
Cabbages	77 (35)	14 (12)
Carrots	110 (50)	19 (16)
Celery	22 (10)	6 (5)
Cucumbers	110 (50)	35 (30)
Dwarf Beans	66 (30)	35 (30)
Lettuces	99 (45)	20 (17)
Onions	66 (30)	12 (10)
Peas	55 (25)	29 (25)
Radishes	13 (6)	4.5 (4)
Salsify	17 (8)	4.5 (4)
Spinach	44 (20)	12 (10)
Tomatoes	44 (20)	9.5 (8)
Zucchini	22 (10)	1.2 (1)

Protection from Environmental Pollution

Steps may need to be taken to protect the garden from environmental pollution, depending on its location. If it is right next to a busy road, near an industrial estate, or in an agricultural area where chemicals are still used intensively, it is advisable to take protective measures:

• A $6^1/_2$ foot (2 meter) wide mixed hedge of native flowering bushes reduces the level of noxious gases considerably. If there is enough space for a 20 foot (6 meter) high hedge, pollution by lead from the road, for example, is reduced to a sixth. The higher the hedge, the more effectively it filters the harmful substances.
• Trees filter dust and pollutants out of the air. Deciduous trees let only half the pollutants contained in the air and rain reach the soil. 50 percent of the dust, soot, and pollutants are trapped by the foliage. In heavily polluted areas, this foliage should be composted separately and only used for decorative and border shrubs.
• A mixed hedge acts as a barrier to salty water splashed up in winter in those parts of the country where the roads are sprinkled with salt to prevent black ice.
• Greenhouses made from glass or plastic sheeting protect the plants from direct precipitation, dust, soot, and spray chemicals from intensive farming.

The Soil Type

It is possible to find out whether a garden has a sandy, loamy, clay, or mixed soil with the following tests:
• With a sandy soil, the sand runs through your fingers when you pick up a handful of earth. The soil cannot be compressed between the hands but falls apart immediately.
• A loamy soil can be crumbled into soft lumps. They hold together but do not stick.
• A clayey garden soil can be compressed between the hands and formed into a lump like modeling clay.
• The proportion of humus can be measured by a simple test: Put some earth in a jar and top it up with water. If, when the earth has settled, the water is clear or only slightly cloudy, the humus content of the soil is low. The more dark particles that can be seen floating in the water, the higher the content of fertile humus.

Indicator Plants

Wild plants give a good indication of the composition of the soil in terms of moisture, acidity and humus content. These indicator plants are an especially accurate pointer on pieces of land which have been lying uncultivated for a long time. But even in a cultivated garden there is always a reason for it if the same weeds keep coming back. A single plant is not a sufficiently reliable pointer. But when a particular group of plants stubbornly keeps reappearing, this can be an important sign. It is then more effective in the long term to improve the soil than to keep weeding and hoeing. But a wild plant is not always indicative of a soil problem. Many of the indicator plants like loose, vital, humus-rich soils best of all: their presence is the biggest compliment an organic gardener can get.

The Soil Test

The most comprehensive information on the composition and condition of the garden soil can be obtained by having a soil test done at a specialized laboratory. These laboratories carry out highly accurate tests and as well as the test results, also give advice on fertilizers and soil improvement. It is important that gardeners mention that they use organic methods when they send in the soil sample. The laboratory will then adapt its suggestions accordingly.

To obtain a complete picture, soil samples should be taken from five to ten different parts of the garden. Sets for taking samples which include full instructions can be bought at all good garden centers.

The Main Nutrients

Garden plants need nutrients in a balanced form. If a nutrient is lacking altogether or present in inadequate amounts, visible deficiencies will appear. A soil test determines which nutrients are present in the garden soil and which are missing.

Nitrogen
Chemical symbol: N

Nitrogen is an important protein component for plants, available in organic compounds in the form of nitrates. These nitrates are produced when proteins of plant or animal origin rot, and are fixed by certain bacteria known as azotobacteria living in the soil or by leguminous plants.

Nitrogen-rich fertilizers: dried blood and horn meal, horn clippings, guano, all types of manure, but particularly poultry, sheep's and goat's manure, manure and stinging nettle liquid fertilizers, green manures containing leguminous plants or young grass.

Phosphorus
Chemical symbol: P, measured as P_2O_5

Phosphorus, present in the soil in the form of phosphoric acid and its salts, the phosphates, is a component of protein. Young plants need phosphorus above all for developing their root network, and older plants need it to produce flowers, fruits and seeds.

Phosphorus-rich fertilizers: bonemeal, guano, poultry manure, rock phosphate, pig's manure, Thomas meal.

Potash
Chemical symbol: K, measured as K_2O

Potash, or more correctly, potassium, is responsible for strong cell structure and for steady growth. Plants well supplied with potash are particularly resistant to animal pests. Fruits and vegetables store well and keep for a long time.
Potash-containing fertilizers: wood ash, poultry, cattle and pig's manure, bonemeal, animal-derived liquid manures, plant-derived liquid manures made from fern and comfrey, leaf compost from fruit trees, sulfate of potash magnesia.

Table of Indicator Plants

Plant	Soil Condition
Annual Mercury	humus-rich, very well-prepared soil
Black Nightshade	high nitrogen content, rich in nutrients
Chickweed	loose, humus-rich soil
Coltsfoot	compacted, wet soil
Creeping Buttercup	compacted, wet soil
Dandelion	high nitrogen content, rich in nutrients
Field Mint	compacted, wet soil
Fumitory	loose, moist soil
Germander Speedwell	loose, nitrogen-rich soil
Goose grass	high nitrogen content, rich in nutrients
Hemp nettle	compacted, wet soil
Hemp-nettle	acid soil
Horsetail	compacted, wet soil
Kew Weed	humus-rich, very well-prepared soil
Meadow Sage	alkaline soil
Medicinal Speedwell	acid soil
Ox eye daisy	compacted, wet soil
Silverweed	highly compacted soil
Sorrel	compacted, wet soil
Speedwell	loose, moist soil
Spurge	humus-rich, very well-prepared soil
Stinging Nettle	high nitrogen content, rich in nutrients
Wild Mustard	high nitrogen content, rich in nutrients
Wild Radish	acid soil

Lime
Chemical symbol: Ca, measured by the pH value

Lime or calcium is an important constituent of the plant's skeleton. Lime fixes acids in the soil and thus raises the pH value, which should be between 6 and 7.5 for most crop plants. Lime aids in the breakdown of organic material.

Lime-containing fertilizers: magnesium, calcium carbonate, fertilizing lime from lime marl, Thomas meal, rock meals, seaweed lime.

Magnesium
Chemical symbol: Mg

Magnesium is the most important element in chlorophyll, the green component of leaves, and is involved in protein formation.

Magnesium-containing fertilizers: ground magnesian limestone, wood ash, seaweed lime, some rock meals, sulfate of potash magnesia.

Trace elements

Iron (Fe), manganese (Mn), copper (Cu), zinc (Zn), molybdenum (Mb), chlorine (Cl), boron (B).

The pH value

The pH (from Latin *potentia hydrogenii*) indicates the degree of acidity of aqueous solutions. The lower the pH value, the more acidic the solution. Water, which is neutral, has a pH of 7, acids have lower values and alkalis have higher values.

The Garden in Equilibrium

Organic gardeners attempt to respect the laws of nature and create a garden microcosm which is as balanced as possible.
The aim is:
A garden
• in which the beneficial insects keep the pests at bay,
• where wild plants are allowed to grow in moderation,
• where insects, butterflies and birds can find food and ample living space,
• where everything blooms and thrives without disease or attack by pests.
A garden in ecological equilibrium.
According to the ecologist's definition, every garden is a "semi unstable ecosystem," in other words, a habitat which, like every field and heath and alpine meadow, has to be carefully tended by man to enable it to maintain its equilibrium.
Amongst the laws of nature which help organic gardeners to keep their gardens in biological equilibrium are the following principles:
• mixing of crops
• crop rotation and fallow soil
• mulching
• loosening, airing, covering, and fertilizing the soil with living plants
• creating new habitats.

Crop Mixing for Healthy Plants

Single crop cultivation is one of man's inventions. This unbalanced form of plant growth is not found anywhere in nature. In a meadow, on the edge of a field or by a stream, very specific plant types live together with very specific animal types. In their special habitat or biotope, they form a biological community or biocenosis. In ecological gardening, each row or bed may have a mixture of plants or the plants may be mixed together in groups to form plant communities of herbs, flowers and vegetables which have a positive influence on each other. This mixing of crops is one of the most important means of keeping the plants healthy. It makes life difficult for pests as they have further to travel between plants. Once the organic grower has developed a feeling for the plant communities, for herbs, flowers and vegetables which can be of benefit to each other, he can create a biocenosis in his own garden.

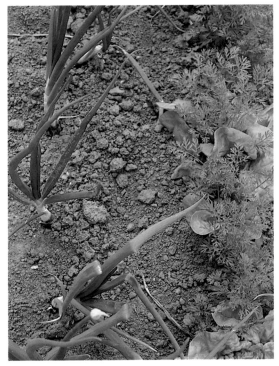

Plants take a like or dislike to each other too. If they are compatible, each enhances the growth and resistance of the other, as with onions, lettuces and carrots in this case.

Green Manure Crops

The most valuable green manure crops are leguminous plants like beans, peas, horse beans, clover, sweet peas, and lupines. They are able to fix atmospheric nitrogen, in other words they collect fertilizer from the air. Cruciferous plants like yellow mustard, summer rape and oil radish loosen the soil right down deep into the ground. They grow rapidly and can still be sown late.
Sunflowers should not be allowed to flower, as they then extract too many nutrients from the soil. They have to be cut back after eight to ten weeks, then they produce plenty of green foliage.
Phacelia or "Bees' Friend," on the other hand, may be allowed to flower as it is an excellent food plant for bees. Spinach is well-suited as a preliminary crop.

Mulching

The Advantages of Mulching

• Less hoeing: The soil no longer has to be mechanically loosened in a mulched bed.
• Less weeding: The mulch layer keeps unwanted wild plants at bay.
• Less watering: The soil water evaporates more slowly so less watering is required.
• Gentle fertilization: Active decomposition by the soil organisms produces valuable clay/humus complexes and nutrients for the plants. The mulch covering releases the fertilizer slowly but constantly.
• When organic material is broken down by the soil organisms, so-called "soil-generated carbon dioxide," is released, providing the plants with an excellent supply of carbon. The plants take up carbon dioxide through holes in the undersides of their leaves. Plants in a mulched bed therefore usually look greener and healthier than ones planted in bare soil.
• Healthy soil life: In an active soil, extra food means a sharp rise in soil activity.

How to Mulch

Mulching takes place in April or May, when the soil has had a good chance to warm up.
• Green mulch material, like lawn cuttings, vegetable waste, comfrey, and fern leaves, has to wilt before it is put on the soil. It is then thinly spread over the earth.
• Coarse compost is scattered in a thin layer and lightly covered with dry material such as straw.
• Chopped straw, hay (not containing wild plant seeds) or reeds can be spread up to 6 inches (15 centimeters) thick on a plant bed which has previously been scattered with a little horn meal or ripe compost.
• The mulch material must not touch seedlings. If the layer gets thinner over the course of the summer, you can simply add more.

Green Manure Crops – Sowing Dates and Characteristics

Plant	Sowing date	Important
Clover Varieties	III–VIII	Nitrogen accumulator
Field Pea and Vetchling	V–VIII	Nitrogen accumulator
Horse Bean	II–VI	Nitrogen accumulator
Lupines	VIII	Nitrogen accumulator
Marigold	III–VI	Counteracts nematodes in the soil
Nasturtium	V–VI	Aphid trap
Oil Radish	VIII	Good soil loosener
Phacelia	V–VIII	Good honey-producing plant, plenty of greenery
Spinach	II–II	Good vegetable from VIII–IX
Summer Rape	V–VIII	Good soil loosener
Sunflower	V–VII	Cut after 8–10 weeks
Sweet Peas	VIII	Nitrogen accumulator
Yellow Mustard	III–IX	Grows extremely quickly

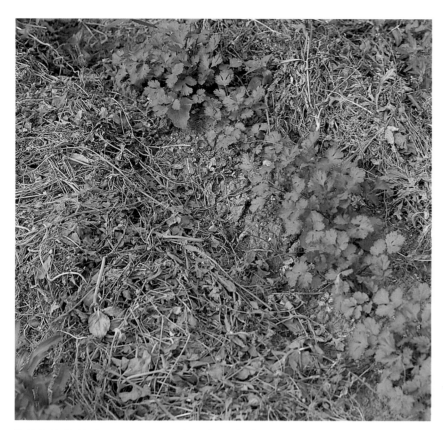

In an organic garden, green manure is an important means of enriching, protecting, and nourishing the soil organisms. The garden soil should never be left bare.

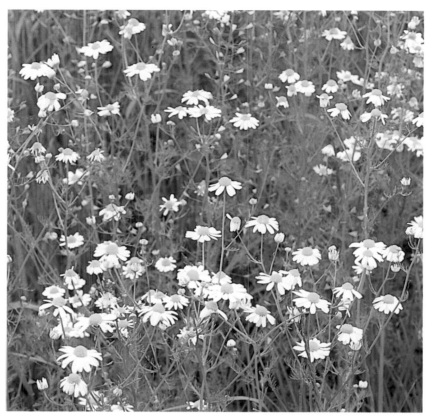

Camomile is another of the indicator plants (see table, p. 401) which show what type of soil one is dealing with. It points to a clay soil.

Crop Rotation for a Healthy Soil

It is a well established fact in agriculture that it is not possible to grow the same crop on the same patch year after year. Every type of plant extracts a certain set of nutrients from the soil and puts into the soil the waste products secreted out through its own roots. Only a few plants, for example tomatoes, are happy to be surrounded by their own root secretions from the previous year. But all plants suffer from a lack of nutrients if they are planted in an exhausted, unbalanced soil.

In an organic garden, plant rotation is based on a three-year cycle of high, moderate and low nutrient-consuming plants. Only a third of the soil is heavily fertilized and planted with very "hungry" plants at any one time. The following year, the same patch is planted with species requiring moderate amounts of nutrients, and the least demanding crops are planted there in the third year.

The three-year cycle can become a four-year cycle with fallowing if the ground is sown exclusively with nitrogen-accumulating green manure plants in the fourth year.

Mulching – a Blanket for the Soil

Exceptionally fertile, humus-rich soil can be found in natural mixed woodland. The soil remains untouched below the layer of leaves and needles, and the microorganisms can carry out their work of producing humus undisturbed.

Organic gardeners imitate this principle when they mulch bare soil. This means they cover the soil with a protective layer of foliage, straw, grass clippings, or organic waste. This protects the soil from downpours, wind and parching sunshine. Microorganisms and earthworms come up to the surface beneath this cover and collect supplies for building up humus.

Green Manures – Living Protection and Nourishment

In nature, deserts are the only places where the ground is constantly bare and uncovered. Elsewhere, any patch of earth which has lost its plant covering for whatever reason acquires a new protective covering in a very short time. Organic gardeners also make sure their plant beds always have a living green covering. Every harvested bed,

every bare patch of soil, is sown with quick-growing green manure plants. They form a living covering which provides just as effective protection as a mulch layer.

Varied Habitats

Foliage under the hedge, stones, stinging nettles, nesting aids for birds and insects, wild plants, and a pile of brushwood in the corner are steps the organic gardener can take to create habitats for the many tiny garden helpers. Beneficial insects will nest here, hedgehogs can hibernate, lizards and toads will find a home here, and birds will have a good place to stay.

The greater the variety of species created by all these different measures, the less susceptible the garden's ecosystem is to disruption. If the garden is in ecological equilibrium, insects will not appear in such numbers that they become pests, and disease carriers will encounter resistant plants which are not so easy to attack.

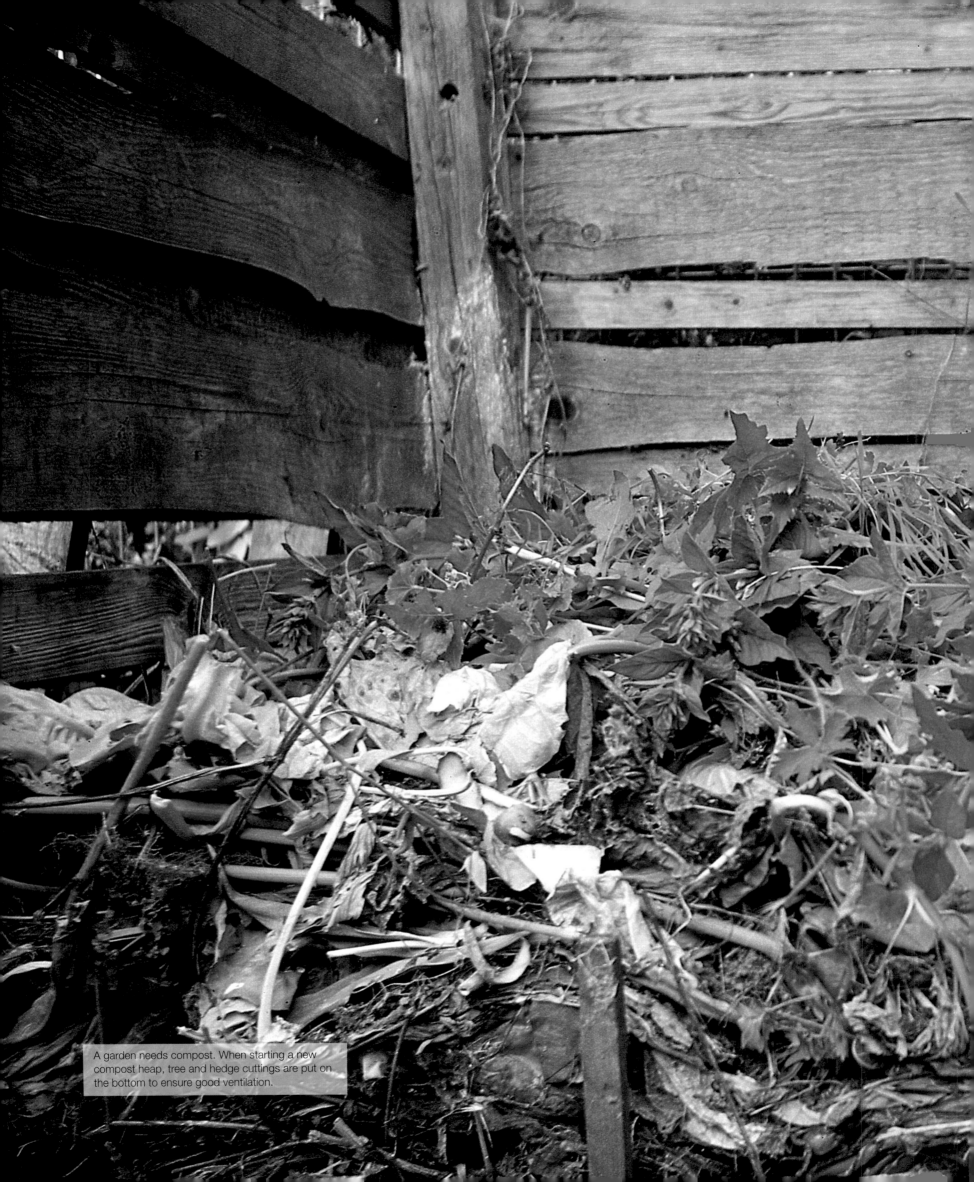

A garden needs compost. When starting a new compost heap, tree and hedge cuttings are put on the bottom to ensure good ventilation.

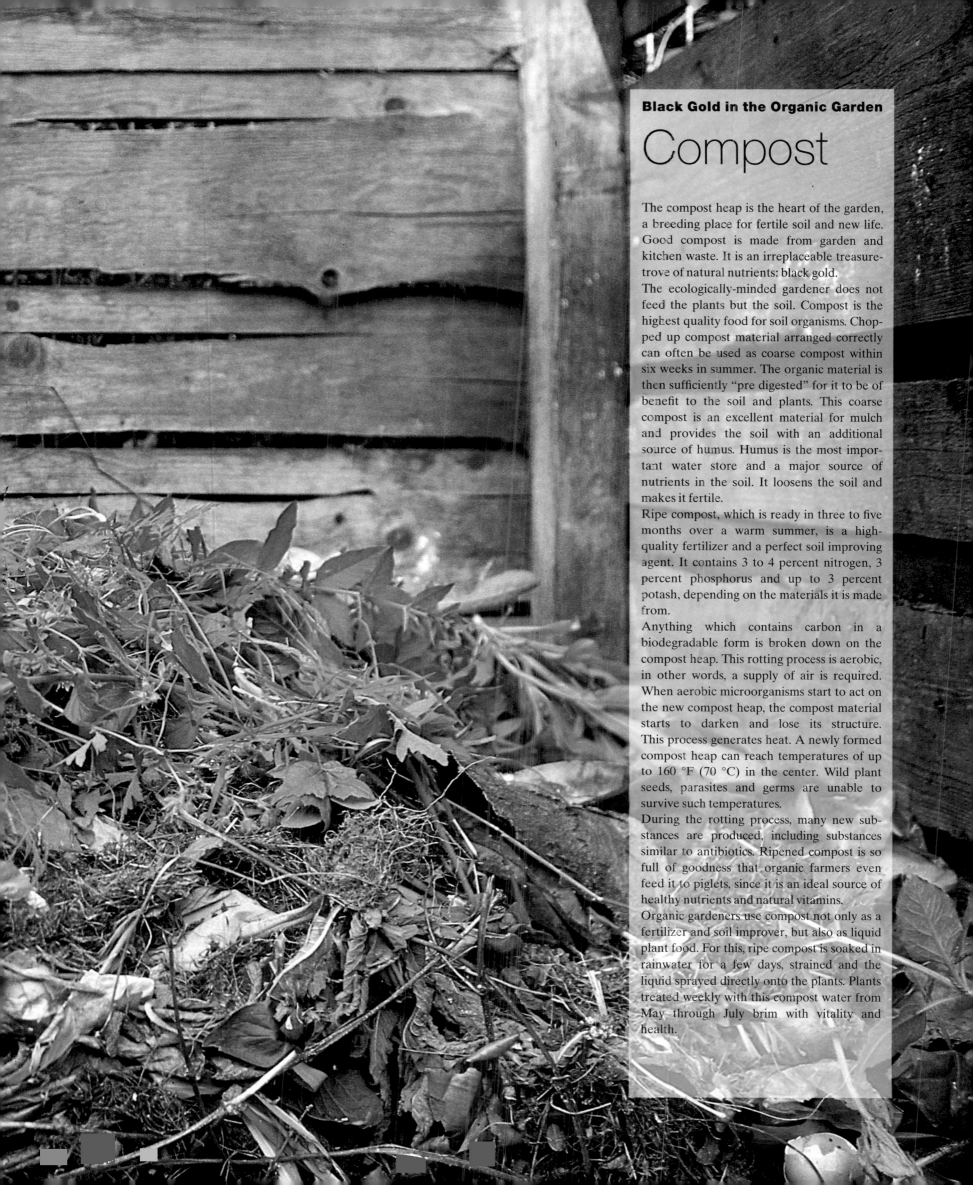

Black Gold in the Organic Garden

Compost

The compost heap is the heart of the garden, a breeding place for fertile soil and new life. Good compost is made from garden and kitchen waste. It is an irreplaceable treasure-trove of natural nutrients: black gold.

The ecologically-minded gardener does not feed the plants but the soil. Compost is the highest quality food for soil organisms. Chopped up compost material arranged correctly can often be used as coarse compost within six weeks in summer. The organic material is then sufficiently "pre digested" for it to be of benefit to the soil and plants. This coarse compost is an excellent material for mulch and provides the soil with an additional source of humus. Humus is the most important water store and a major source of nutrients in the soil. It loosens the soil and makes it fertile.

Ripe compost, which is ready in three to five months over a warm summer, is a high-quality fertilizer and a perfect soil improving agent. It contains 3 to 4 percent nitrogen, 3 percent phosphorus and up to 3 percent potash, depending on the materials it is made from.

Anything which contains carbon in a biodegradable form is broken down on the compost heap. This rotting process is aerobic, in other words, a supply of air is required. When aerobic microorganisms start to act on the new compost heap, the compost material starts to darken and lose its structure. This process generates heat. A newly formed compost heap can reach temperatures of up to 160 °F (70 °C) in the center. Wild plant seeds, parasites and germs are unable to survive such temperatures.

During the rotting process, many new substances are produced, including substances similar to antibiotics. Ripened compost is so full of goodness that organic farmers even feed it to piglets, since it is an ideal source of healthy nutrients and natural vitamins.

Organic gardeners use compost not only as a fertilizer and soil improver, but also as liquid plant food. For this, ripe compost is soaked in rainwater for a few days, strained and the liquid sprayed directly onto the plants. Plants treated weekly with this compost water from May through July brim with vitality and health.

The Compost Site

Compost, like an incubator, needs warmth and protection from the wind. A place half shaded by bushes, sheltered from the wind and out of direct sunlight is ideal.

A compost bin (this is what the container is called) should be 4 to 6½ feet (1.20 to 2 meters) wide and as long as required. A compost bin measuring 6½ by 10 feet (2 by 3 meters) is large enough for a garden covering 120 square yards (100 square meters). In larger gardens, the compost site can take up as much as 8 to 10 percent of the garden area. The more space is allowed for the compost, the easier it is to keep it in order. It then becomes the garden's own humus factory.

It has proved useful in practice to have two bins and one collecting place if there is sufficient space for this. The raw material for composting is best kept in a well-aired container until enough has been collected to warrant setting up a bin.

The Compost Material

All organic material from the household and garden can be composted: vegetable waste, wilted flowers, weeds which have been dug up, grass clippings, chopped-up twigs, egg shells, coffee grounds, tea leaves, paper and cardboard without a glossy finish or colored print. The organic material has to be in small pieces for it to rot quickly. Paper therefore has to be torn up and cardboard cut up into small pieces, and plant stems are cut down into handy 4 inch (10 centimeter) lengths with secateurs or with an axe and chopping block. Cabbage stalks and very hard plant stems can be crushed with a hammer. Bulky vegetable waste, branches and plants which have finished flowering can also be chopped up easily with a garden shredder (see p. 411).

Making Compost, Layer by Layer

Compost is made by adding layer upon layer, like a gateau. Chopped up tree and hedge cuttings form the bottom layer. They ensure the compost is well ventilated. Then all the remaining organic material is mixed thoroughly, so that soft plant matter is mixed with woody and dry with moist.

The well mixed composting material is spread over the coarse material in the base of the bin in layers a few inches thick. A thin layer of powdered seaweed lime or rock meal is added between each layer. This improves the quality of the compost, soaks up excess moisture, acts as a buffer for any acids produced, and absorbs smells. If a lot of the material is dry and low in nitrogen, some horn, blood and bone meal can be scattered over. Manure from organic farms, stables or small animals can be mixed directly into the compost material in small amounts or spread in thin layers between the layers of garden waste.

To help it get going, a few shovelfuls of good garden soil or some ripe compost full of micro-organisms are added.

When the compost heap is built up, all the material should be uniformly moist. If dry materials like paper or straw are included, the compost must be watered with rain water or diluted plant manure after it has been loaded into the compost bin.

A Good Climate for Compost

The microorganisms need water, air and warmth to be able to accomplish their enormous task of devouring and digesting the compost material.

The carefully incorporated coarser material like tree and hedge cuttings ensures there is adequate ventilation from the outset.

Rainfall is not a very regular or reliable source of water. In winter and in rainy summers, the compost has to be protected from too much water. In the hot summer months, on the other hand, the compost heap has to be thoroughly watered once a week.

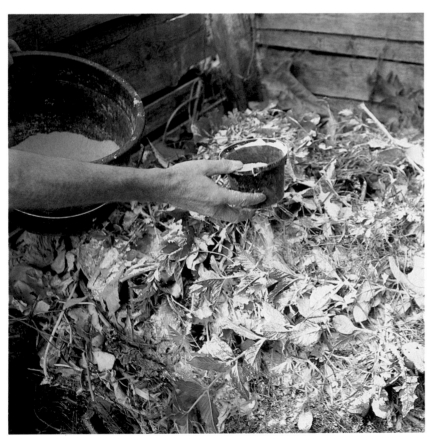

Ideally, a little seaweed lime or rock meal should be scattered on top of each layer of organic material to enrich the compost.

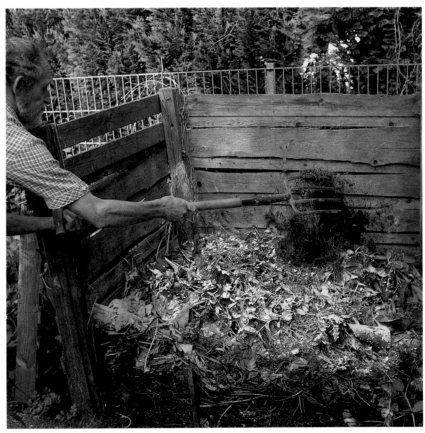

This is then covered with a new layer of chopped, well-mixed garden and kitchen waste. It should be spread in an even layer.

Hot Phase in the Compost Heap

Microorganisms heat the freshly laid compost heap to temperatures of up to 160 °F (70 °C). It is highly acidic during this phase: pH 4.5 to 5. The hotter it gets, the more alkaline it becomes: up to pH 8.5. A well structured compost heap will retain its heat for four to five days, then it starts to cool down. Now the pH comes closer to the plant-compatible neutral level of pH 7.5, and the compost heap gains some new inhabitants. It is now cool enough for compost worms. These earthworms, which are specially adapted to feed on relatively fresh green matter, cannot tolerate the initial acidity or heat. When they get to work, the ripening phase begins. Compost worms can easily be distinguished from ordinary earthworms in the garden soil as they are smaller, thinner and red.

Sweet-smelling Compost in Three Months

If the compost is prepared properly, it is ready for use as a plant-compatible, nutritious mulch material after just six weeks in summer. It is transformed into fertile material smelling of forest earth in three to five months. Coarser sticks and stems will still be recognizable – they can be taken out and put on the next heap. Compost does not normally need to be forked over, but for anyone who has the time to do so, the compost will be ready a few weeks earlier.

If compost is left for a while, the mineralization, or breakdown of organic substances to inorganic components, continues. This process can last for up to three years. However, complete mineralization is not desirable in an organic garden as composted earth of this sort hardly provides any food for the soil organisms.

The Compost Ripeness Test

To discover whether the compost is ripe and plant-compatible, the cress test can be carried out. Cress seeds are sprinkled onto a dish containing compost and moistened. If they have germinated after three to five days and look green and juicy, the "black gold" is ready. If the cress is yellow and germinates unevenly or not at all, the compost has not yet completely ripened.

As an alternative to a homemade compost bin, gardening stores sell kits for making composting containers in a wide range of shapes and materials.

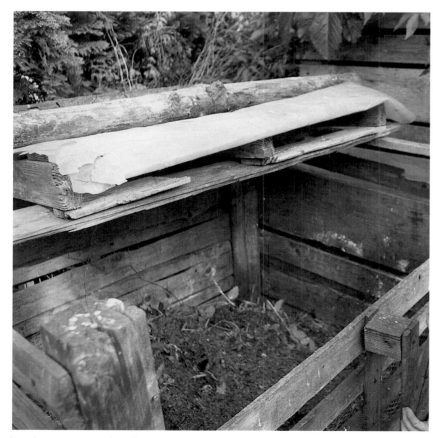

It makes sense to wait until the compost bin is well over half full before nailing down the lid.

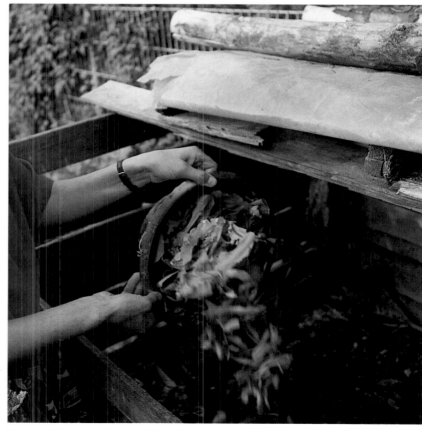

The smallest material is added last. Provided the composting material is now kept moist and the sun keeps it warm, the compost will be ripe in a few months.

Planned in Harmony with Nature

In organic gardening, nature is gently guided in a certain direction. It is therefore essential for each plant to be planted in a suitable place. It will only be able to grow into a good, sturdy plant if the soil, light, temperature, and wind conditions are right.

A cultivation plan gives a good overview of the gardening tasks ahead and helps prevent mistakes. A plan of this sort can be drawn up for plant beds and borders, and next summer's glorious floral display can be thought out half a year in advance. But it is particularly important to have a cultivation plan for the vegetable garden. Crop mixing and rotation should be carefully planned to enable the garden soil and crops to develop healthily.

The vegetable garden will thrive best in the sunniest part of the garden. To produce the plan, the vegetable beds are drawn to scale on a large sheet of squared paper. This basic plan can be photocopied and used again each year. The crops just move along a section each year.

A three-year crop cycle is simple and labor-saving. It is devised based on the nutrient requirements of the individual crops. They are classed as high, moderate and low nutrient-consuming plants, depending on their requirements. The vegetable patch is now divided into three sections.

• In the fall, the soil in the first section is covered with a thick layer of rotten manure or compost and rock meal. In the spring, the high nutrient consumers like cabbage varieties, potatoes, celery, leeks, cucumbers, and pumpkins are planted in this section. These vegetables can also be given a liquid plant manure made from fermented stinging nettles and fern as a top dressing during the vegetation period.

This organic garden has been well thought out, as various different species have been mixed in together and grow happily alongside each other.

Partner Crops

Plant	Good companion plant	Bad companion plant
Cabbage	Lettuces, tomatoes, potatoes, peas, leeks	Onions, leeks
Carrots	Onions, leeks, peas, tomatoes	
Celery	Cabbage, cucumbers, tomatoes, dwarf beans	Lettuces, potatoes
Cucumbers	Lettuces, beans, peas, leeks, celery, cabbage	Tomatoes, radishes, early potatoes
Dwarf beans	Cucumbers, celery, lettuces, tomatoes, potatoes	Onions, leeks, peas, fennel
Fennel	Lettuces, cucumbers, peas	Beans, tomatoes
Leeks	Carrots, tomatoes, onions, cabbage	Beans, peas, red beet
Lettuces	All vegetables except celery	Celery
Onions	Carrots, lettuces, cucumbers	Potatoes
Peas	Lettuces, cabbage, fennel, cucumbers, carrots	Beans, potatoes, onions, leeks
Potatoes	Peas, cabbage, dwarf beans, spinach	Pumpkins, tomatoes, celery, cucumbers, onions
Radishes	Cress, lettuces, tomatoes, cabbage, beans	Cucumbers
Salsify	Lettuces, leeks	
Spinach	Beans, radishes, cabbage, potatoes	Not as an early crop before red beet
String beans	Lettuces, celery, potatoes	Onions, fennel, peas
Tomatoes	Lettuces, radishes, carrots, celery, spinach	Cucumbers, peas, potatoes, fennel
Zucchini	String beans, onions, lettuces	Potatoes

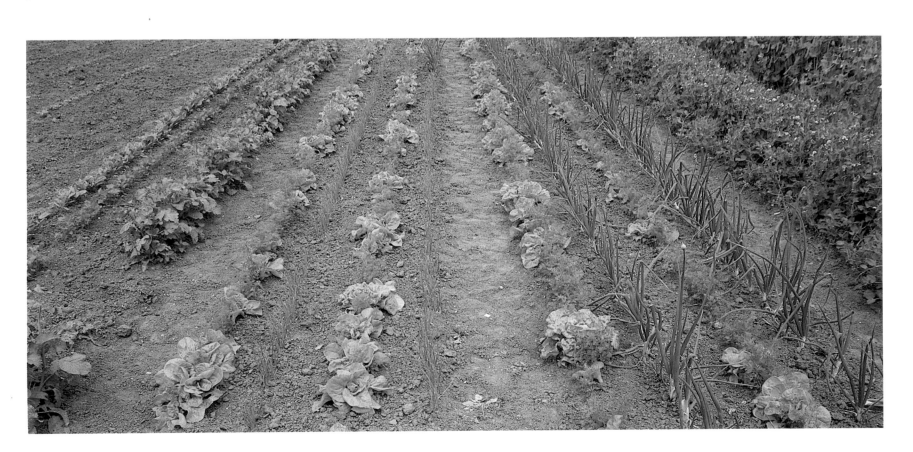

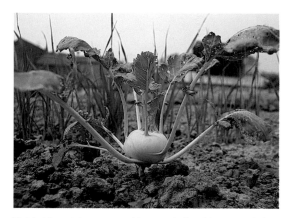

Kohlrabi, potatoes, pumpkins, and all cabbage varieties are examples of high nutrient consumers, which demand soil beds that are well fertilized with manure and compost.

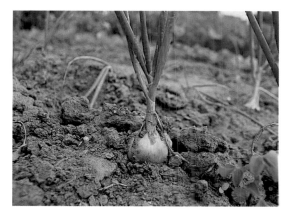

Onions, carrots, bell peppers, and lettuces are amongst the moderate nutrient consumers, which will take the place of the high consumers in the second year

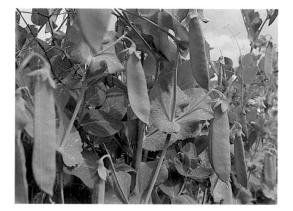

Beans, peas and herbs are content to occupy the bed in the third year, but in the fourth year, only leguminous plants are sown to give the soil a chance to recover.

• The following fall, the second section is heavily enriched, and the high nutrient consumers are moved to this section. There is now room in the first section for moderate nutrient consumers like carrots, red beets, onions, radishes, bell peppers, and lettuces. They have more modest requirements, but still need a layer of nutritious compost by way of preparation and some liquid plant fertilizer as a top dressing during the summer.

• In the third year, the undemanding low nutrient consumers can be planted in the first section. Apart from a little compost, they do not need any fertilizer. The peas, beans, cooking herbs, and medicinal herbs would not tolerate too many nutrients.

• The three year cycle can become a four year cycle if the garden is already divided into four sections. The soil last used for the low nutrient consumers is sown only with nitrogen-accumulating leguminous plants in the fourth year. If the soil is infested with, for example, nematodes or root eelworms, marigolds and French marigolds can be mixed in with the leguminous plants as a living soil remedy. They will drive out the soil pests.

Perfectly Planned Mixed Cultivation

In organic gardening, a mixture of plants is always cultivated. Several species are either positioned next to each other in rows in the same bed, or different plant types are combined within each row.

Mixed cultivation keeps plants healthy. In a monoculture, potato bugs, ants or greenflies do not have far to go from one plant to the next. Pathogenes are spread from plant to plant in just a breath of wind. Mixed cultivation, on the other hand, makes life difficult for pests. They have to cover long distances, encounter plants which they cannot "smell" and animals who are their natural enemies. Diseases spread less rapidly because of

the large distances between plants of the same species. And the soil is not exhausted over a large area by a single plant species. If a sensible crop rotation cycle is maintained, the soil is ready and healthy enough to be cultivated again the next season.

When considering which plants should be allowed to grow in immediate proximity to each other, the mutual compatibility of the plants is an important deciding factor. It is also important that the mixed crops protect and shade the soil for as long as possible and that the plants do not obstruct each other. Tall, thin plants like leeks grow well next to carrots, which above all need plenty of space under the ground, whilst, above the ground, their fine, feathery leaves provide shade.

Plants affect each other with their root excretions (phytoncides) and with gaseous substances like essential oils which they secrete from their leaves. The effects of the phytoncides are very varied. Some are directly poisonous to other plants, whereas others have a positive effect on the microorganisms or fungi which their neighbor needs to survive. If plants are happy being next to each other, the yields will be higher and the plants healthier. But if neighboring plants cannot "smell" each other, harvests are small or one species might even fall sick.

By way of example, in a bed of high nutrient consuming plants, the adjacent plant rows could be arranged as follows:
• Cress, radishes
• Cabbage varieties
• Iceberg lettuce
• Cabbage varieties
• Radishes, cress

A bed of moderate nutrient consuming plants might look like this:
• Radishes, cress
• Cutting-lettuces, red and green
• Kohlrabi

Crop Rotation in a Four Year Cycle

Year 1:
High consumers
Cabbage varieties, potatoes, celery, leeks, cucumbers, pumpkins
Fertilizer: manure, compost, rock meal, liquid plant manure

Year 2:
Moderate consumers
Carrots, red beets, onions, radishes, bell peppers, lettuces
Fertilizer: compost, liquid plant manure

Year 3:
Low consumers
Peas, beans, cooking and medicinal herbs
Fertilizer: compost

Year 4:
Leguminous plants
Horse beans, lupines, vetchling, sweet peas
Fertilizer: none

Then start from the beginning again.

• Early cabbage lettuces
• Kohlrabi
• Cutting-lettuces, red and green
• Radishes, cress

And an example of a low nutrient consuming plant bed is as follows:
• Dwarf beans, savory
• Red beets
• Dwarf beans
• Red beets
• Dwarf beans, savory

409

Gardening Equipment

A fork, pigtooth, hoe, rake, trowel, watering can, and good secateurs are the basic tools an organic gardener will need. For a large garden, it is worth getting hold of other items which can speed up garden work.

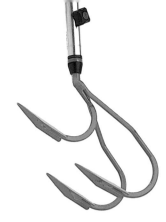

Spade

In organic gardening, the spade is mainly used for laying paths, high beds and sloping beds, and for working with compost. Good spades have a one-piece blade and socket made of stainless steel, with a blade as sharp as a knife. The handle should be made of polished or varnished wood or unbreakable plastic.

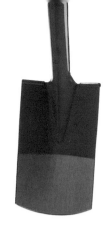

Claw Hoe

The claw hoe has four strong downward-pointing prongs. It is very useful for loosening, leveling, separating large clumps of earth, and lifting or incorporating manure or compost.

Practical Garden Tools

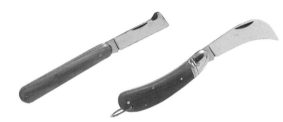

Knives

General purpose garden knives are suitable for harvesting vegetables, taking cuttings and preparing grafts. Knives for cuttings have a straight blade and have many different uses. The blade of a grafting knife has a protrusion on the end which is used for removing the bark during grafting. A pruning knife has a curved blade. It is ideally suited for cutting branch stumps cleanly when a tree is pruned.

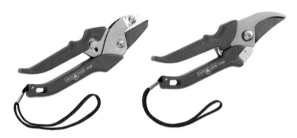

Secateurs

Long-handled branch secateurs cut branches or woody stems $1/2$ to 1 inch (1 to 3 cm) thick. The long handles and good levering action make cutting easier. Rose secateurs can cut thick, woody stems up to $1/2$ inch (1 cm) thick, as well as leafy stems and shoots of any thickness. Rose cutters must be comfortable to hold, and must cut cleanly and accurately without crushing the stems. Hedge clippers are available in manual, electric or motor-powered versions. Battery-powered devices are practical and quiet.

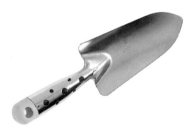

Planting Tools

Planting trowels must be strong, and preferably made of polished high-grade steel. A rounded wooden handle is particularly comfortable to hold. Trowels with engraved plant depth markings are practical. Bulb planters usually have marks of this sort. The round, hollow metal part is pushed as far down into the soil as the bulbs need to be planted. The earth can easily be lifted out because this special tool is hollow inside. A wooden planting stick or a metal planting rod with a bent handle are used when making holes for seedlings.

Compression Sprayer

A compression sprayer is used in an organic garden to sprinkle teas and infusions finely and evenly. It is important to have a model which comes with larger nozzles and a bio-sieve as accessories, so that plant infusions, compost extracts and lime mixtures can be sprayed without difficulty.

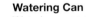

Watering Can

Watering cans made of plastic are light and inexpensive. Zinc cans are particularly attractive and last for decades. Cans with an extra long spout are handy for the greenhouse.

Sowing Wheel

There are many different types of hand sowing devices, ranging from the simple plastic trowel with inserts with differently spaced holes, to small wheels or drums which can be attached to a handle, and four-row sowing machines which are worthwhile for larger gardens.

Rake

Metal rakes with as large a width as possible are used for smoothing over seed drills and beds and raking up leaves and grass cuttings. A wooden rake is better for long meadow grass as it does not get caught up in the long grass.

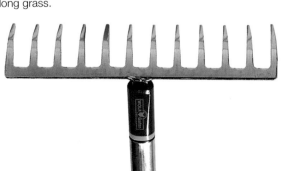

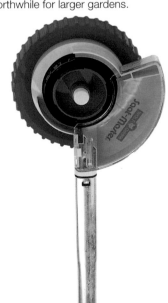

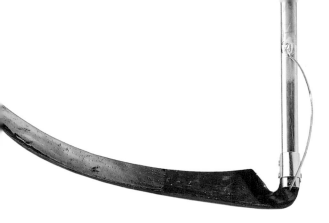

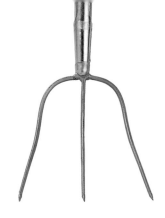

Scythe

A good scythe is important for a flowering meadow, but is also useful for cutting stinging nettles and wild plants by the edge of a wood or path. It is sometimes possible to find courses where one can learn every aspect of correct scythe handling, from mowing to sharpening. A hand sickle is sufficient for smaller areas.

Hoe

Hoes are used to remove wild plants, loosen the soil and make seed drills. Dutch hoes have a chisel-like blade and require quite a lot of strength. Beater hoes cut through weed roots just below the surface of the ground and loosen the soil without too much effort. The draw hoe or leaf hoe is also easy to handle. The scuffle hoe or push hoe is ideal for weeding. A practical idea is a multi purpose handle to which a wide range of attachments can be fixed, as required.

Hay Fork

A sturdy hay fork with sharpened prongs is ideal for distributing mulch material, turning the hay in a field, piling up brushwood, and much more.

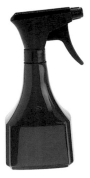

Powder Puffer

A plastic powder puffer distributes rock meal in a fine layer over cabbages, tomatoes and fruit bushes to protect against caterpillars and hungry birds.

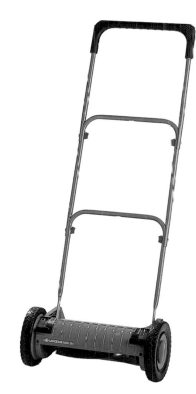

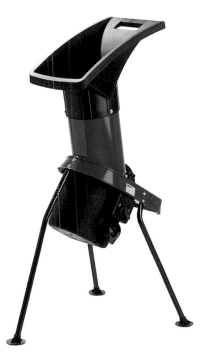

Chopper

Even a hand chopper can cut up big branches without trouble. For larger gardens, a motorized unit may be worthwhile. Exceptionally quiet choppers are allowed to bear the "environment-friendly" label. The most powerful choppers are swing-hammer mills which not only chop up the material but also shred it so it breaks down very rapidly when composted. Always wear protective goggles when using a chopper.

Flame Guns

Flame Guns keep wild plants under control. These devices, which are powered by gas or electricity, depending on the model, use a naked flame or an infrared radiator. It is guided slowly over paths or beds affected by weeds, and the unwanted plants are heated to about 160 °F (70 °C) and die. Models range from light, portable hand units to agricultural units which are mounted on a tool carrier or trailer.

Lawnmower

For a small area of grass, a hand mower is sufficient, preferably a rotary bladed mower which cuts very cleanly. Mulch mowers are useful for larger areas of lawn. The grass clippings are automatically cut up small and are left on the lawn as fertilizer. A motor mower which can cut long grass without getting blocked is useful for large fields.

Digging Fork

A digging fork has four flat steel prongs. It is essential for loosening the soil, applying compost, harvesting root vegetables etc. Organic digging forks have long, rod-like prongs which are easy to push into the soil. They are triple the width of standard forks and are designed only for loosening and airing the soil.

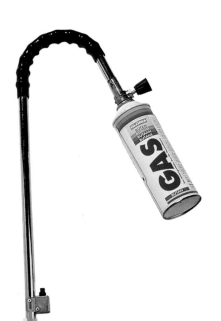

Cultivator

This tool, possibly the most important one in the organic garden, is available with three or five teeth, rigid or sprung. At the end of each tooth is a lance-like shovel, the duckfoot. The cultivator loosens hard earth and breaks it up. A cultivator with one tooth is called a pigtooth.

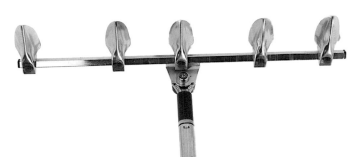

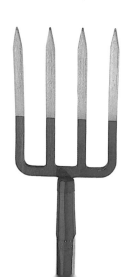

Gentle Deterrents for Pests and Diseases

Working Without Chemicals

When trouble is looming in the organic garden, if for example weather conditions are bringing on a plague of pests, manual work and gentle deterrent measures can solve garden problems quickly and without toxic chemicals:

• In the event of infestation by potato bugs, caterpillars, snails, cockchafers, or greenfly, the quickest solution is to gather in the yield and shake off the pests.

• Affected parts of the plant can be cut off as a first aid measure in the case of fungal diseases like raspberry stem disease, brown rot in pomaceous and pitted fruits and leaf curl in peaches.

• Lime bands can be tied around fruit trees from September, before the winter moth caterpillars crawl into the trees.

• Cherry fly traps made of yellow plastic coated with special lime are hung in the cherry tree before the fruits begin to ripen.

• Snail barriers made of bent metal help deter hungry mollusks. Sharp sand, wood ash or barley chaff also slow them down.

• Trap crops like halved potatoes attract wireworms.

• Clay paint frees fruit trees of harmful insects. For this, clay is mixed to a homogenous liquid with cold horsetail tea and, where available, with fresh cow's manure and brushed on to the tree trunk. Clay, when diluted and sprayed over berry bushes, spoils birds' appetite for the young buds.

• Vegetable nets protect the plants from birds and vegetable flies and can even keep mice at bay.

• Dusting with rock flour, wood ash or seaweed lime prevents fungal diseases, counteracts aphids and flea beetles and deters slugs and snails.

• For teas and infusions, plant parts are soaked in water in an enameled cooking vessel for 24 hours. The mixture is then

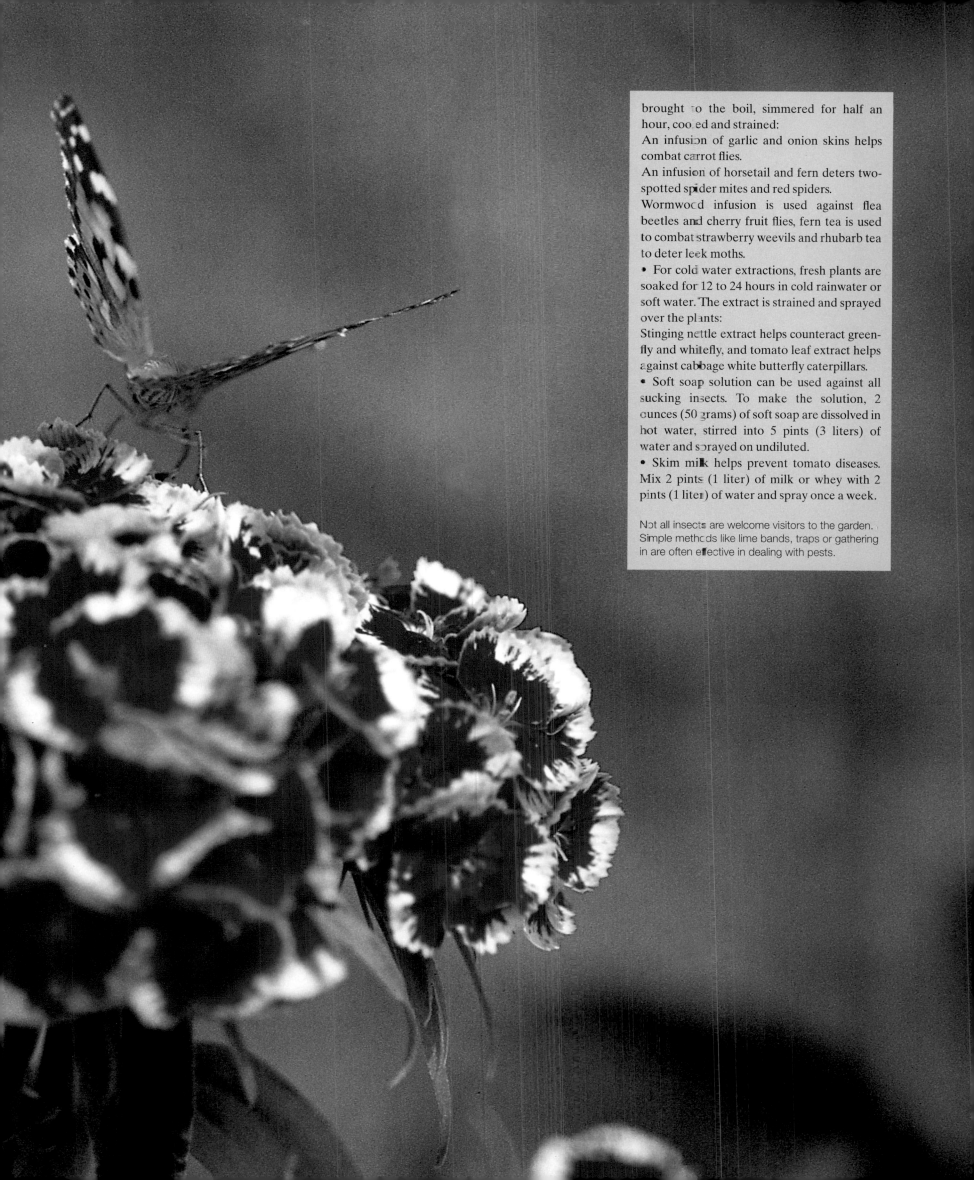

brought to the boil, simmered for half an hour, cooked and strained:

An infusion of garlic and onion skins helps combat carrot flies.

An infusion of horsetail and fern deters two-spotted spider mites and red spiders.

Wormwood infusion is used against flea beetles and cherry fruit flies, fern tea is used to combat strawberry weevils and rhubarb tea to deter leek moths.

• For cold water extractions, fresh plants are soaked for 12 to 24 hours in cold rainwater or soft water. The extract is strained and sprayed over the plants:

Stinging nettle extract helps counteract green-fly and whitefly, and tomato leaf extract helps against cabbage white butterfly caterpillars.

• Soft soap solution can be used against all sucking insects. To make the solution, 2 ounces (50 grams) of soft soap are dissolved in hot water, stirred into 5 pints (3 liters) of water and sprayed on undiluted.

• Skim milk helps prevent tomato diseases. Mix 2 pints (1 liter) of milk or whey with 2 pints (1 liter) of water and spray once a week.

Not all insects are welcome visitors to the garden. Simple methods like lime bands, traps or gathering in are often effective in dealing with pests.

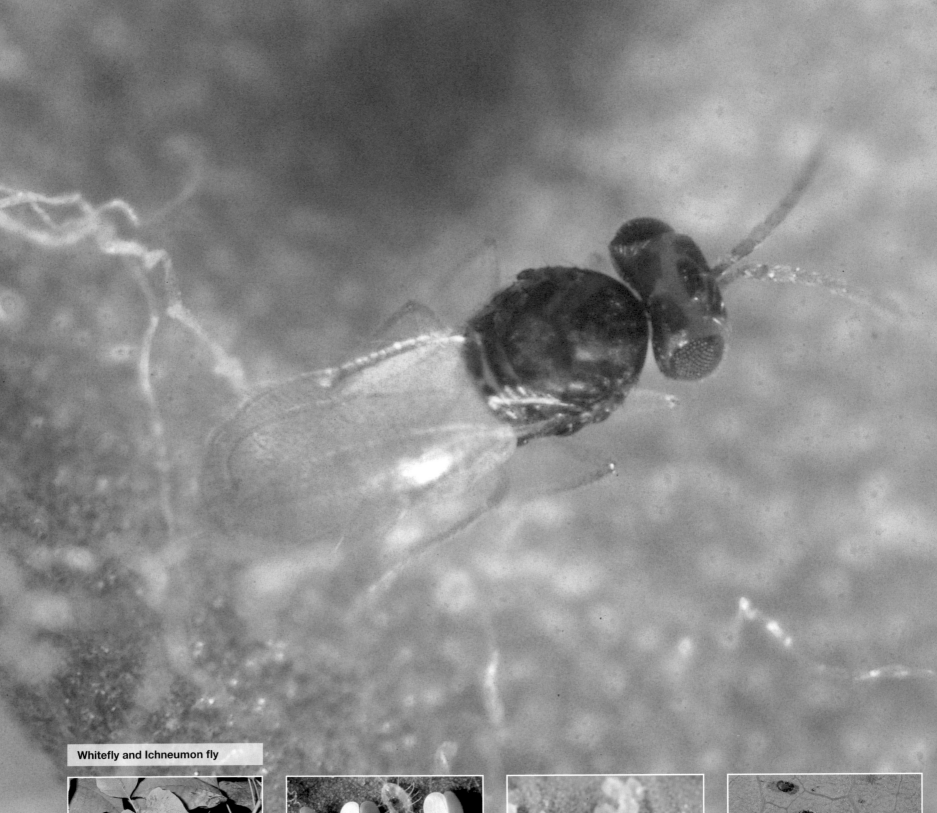

Whitefly and Ichneumon fly

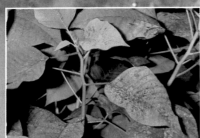

Whitefly infestation leaves severe honey dew markings on the leaves of the poinsettia – a result of it being robbed of its nutrients.

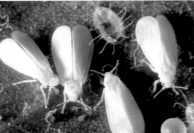

The greenhouse whitefly (1.5 to 2 mm in length); empty nymph shells and drops of honey dew can be found only on the undersides of the leaves.

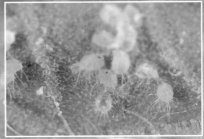

Whiteflies in their first growth phase as nymphs are hardly visible to the naked eye. These are closely related to the greenfly.

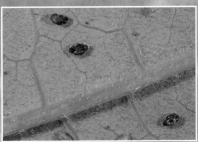

The whitefly nymphs attacked by the ichneumon fly turn black. Nymphs of another strain of whitefly go transparent.

Dr Reinhard Albert

Beneficial Organisms and Pests

Pests can be a big problem in the garden. Greenfly on lettuces and beans, apple and cherry trees, and roses, or caterpillars on cabbages occur more frequently than gardeners would like, and cause damage both to plants and fruits. In the garden, the pest's natural enemies like titmice and other insect-eating birds, ichneumon flies, predator mites, spiders, and others, the so-called beneficial organisms, appear. (All animals in an ecosystem have a function. The subjective terms "beneficial organism" and "pest" are used here only for the sake of simplicity.) How quickly the number of pests in the garden is reduced depends on the degree of infestation, and the size and growth rate of the population of beneficial organisms. Beneficial organisms often become active very early on and get the infestation under control before the gardener notices that there is a problem. But from time to time, organic gardeners are obliged to take control of the situation using infusions and extractions.

The favorable climatic conditions in greenhouses mean that pests are a serious problem because they can grow at such a rapid rate. Greenfly, whitefly and sometimes also mealy bugs and other coccids extract the nutrients from plants and produce sweet honey dew. Black mold becomes established here, contaminating the plants and fruits and attracting ants.

Ants can actively spread pest infestation, protecting them against the various beneficial organisms. For example, they bite off the wings of female greenflies of the species which produce honey dew, thereby forcing them to stay on the plant. They then spread these unwinged creatures on to other plants. As their reward, the ants can feed on the greenfly's secretions, the honey dew, which they take from the greenflies via the wax glands. Soldier ants drive away or catch the ant's natural enemies. Some of the rivals have adapted themselves to this. Larvae and adults of the predatory gall midge *Aphidoletes aphidimyza* are not recognized as enemies either by ants or by greenfly. The ichneumon fly *Lysiphlebus testaceipes* successfully disguises itself using a greenfly smell.

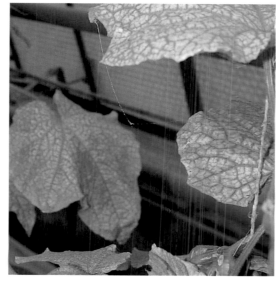

Cucumbers and string beans come under attack from two-spotted spider mites. Here you can see a female two-spotted spider mite of the *Tetranychus urticae* species with eggs under a cucumber leaf (left-hand edge).

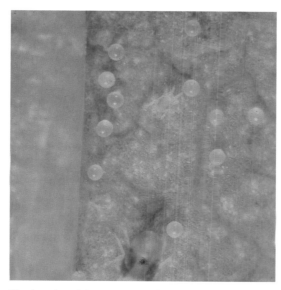

The females of the two-spotted spider mites, which become red spiders in winter, lay about 100 eggs in their 14 day existence.

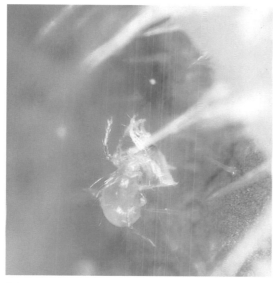

A female predator mite (*Phytoseiulus persimilis*), about 0.5 mm in length, sucks out a two-spotted spider mite. It eats 5 adult or 20 young insects or eggs a day.

Vegetables cultivated in greenhouses in central Europe during the summer season, like cucumbers, tomatoes, beans, and eggplants can come under attack from whitefly of the *Trialeurodes vapoariorum* species and from greenfly species like *Aphis gossypii* or *Aphis fabae, Aulacortum solani, Macrosiphum euphorbiae,* or *Myzus persicae.* Greenfly are also a problem on bell pepper plants. There are also other pests which can destroy the plant altogether. For example, two-spotted spider mites like *Tetranychus urtiae* suck out individual cells on the undersides of leaves. This can cause the whole leaf to die. Thrips damage leaves in a similar way, but also cause severe damage to fruits by blocking the pores. They also pass on viruses harmful to plants. The larvae of the leaf miner tunnel into leaves, and butterfly caterpillars devour whole leaves (see the tables of primary and secondary pests for cucumber and tomato crops on p. 416).

In the past, in bio dynamic or organic cultivation, everything often had to be replanted from scratch after a severe pest attack in the greenhouse. In conventional cultivation, pests are combated with insecticides and acaricides. Excessive use of pesticides can then cause even greater problems as the pests start to develop a resistance to these chemicals. And pesticides often leave residues on the fruits and vegetables. Furthermore, only a few fungicides and very few insecticides have been shown to be effective for cultivation under glass and the latter have not been tested on every type of vegetable crop. This shortfall in chemical plant protection is largely due to a lack of interest on the part of the industry, which does not want to carry out expensive trials for crops which are only grown on a relatively small scale.

This gap in the pesticide market, which has widened steadily over the last few years, has given gardeners a good opportunity to combat pests by organic means, and especially using beneficial organisms.

Large photograph, left: Useful insect or pest? The answer depends on your point of view.

Organic Pest Control

Organic pest control means the use of organisms and viruses which have been collected and reproduced expressly for the purpose of controlling pest populations in order to protect plants, animals and humans. In simple terms this means that pests are combated not with chemicals but with their own natural enemies.

Biological pest control in itself is a strategy people have been aware of for a long time. A well-known example is the introduction of the cat in central Europe as a replacement for the marten, which was common at that time, to rid the house and barn of rodents. The use of beneficial organisms also has a long history in greenhouse cultivation. The ichneumon fly *Encarsia formosa* was bred and used in commercial greenhouses and botanical gardens in Great Britain back in the 1930s for combating the whitefly *Trialeurodes vaporariorum*. The Second World War and the invention of modern insecticides put an end to this practice. But since the end of the 1960s, beneficial organisms have been used ever more widely in western Europe for vegetable crops grown under glass.

Pests do not affect all crops equally. Cucumber plants, for example, are attacked by two-spotted spider mites, whitefly, greenfly, and the Californian flower thrips and five rival organisms have to be used regularly and simultaneously over a large area. Tomatoes, on the other hand, only have one primary pest – whitefly – which has to be dealt with virtually everywhere tomatoes are cultivated.

The use of beneficial organisms provides considerable advantages for gardeners and consumers, but it can also entail disadvantages for gardeners (see summary above). There will always be difficult situations and unfavorable conditions. During prolonged cool or otherwise very warm weather, the climatic requirements of many useful organisms are not met or are exceeded, so the pests can continue to multiply. For example, in the height of summer, bugs can cause severe damage to cucumbers while unchecked by natural enemies.

The sometimes considerable cost of introducing beneficial organisms is a further disadvantage for the gardener. These increased costs are not repaid

Organic Protection for Cucumbers

Primary Pests

Pest	Counter-organism	Additional measures
Two-spotted spider mite	*Phytoseiulus persimilis* *Amblyseius californicus*	Limed yellow and blue panels for pest monitoring
Whitefly	*Encarsia formosa*	
Greenfly	*Chrysoperta camea* *Aphidoletes aphidimyza* *Aphidius colemani* *A. matricariae, A. ervi*	*C. camea* for home treatment
Thrips	*Amblyseius barkeri* *A. cucumeris* *Orius sp.*	

Secondary Pests

Pest	Counter-organism	
Mining flies	*Diglyphus isaea* *Dacnusa sibirica*	
Caterpillars	*Bacillus thuringiensis*	

Organic Protection for Tomatoes

Primary Pests

Pest	Counter-organism	Additional measures
Whitefly	*Encarsia formosa* *Macrolophus caliginosus*	Limed yellow panels

Secondary Pests

Pest	Counter-organism	Additional measures
Greenfly	*Aphelinus abdominalis* *Chrysoperla carnea* *Aphidoletes aphidimyza* *Aphidius colemani* *A. matricariae, A. ervi*	Limed yellow and blue panels for pest monitoring *C. camea* for home treatment
Thrips	*Amblyseius barkeri* *A. cucumeris* *Orius sp.*	
Two-spotted spider mite	*Phytoseiulus persimilis* *Ablyseius californicus*	
Mining fly	*Diglyphus isaea* *Dacnusa sibirica*	
Caterpillars	*Bacillus thuringiensis*	
Bumble bees	*Bombus terrestris*	For pollination

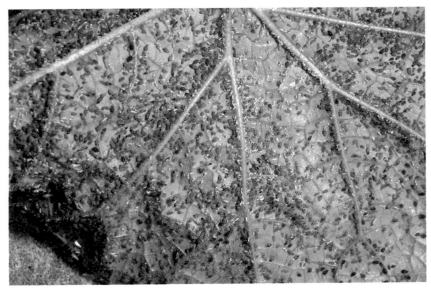

Severe infestation by the cotton greenfly *Aphis gossypii* under a cucumber leaf. The resulting damage is similar to that produced by whitefly. The white shells of the greenfly are also found on the upper surface of the leaf.

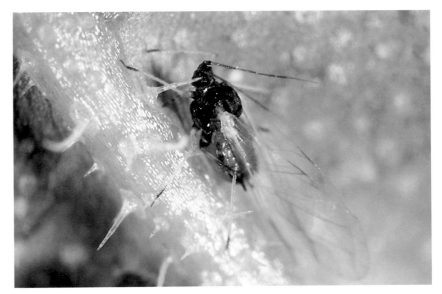

Winged female of the cotton greenfly which produces 3 to 6 nymphs per day in summer. These produce young of their own after just a week. An easy meal for beneficial insects.

by retail chains because of the need to keep up with international competition and the price-consciousness of the customers. However, organic greenhouse cultivation would not be possible today without the use of these small helpers from the natural world. They have proved their worth particularly in the protection of crops like tomatoes, bell peppers, eggplants, and beans. And beneficial organisms are used to protect other crops too. In Germany, for example, almost 15,000 acres (6,000 hectares) of corn fields are protected from the European corn borer *Ostrinia nupilalis* by the two-spotted spider mite *Trichogramma evanescens*. Other Trichogramma species are used by private gardeners to combat fruit moths on apple and plum trees. In cabbage cultivation, individual farms have successfully used ichneumon flies against various destructive types of butterfly. But this organic method is between two and ten times more expensive than chemical plant protection, depending on the crop and form of cultivation. However, it is being employed increasingly for ornamental plants, particularly poinsettia and other pot plants, as well as for indoor plants.

It is possible, to a limited extent, to make use of beneficial organisms in a private organic garden. Beneficial organisms can be encouraged by installing nesting boxes for birds and creating shelter for small mammals, earwigs, ichneumon flies, lacewings and predator mites. Organic control of the larvae of the black vine weevil with insect-pathogenic nematodes of the *Heterorhabditis* and *Steinernema* families is an effective. proven method. Attempts at using lacewing larvae to combat greenfly or using predator mites of the *Phytoseiulus persimilis* species to combat two-spotted spider mites on short plants like strawberries, raspberries and gooseberries have also been successful.

In all, 42 species of beneficial organism are available from specialist breeders and dealers in western European countries at present. These will counteract all pests affecting greenhouse crops with the exception of root aphids, bugs, cicadas, slugs, and snails. But there will soon also be environmentally compatible ways of dealing with slugs in the garden and greenhouse in the form of new slug pellets and an anti slug nematode, which works on field slugs.

The costs of beneficial organisms vary greatly. The useful organisms for indoor plants are extremely expensive. But, as we have seen in the last two years, much can be achieved with a little patience and a small quantity of the useful organism.

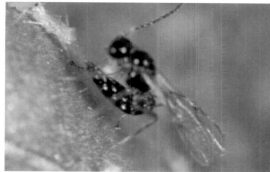

The 2 millimeter long ichneumon *Aphidius maticariae* lays its eggs in greenflies, which are eaten by the larvae.

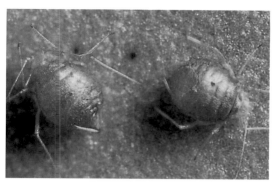

Only the brown-colored shells of the greenflies remain. The ichneumon larvae pupate inside.

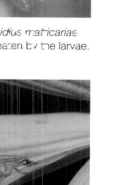

The lacewing *Chrysoperla carnera* which feeds only on honey dew and pollen produces larvae with an extremely big appetite.

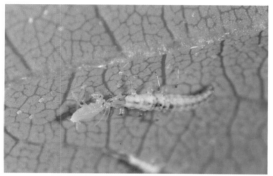

The lacewing larva devours or kills between 200 and 500 greenflies in the 10 to 20 days before it pupates.

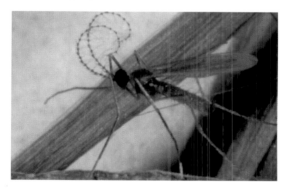

The 2 millimeter long, nocturnal predator gall midge *Aphidoletes aphidimyzia* often sits, unharmed, in spiders' webs during the day.

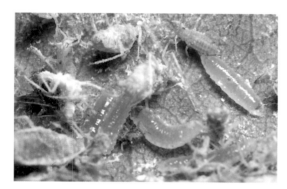

The females lay 100 to 150 eggs, from which the larvae hatch after a week. They each suck out 20 to 50 greenflies; ir expensive to breed.

Advantages and Disadvantages of Biological Pest Control for Greenhouse Vegetables

Advantages of using beneficial organisms	Disadvantages of using beneficial organisms
▼	▼
Beneficial organisms are distributed simply, and rapidly without using machines	Necessary to check for presence of pest and of beneficial organisms
▼	▼
Beneficial organisms are obtainable quickly and as a high quality product from the producers	Beneficial organisms have to be borne in mind when carrying out cultivation procedures like pruning or thinning out shoots and leaves
▼	▼
No harmful effects on users, soil, plants, fruit, or vegetables caused by chemicals or their residues	Knowledge of the biology of the pests and opportunities for biological control required
▼	
Kind to spontaneously occurring useful organisms No delays for cultivation procedures or harvesting	
▼	
Yields between 5 and 10% higher as the flowers are not damaged and the plants grow better	

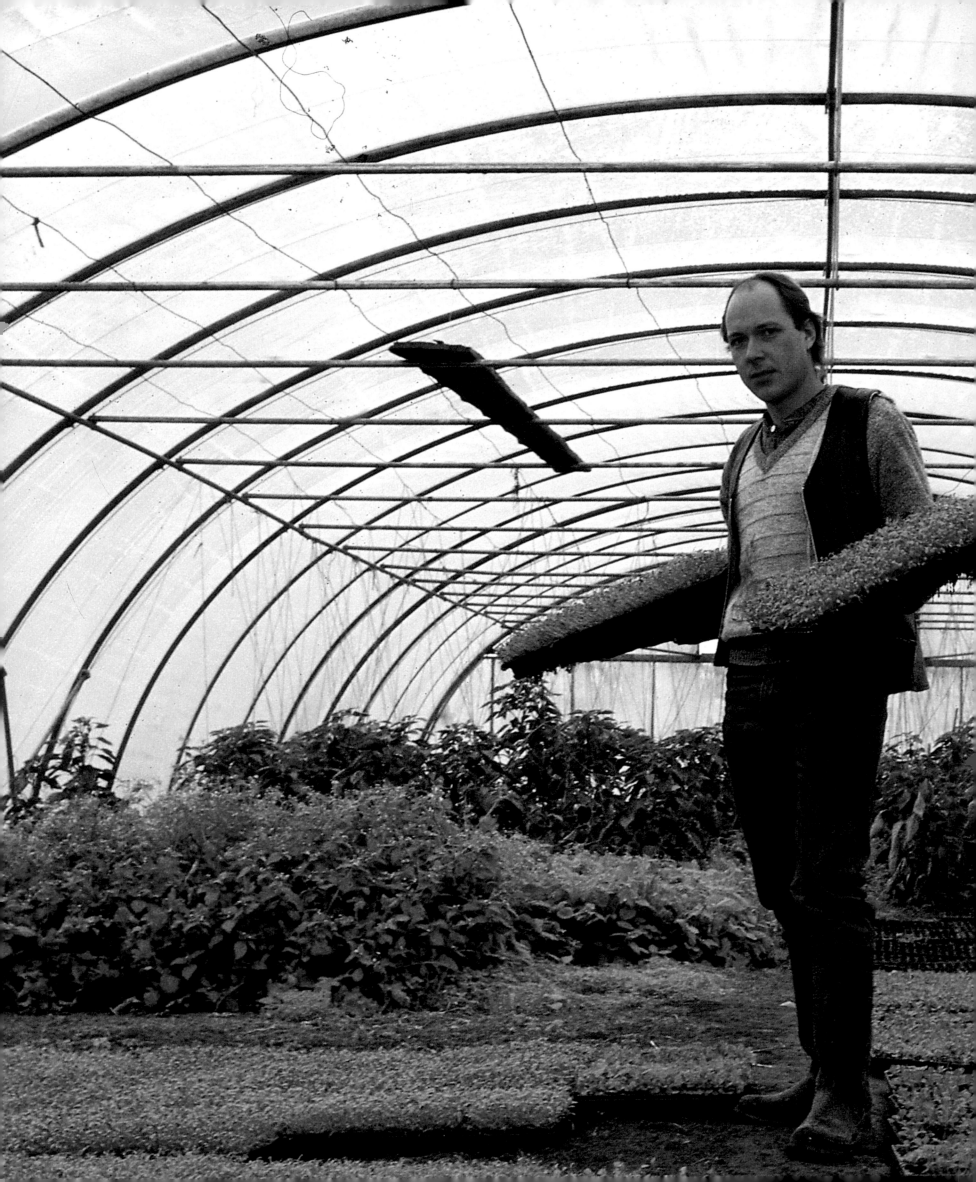

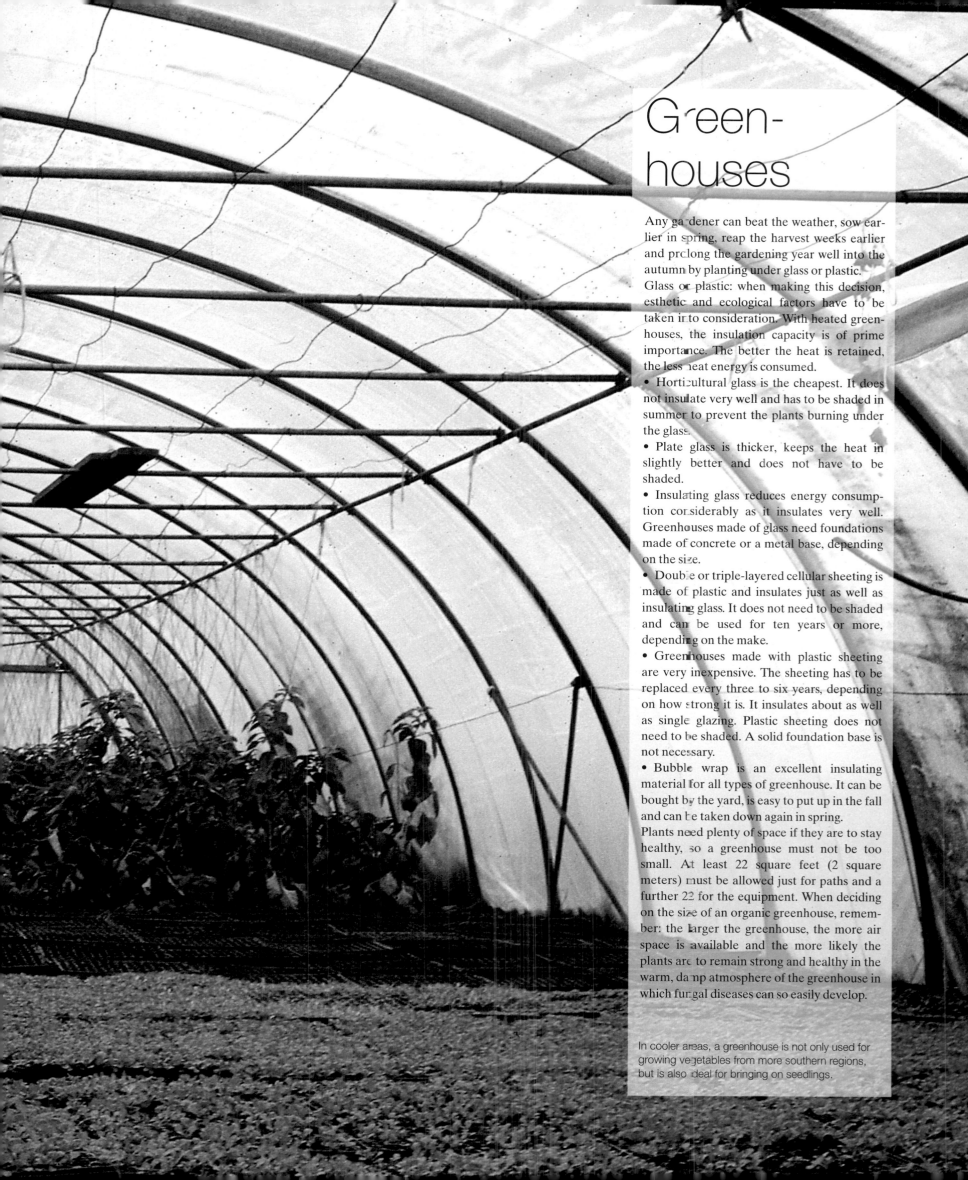

Green-houses

Any gardener can beat the weather, sow earlier in spring, reap the harvest weeks earlier and prolong the gardening year well into the autumn by planting under glass or plastic.

Glass or plastic: when making this decision, esthetic and ecological factors have to be taken into consideration. With heated greenhouses, the insulation capacity is of prime importance. The better the heat is retained, the less heat energy is consumed.

• Horticultural glass is the cheapest. It does not insulate very well and has to be shaded in summer to prevent the plants burning under the glass.

• Plate glass is thicker, keeps the heat in slightly better and does not have to be shaded.

• Insulating glass reduces energy consumption considerably as it insulates very well. Greenhouses made of glass need foundations made of concrete or a metal base, depending on the size.

• Double or triple-layered cellular sheeting is made of plastic and insulates just as well as insulating glass. It does not need to be shaded and can be used for ten years or more, depending on the make.

• Greenhouses made with plastic sheeting are very inexpensive. The sheeting has to be replaced every three to six years, depending on how strong it is. It insulates about as well as single glazing. Plastic sheeting does not need to be shaded. A solid foundation base is not necessary.

• Bubble wrap is an excellent insulating material for all types of greenhouse. It can be bought by the yard, is easy to put up in the fall and can be taken down again in spring.

Plants need plenty of space if they are to stay healthy, so a greenhouse must not be too small. At least 22 square feet (2 square meters) must be allowed just for paths and a further 22 for the equipment. When deciding on the size of an organic greenhouse, remember: the larger the greenhouse, the more air space is available and the more likely the plants are to remain strong and healthy in the warm, damp atmosphere of the greenhouse in which fungal diseases can so easily develop.

In cooler areas, a greenhouse is not only used for growing vegetables from more southern regions, but is also ideal for bringing on seedlings.

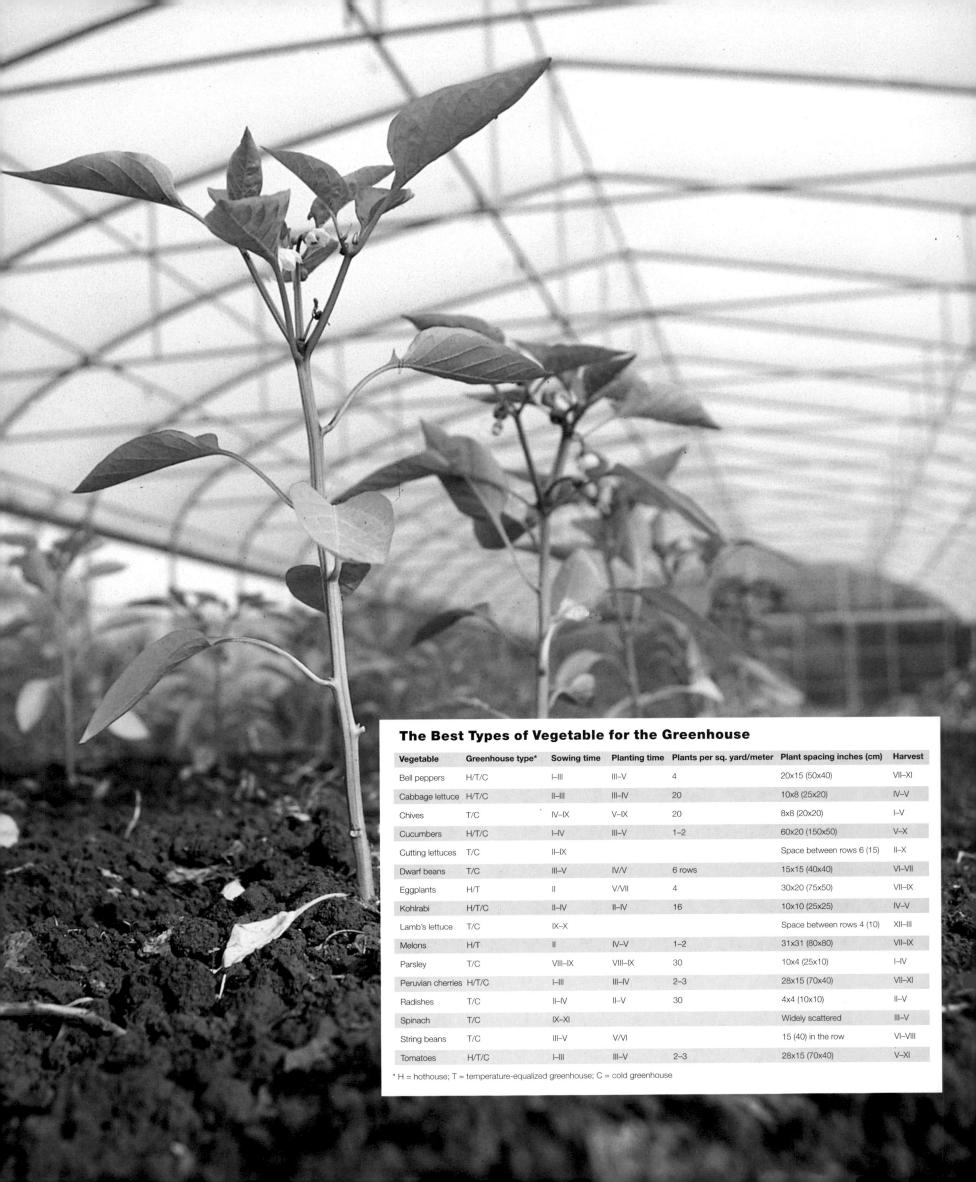

The Best Types of Vegetable for the Greenhouse

Vegetable	Greenhouse type*	Sowing time	Planting time	Plants per sq. yard/meter	Plant spacing inches (cm)	Harvest
Bell peppers	H/T/C	I–III	III–V	4	20x15 (50x40)	VII–XI
Cabbage lettuce	H/T/C	II–III	III–IV	20	10x8 (25x20)	IV–V
Chives	T/C	IV–IX	V–IX	20	8x8 (20x20)	I–V
Cucumbers	H/T/C	I–IV	III–V	1–2	60x20 (150x50)	V–X
Cutting lettuces	T/C	II–IX			Space between rows 6 (15)	II–X
Dwarf beans	T/C	III–V	IV/V	6 rows	15x15 (40x40)	VI–VII
Eggplants	H/T	II	V/VII	4	30x20 (75x50)	VII–IX
Kohlrabi	H/T/C	II–IV	II–IV	16	10x10 (25x25)	IV–V
Lamb's lettuce	T/C	IX–X			Space between rows 4 (10)	XII–III
Melons	H/T	II	IV–V	1–2	31x31 (80x80)	VII–IX
Parsley	T/C	VIII–IX	VIII–IX	30	10x4 (25x10)	I–IV
Peruvian cherries	H/T/C	I–III	III–IV	2–3	28x15 (70x40)	VII–XI
Radishes	T/C	II–IV	II–V	30	4x4 (10x10)	II–V
Spinach	T/C	IX–XI			Widely scattered	III–V
String beans	T/C	III–V	V/VI		15 (40) in the row	VI–VIII
Tomatoes	H/T/C	I–III	III–V	2–3	28x15 (70x40)	V–XI

* H = hothouse; T = temperature-equalized greenhouse; C = cold greenhouse

Gardening Under Glass and Plastic

The Bedding Soil
Greenhouse earth needs to be well looked after. Ideally, an inch-thick layer of well-rotted compost should be added each year and rock meal should be used as a long-term fertilizer and soil improver. A thin layer of mulch, which is renewed frequently, keeps down moisture losses and reduces the need for watering.

Seeds and Seedlings
For greenhouse crops, it is advisable to use varieties intended specifically for cultivation under glass. They are better suited to the light conditions and are resistant to typical greenhouse diseases.

Preventive Plant Protection
• Horsetail infusion is poured over the greenhouse earth in spring and sprayed repeatedly over the plants and soil during the vegetation period.
• Skim milk sprays also have an anti fungal effect.
• Plants which do not tolerate high air humidity well, like tomatoes, are regularly scattered with rock meal.
• Beneficial organisms can be used under glass and plastic by private and commercial gardeners alike. Here are a few examples:
Gall midge larvae feed on greenfly. Gall midges can be obtained in pupa form, and embedded in damp peat which can be piled in small heaps underneath the affected plant.
Ichneumon flies lay about 50 eggs per female. They help counteract whitefly.
Predator mites are bright, gleaming red. They feed on two-spotted spider mites. Predator mites are used on bean leaves.
The common lacewing lays its eggs in thread-like strings about 1/4 inch (5 millimeters) long. The larvae feed on greenfly.
(See section Beneficial Organisms and Pests, p. 412 ff.)

Accessories for the Organic Greenhouse

Ventilation is important for plants if they are to remain healthy without pesticides. Two roof windows and a gable door are the minimum requirement. The more air vents, the better, as they enable the greenhouse to be ventilated without causing drafts. Drafts can cause some plants, for example cucumbers and string beans, to become infested with two-spotted spider mites. Roof and side vents along the entire length of the greenhouse are available for larger, commercial sized greenhouses. Healthy movement of the air can be achieved with a ventilator – from an ecological point of view this should ideally be a solar model powered by solar cells. Automatic window openers which work without electricity by means of an expansion liquid help prevent ventilation mistakes.
A dividing wall can be built in larger greenhouses to create different climate sections. This is

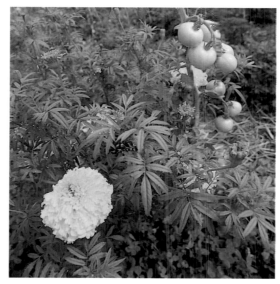

It is not just tomatoes that thrive under glass – flowers also give a splash of color.

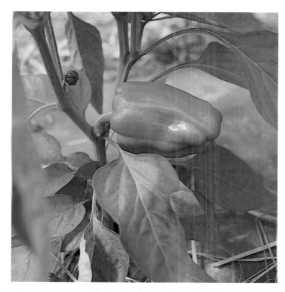

Bell peppers need plenty of warmth and light, especially if they are to turn red.

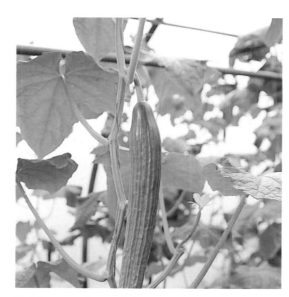

Only in warm climates is it possible to grow such lovely cucumbers without a greenhouse.

important, for example, when cucumbers and tomatoes are being cultivated together: cucumbers like high air humidity but tomatoes do not. A hygrometer is used to measure the air humidity in the greenhouse. This is important to prevent fungal diseases. Watering systems like sprinklers save water and keeps plants healthy, while very thin hoses controlled manually or by automatic valves direct the water to the area of the plant roots. When choosing stands and shelves, the main factor to consider is whether they allow adequate air circulation.

Greenhouse Heating
Organic gardeners like to keep their consumption of electricity and fossil fuels as low as possible. To maintain a steady temperature in a well insulated greenhouse, a small heater, a fan heater or an economy gas burner are quite sufficient. The Beta Solar heat accumulator provides solar heating without electricity. Black plastic hoses full of water are laid between the plant rows a foot (30 centimeters) apart. They store energy from the sun during the day and release it in controlled amounts at night. This is usually enough to protect plants from night-time frosts in spring.
Whether to use heating and what type to choose depends on the plants you are planning to grow:
• A hothouse has a minimum temperature of 55 °F (13 °C) year in, year out, and is suitable for breeding delicate special plants like orchids, foliage and flowering plants. It uses the most energy.
• A temperature-equalized greenhouse can drop to a minimum temperature of 41 °F (5 °C) at night and so remains protected from frost. Subtropical plants can be put here for the winter, vegetables can be cultivated and young plants brought on in the lighter months of fall and early spring.
• No heating at all is used in a cold greenhouse. Sun-loving vegetables and lettuces can grow here from the spring onwards, and frost-resistant ones can be grown here in winter.

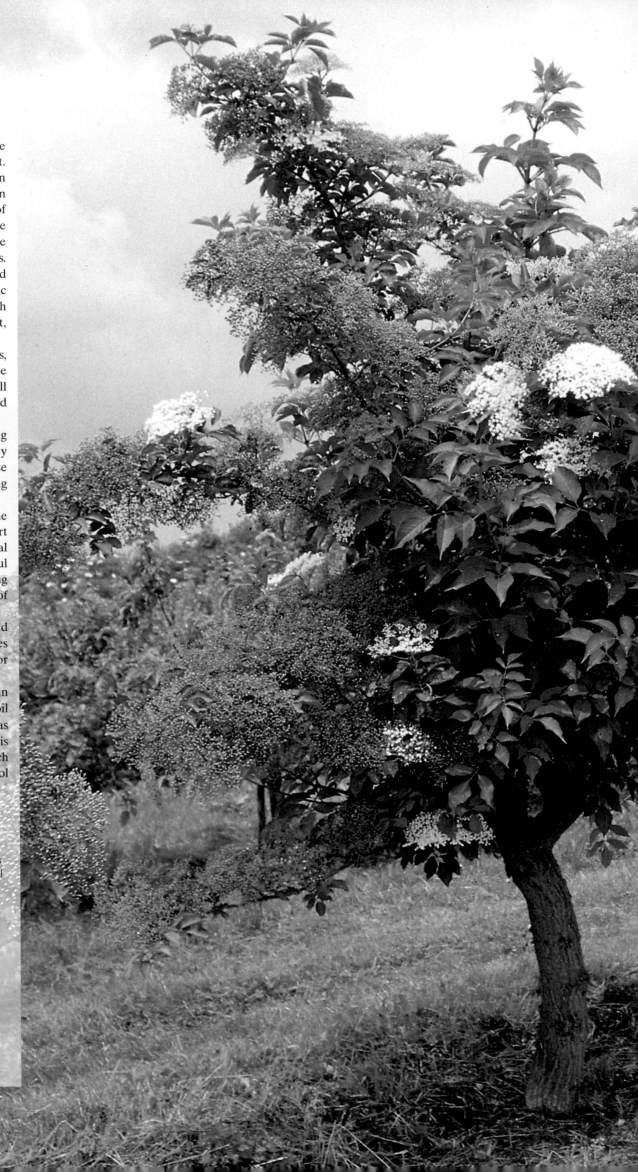

Fruit from Shrubs, Bushes and Trees

The fruit tree's natural habitat is on the edge of a wood where there is plenty of light. Berries, on the other hand, originally grew in the pale shade of deciduous trees and in clearings in the wood. Knowing the origin of the fruit plants means gardeners can arrange their fruit gardens in accordance with the natural needs of the shrubs, bushes and trees. If the soil and light conditions are right and the plants are carefully tended by organic means, they will remain in the peak of health and will produce rich harvests of sweet, aromatic fruits.

Fruit trees have different requirements, depending on their size. They can be classified, for example, as spindle bushes, wall plants, shrub trees, half-standard, or standard trees.

• Small-crowned trees with slow-growing rootstock are good for small gardens. They are convenient for fruit-picking and cease bearing fruit after 15 to 25 years, depending on the variety.

• Half-standard and standard trees, on the other hand, take a long time before they start to bear fruit. These trees will last several generations, with strong growth and plentiful yields. Trees like these are biotopes brimming with thousands of different species of organisms from the root to the crown.

• Fruit trees need full sunshine. The tree-grid above the roots and beneath the branches should be carefully tended and mulched or sown with medicinal herbs.

• Berry bushes and shrubs can thrive even in the half-shade. They have important soil requirements: many are happiest in a soil as acidic as their native soil, the forest floor. It is especially important to have a layer of mulch around all the bushes. This keeps the soil cool and moist.

Berries

Strawberries
Strawberries are planted in July or August in rows 1 foot (30 centimeters) apart. Straw or wood wool is scattered between the rows as a mulch layer. The runners of thriving mother plants can be removed and rooted in the soil. The plants are fertilized after the harvest with plenty of ripe compost.

Raspberries
Raspberries are planted in rows 20 inches (50 centimeters) apart. The stems need support wires to hold on to. The soil should be slightly acidic (pH 5). After the harvest, spent stems are cut down to just above ground level.

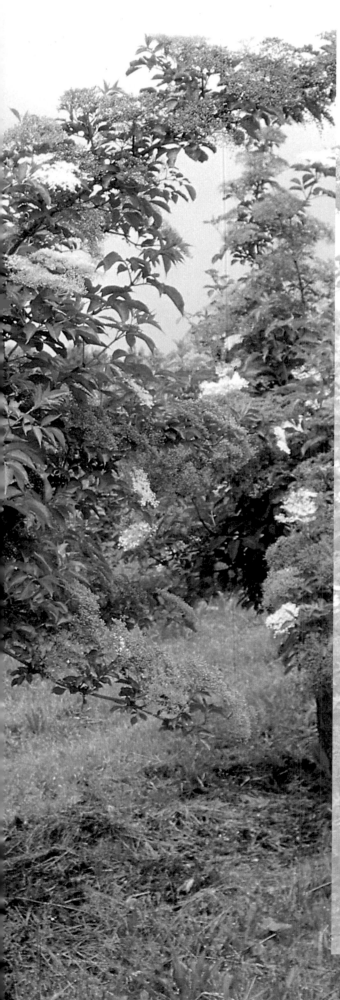

Blackberries

Blackberries on prickly bushes have a better flavor, but those on less prickly ones are not as painful to pick. The bushes must be planted 6 feet (2 meters) apart. Spent stems are cut off after the harvest.

Red, white, and black currants

Red, white, and black currants can bear fruit even in the half-shade. They produced fruit on two and three year old stems. The bush can have eight to twelve main stems. Dark, older branches are cut off just above ground level in the fall. Two or three new shoots are allowed to grow each year.

Gooseberries

Gooseberries have the same requirements as red and black currants: good garden soil (pH 7), wood ash and compost as fertilizer and a mulch covering of comfrey or fern leaves.

Blueberries

Some garden blueberry varieties can grow to over three feet (1 meter) in height. They only like acidic soils (pH 4.3 to 5.5). They are mulched with leaf compost, sawdust or tree needles. Blueberry bushes are pruned and thinned out each year.

Pomaceous Fruit

Apples

Apple trees exist as half-standard and standard trees. These tall trees traditionally grow in large organic gardens and orchards. The crowns of old apple trees are amongst the most varied habitats in the garden.
Spindle bushes and shrub trees are suitable for small gardens. Apart from new, disease-resistant trees, the main varieties available are old ones which are ideally adapted to the soil and climate and produce apples with a wonderful flavor. The earliest variety, the early dessert apple is ripe in July. Varieties suitable for storage like russet or winter rambour can be stored from November until the early summer.
Apple trees need a second tree nearby as a pollen provider. No digging should be done beneath the tree foliage as apple trees have a very flat root system. A layer of leaves and compost is good for the tree.

Pears

Pear trees grow upwards and do not overhang as much as apple trees. They are most suitable as wall fruit. The long taproots of established trees extract water from deep down, even in times of drought. Pear trees also need a second tree as a pollen donor.

Quinces

Can be planted as part of a mixed hedge or as a free-standing tree. It is usually available as a shrub tree. Apple and pear quinces, which are long, round fruit, can only be eaten cooked. They are excellent for making delicious jellies. Quinces are self-pollinating.

Pitted Fruits

Peaches

Peaches do best in a wine-growing climate. They bear fruit on one year old branches and have to be pruned every year. The actual fruit stems – branches with flowers and woody buds – are cut in half. The false fruit stems, which only bear flower buds, are cut back to leave just one or two nodes. Shoots which only have leaf buds are cut back to leave three to five nodes.

Greengages, Mirabelles

Greengages and mirabelles have the same requirements as regards location and soil: they thrive anywhere, but need more warmth than the undemanding plum. There needs to be another pitted fruit tree nearby for pollination.

Sour Cherries

Sour cherries grow on one year old wood. The spent branches are cut back every year, and only one new, young shoot is left. If this is not done regularly, the tree will only flower and bear fruit on the tips of the branches.

Sweet Cherries

It can take up to eight years after planting before sweet cherry trees start to bear fruit. Waterlogged soil is not good for the trees. Cherries are sensitive to acidity in the soil, which causes deep splits in the fruit. Regular additions of lime are important. Cherries need a second tree as a pollen provider.

Plums

They are available as half-standard and standard trees, and early and late varieties. It is important to select a variety in which the fruit flesh detaches easily from the stone. Some varieties are self-pollinating and some are not.

Nuts

Hazelnuts

There are certain varieties of hazelnut bush which produce extra large nuts. The catkin blossom on hazelnut bushes is one of the first food sources for bees in the spring. The plants have to be spaced 10 feet (3 meters) apart, as bushes of this sort can grow very large. Hazelnuts do not self-pollinate, but release pollen into the wind. If there is not another hazelnut bush nearby, two bushes must be planted together. Hazelnut plants do not have any special requirements as regards the soil and location. If they are thinned out in the fall, leaving six thick main branches, the bushes will give a long, plentiful harvest. Hazelnut bushes with green foliage and blood hazel bushes with dark red foliage are available.

Walnuts

The walnut tree used to be a traditional garden tree. Organic gardeners with plenty of space particularly like to plant walnut trees because the odor of the leaves keeps mosquitoes at bay. In areas with a mild climate, the tree grows up to 65 feet (20 meters) tall and develops an overhanging crown. It can be 15 years before the first walnuts appear. Anyone wanting to avoid the wait should pick a variety with a less spreading rootstock which bears nuts earlier. Unfortunately, these trees are not very frost-resistant. They are particularly suited to a wine growing climate. Collecting in the walnut harvest is a simple matter: when they are ripe, the green shells open and the nuts fall to the ground.

Background: Elders are robust bushes which grow up to 33 feet (10 meters) tall. Apart from their healthy berries, the flowers have various uses and the leaves are suitable for tea.

Herbs from the Garden

Flavorings and Remedies

As this gallery of herbs shows, there are many more than just the three or four herbs usually used in cooking and in bouquet garni. It is worth expanding one's repertoire and livening up dishes with new and different aromatic accents.

But herbs can also be used for health purposes. The valuable elements they contain stimulate the body in a natural way. Pleasant and mildly medicinal teas (see p. 241) can be prepared from most herbs. As regards growing requirements, most herbs are undemanding and easy to look after. They normally need plenty of sunshine to enable their essential oils to develop fully.

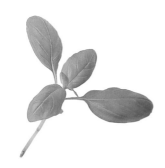

Basil
Basil is grown on the window sill. As it requires light to germinate, it must not be covered with earth after sowing. It can be planted outdoors or in the greenhouse from the end of May. Basil goes with tomatoes, mutton, lamb, and white beans.

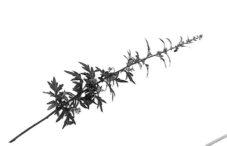

Mugwort
The perennial mugwort can grow up to 5 feet (150 cm) tall. The buds are cut off and dried shortly before they start to open. Mugwort is aromatic and slightly bitter, aids digestion and goes with fatty meats, goose, duck, roast mutton, and roast pork.

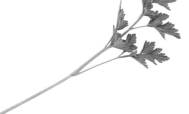

Flat-leafed Parsley
The particularly aromatic flat-leafed parsley, like the crinkly-leafed varieties, is sown from March onwards in rows 4 to 6 inches (10 to 15 cm) apart. Flat-leafed parsley can be picked at any time and can be dried or frozen. It grows wild in southern Europe.

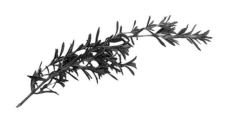

Savory
The annual savory plant is sown outdoors in mid-May. Fresh leaves can be picked throughout the summer or dried. Mountain or winter savory has a particularly strong flavor and is one of the typical Provençal herbs.

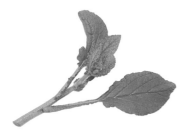

Borage
Borage or cucumber herb grows up to 2 feet (60 cm) in height. It is sown in April spaced 10 inches (25 cm) apart. The young leaves, which have a cucumber-like flavor, are served fresh with salads, vegetables of the cabbage family and remoulades. Borage cannot be preserved.

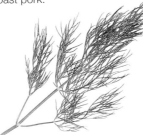

Dill
Dill is sown outdoors in April in rows 10 inches (25 cm) apart. Additional seeds can be sown at four week intervals to ensure a constant supply of fresh leaves. The fresh leaf tips go with salads and sauces. The seeds are used for pickled cucumbers and fish. Dill can be dried or frozen.

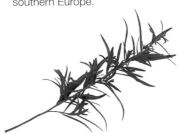

Tarragon
Aromatic German tarragon can only be grown as a pure variety from cuttings. Leaves and shoot tips can be picked continuously, but are not good for drying. Tarragon is suitable for herb vinegar, marinades, salads, sauces, and soups.

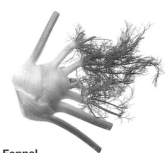

Fennel
This quick-growing herb which grows wild in warm climates has very aromatic, fine, feathery leaves with a flavor similar to aniseed. Goes particularly well with fish. The seeds are also used as a flavoring for marinades and pickled vegetables. The leaves have a less intense flavor.

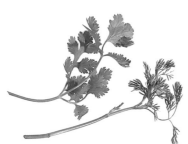

Chervil
Chervil, with its aniseed-like, sweetish flavor, is picked before it flowers, when it is about a foot (30 cm) tall. Chervil is always used fresh in soups, white and green sauces and salad dressings. It cannot be preserved.

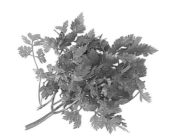

Cilantro
Whilst in northern Europe, its peppercorn-sized seeds (known as coriander) are dried and used in baking, in the south, the very distinctive flavor of its leaves makes it popular for salads, couscous or with ground meat.

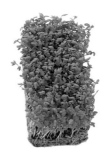

Cress
Cress can be cut just a week after sowing, mixed into salads or eaten in sandwiches. The disinfecting mustard oils it contains make it very aromatic. Cress cannot be preserved.

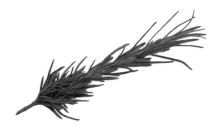

Lavender
Lavender, with its enchanting flowers, is an excellent honey-producing plant. Young leaf tips go well with fish, lamb and poultry. The fragrant flowers are bundled, dried and used for pot pourris and in lavender bags for scenting clothes.

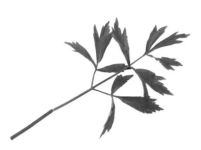

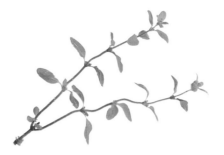

Bowles mint

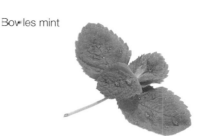

Cat mint

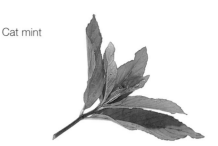

Lovage
This perennial plant can grow up to 6½ feet (2 meters) in height. Tender leaves and shoots can be cut throughout the whole of the vegetation period and used fresh in soups, sauces and salads. This diuretic herb also makes an excellent soup flavoring when dried.

Marjoram
The annual marjoram plant is sown after mid-May and only dusted very thinly with earth. Three seedlings at a time are then planted out at the end of May. For drying, the plant is cut off above the soil just before it comes into flower, tied in bunches and hung up.

Mint
All mint varieties are perennial and, if possible, should have a bed to themselves as they tend to run wild. There is a huge selection of varieties: peppermint, True Mitcham mint, apple, pineapple, orange, spice, and curly mint can be used fresh or dried as a flavoring or a stomach-soothing medicinal tea.

Peppermint

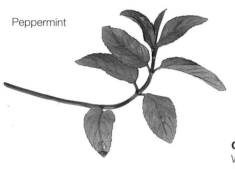

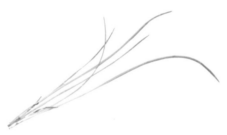

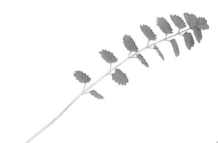

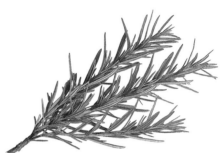

Oregano
Wild marjoram, known as oregano, has a stronger flavor and is perennial. It is cut just before it flowers and dried. It has a more powerful aroma dried than fresh and is used for flavoring pizzas and other southern dishes.

Burnet Saxifrage
This perennial plant grows up to 2 feet (60 cm) tall. The leaves, rich in vitamin C, can be picked fresh at any time. Burnet saxifrage goes with salads, soups, fish, and vegetables. It cannot be preserved.

Rosemary
It needs a sunny location sheltered from the wind, with a soil poor in nutrients. Rosemary can be sown under glass from February onwards or grown from cuttings. Rosemary leaves go with game, meat and poultry.

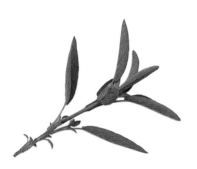

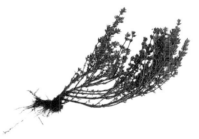

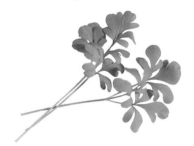

Sage
This perennial plant grows up to 20 inches (50 cm) tall. Sage can be used sparingly fresh or dried with goose, duck, pork, or mutton, and also as sage butter with pasta. Sage tea helps combat inflammation of the throat or gums.

Chives
Chives need a good garden soil and a regular supply of compost. They are propagated by dividing old plants and can be frozen. A special variety is garlic chives, which has an intense flavor.

Thyme
Just before they flower, the stems are cut off a hand's width above the ground and hung up to dry. Thyme goes with meat, sausage, sauces, and poultry. It has disinfectant properties and is made into a tea for coughs and throat infections. Lemon thyme is a special variety.

Common Rue
This perennial plant grows 2½ feet (80 cm) tall and needs direct sunlight. Common Rue, also known as Herb of Grace is a very old medicinal herb, which is used in sauces or herb vinegar. It aids digestion and stimulates the appetite.

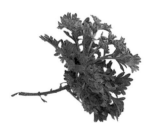

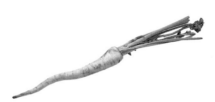

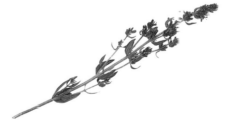

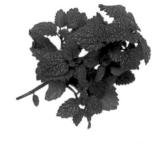

Wormwood
Bitter wormwood is a perennial shrub which grows 5 feet (150 cm) tall. It has the same requirements as mugwort. The leaves go with game, meat or casseroles and can be dried. It grows extensively in the wild in southern Europe.

Turnip-rooted Parsley
Turnip-rooted parsley is sown in rows from late March onwards. It needs constant moisture and compost for nutrients and must be dug up before the first frost, the leaves cut off and the roots covered in sand as supplies for the winter.

Hyssop
The leaves and young shoots are gathered fresh throughout the whole summer. For drying, cut off the stems a hand's width above the ground before they flower and hang them up. Hyssop, which aids digestion, is good in marinades, herb vinegar and salads.

Lemon Balm
The fresh leaves and shoot tips can be cut at any time. To gather supplies for the winter, pick the leaves shortly before the plants come into flower and dry them. The fine lemon flavor goes with salads, herb butter, soups, farmer's cheese, and desserts.

The Herb Garden

Fragrant flavoring and medicinal herbs, which can thrive either in a separate herb garden or mixed in amongst the flowers and vegetables, are an important part of every organic garden. Herbs are indispensable as flavorings, for teas and ointments, or as additions to the liquid manure tub. They are also essential in attracting a wide variety of living organisms to the garden: moths, bees and countless insects find food, a breeding ground, and hunting territory here.

Tips for the Herb Garden

• Herbs can be grown from seed, but it is simpler to buy delicate cooking and medicinal herbs as young plants.

• When fermented together with stinging nettles in rainwater, herbs produce a healing liquid manure after 10 to 14 days which is good for the soil and plants.

• Do not over-fertilize the herb garden: too much nitrogen causes the plants to grow excessively. They develop thick foliage and lose their flavor. A little ripe compost is sufficient for preparing the beds in the spring, and provides enough nutrients for the herb plants.

• Many herbs can be propagated by taking cuttings in August or September. Fresh, non-woody shoot tips are cut off with a sharp knife and put in pots filled with unenriched soil with added sand, propagation soil or fine clay granules. They will soon take root if kept warm and moist and can be planted out the following spring. Lavender, hyssop, rosemary, sage, and thyme can be grown in this way.

• As well as the herbs which have been sown and planted, there may also be room for a wild herb corner in the herb garden. The golden St. John's wort, the white or blue flowers of the comfrey plant and the true camomile act as a magnet to butterflies and bees.

• Note that stinging nettles multiply at great speed. If you want to grow stinging nettles in a corner, it is best to grow them in a buried pot with no bottom, to keep their root growth under control. This is also a good way of keeping horseradish and mint from spreading.

The Best Sites for Herbs

Many herbs need sunshine and a light, porous soil, as they come from the Mediterranean. Others originate from northern Europe. A herb garden should therefore provide different conditions:

• a bed for herbs which grow in good garden soil;
• one for those which prefer a sandy, porous substrate;
• nutrient-rich soil for the more hungry herbs;
• a bed with naturally moist soil.

The Herb Spiral

A good way of providing the specific requirements of each herb within a very small area is with a herb spiral. In a sunny area about $6^1/_2$ feet (2 meters) in diameter, a spiral-shaped dry wall, 30 inches (80 cm) high in the middle, is built from natural stones and earth.

A tiny pond is made at the flat end of the spiral.

Rosemary, thyme, oregano, and lavender thrive at the top of the spiral where it is sunny and dry and the soil low in nutrients.

Sand, gravel and topsoil are added a little further down. Rue and sage will grow here.

The third level consists of sand, garden soil and ripe compost. Basil, marjoram, cilantro, burnet saxifrage, tarragon, hyssop, and lemon balm can be planted here.

The fourth section of the herb spiral is filled with garden earth and ripe compost. Parsley, chives, chervil, and lovage do particularly well here.

And finally, the end of the spiral by the small pond is the best place for watercress, peppermint and apple mint which like the nutritious garden soil.

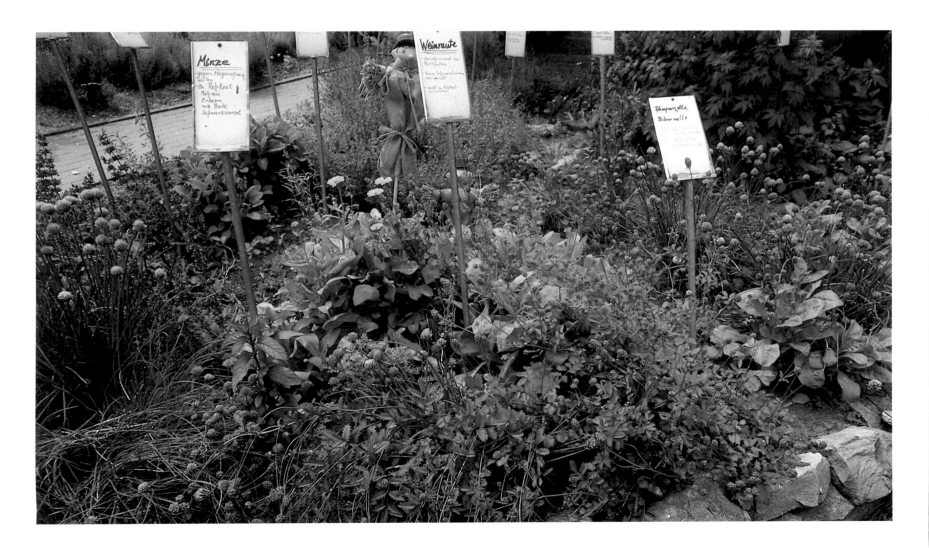

Herbs – Perfect Neighbors for Fruit, Flowers, and Vegetables

Herbs, with their rich store of essential oils, work wonders when planted next to fruit, vegetables and flowers. They strengthen the flavor, deter pests with their aroma and promote growth. Herbs have a similar effect when dried and scattered on the ground next to crop plants or fermented and poured over the soil as a liquid manure.

Preserving Herbs

Drying

Herbs for drying are cut before or while they are in flower on a sunny day in the late afternoon. The sprigs are tied in small bunches and hung upside

Uses for Herbs in the Garden

Borage
Protects lettuces and strawberries from aphids.
Caraway
Flavor-enhancer for cabbages, cucumbers and potatoes.
Camomile
Can be allowed to grow anywhere in the garden as it has a beneficial effect on the soil. Keeps pests away from cabbages, leeks, onions, and celery.
Chervil
Improves the flavor of lettuces and tomatoes.
Chives
Keeps pests away from salsify, carrots, red beets, and lettuces.
Cilantro
Discourages pests from attacking cabbages, cucumbers and carrots.
Cress
Gives radishes a full, delicate flavor.
Dill
Strengthens the flavor of cucumbers, lettuces and peas. It deters cabbage white butterflies and vegetable flies from laying eggs on all kinds of cabbages and on carrots.
Garlic
Intensifies the flavor of strawberries, cucumbers, tomatoes, and carrots. Garlic planted in flower beds, under trees and between roses deters voles and keeps flowers and trees healthy.
Lavender
Drives away ants when planted between roses.
Marigold
Compatible with all vegetables; keeps the soil healthy.
Mugwort
Keeps cabbage white butterflies away from all cabbage varieties.
Nasturtium
Attracts greenfly when planted under trees. It also keeps radishes, potatoes and tomatoes free of pests.
Parsley
Helps tomatoes to grow better.
Sage
Intensifies the flavor of fennel, lettuces and red beet.
Savory
Improves the flavor of dwarf and string beans, red beets and onions. Its fragrance keeps bean flies and aphids at bay.

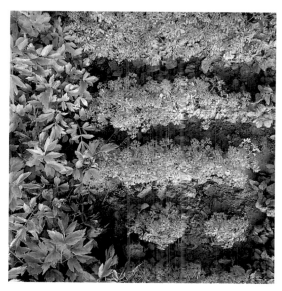

Lovage, common rue and balm are three useful perennial herbs which, unfortunately, are not widely used.

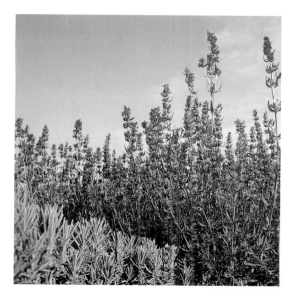

Lavender and rosemary give gardens a hint of the Mediterranean, attract bees and deter pests.

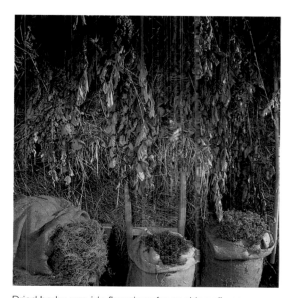

Dried herbs provide flavorings for cooking all year round, but they can also be used in the garden.

down to dry in a shady, airy place. When the herbs are so dry that they rustle, they are taken down and the leaves removed from the stems. The herbs are put into jars and stored in a cool, dark place.

Suitable herbs: savory, hyssop, thyme, lavender, wormwood, mugwort, oregano, peppermint, lovage, parsley, marjoram.

Herb Seeds
Herbs whose main flavoring potential is in the seeds are allowed to ripen fully. Before the seeds fall the seed pods are cut off and left to dry on clean brown paper. When the seeds are completely dry, they are shaken out of the pods, put in screw-top jars and stored in a cool, dry place.
Suitable herbs: dill, coriander, fennel, caraway, aniseed.

Freezing
Herbs for freezing are washed, chopped and spread out flat to be frozen. Once hard, they are put in bags and can later be taken out of the freezer in portions. Herb mixtures, for example for salad dressings, can also be chopped and mixed together with lemon juice in ice cube containers. Do not salt!
Suitable herbs: chives, dill, parsley.

Salting
Chop the herbs finely, weigh them and mix them with an equal weight of coarse salt. The herb/salt mixture is put in small screw-top jars and stored in a cool, dark place. Salted herbs taste good separately or in a mixture in salad dressings and soups.
Suitable herbs: celery, dill, basil, parsley.

Preserving in Oil or Vinegar
Fine herb vinegars and spice oils capture the whole flavor of the herb garden. Vinegar or oil is poured over the fresh herbs until they are completely covered. Leave to marinate for at least six weeks before sampling.
Suitable herbs: rosemary, dill, garlic, thyme, tarragon.

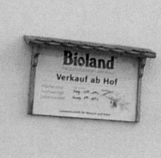
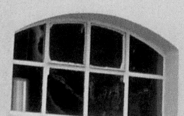

Claudia & Reinold Fischer

Farming

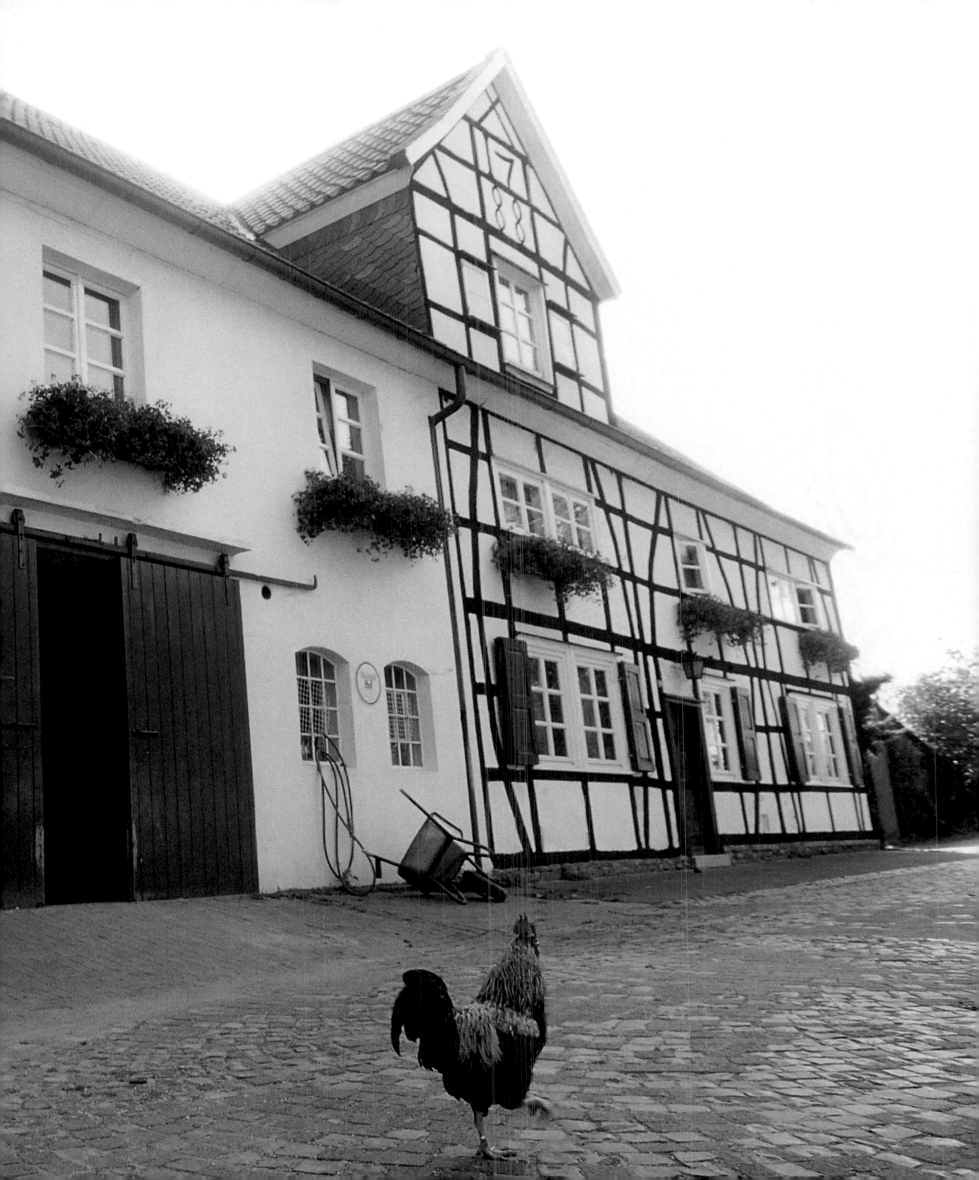

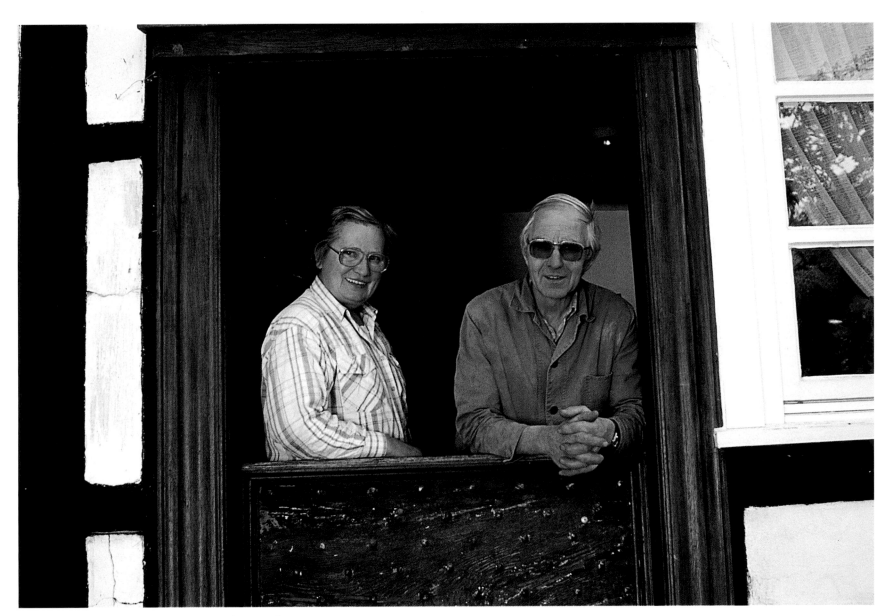

Siegfried and Maria Kuhlendahl are seen as pioneers of organic farming in Germany. They realized early on that using agricultural chemicals has negative effects on the environment.

Previous double page: The Kuhlendahls' beautiful old farm near Wiesbaden, Germany.

Ripe cornfields dotted with wild flowers, field borders awash with red poppies, cornflowers and chamomile – an organic farmer's fields are full of the flowers and colors which are signs of a natural farming process.

No organic farmer would ever dream of destroying wild flowers. 13 different types of insect on average live off every type of wild plant found in the fields. Organic farmers are well aware of this and use these tiny helpers to assist them in their battle against pests, which shows that organic farmers think and work on a level that takes the whole of their environment into account. Every organically run farm has to be seen as a living organism. Soil, plants, animals, and humans: every part of the structure has its own function in this dynamic system of interrelationships. Crop rotation, ecologically sound fertilization methods that do not pollute ground water, mechanical as opposed to chemical weed control – these all form part of a complex system of environmental measures designed to complement each other. The main goal for organic farmers is to sustain a healthy farm organism, to keep the natural cycles intact and to ensure that the soil remains fertile. Maximizing crop yields and profits is not an issue; the overriding aim is to produce highly nutritious and healthy foodstuffs at as little cost to the environment as possible.

This farming process is largely self-sufficient, which means that consumption of non renewable supplies of energy and raw materials is kept to a minimum. Living soil produces healthy plants, and natural pastures and spacious barns provide the food and living space needed for proper animal care. In organic farming, synthetic chemicals like pesticides or nitrogen fertilizers, plant treatment, preservation, protection and ripening agents, hormones and growth enhancers all become superfluous.

As a logical consequence, organic farmers oppose the use of genetic engineering in farming. They also offer a globally responsible contribution towards solving the problem of hunger in the developing world. Organic farmers appreciate that any animal feed imported from developing countries has been produced at the expense of foods urgently required for basic local needs, which is why this type of feed is never used in organic farming.

Organic Farming

Organic farming is based on clear, rational principles. Natural resources are used as sparingly as possible, soil fertility is nurtured and any pollution of the soil, water, air, or environment is purposely avoided.

However, individual organic farmers are not left to act at their own discretion. Originally, associations of organic farmers in Europe drew up various guidelines setting out what an organic farmer may and may not do. Later, several countries drew up their own basic guidelines aimed at establishing minimum standards throughout organic farming. In addition, the European regulation on organic farming of June 1991 imposes specific regulations concerning plant products (see Appendix).

Organic farming developed historically from two main schools of thought: bio dynamic farming and bio-organic farming. The former has a longer tradition, as it is based on a course given in 1924 by Rudolf Steiner, the founder of anthroposophy. This philosophy does not investigate life processes on a purely materialistic level, but, for instance, incorporates astral constellations. The whole farm is considered an organic entity. Bio organic farming was founded after the Second World War by Dr. Hans Müller from Switzerland. The scientific background was provided by the medical doctor and lecturer Dr. Hans Peter Rusch, who was primarily interested in increasing natural soil fertility by stimulating the life forms present in the soil.

Modern organic farming has come a long way since then and developed in many different ways. There is much more to organic farming than simply omitting artificial fertilizers and pesticide sprays. Organic farmers take a whole range of practical measures that both complement each other and make each other necessary. These range from varied crop rotation to special processes which minimize fertilizer losses, weed control without the use of chemicals, and proper animal husbandry. Organic farmers work closely with nature, not against it. This is most successful where the processes employed on a farm most closely resemble those found in nature. The ideal situation is a mutually advantageous, cyclic process which benefits both the farmer and the end consumer who is looking for healthy farm products.

Conventional versus Organic Farming

Conventional Farming
Incomplete cycles; damage to the environment; high dependency on external suppliers

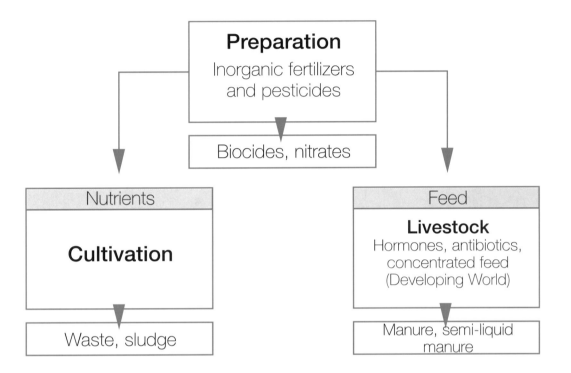

Organic Farming
Complete cycles; improvement of soil structure and water resources, no pollution of water, clean-up of the landscape

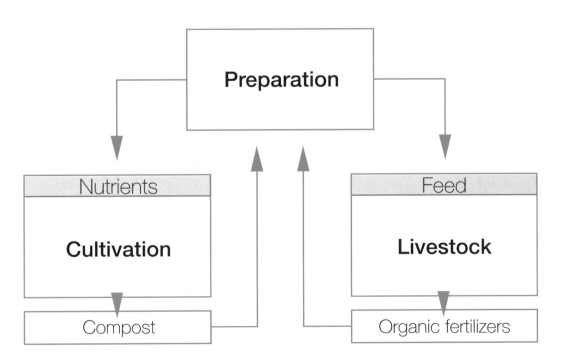

The Farming Cycle

A successful farming cycle not only follows nature, but strives to become part of it. The soil nourishes the crops, the crops feed the animals, and the animals fertilize the ground. An organic farm needs to be as self-sufficient as possible. This means:

• As little as possible should be bought externally, and then only from organic farms;
• Animal feed should be produced on the farm itself;
• The soil should be fertilized with manure produced by the animals kept on the farm, vegetable waste or leguminous plants;
• The entire working structure should be designed to be varied enough to support a wide variety of life forms.

Crops and livestock must be suited to the soil and climate, and the number of animals kept must not exceed the limits of what the land can support.

Varied Crop Rotation

One of the roles of organic farming associations is to advise farmers on crop rotation. Crop rotation takes on a different form for each farm, and should be as varied as possible, whilst taking the particular conditions at the farm into account. A sensible rotation includes cereals, root crops, field vegetables, and leguminous plants. Factors such as climate, soil, farm size, available machinery, and buildings are just as important as the farm manager's personal skills and preferences. Varied crop rotation not only prevents the nutrients in the soil from being exhausted, but provides a wealth of crops to match any natural variety. Finally, this varied production ensures a food supply for all the livestock kept on the farm, thus completing the farm's own cycle.

Soil Care

Every organic farmer works hard to look after the soil and keep it fertile. The secret behind proper cultivation of the soil is to loosen the subsoil and to turn over a shallow layer of topsoil. By doing this, the soil remains layered, with each organism in its proper layer. Rough plowing with heavy machinery and intensive use of chemicals often destroy this system of layering, effectively killing off the soil in the long term.

Organic farmers also pay great attention to nourishing the soil organisms which process organic material into nutrients that can be absorbed by plants. This means that by mulching and fertilizing the ground with green manures, the farmer is effectively feeding the soil, not the plants – a natural approach that reflects natural processes.

Chemical-free Farming

The use of chemical or artificial pesticides, fertilizers, plant treatment, preservation, protection and ripening agents, hormones, and growth accelerators is forbidden in organic farming. Organic farmers exclusively use natural substances. For instance, instead of spraying crops with inorganic nitrogen fertilizer, a farmer can sow leguminous plants such as lupines, sweet peas or clover as intercrops. These are capable of absorbing atmospheric nitrogen and fixing it in their root tubers.

Modern organic farming is, in many respects, a continuation of pre industrial farming, which relied on methods derived from centuries of experience. This experience teaches us that there is an effective natural solution for any problem that may arise.

Useful "Weeds"

Organic farmers prefer to call weeds "wild plants." These particularly sturdy and adaptable plants simply have the misfortune to get in the farmer's way. Whenever they do actually threaten crops their numbers can be reduced to a tolerable level, but this should be done without the use of chemicals, usually by hoeing. Wild plants that are left to grow in the right places can reduce the risk of erosion, promote soil life, and provide a habitat and food for useful insects. Any plants that have been hoed out can be used as mulch.

Wild hedgerows offer ideal living conditions for wild plants, which in turn bring benefits to small animals and insects. Useful insects, soil organisms and crop health can also be stimulated by undercropping or intercropping with mixed crops or by sowing covering crops, which has the same effect as a covering of wild plants.

Animal Husbandry

Pigs are lively and playful, cows prefer to spend all day grazing in the meadow, and chickens love to scratch and peck around in sand. Organic farmers try to meet the natural needs of their animals as fully as possible. It is forbidden to administer any prophylactic medication to increase production, and livestock raised on organic farms are fed on homegrown, highly nutritious feed. Feed imports from developing countries are boycotted as a gesture of solidarity with the farmers there. The number of animals that can be kept per acre of farmland is restricted.

Making the Grade: the Transition to Organic Farming

If a farmer wishes to convert to organic farming, he will receive support from a consultant who will work out a transition plan together with him. The farmer then officially undertakes to adhere to the guidelines of the relevant associations. Three to five years may pass before the status of 'organic farm' is awarded.

The Inspection Scheme

The European directive on organic farming and the association guidelines form the basis of the inspection system. An inspector, who is an independent expert, may visit the farm at any time without prior notice. The inspector will be familiar with the local soil quality, previous crops and regional weather conditions, and will check fields, grasslands, woodlands, vineyards, barns, farm buildings, and the book keeping. He will also take an interest in animal feed and fertilizers, stables and animal health, crop growth and quality, and the presence of wild plants and whether they are controlled in an environmentally friendly way. There must be no evidence of artificial fertilizers or chemical pesticides – not even an old fertilizer bag or container may be used or found on the premises. It is particularly important to monitor the book-keeping. Every bill and every delivery note is checked to make sure that nothing unauthorized has been purchased, and also to check that the crop yield is exactly in line with what are deemed to be appropriate levels of production on an organic farm of a given size. Any "black sheep" that are discovered can expect a variety of sanctions to take effect, ranging from simple recommendations through formal warnings to immediate loss of status. However, according to the associations' figures, the number of genuine "black sheep" make up less than one percent of all organic farms.

Rejuvenating the Soil

More and more farmers are realizing that their soil is becoming increasingly compressed and infertile, which is a clear indication that the soil is lifeless. Only roots and micro and macroorganisms can penetrate the ground and create a vast wealth of microscopic channels, through which oxygen and energy-generating organic substances and water can enter the soil. And only microbes and bacteria can convert the minerals that are found deeper down in the soil into a form that can be absorbed by plants. When starting from scratch it is a good idea to loosen the soil very carefully. However, the plants play the most important role initially, because the space and organic matter that the microorganisms need can only be provided if the ground is thoroughly penetrated with roots. It is essential for further recovery of soil life that the surface stays completely covered. This can be achieved as part of the crop rotation, by sowing plants after the main crop has been harvested, or by spreading mulch, compost or manure. Growing a wide variety of plants in the soil produces a richer soil life and a naturally more fertile ground.

Natural Preparations

Organic farmers understand the biological links in farming. However, bio dynamic farmers go a step further and take other considerations into account when planning their everyday work. Following the teachings of Rudolf Steiner, they believe that enormous forces of biological energy can be captured inside tiny particles of matter. These forces are radiated onto the earth from space and the stars, and on earth they can be stored both organically and in minerals. Bio dynamic farmers now want to make use of these hidden forces once again.

Compost and spray preparations play an important part in this. Anyone can prepare these natural compounds themselves. The compost preparation is made from medicinal herbs like stinging nettles, yarrow, chamomile, oak bark, dandelion, and valerian. Both the compost and the spray preparation, which is made from cattle manure or quartz, are buried in the ground for a part of the year where they absorb cosmic and terrestrial forces.

In order to activate the forces that are concentrated in these preparations, the substances are stirred with lukewarm rainwater for a whole hour without interruption.

Automatic stirring machines are available for this purpose, but it is preferable to do the work by hand. In this highly diluted form, the preparations are ready to be sprayed on the fields. These methods could be described as a type of "homeopathy for the soil, farm manure and plants," as the potency of the diluted preparations is similar to those used in homeopathic medicine. Farmers who work bio dynamically have rarely had much success from applying a single preparation alone. The different preparations all need to be combined, and each one applied at its correct point in a harmonious farming cycle, to have the desired effect of transferring this dynamism into the life cycles.

Bio dynamic Spray Preparations: Horn Manure and Horn Gravel

Followers of anthroposophy believe that a special preparation of horn manure can strengthen terrestrial force fields. It is believed that once it has been filled into a cow's horn and buried in the ground, this preparation can condense and retain the forces existing in the soil during winter. As fall begins, good, well-formed manure is collected from dairy cattle – from the pasture if possible – and pressed firmly into horns previously shed by the cows. The horns are then buried in the soil,

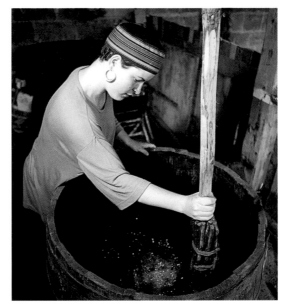

Cosmic energy is passed onto the matured horn manure by mixing it with water and stirring it vigorously for an hour.

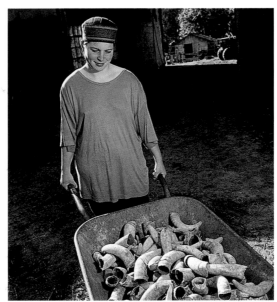

The undamaged cow horns are cleaned and can be re-used up to five times.

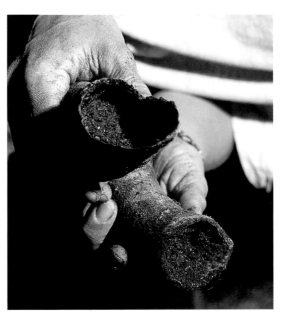

Horn with a well matured, dark preparation.

where they remain until spring. If the process is successful, then what was rather smelly manure in the fall has transformed into a dark substance with a pleasant odor of woodland soil.

The horns are then either left in the ground together with their contents until they are used, or they can be stored in earthenware pots. This preparation is believed to pass on concentrated, revitalizing strength to the soil, and, in particular, is thought to encourage root and shoot growth. The horn manure preparation is applied before the seeds are sown. Before it is spread on the fields it is stirred in lukewarm rainwater for an hour. The mixture is stirred concentrically from the outside inwards with a birch besom until a funnel shape forms. Then the mixture is stirred in the opposite direction, again until a deep hole forms in the middle, and so forth for an hour. The liquid is then strained and sprayed onto the fields, either using a rear-mounted tractor sprayer or knapsack sprayer or, if the area to be sprayed is very small, using a hand spray or hand brush.

Horn manure has a counterpart in harnessing the flow of cosmic forces: horn gravel. Rock crystals, crystalline quartz or potassium feldspar are ground into a fine powder which is then mixed with rainwater into a semi solid paste and again filled into cow horns. The horns are buried in late spring in a sunny spot and left there for the summer. In late fall the mixture is ready for use or storage in a glass container, again in a sunlit place. This preparation is also stirred in lukewarm rainwater for an hour prior to use. Horn gravel can be used for the following applications:
• on grain, as soon as the ear becomes visible on the stalk;
• on root crops, once the green part of the plant has grown to hand height;
• on leguminous plants, once the first few buds have developed;
• on forage plants, as soon as an even carpet of leaves about 4 inches (10 centimeters) high has formed;
• on vegetables like cabbages, once the inner leaves have started to turn inwards, and on fruit before they start to flower.

The required amounts per hectare (about half an acre) are: 9–13 gallons (40–60 liters) of water and 9–11 ounces (250–300 grams) of horn manure or 1 teaspoon (4 grams) of horn gravel.

Compost Mixtures

The special compost mixtures are designed to stimulate both soil and compost, and to activate soil life. Certain plant preparations are used for this purpose in bio-dynamic farming:

Yarrow (*Achillea millefolium*) flowers are hung up inside the bladders of red stags in the sun for the whole summer. Afterwards they are buried for the winter. This preparation is believed to aid nitrogen and potassium processes in the soil.

Scented Mayweed (*Chamomilla recutita*) petals are packed into a cow's small intestine, and again